GW00778110

EQUINE INFECTIOUS DISEASES V

EQUINE INFECTIOUS DISEASES V

Proceedings of the Fifth International Conference

Edited by DAVID G. POWELL

THE UNIVERSITY PRESS OF KENTUCKY

The University of Kentucky Equine Research Foundation provided financial support for the Fifth International Conference and for the publication of these proceedings.

The organization of the Fifth Conference was undertaken in a most capable manner by Ms. Donna Hall and her colleagues of the Special Programs Department, University Extension, University of Kentucky. The Scientific Review Committee, composed of John T. Bryans, George P. Allen, William H. McCollum, and Peter J. Timoney of the Department of Veterinary Science, University of Kentucky, provided invaluable assistance in the evaluation of manuscripts submitted for presentation to the conference. Sharon Ihnen was a most meticulous and conscientious technical editor who considerably enhanced the presentation of many of the contributions.

Scholarly publisher for the Commonwealth, serving Bellarmine College, Berea College, Centre College of Kentucky, Eastern Kentucky University, The Filson Club, Georgetown College, Kentucky Historical Society, Kentucky State University, Morehead State University, Murray State University, Northern Kentucky University, Transylvania University, University of Kentucky, University of Louisville, and Western Kentucky University.

Editorial and Sales Offices: Lexington, Kentucky 40506-0336

Library of Congress Cataloging-in-Publication Data

Equine infectious diseases V: proceedings of the Fifth International Conference / edited by David G. Powell.

p. cm.
Bibliography: p.
Includes index.
ISBN 0-8131-1676-7
1. Horses—Infections—Congresses. I. Powell, David G., 1942- II. International Conference on Equine Infectious Diseases (5th : 1987: Lexington, Ky.)
SF951.E56 1988
636. 1′08969—dc19 88-27670

This book is printed on acid-free paper meeting the requirements of the American National Standard for Permanence of Paper for Printed Library Materials.
∞

Contents

Herpes

Infections of the Reproductive System

Vector-Borne Diseases

Introduction

The Fifth International Conference on Equine Infectious Diseases took place in Lexington, Kentucky, on October 7-10, 1987, in association with the opening of the Maxwell H. Gluck Equine Research Center, which now houses the Department of Veterinary Science of the University of Kentucky. An interval of eleven years had elapsed since the fourth conference in Lyon, France. In the time since, a number of previously unknown diseases have been recognized among the equine population, including contagious equine metritis (CEM), Lyme disease, and Potomac horse fever. Papers on these diseases are included in the proceedings of the fifth conference. Because of the enthusiastic response of contributors, who submitted more than one hundred abstracts for presentation at the meeting, a poster session was added to the program. Conference participants commented on the excellence of the poster presentations, which certainly contributed to the overall success of the meeting.

The scientific proceedings were divided into seven sessions: influenza, herpesviruses, strangles and other respiratory infections, infections of the reproductive system, vector-borne diseases, gastrointestinal infections, and a general session covering a variety of topics. The papers were submitted for external review prior to publication and changes were made as recommended by the reviewers and the scientific committee.

In the first session, on strangles and other respiratory diseases, three papers discussed equine arteritis virus (EAV) and three dealt with streptococcal infections. The papers on EAV, presented by research workers from the Department of Veterinary Science at the University of Kentucky, reflected the considerable scientific and industry concern generated by the 1984 outbreak of the disease among Thoroughbreds. Todd Murphy described the technique of oligonucleotide fingerprint analysis to examine genomic variation among isolates of EAV from North America and Europe. His results indicated a high degree of homology between isolates from epidemiologically unrelated outbreaks, confirming earlier cross-immunization studies. The relationships among fingerprint heterogeneity, antigenic variation, and pathogenicity are as yet undefined, promising to be a fruitful area for further research.

The second paper from the Kentucky group, presented by William McCollum, described the results of an EAV challenge study. Although no clinical signs were detected in vaccinated mares, the antibody response was significant, and for a short period challenge virus was recovered in small amounts from the nasopharynx and blood of vaccinated mares. The amount of virus eliminated by vaccinated mares was sufficient to establish infection in one of seven in-contact, nonvaccinated mares. These results, which corroborate considerable field data compiled since 1984, indicate that vaccination of mares prior to breeding to an EAV-shedding stallion confers clinical protection and significantly reduces dissemination of the virus.

The third paper on EAV, by Peter Timoney, examined the safety of a commercial modified live vaccine that has been used extensively in Kentucky since 1984 in the stallion. No significant changes in sperm quality were noted, apart from a temporary reduction in sperm numbers. Vaccine virus was isolated sporadically from blood and nasopharynx but not from semen or urine. Neither aerosol nor venereal transmission of vaccine virus was observed, confirming the safety of vaccine for the stallion. The three papers furnish ample evidence of how an intensive, well-organized research program can help solve problems that inevitably arise during and following major disease epizootics.

Two papers investigated strangles. The first, by John Timoney from Cornell University, described a natural outbreak of strangles in a herd of ponies and investigated the duration of shedding of *Streptococcus equi*. *S. equi* was repeatedly isolated from the soft palate and tonsilar region of ponies that were experimentally challenged via the intranasal route. The second paper, by Jorge Galán from Washington University, St. Louis, Missouri, introduced the technique of transfusing the gene coding for the M protein of *S. equi* into avirulent strains of *Salmonella typhimurium*. The M protein gene was expressed at high levels in the resulting recombinant. Further studies are underway to test the recombinant in horses and to stimulate a generalized secretory immune response against *S. equi* infection. This development, certainly exciting in the context of controlling equine infectious disease, offers a possible alternative to the conventional approach to vaccination, which in the case of strangles is less than adequate.

The final paper in this session, presented by Mary Mackintosh from the Animal Health Trust, Newmarket, reported the isolation of *S. pneumoniae* capsule type 3 from cases of respiratory disease among Thoroughbred horses in training in England. It should not be forgotten that certain bacteria, acting as opportunistic pathogens, may invade the respiratory system after initial viral infection and prolong the course of disease, thereby hindering the recovery of the animal and its ability to perform to full potential.

The influenza session comprised eight papers, emphasizing the extensive research interest in this group of viruses. The paper by Yoshihiro Kawaoka, of the World Health Organization influenza reference center at St. Jude Children's Research Hospital, Memphis, Tennessee, summed up results of a sophisticated study of the identity and origin of the most recent major equine influenza outbreak. The epizootic, which occurred at Thoroughbred racing and breeding centers in South Africa during December 1986 and the early part of 1987, was of particular interest in that the South African equine population was one of only two worldwide that had not previously been exposed to influenza viruses, the other virgin area being Australia and New Zealand. The South African virus was shown to be similar to equine-2 influenza A viruses circulating among the horse population of the United States at the time of the outbreak. The findings underlined the considerable impact that international air transport of horses can have on the spread of equine infectious disease. Horses from the United States in either the incubation or the acute phase of infection had been transported by air from the United States via Canada and placed in quarantine in South Africa during December 1986. They infected other horses in the quarantine station, which were then released into the general equine population, disseminating influenza virus over a wide area. Using similar molecular technology, Rodney Daniels, of the National Institute for Biological Standards and Control in London, presented an elaborate study of antigenic drift among equine-1 influenza A viruses isolated between 1956 and 1977. The 16 equine-1 influenza A strains examined fell into distinct antigenic groups, spanning the periods 1956-63 and 1964-77. The major antigenic drift between 1963 and 1964 may have been due either to interspecies transmission or to a minor mutation that gave an infectious advantage.

Three papers in the influenza session discussed techniques for improving the isolation of virus, the measurement of local and cell-mediated immunity, and the standardization of influenza vaccines. The three papers represented some of the results of collaborative research by several institutes in England, including the Equine Virology Unit of the Animal Health Trust and the National Institute for Biological Standards and Controls. Frank Cook presented evidence that equine-2 influenza A virus from the same clinical sample exhibited different properties when isolated in embryonated eggs than it did in tissue culture. Such differences raise questions about the most suitable methods of virus isolation for epidemiological studies, preparation of diagnostic reagents, and antigens for inclusion in vaccines. Duncan Hannant studied the local antibody response in the respiratory tract following equine-2 influenza A infection and vaccination, and made some preliminary observations on the cell-mediated response to natural infection. The obvious need for a reliable in vitro potency test for equine influenza vaccines was cogently addressed by John Wood in discussing the single radial immunodiffusion (SRD) test for measuring hemagglutinin; the test is the accepted international standard for human influenza vaccines. When SRD reagents to the hemagglutinin of both equine-1 and -2 were used to measure the hemagglutinin content of available vaccines, a good correlation was observed between vaccine content and postvaccination antibody responses in the horse. If international standardization is to be achieved, the variety of equine influenza antigens in vaccines must be limited by incorporating only those strains that are of current epidemiological significance.

However, other components of the virus beside the hemagglutinin antigen also stimulate protection. Two papers addressed this issue with preliminary reports on alternative approaches to inactivated vaccines. It is recognized that the surface glycoproteins hemagglutinin and neuraminidase of the influenza virus stimulate protective B-cell activity, aided by the cytotoxic T-lymphocyte response (CTL). However, vaccines containing inactivated surface glycoproteins stimulate immunity of only short duration, which must be renewed by frequent booster vaccinations, and the vaccines cannot stimulate a CTL response, which occurs only following natural infection. To remedy this deficiency, studies in laboratory animals have demonstrated that live virus vaccinia recombinants containing human hemagglutinin are capable of inducing a CTL response.

Vaccinia recombinants containing the hemagglutinin and neuraminidase of both equine-1 and -2 influenza A viruses were prepared by Beverly Dale and her colleagues at California BioTechnology, who reported preliminary findings on circulating antibody responses when the recombinants were administered to horses. Lucinda Lamb from Cornell University reported the results of challenge studies in ponies that had received a temperature-sensitive influenza A virus derived by fusing human influenza A virus with equine-1 influenza A virus. Temperature-sensitive mutants are restricted in replicating at normal body temperature but can replicate successfully at the lower temperatures found in the upper respiratory tract. These mutants are thus capable of stimulating a local and systemic response without causing overt disease. The final paper, by Eric Plateau and his colleagues from France, reported a conventional study of the circulating hemagglutination inhibition antibody response in various groups of horses, following the administration of different vaccines at varying intervals of time.

The five papers describing recent studies on equid herpesvirus-1 (EHV-1), as well as another paper reporting an equid herpesvirus-3–like donkey isolate, reflected the current thrust of molecular biology in contemporary herpesvirus research. The six papers exemplified, in a clear and relevant fashion, how new and sophisticated research methods—such as monoclonal antibodies, recombinant DNA techniques, and immunoassays for cell-mediated immunity—are being brought to bear upon the resolution of critical, technically complex problems associated with herpesvirus infection of the horse.

Significantly, three of the six manuscripts—presented by George Allen from the University of Kentucky, James Whalley from Macquarie University, Australia, and Neil Edington of the Royal Veterinary College, London—dealt with an area crucial to control of EHV-1 infections by immunoprophylactic intervention: characterization of the equine immune response to EHV-1 infection and of the viral antigens that elicit such immune responses. The other two papers on EHV-1, by Ann Cullinane of Glasgow University, Scotland, and Alice Robertson of Louisiana State University, described investigations aimed at the molecular characterization of the genome of EHV-1 and the viral strategy for expressing the genetic information carried by the that genome during infection of cells. The sixth paper on herpesvirus, by Robert Jacob of the University of Kentucky, established the intermediate evolutionary and taxonomic status of an isolate of equine herpesvirus recovered in 1974 from the nares of a donkey foal.

Of notable significance among the results of research on EHV-1 were the determination, for the first time, of the complete nucleotide sequence of an EHV-1 gene that encodes for a major glycoprotein antigen (gp14), and the identification and characterization of the antigenic epitopes of another major glycoprotein antigen (gp13) of EHV-1 with a panel of 42 monoclonal antibodies. Restriction endonuclease cleavage fragment maps were constructed for subtype 2 isolates of EHV-1, and genetic colinearity between the genomes of the two EHV-1 subtypes was subsequently demonstrated. Equine cytotoxic T-lymphocytes with specificity for EHV-1–infected target cells were shown to be "genetically restricted," reacting only to target cells bearing histocompatibility antigens identical to those of the effector T-cells. Research has also identified the transcriptionally active subregions of the EHV-1 S-region, and of the individual viral messenger RNAs transcribed from that region of EHV-1 DNA.

Of the six papers in the session on reproduction, four dealt with specific diseases of the reproductive tract: contagious equine metritis (CEM), equine viral arteritis (EVA), and leptospirosis. A fifth paper reviewed 200 cases of placentitis, and the sixth investigated the humoral response of the uterus following experimental bacterial infection. Suzanne Neu from the University of Kentucky Department of Veterinary Science, continuing the extensive investigation of EVA at the university since the 1984 outbreak, described an experimental study in which stallions were inoculated with equine arteritis virus and then monitored for evidence of persistent infection. During the acute phase, EAV was recovered from the nasopharynx, urethra, semen, urine, and buffy coat, but not from most other sites in the body, by 40 days postinoculation. However, the majority of stallions continued to shed equine arteritis virus in the semen beyond 56 days. Virus was most frequently isolated from the vas deferens and bulbourethral glands. The critical role of the carrier, or shedding, stallion in perpetuating equine viral arteritis among the equine population was verified.

One of the major diseases that have emerged since the last conference is contagious equine metritis. Since CEM was first recognized in 1977 and the etiological agent identified and named *Taylorella equigenitalis*, significant progress has been made in its diagnosis, treatment, and control. Cases are still being diagnosed in Japan and France, and import regulations are strict worldwide, to control the spread of the disease. When CEM was first reported in Europe, one of the characteristic clinical features was copious vaginal discharge. As time passed and other outbreaks were reported, this symptom became less characteristic, with very little discharge or none at all being observed. Takumi Kanemaru and his colleagues from the Equine Research Institute, Japan, reported a study in which two colonial variants (large and small) of *T. equigenitalis*, isolated from field cases of CEM in Japan, were inseminated selectively into groups of mares. Mares given the large variant developed obvious clinical signs but there were no signs in the mares that received the small variant—a difference that may explain the variation in clinical signs observed during field outbreaks. A second paper on CEM, presented by Chihiro Sugimoto from the National Institute for Animal Health in Japan, described the characterization of the outer membrane of *T. equigenitalis*. Such detailed molecular studies can assist in the development of more effective methods to diagnose CEM.

The role of Leptospira organisms as a cause of disease in the horse has received scant attention in the past, due in part to the difficulty in culturing the organism. Leptospirosis has been implicated as a cause of acute and chronic disease, characterized by a variety of signs, including jaundice, abortion, premature foaling, and periodic ophthalmia. John O'Brien from the Veterinary Research Laboratories in Northern Ireland described the isolation of several serogroups of *Leptospira interrogans* from aborted fetuses and fatal cases of jaundice in very young foals. His findings, indicating a high rate of isolation, should certainly stimulate others to investigate the role of this spirochete as an equine pathogen.

A most comprehensive review of 200 cases of placentitis examined at the Animal Health Trust, Newmarket, between 1969 and 1987 was presented by Katherine Whitwell. A wide range of bacteria and fungi were isolated from placentitis cases, with streptococci and aspergillus being the most frequent organisms cultured. Macroscopic and microscopic lesions in the placentae and fetuses were described, as well as the clinical signs observed in the mare and the consequent breeding history. The final paper in the session, by Elaine Watson from the University of Bristol, described a study of the local humoral response of the uterus to bacterial infection, and the influence of ovarian hormones on that response.

The session on vector-borne diseases took a look at the old as well as giving a glimpse of the new. Two papers from Louisiana State University provided molecular and epizootiological data on equine infectious anemia virus (EIAV), a long-time foe. Since EIAV is closely related to the acquired immunodeficiency syndrome (AIDS) virus, the intensive research currently underway on the disease in humans will inevitably improve our knowledge of EIAV. Conversely, equine infectious anemia provides an excellent animal model to improve the understanding of AIDS, especially in terms of the humoral and cell-mediated responses to infection. A study of eastern equine encephalomyelitis from the University of Florida suggested improvements in the current vaccination program. Three other papers in the session described studies of two diseases that have only recently been recognized in the horse population of the United States. Lyme disease, or borreliosis, a zoonosis first recognized in the human population in the mid-1970s, has since been diagnosed in several animal species, including the horse. Potomac horse fever has aroused considerable passions since its recognition in Maryland in the late 1970s. Isolation of the causal agent in 1984 was a considerable step toward eventual control.

The paper by Lane Foil of Louisiana State University provided an exceptionally clear and concise view of the current knowledge of mechanical-vector transmission of EIAV. The probability of transmission by tabanid insects, primarily horse flies and deer flies, depends on the clinical status and corresponding viremia of positive horses and on the amount of blood transferred between positive and negative horses. The volume of blood transferred is influenced by the distance that separates infected and susceptible animals from the tabanid population, and by the kinds of tabanid species present in the area. These observations have considerable bearing on management practices and statutory regulations for the control of EIAV.

Until recently the agar gel immunodiffusion, or Coggins, test and the horse inoculation test were the only approved methods of diagnosing EIAV. Charles Issel from Louisiana State University compared three serological tests to detect antibody to EIAV in equine sera. When the conventional agar gel immunodiffusion gave equivocal or negative results, competitive-ELISA and Western immunoblot proved more sensitive, suggesting a better approach to detecting the EIAV carrier horse.

As the result of an increase in the incidence of eastern equine encephalomyelitis among vaccinated young horses in Florida, Paul Gibbs and his colleagues from the University of Florida undertook a serological study of foals, monitoring the level of maternally derived antibody and the response to vaccination. They observed that passive antibody derived from the mare did not interfere with vaccination at three and four months. At 10 months, however, hemagglutination inhibition antibody levels had fallen considerably despite vaccination. The remedy proposed was vaccination of foals at three, four and six months of age, followed by revaccination at six-month intervals.

The variable clinical signs of Potomac horse fever, which has now been recognized in more than 30 of the United States, include fever, depression, and severe watery diarrhea, which occasionally leads to laminitis and death. In 1984 the causal agent was identified as a previously unrecognized rickettsia, which was named *Ehrlichii risticii*. The mode of transmission is not known, but based on epidemiological grounds and on the behavior of other Ehrlichia species, the disease is suspected of being vector-borne. Miodrag Ristic and his colleagues from the University of Illinois described a series of studies in which ponies were administered two doses of an inactivated *E. risticii* vaccine and challenged with *E. risticii* four weeks after the second dose. Clinical signs observed in vaccinates were slight and of short duration compared with the signs in challenge control ponies. The vaccine received a conditional U.S. Department of Agriculture license in the summer of 1987, but its effectiveness in the field has still to be proven. Jacqueline Dawson, also from the University of Illinois, reported the isolation of *E. risticii* from the seven-month-old fetus of a mare that had been inoculated with the organism at three months of pregnancy. This unique observation, along with the finding of antibody in the sera of several live foals before nursing, suggests that the organism may cross the placental barrier and invade the fetus.

Lyme disease, a multisystem inflammatory disease caused by the spirochete *Borrelia burgdorferi*, is transmitted by ixodid ticks to humans and domestic animals from wild mammals such as deer. The disease is manifest in humans by a primary skin lesion, followed in some cases by arthritis, neuralgia, and cardiac problems; it occurs most often in the Northeast, the Midwest, and the western United States. Elizabeth Burgess from the University of Wisconsin reported an outbreak of abortion and foal mortality in 1986 among a small herd of Appaloosa mares in an area of Wisconsin known to be endemic for Lyme disease. Of seven mares bred in 1985, only one delivered a foal that was still alive at the end of 1986. Based on isolation of Borrelia from the kidneys of dead foals, and on antibody titers to *B. burgdorferi* in both the mares and foals, it was suggested that in utero infection had occurred, resulting in abortion and foal mortality. If confirmed, this observation points to yet another agent of fetal loss in the pregnant mare.

The gastrointestinal session comprised four papers: two on salmonella, a third reporting an association between *Clostridium difficile* and foal diarrhea, and the fourth a challenge study of foals with rotavirus. Gihei Sato and his colleagues from the Obihiro University in Japan discussed in considerable detail the technique of plasmid profile analysis to investigate strains of *S. typhimurium* isolated from horses in the Hokkaido region between 1976 and 1985. Three distinct profiles were recognized, two of them found also in strains isolated from cattle in the same area. With the exception of a few isolated during 1976, all the equine strains were multiresistant to antibiotics, as were the cattle strains. The data suggested that the source of equine infection was calves in which the problem had existed for a long time.

The paper by David Powell and his colleagues from the University of Kentucky discussed a retrospective epidemiological study of salmonella infection among the equine population of central Kentucky during 1985 and 1986. *Salmonella saint-paul* was the serotype most frequently isolated, although results from the previous four years indicated a frequent change in the predominant serotype. The majority of *S. saint-paul* isolates belonged to a single plasmid type, suggesting a common source of infection. The very high degree of antibiotic resistance reflected the extensive, frequent use of a wide range of antimicrobial agents to treat foal diseases.

A concise paper by Robert Jones of Colorado State University reported the isolation of *Clostridium difficile* and its cytotoxin from the feces of foals with diarrhea. Two clinical syndromes were observed: a fatal hemorrhagic, necrotizing enterocolitis and a severe watery diarrhea. The experimental reproduction of the disease is strong evidence of another pathogen to add to the list of agents causing foal diarrhea. The final paper in this section was a detailed experimental study of rotavirus infection presented by William Higgins from Cornell University. Foals developed signs of the disease following administration of cell culture–propagated virus. Little correlation was observed between the level of circulating neutralizing antibody and the protection against clinical signs. The results suggested a continuous circulation of virus through the asymptomatic mare, the environment, and the susceptible foal.

The general session at the end of the conference included two papers from Japan, the first by Hiroshi Sentsui from the National Institute of Animal Health, who investigated the mechanism by which EIAV induces anemia in the horse. He suggested that the lysis of red cells by EIAV was complement-dependent, involving phagocytosis by macrophages and polymorphonuclear cells. Takeo Sugiura from the Equine Research Institute reported the results of a seven-year study to determine the prevalence of antibodies to viral respiratory pathogens among racehorses in Japan. When paired sera were examined from over 4,000 horses that experienced pyrexia between 1980 and 1986, evidence of infection by equine rhinopneumonitis, equine rhinovirus type 1, rotavirus, and equine adenovirus was observed.

Ewan Chirnside from the Animal Health Trust, Newmarket, described the production of monoclonal antibodies to equine arteritis virus and evaluated use of the antibodies as a diagnostic tool; ultimately, the technique may be capable of distinguishing between horses acquiring natural infection and those that have received live EAV vaccine. The presentation by Andrew Clarke from the University of Bristol examined the role of the environment in the disease process. Air hygiene and ventilation rates were compared in two contrasting stable environments, and their influence on the prevalence of lower respiratory tract disease among stabled horses was evaluated by endoscopy during an episode of EHV-1 infection. Increases in mucopus were observed in the trachea of horses during an outbreak of EHV-1, with larger amounts found in horses housed in poorly ventilated stables. Heinz Gerber from Bern University, Switzerland, presented equine family data and population data demonstrating that the chromosome segment containing genes for equine lymphocyte antigens also includes genes for susceptibility to sarcoid turmors. Sarcoid tumors are of probable viral etiology, but this study demonstrated a strong genetic component of susceptibility that would allow unaffected susceptible horses to be distinguished from nonsusceptible siblings. Susceptibility to sarcoid tumor joins the small group of genetic diseases of the horse that have been characterized in family studies.

Even bearing in mind the length of time that had elapsed since the last assembly, the highlights of the fifth conference are impressive. Several papers discussed the application to equine disease of sophisticated techniques in molecular biology that were originally developed in research on human disease. Whether these will prove of value in the diagnosis and eventual control of a variety of equine infectious diseases, only time will tell. Since the research effort over the last decade has tended to concentrate on viral diseases such as equine infectious anemia, EHV-1, and influenza, it was particularly gratifying to see a number of papers concentrate on bacterial problems such as strangles, CEM, leptospirosis, and salmonellosis.

Although the number of workers active in research on equine infectious disease is still small, it has in fact risen, especially in the United States, Japan, and the United Kingdom. The recognition by the equine industry of the adverse economic impact of disease on the horse population has stimulated a greater awareness of the need for research. Whilst the number of research workers is small, their motivation and enthusiasm is considerable, as reflected by the quality of the presentations at the Fifth Conference. It will be intriguing to attend the Sixth Conference in Cambridge, England, during 1991 to observe further progress, as well as the new areas of scientific endeavor embarked upon.

Strangles & Other Respiratory Infections

Analysis of Genetic Variation among Strains of Equine Arteritis Virus

Todd W. Murphy, Peter J. Timoney, and William H. McCollum

SUMMARY

Genomic variation among 14 isolates of equine arteritis virus was investigated using the oligonucleotide fingerprinting technique of Dewachter and Fiers. Comparisons of the fingerprints produced by five isolates from the 1984 Kentucky epizootic of equine viral arteritis have demonstrated homologies ranging from 79% to 97%. Comparisons of the fingerprints of eight recently isolated and epidemiologically distinct strains of equine arteritis virus from North America have revealed homologies ranging from 88% to levels that were not determinable. When the fingerprints of the prototype Bucyrus strain and a strain isolated in Europe in 1968 were compared with the eight recent North American isolates, the level of homology with the recent North American isolates was consistently higher for the Bucyrus strain than for the European strain. One of the recently isolated North American strains of equine arteritis virus demonstrated little or no fingerprint homology with any of the other strains examined in this study. The significance of the differing levels of fingerprint homology with regard to differences in antigenicity and pathogenicity has yet to be determined.

INTRODUCTION

Equine arteritis virus (EAV) was first recognized as a specific viral entity following investigation of an epizootic of abortion on a Standardbred farm in Bucyrus, Ohio, in 1953 (Doll et al. 1957). Since then, the virus causing the infection has been isolated in Switzerland (Burki 1965), Austria (Burki 1970), Poland (Golnick & Michalak 1979), the United States (McCollum & Swerczek 1978; Timoney 1985; Traub-Dargatz et al. 1985; McCollum & Timoney, unpublished data), and Canada (Timoney, personal communication). Clinical signs of equine viral arteritis (EVA) commonly include fever, edema of the legs and of the scrotum and prepuce in stallions, rhinitis, conjunctivitis, and abortion in pregnant mares. Horses infected with EAV may display all, some, or none of these clinical signs. Pottie (1888) was one of the earliest to describe a clinically similar condition of horses known as "epizootic cellulitis-pinkeye" or "equine influenza."

Currently, EAV is the only recognized member of the genus *Arterivirus* in the family Togaviridae (Westaway et al. 1985). The spherical enveloped virion has a diameter of 60 nm ± 13 nm with an isometric core of 35 nm (Horzinek 1981). The genome is a single-stranded 48S polyadenylated RNA (Van der Zeijst et al. 1975).

Seroepidemiological surveys conducted in North America, Europe, and Africa (McCollum & Bryans 1973; McGuire et al. 1974; Moraillon & Moraillon 1978; Timoney & McCollum, unpublished data) have revealed widespread prevalence of antibodies against EAV in horse populations in different parts of the world. In surveys conducted of North American Standardbreds and Thoroughbreds by McCollum and Bryans (1973) and Timoney and McCollum (unpublished data), a much higher percentage of Standardbreds tested positive for EAV antibodies than Thoroughbreds in an equivalent population. Similar studies have disclosed differences in sero-prevalence of antibodies between breeds in Africa and Europe (McGuire et al. 1974; Moraillon & Moraillon 1978), with certain Thoroughbred populations having a higher prevalence of antibodies than those reported in the United States.

Investigation of the carrier state of this disease has identified a number of stallions currently shedding EAV in the semen (Timoney et al. 1986). These carrier stallions belong to Thoroughbred, Standardbred, Arabian, and Tennessee Walking Horse breeds.

All isolates of EAV tested to date cross-react with equine antiserum against the prototype Bucyrus strain of the virus. No major antigenic variation has yet been demonstrated between isolates of geographically and temporally distant origins. Using the complement fixation test, Fukunaga and McCollum (1977) have, however, demonstrated minor antigenic differences between virulent Bucyrus, avirulent Bucyrus, Bibuna, and Vienna strains of the virus using homologous and heterologous equine antisera. When the disease is caused by the Vienna, Bibuna, and Red Mile (Kentucky, 1978) strains of EAV, Burki (1970) and McCollum and Swerczek (1978) have commented on the variation in severity of clinical signs when compared with those of the virulent Bucyrus strain of the virus. Reproducible differences, both in growth characteristics of cell culture and in concentration of virus shed in the semen, have been demonstrated with respect to the strains of EAV shed by different carrier stallions (Timoney et al. 1987).

The present study was undertaken to investigate the genomic heterogeneity among strains of EAV using the oligonu-

---

Maxwell H. Gluck Equine Research Center, University of Kentucky, Lexington, Kentucky. Published as paper No. 88-4-28 by permission of the Director, Kentucky Agricultural Experiment Station.

cleotide fingerprint technique of DeWachter and Fiers (1972) as modified by Lee and colleagues (1979). This procedure was shown by Young and others (1981) to be useful in detecting genetic variation between virus strains up to a 5% level. Variations exceeding 5% in fingerprint patterns are virtually uncorrelatable. This technique of genomic analysis allows comparison of closely related strains and differentiation between strains of greater genetic diversity.

Specific objectives of this study were to determine: 1) the similarity between isolates of EAV from horses infected during the 1984 Kentucky epizootic of EVA; 2) the homology among isolates of the virus from North American carrier stallions and from recent North American epizootics of the disease; 3) the genetic relationship between pre-1984 isolates of North American and European strains of EAV and more recent North American isolates of the virus.

METHODS AND MATERIALS

Virus strains. A total of 14 strains of EAV representing nine epidemiologically unrelated sources were studied. Respective origins, dates of isolation, and passage histories in cell culture and in the horse are given in Table 1. All isolates had been serologically confirmed as EAV in a one-way serum neutralization test (McCollum 1970) using convalescent horse serum against the prototype Bucyrus strain of the virus. The strains comprised clinical isolates as well as strains isolated from the semen of inapparently infected long-term carrier stallions.

Cell culture. The cell culture stocks in the study were equine dermis, EC1D, NBL-6 (George Allen, University of Kentucky) and a continuous rabbit kidney cell line, RK-13, (ATCC 16. ccl-37) [American Type Culture Collection, Rockville, Md.].

Other reagents. The following enzymes were used: Proteinase K (Mannheim-Boehringer, Indianapolis, Ind.); Ribonuclease T-1 (Calbiochem, San Diego, Calif.); T-4 polynucleotide kinase (Pharmacia Biotechnologies Group, Piscataway, N.J.). Other materials included gamma-labeled ^{32}P-ATP (New England Nuclear Research Products, Boston, Mass.) and purified yeast tRNA and purified rabbit globin mRNA (Bethesda Research Laboratories, Gaithersburg, Md.).

Cell culture procedures and virus production. EC1D and RK-13 cell cultures were propagated as described by McCollum (1969). Isolations of virus from semen samples were attempted using the method of Timoney and colleagues (1986). High-titered seed virus stocks of each isolate were produced following two to four serial passages in a permissive cell culture system. While greater yields of virus were produced using EC1D cell culture, certain isolates of EAV did not replicate well in them. Large-volume virus stocks were produced by inoculating 12 to 18 150-cm^2 flasks of either EC1D or RK-13 cell cultures with seed preparations of each isolate using multiplicities of infection (MOI) ranging from 0.01 to 2 plaque-forming units (PFU) per cell. A 2-ml inoculum was allowed to adsorb for 2 hr, after which 25 ml of MEM with 2% FBS was added. Cell cultures were incubated for two to six days at 37°C, and the infective tissue culture supernatants were harvested when approximately 60% cytopathic effect (CPE) was evident.

Virus purification. Virus was purified from the infective tissue culture supernatants using the techniques of Trent and Grant (1980).

RNA extraction. Viral RNA was extracted using a modification of the procedure of Monath and colleagues (1983). The purified virus was suspended in 200µl of TNE buffer (20 mM Tris-HC1:1 mM EDTA:15 mM NaC1; pH 8.0) and allowed to stand overnight at 4°C. After overnight solubilization, 40 µg of Proteinase K was added and the mixture incubated at 37°C for 15 min. To this, 20 µl of 10% sodium dodecyl sulfate (SDS) was added, and the mixture was incubated at 56°C for 30 min. The solution was extracted twice with equal volumes of phenol:chloroform:isoamyl alcohol. The first organic phase was reextracted with TNE buffer. The final aqueous phase was washed with ether and precipitated with 2.5 volumes of 100% ice-cold ethanol and 40 µl of 3-M sodium acetate. The precipitated RNA was pelleted by centrifugation at 14,000 rpm for 30 min at 4°C in an Eppendorf microfuge (Eppendorf Geratebau, Hamburg). The pellet was resuspended in distilled water, stored at −70°C until digested, and labeled.

RNA digestion and 5′ end labeling. The procedure used was a modification (Trent et al. 1983) of that described by Pedersen and Haseltine (1980).

Two-dimensional electrophoresis. The oligonucleotides were separated using a modification (Lee et al. 1979) of the technque of DeWachter and Fiers (1972). The bromophenol blue dye marker was allowed to electrophorese 24 cm in each dimension, and the citric acid buffer added to the first-dimension gel was pH 2.13. The characteristics of the resulting gels optimized the interpretation of the oligonucleotide fingerprints produced. The gels were wrapped in cellophane and frozen at −70°C. Autoradiographs were made using Kodak X-omat photographic plates. Exposure times ranged from 6 to 20 hr.

Interpretation of autoradiograph. The study compared the fingerprints of isolates that were epidemiologically unrelated as well as representatives of related isolates. Approximately 30 (27-32) of the largest oligonucleotides on each autoradiograph were numerically designated, mapped, and used

Table 1. Histories of isolates of equine arteritis virus

Isolate	Isolation data			Associated with		Passage	
	Date	Breed[a]	Location	Epizootic	Abortion	History[b]	
Bucyrus	11/01/53	STB	Ohio	Yes	Yes	Horse	p^8
						RK-13	p^2
Vienna	—/—/68	STB	Austria	Yes	No	HK	p^2
						ED	p^2
						RK-13	p^2
84KY-Al	5/12/84	TB	Kentucky	Yes	No	RK-13	p^2
84KY-A2	6/11/84	TB	Kentucky	Yes	No	RK-13	p^2
84KY-A3	6/14/84	TB	Kentucky	Yes	No	ED1D	p^2
84KY-A4	6/14/84	TB	Kentucky	Yes	No	ED1D	p^2
84KY-A5	6/14/84	TB	Kentucky	Yes	No	ED1D	p^2
85KY-B1	4/29/85	TB	Kentucky	No	No	EC1D	p^3
85KY-C1	5/09/85	TB	Kentucky	No	No	ED1D	p^3
85KY-D1	5/22/85	TB	Kentucky	No	No	ED1D	p^3
86NY-A1	4/01/86	TB	New York	No	No	ED1D	p^3
86NY-B1	7/01/86	TB	New York	No	No	EC1D	p^3
86AB-A1	11/25/86	TB	Alberta	Yes	Yes	RK-13	p^3
87AR-A1	4/07/87	Ara	Arizona	Yes	Yes	RK-13	p^3

[a] STB = Standardbred; TB = Thoroughbred; Ara = Arabian.

[b] RK-13 = rabbit kidney; HK = horse kidney; ED = equine dermis; EC1D = equine dermis (NBL-6)

to assess homology between fingerprints. The upper regions of the autoradiographs consisted of short oligonucleotides that consistently formed a fan-like pattern. When aligning two fingerprints to be compared, the fan-like pattern was found to be a more useful reference than either the bromophenol or xylene cyanol dye migration points. To minimize subjectivity in interpreting oligonucleotide homologies, reciprocal cross-comparisons were used. First, percentages of homology were determined sequentially, using each strain as a reference standard against which the fingerprints of all other strains were compared. A cross-comparison was based on the two percentages of homology generated by reciprocal comparison. (For example, in a cross-comparison between 85KY-A1 and 86NY-A1, the fingerprint of the 85KY-A1 strain was compared using the fingerprint of the 86NY-A1 strain as a reference standard. Then the 86NY-A1 fingerprint was compared using the 85KY-A1 strain as the reference standard). Homology determinations for 84KY-A strains and for recent isolates of EAV were carried out using this cross-comparison procedure. If major discrepancies were recorded between percentage homologies, the cross-comparisons were repeated. When recent isolates were compared with the earlier isolates of EAV (i.e., Bucyrus and Vienna), the only homologies determined were those derived when the Bucyrus and Vienna strains served as reference standards.

RESULTS

Oligonucleotide homology among five isolates from 1984 Kentucky epizootic. Five isolates of EAV obtained during the first eight weeks of the epizootic in Kentucky were fingerprinted and compared. The fingerprint of the first strain to be isolated (84KY-A1) is shown in Figure 1D, and the corresponding map outlines the locations and numerical designations of the large oligonucleotides (Fig. 1A). The frequency of occurrence of each of the labeled oligonucleotides among the 84KY-A isolates is given in Figure 1B. The results of cross-comparisons for all the 84KY-A isolates are expressed as percentages of homology between the strains (Table 2). Discrepancies in the percentage of homology on reciprocal comparison between strains presumably arose due to the presence of other oligonucleotides in the region used for comparison. (For example, in the comparisons of 84KY-A1 and 84KY-A4, the use of 84KY-A1 as the reference standard yielded 97% homology, while the homology was 94% when 84KY-A4 served as the reference standard. In this case, the 84KY-A4 fingerprint had one extra oligonucleotide, which lowered the homology by 3 percentage points when the 84KY-A4 strain was used as the reference standard. In subsequent comparsons, more pronounced differences, up to 10%, were observed.)

A total of 28 of the 32 oligonucleotides mapped for 84KY-A1 were present in all the 84KY-A isolates. Only one oligonucleotide was unique to the 84KY-A1 isolate. It migrated slightly faster in both the first and second dimensions than an oligonucleotide that was found in all the other 84KY-A isolates but was lacking in A1. The spot unique to A1 probably arose from the loss of one nucleotide base. Percentage homology between isolates ranged from a low of 79% to a high of 97%. The greatest divergence occurred between two strains isolated four and one-half to six weeks after clinical recovery of the respective horses. The 84KY-A1 isolate demonstrated over 90% homology in all comparisons when it was used as the reference standard.

Fig. 1A

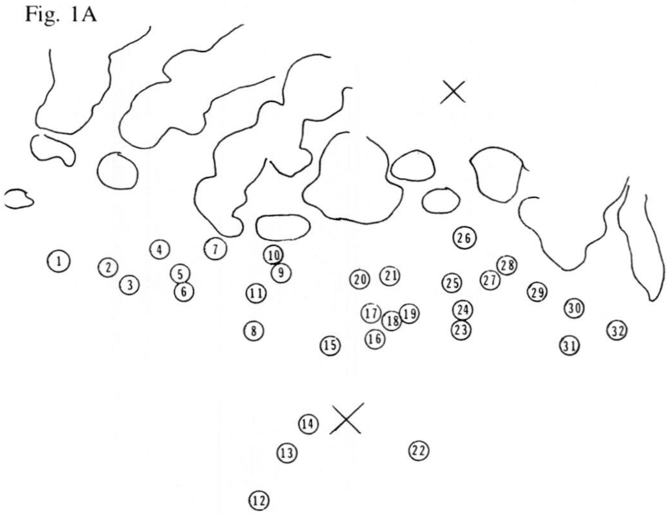

Fig. 1B

84KY-A1

Olig. no.	OF	Olig. no.	OF
1	4/4	17	4/4
2	4/4	18	4/4
3	4/4	19	4/4
4	4/4	20	4/4
5	4/4	21	4/4
6	4/4	22	4/4
7	3/4	23	4/4
8	4/4	24	4/4
9	4/4	25	4/4
10	4/4	26	3/4
11	4/4	27	4/4
12	4/4	28	4/4
13	3/4	29	4/4
14	0/4*	30	4/4
15	4/4	31	4/4
16	4/4	32	4/4

Olig. no. = oligonucleotide number; OF = occurrence frequency.

Fig. 1C

84KY-A1

Olig. no.	OF	Olig. no.	OF
1	4/6	17	3/6
2	3/6	18	4/6
3	5/6	19	4/6
4	4/6	20	4/6
5	5/6	21	2/6
6	4/6	22	5/6
7	4/6	23	3/6
8	4/6	24	3/6
9	2/6	25	4/6
10	5/6	26	2/6
11	4/6	27	5/6
12	4/6	28	3/6
13	4/6	29	4/6
14	1/6	30	5/6
15	4/6	31	4/6
16	2/6	32	4/6

Olig. no. = oligonucleotide number; OF = occurrence frequency.

Fig. 1D

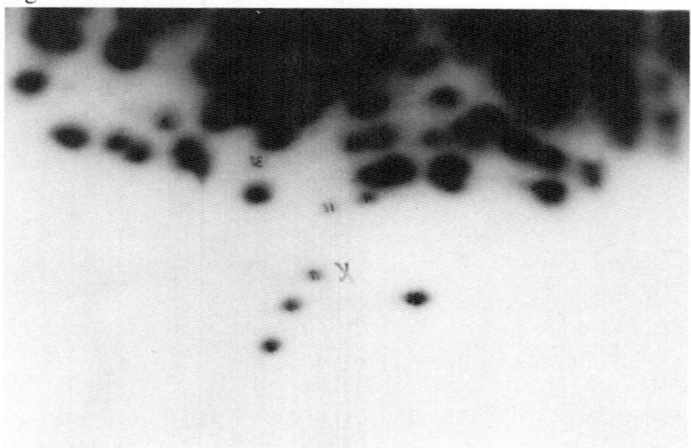

Fig. 1. A. Numerical designation of significant oligonucleotides of 84KY-A1 isolate. B. Occurrence frequencies of numerically designated oligonucleotides in comparisons with other isolates of 1984 Kentucky epizootic. C. Occurrence frequencies of numerically designated oligonucleotides in comparisons with other recent isolates of EAV. D. Fingerprint of 84KY-A1 isolate.

Table 2. Percentages of homology in oligonucleotide fingerprint comparisons for isolates of equine arteritis virus from 1984 Kentucky epizootic

	Reference standard				
Isolate	84KY-A1	84KY-A2	84KY-A3	84KY-A4	84KY-A5
84KY-A1	—	85%	88%	94%	88%
84KY-A2	91	—	91	85	79
84KY-A3	94	91	—	94	97
84KY-A4	97	82	88	—	91
84KY-A5	97	85	97	97	—

Homology among eight recent North American strains. Eight North American strains of EAV isolated between 1984 and 1987 including one from the 1984 Kentucky epizootic, were fingerprinted, mapped, and numerically labeled (Figs. 1A-7A and 8). The frequency of occurrence of the numerically labeled oligonucleotides (Figs. 1A-7A) in the other recent isolates is shown in Fig. 1C and Figs. 2B-7B. The percentages of homology based on cross comparisons of seven of the recent isolates of EAV are given in Table 3. The eighth isolate was excluded from comparisons because of the radically different oligonucleotide pattern it produced (Fig. 8). (Repeat fingerprints of 85KY-D1 yielded identical results.)

Between seven and 18 of the large oligonucleotides were highly conserved among the seven recent isolates in this study (Figs. 1C and 2B-7B). Very few oligonucleotides seemed to be unique to any single isolate. The range in the number of highly conserved oligonucleotides may be a reflection of the subjective nature of both map generation and fingerprint comparison.

Results of cross comparisons (Table 3) between recent isolates revealed a wide range of homology. The two New York strains (86NY-A1 and 86NY-B1) had a high degree of homology, as did three of the Kentucky strains (84KY-A1, 85KY-B1, and 85KY-C1). The Canadian strain (87AB-A1), though demonstrating 78% homology with 84KY-A1, had consistently lesser homology when compared with the New York strains and with other Kentucky strains of the virus. Except for strain 85KY-D1, the 87AR-A1 isolate was found to have the least degree of homology on comparison with all other recently isolated strains of EAV.

Homology among European and North American strains of EAV. Two earlier isolates of EAV, the prototype Bucyrus strain and the Vienna strain, were fingerprinted and the large oligonucleotides were mapped and given numerical designations (Figs. 9A and 10A). Cross-comparisons were made between fingerprints of the Vienna and Bucyrus strains, while only one-way comparisons were made with recently isolated strains of EAV, using Vienna and Bucyrus strains as reference standards. The frequencies of occurrence of the numerically labeled oligonucleotides in the fingerprints of the Bucyrus and Vienna strains and recently isolated strains of EAV are given in Figs. 9B and 10B; occurrence of the

Table 3. Percentages of homology in oligonucleotide fingerprint comparisons for recent North American isolates of equine arteritis virus

	Reference standard						
Isolate	84KY-A1	85KY-B1	85KY-C1	86NY-A1	86NY-B1	86AB-A1	87AR-A1
84KY-A1	—	71%	82%	76%	67%	68%	48%
85KY-B1	78	—	86	85	73	54	52
85KY-C1	78	84	—	76	73	68	48
86NY-A1	78	84	79	—	80	64	59
86NY-B1	78	81	89	88	—	71	56
86AB-A1	78	48	75	61	63	—	56
87AR-A1	56	42	43	49	53	46	—

oligonucleotides in the other pre-1984 strain was also noted. Eleven oligonucleotides from the Bucyrus strain were highly conserved in the fingerprints of recent North American strains, as were 10 oligonucleotides from the Vienna strain. Bucyrus had one unique oligonucleotide while Vienna had two.

In comparisons using the Bucyrus strain as the reference standard (Table 4), a moderate degree of homology was observed with strains 84KY-A1, 85KY-C1, 86NY-A1, 86NY-B1, and 86AB-A1. A lesser degree of homology was present between the Vienna, 85KY-B1, and 87AR-A1 strains. When the Vienna strain was used as the reference standard, the percentages of homology were considerably lower in comparisons with 84KY-A1, 85KY-C1, 86NY-A1, and 86NY-B1 strains of EAV. Only 86AB-A1 demonstrated greater than 60% homology when compared with the Vienna strain.

DISCUSSION

Two important factors to be considered when interpreting the oligonucleotide homology data presented in this study are the sensitivity of the oligonucleotide fingerprinting technique, and the disparate nature of the isolates analyzed. Young and colleagues (1981) calculated the relationship between known nucleotide base sequence divergence and oligonucleotide fingerprint homologies. A 5% sequence divergence resulted in a 50% fingerprint homology in both computer simulations and in actual oligonucleotide fingerprints, while a 10% sequence divergence produced less than 30% homology. With between 5% and 15% of the genome represented in the oligonucleotides, two viral isolates with less than 1% nucleotide base sequence divergence between their genomes would be expected to produce slightly different oligonucleotide fingerprints (Kew et al. 1984). Considering the well-documented plasticity of the RNA genome (Holland et al. 1982) and the diversity of epidemiological origins of the EAV isolates fingerprinted, a high degree of genetic divergence was expected. While this expectation was confirmed to a certain extent, an unexpectedly high degree of homology was also demonstrated between isolates that—as far as could be determined—were epidemiologically unrelated.

The differences in fingerprint homologies among isolates obtained during the 1984 Kentucky epizootic of EVA emphasized the heterogenity inherent in the RNA genome. Though isolated from horses on the same premises within a period of only 32 days, complete fingerprint homology was not demonstrated between any two isolates. There was evidence that considerable heterogenity was generated in some of the 84KY-A isolates over a relatively short period of time.

In sharp contrast to the heterogenity of the closely related 84KY-A isolates was the level of homology among isolates that were geographically and temporally disparate, namely 84KY-A1, 85KY-B1, 85KY-C1, 86NY-A1, 86NY- B1, and to a lesser extent 86AB-A1. These isolates though epidemiologically unrelated and in some cases geographically separate in origin, demonstrated 65% to 89% fingerprint homology. Based on the calculations of Young and colleagues (1981), the nucleotide sequence divergence appears to be less than 3%. A similar finding was the 71% fingerprint homology demonstrated between the prototype Bucyrus strain of EAV and two recent isolates of the virus. It appears that the genome of EAV can remain highly conserved over extended periods of time. Morita and Igarashi (1984) working with Getah virus isolates of analogous temporal and geographic relationships, demonstrated corresponding levels of homology.

The greatest degree of genomic variation was demonstrated between the Vienna, 85KY-D1, and 87AR-A1 isolates of EAV. This heterogenity might be expected of the Vienna isolate in view of its unique geographic and temporal characteristics, and perhaps indicates a very distant epidemiological link. Based on circumstantial evidence, the 87AR-A1 isolate was probably introduced recently into the United States from Europe. This fingerprint type may be representative of the European equivalent of the Bucyrus strain of EAV. The radically different fingerprint produced by the 85KY-D1 isolate would indicate that the EAV genome is capable of a considerable degree of genomic variation. Due to limitations in the oligonucleotide fingerprinting, it was not possible to assess the actual relationship of the 85KY-D1 isolate to other isolates of EAV. As more isolations of EAV are made from additional carrier stallions, the prevalence of this fingerprint type may become apparent.

Fig. 2A

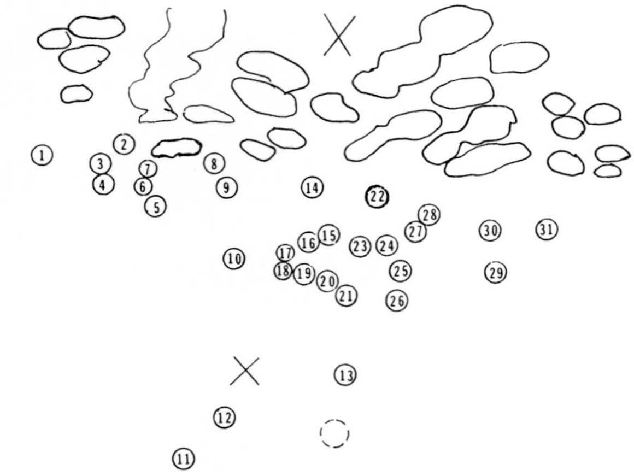

Fig. 2. A. Numerical designation of significant oligonucleotides of 85KY-B1 isolate. B. Occurrence frequencies of numerically designated oligonucleotides in comparisons with other recent isolates of EAV.

Fig. 2B

85KY-B1

Olig. no.	OF	Olig. no.	OF
1	4/6	17	4/6
2	5/6	18	3/6
3	4/6	19	5/6
4	5/6	20	5/6
5	3/6	21	1/6
6	4/6	22	6/6
7	3/6	23	2/6
8	5/6	24	5/6
9	4/6	25	4/6
10	2/6	26	4/6
11	5/6	27	5/6
12	5/6	28	6/6
13	1/6	29	6/6
14	5/6	30	6/6
15	5/6	31	3/6
16	2/6		

Olig. no. = oligonucleotide number; OF = occurrence frequency.

Fig. 3A

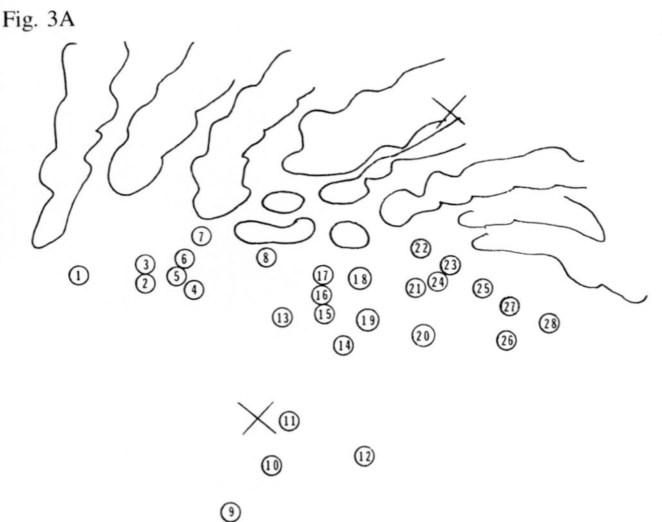

Fig. 3. A. Numerical designation of significant oligonucleotides of 85KY-C1 isolate. B. Occurrence frequencies of numerically designated oligonucleotides in comparisons with other recent isolates of EAV.

Fig. 3B

85KY-C1

Olig. no.	OF	Olig. no.	OF
1	5/6	15	5/6
2	5/6	16	4/6
3	2/6	17	3/6
4	5/6	18	6/6
5	6/6	19	6/6
6	3/6	20	5/6
7	5/6	21	6/6
8	5/6	22	5/6
9	4/6	23	5/6
10	5/6	24	5/6
11	4/6	25	3/6
12	5/6	26	6/6
13	2/6	27	4/6
14	2/6	28	5/6

Olig. no. = oligonucleotide number; OF = occurrence frequency.

Fig. 4A

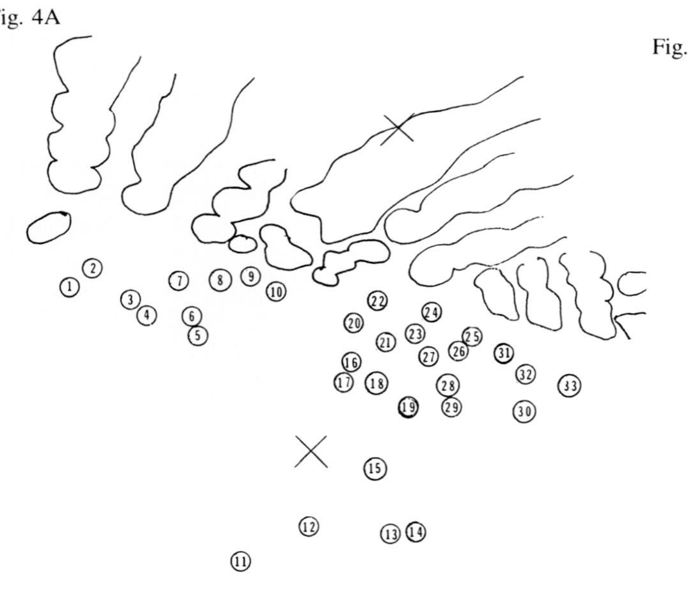

Fig. 4. A. Numerical designation of significant oligonucleotides of 86NY-A1 isolate. B. Occurrence frequencies of numerically designated oligonuceotides in comparisons with other recent isolates of EAV.

Fig. 4B

86NY-A1

Olig. no.	OF	Olig. no.	OF
1	5/6	18	5/6
2	1/6	19	3/6
3	5/6	20	2/6
4	4/6	21	6/6
5	5/6	22	3/6
6	5/6	23	2/6
7	4/6	24	6/6
8	6/6	25	6/6
9	4/6	26	5/6
10	6/6	27	5/6
11	6/6	28	3/6
12	4/6	29	5/6
13	5/6	30	6/6
14	1/6	31	4/6
15	2/6	32	5/6
16	4/6	33	5/6
17	5/6		

Olig. no. = oligonucleotide number; OF = occurrence frequency.

Fig. 5. A. Numerical designation of significant oligonucleotides of 86NY-B1 isolate. B. Occurrence frequencies of numerically designated oligonucleotides in comparisons with other recent isolates of EAV.

Fig. 5A

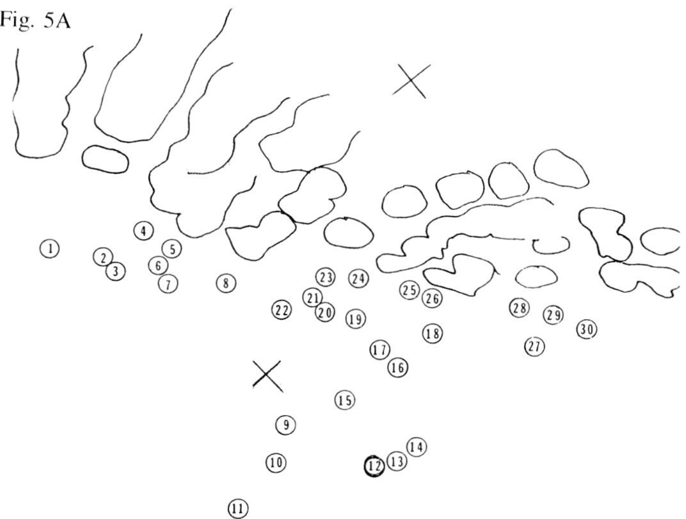

Fig. 5B

86NY-B1

Olig. no.	OF	Olig. no.	OF
1	6/6	16	3/6
2	6/6	17	2/6
3	4/6	18	6/6
4	4/6	19	6/6
5	4/6	20	5/6
6	6/6	21	4/6
7	4/6	22	3/6
8	3/6	23	3/6
9	5/6	24	6/6
10	4/6	25	6/6
11	4/6	26	2/6
12	3/6	27	5/6
13	2/6	28	4/6
14	1/6	29	5/6
15	0/6	30	4/6

Olig. no. = oligonucleotide number; OF = occurrence frequency.

Fig. 6. A. Numerical designation of significant oligonucleotides of 86AB-A1 isolate. B. Occurrence frequencies of numerically designated oligonucleotides in comparisons with other recent isolates of EAV.

Fig. 6A

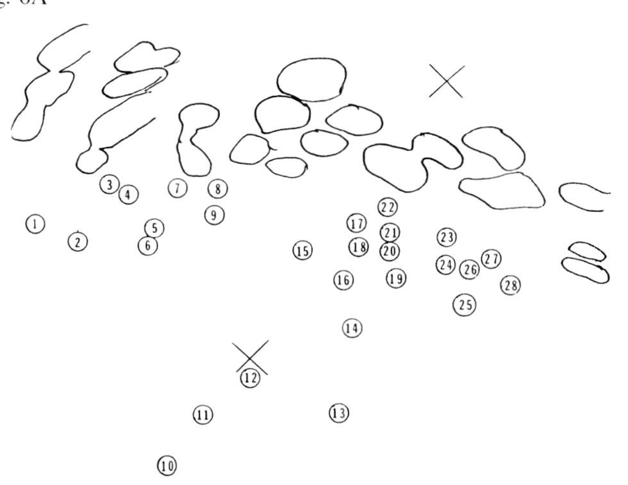

Fig. 6B

86AB-A1

Olig. no.	OF	Olig. no.	OF
1	4/6	15	5/6
2	1/6	16	6/6
3	2/6	17	2/6
4	3/6	18	0/6
5	6/6	19	6/6
6	5/6	20	4/6
7	6/6	21	1/6
8	4/6	22	5/6
9	3/6	23	5/6
10	2/6	24	1/6
11	4/6	25	6/6
12	5/6	26	4/6
13	5/6	27	1/6
14	2/6	28	4/6

Olig. no. = oligonucleotide number; OF = occurrence frequency.

Fig. 7. A. Numerical designation of significant oligonucleotides of 87AR-A1 isolate. B. Occurrence frequencies of numerically designated oligonucleotides in comparisons with other recent isolates of EAV.

Fig. 7A

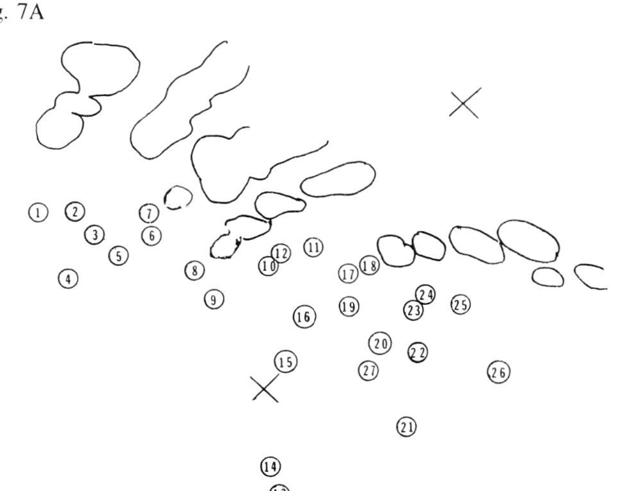

Fig. 7B

87AR-A1

Olig. no.	OF	Olig. no.	OF
1	4/6	15	4/6
2	2/6	16	0/6
3	5/6	17	4/6
4	2/6	18	1/6
5	3/6	19	2/6
6	4/6	20	5/6
7	5/6	21	6/6
8	3/6	22	1/6
9	4/6	23	2/6
10	1/6	24	6/6
11	1/6	25	6/6
12	3/6	26	4/6
13	3/6	27	6/6
14	0/6		

Olig. no. = oligonucleotide number; OF = occurrence frequency.

Fig. 8. Fingerprint of 85KY-D1 isolate (right), graphically represented. (Due to high degree of heterogeneity observed between this fingerprint and all other fingerprints, the 85KY-D1 isolate was excluded from all comparisons.)

Fig. 9. (below) A. Numerical designation of significant oligonucleotides of the prototype Bucyrus strain. B. Occurrence frequencies of numerically designated oligonucleotides in comparisons with recent isolates of EAV, and presence or absence of the oligonucleotides in the Vienna strain.

Fig. 10. (bottom) A. Numerical designation of significant oligonucleotides of the Vienna strain. B. Occurrence frequencies of numerically designated oligonucleotides in comparisons with recent isolates of EAV, and presence or absence of the oligonucleotides in the Bucyrus strain.

Fig. 8

Fig. 9A

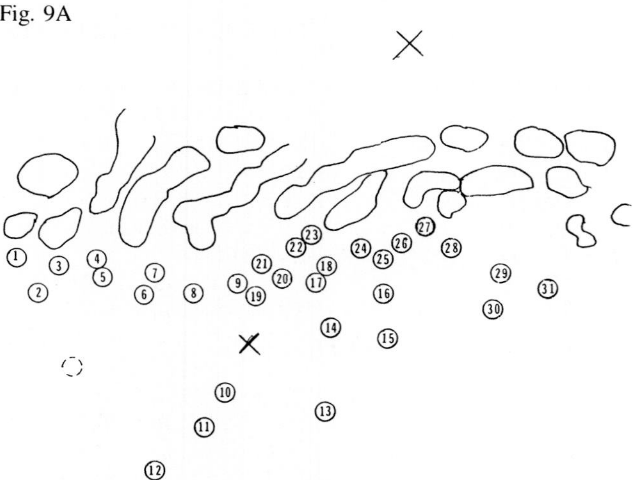

Fig. 9B

Bucyrus

Olig. no.	OF	Vienna	Olig. no.	OF	Vienna
1	5/7	Y	17	6/7	N
2	4/7	Y	18	3/7	N
3	5/7	N	19	1/7	Y
4	7/7	N	20	7/7	N
5	6/7	Y	21	3/7	Y
6	0/7	N	22	4/7	Y
7	2/7	Y	23	5/7	Y
8	4/7	N	24	6/7	Y
9	3/7	Y	25	4/7	Y
10	4/7	N	26	6/7	Y
11	5/7	N	27	5/7	N
12	6/7	N	28	6/7	N
13	3/7	Y	29	6/7	N
14	5/7	Y	30	6/7	N
15	2/7	Y	31	4/7	N
16	7/7	Y			

Olig. no. = oligonucleotide number; OF = occurrence frequency.

Fig. 10A

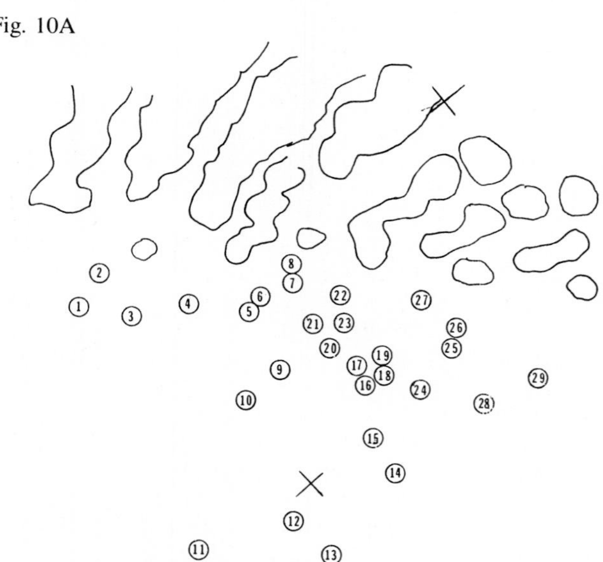

Fig. 10B

Vienna

Olig. no.	OF	Bucyrus	Olig. no.	OF	Bucyrus
1	2/7	N	16	2/7	Y
2	2/7	Y	17	5/7	Y
3	4/7	Y	18	2/7	Y
4	6/7	Y	19	2/7	Y
5	0/7	N	20	3/7	N
6	6/7	Y	21	5/7	Y
7	3/7	Y	22	6/7	Y
8	6/7	Y	23	3/7	N
9	1/7	N	24	6/7	N
10	0/7	N	25	7/7	Y
11	6/7	N	26	7/7	N
12	4/7	Y	27	7/7	Y
13	1/7	N	28	4/7	Y
14	2/7	N	29	6/7	Y
15	2/7	N			

Olig. no. = oligonucleotide number; OF = occurrence frequency.

Table 4. Percentages of homology in oligonucleotide fingerprint comparisons for historic and recent North American isolates of equine arteritis virus

	Reference standard	
Isolate	Bucyrus	Vienna
Bucyrus	—	59%
Vienna	52	—
84KY-A1	68	52
85KY-B1	55	55
85KY-C1	71	59
86NY-A1	71	55
86NY-B1	74	38
86AB-A1	65	66
87AR-A1	52	52

There appeared to be greater than 90% conservation of the genome with respect to the strains of EAV compared in this study. The lack of complete homology may be correlated with the variation in pathogenicity observed among different strains of EAV, and the responses they elicit in the horse (Burki 1970; McCollum & Swerczek 1978). It may also be reflective of minor antigenic differences demonstrated using the complement-fixation test (Fukunaga & McCollum 1977). The high level of homology is consistent with the results of earlier cross-immunization studies in which horses infected with five North American and one European strain were protected against subsequent challenge with the Bucyrus strain (McCollum 1969), indicating the probable existence of only one serotype. It is not clear whether cross-immunity in the horses investigated resulted from conservation of epitopes in all the investigated strains of EAV, or whether various epitopes are shared but no epitope is common to all these strains. This is especially pertinent in attempts to develop a subunit vaccine.

Factors affecting the degree of virulence displayed by a particular strain of EAV are currently unknown. Amount of challenge virus and route of exposure are important (McCollum, personal communication), but they are not the sole determinant. The highly virulent Bucyrus strain seems to have arisen through random mutations of the viral genome. Its virulence was attenuated successfully by multiple passages in tissue culture (Doll et al. 1968; McCollum 1969). Changes in virulence were detectable by the thirtieth passage when only minor fingerprint heterogenity was detected (Murphy, Timoney & McCollum, unpublished data). There was no indication from fingerprint data derived in this study that any relationship existed between pathogenicity and percentage homology with the Bucyrus strain.

The results of this study have demonstrated genomic variation between most of the isolates of EAV investigated. The existence of a high degree of genomic conservation was also established between distantly related isolates. The significance of genomic homology and genomic heterogenity as they relate to both antigenic variation and biological properties, especially pathogenicity, remains to be determined. Further studies will be necessary to determine the distribution of fingerprint types such as the 85KY-D1; the relationship between fingerprint heterogenity, antigenic variation, and pathogenicity; and the significance of the highly conserved oligonucleotides with regard to conservation of antigenic epitopes.

ACKNOWLEDGMENTS

The authors gratefully acknowledge Wayne Roberts (University of Kentucky), Dr. Edward Dubovi (Diagnostic Laboratory, New York State College of Veterinary Medicine, Cornell University), Dr. George Paff-Vid (Reference Laboratory, Alberta Agriculture, Edmonton, Alberta) and Dr. Kent Holm (Scottsdale, Arizona).

REFERENCES

Burki, F. (1965) Eigenschaften des virus der equinen arteritis. *Pathol. Microbiol.* **28**, 939-49.

———. (1970) The virology of equine arteritis. *Proc. 2d Int. Conf. Equine Infect Dis.*, pp. 125-29.

Dewachter, R., and Fiers, W. (1972) Preparative two-dimensional polyacrylamide gel electrophoresis of ^{32}P-labeled RNA *Analyt. Biochem.* **49**, 1874-97.

Doll, E.R.; Bryans, J.T.; McCollum, W.H.; and Crowe, M.E.W. (1957) Isolation of a filterable agent causing arteritis of horses and abortion by mares. Its differentiation from the equine abortion (influenza) virus. *Cornell Vet.* **47**, 3-41.

Doll, E.R.; Bryans, J.T.; Wilson, J.C.; and McCollum, W.H. (1968) Immunisation against equine viral arteritis using modified live virus propagated in cell cultures of rabbit kidney. *Cornell Vet.* **47**, 3-41.

Fukunaga, Y., and McCollum, W.H. (1977) Complement fixation reactions in equine viral arteritis. *Am. J. Vet. Res.* **38**, 2043-46.

Golnik, W., and Michalak, T. (1979) Cases of equine arteritis virus infections in horses in Poland. *Medycyna Wet.* **35**, 605-6.

Holland, J.J.; Spindler, K.; Horodyski, F.; Grabau, E.; Nichol, S; and Vande Pol, S. (1982) Rapid evolution of RNA genomes. *Science* **215**, 1577-85.

Horzinek, M.C. (1981) *Nonarthropod-borne Togaviruses*. Academic Press, London.

Kew, O.M.; Nottay, B.K.; and Obijeski, J.F. (1984) Applications of oligonucleotide fingerprinting to the identification of viruses. In *Methods in Virology*, Vol. 3, pp. 41-84. Academic Press, New York.

Lee, Y.F.; Kitmura, N.; Nomoto, A.; and Wimmer, E. (1979) Sequence studies of poliovirus RNA. V. Nucleotide sequence complexities of poliovirus type 1, type 2 and two type 1 defective interfering particles RNAs and fingerprint of poliovirus type 3 genome. *J. Gen. Virol.* **44**, 311-22.

McCollum, W.H. (1969) Development of a modified virus strain and vaccine for equine viral arteritis. *J. Am. Vet. Med. Assoc.* **155**, 318-22.

———. (1970) Vaccination for equine viral arteritis. *Proc. 2d Int. Conf. Equine Infect. Dis.*, pp. 143-51.

McCollum, W.H., and Bryans, J.T. (1973) Serological identification of infection by equine arteritis virus in horses of several countries. *Proc. 3d Int. Conf. Equine Infect. Dis.*, pp. 256-62.

McCollum, W.H., and Swerczek, T.W. (1978) Studies of an epizootic of equine viral arteritis in racehorses. *J. Equine Med. Surg.* **2**, 293-99.

McGuire, T.C.; Crawford, T.B.; and Henson, J.B. (1974) Prevalence of antibodies to herpesvirus type 1 and 2, arteritis and infectious anemia viral antigens in equine serum. *Am. J. Vet. Res.* **35**, 181-85.

Monath, T.P.; Kinney, R.M.; Schlesinger, J.J.; Brandriss, M.W.; and Bres, P. (1983) Ontogeny of yellow fever 17D vaccine: RNA oligonucleotide fingerprint and monoclonal antibody analyses of vaccines produced world-wide. *J. Gen. Virol.* **64**, 627-37.

Moraillon, A., and Moraillon, R. (1978) Results of an epidemiological investigation on viral arteritis in France and some other European and African countries. *Ann. Rech. Vet.* **9**, 43-45.

Morita, K., and Igarashi, A. (1984) Oligonucleotide fingerprint analysis of strains of getah virus isolated in Japan and Malaysia. *J. Gen. Virol.* **65**, 1899-1908.

Pedersen, S.K., and Haseltine, W.A. (1980) A micromethod for detailed characterization of high molecular weight RNA. In *Methods of Enzymology*, Vol. 65, pp. 680-87. Academic Press, New York.

Pottie, A. (1888) The propagation of influenza from stallions to mares. *J. Comp. Path.* **1**, 37-38.

Timoney, P.J. (1985) Clinical, virological and epidemiological features of the 1984 outbreak of equine viral arteritis in the Thoroughbred population in Kentucky. *Proc. Grayson Found. Int. Conf. Thoroughbred Breeders Orgs. on EVA*, pp. 24-33.

Timoney, P.J.; McCollum, W.H.; Roberts, A.W.; and Murphy, T.W. (1986) Demonstration of the carrier state in naturally acquired equine arteritis virus infection in the stallion. *Res. Vet. Sci.* **41**, 279-80.

Timoney, P.J.; McCollum, W.H.; Murphy, T.W.; Roberts, A.W.; Willard, J.G.; and Carswell, G.D. (1987) The carrier state of equine arteritis virus infection in the stallion with specific emphasis on the venereal mode of transmission. *J. Reprod. Fert. Suppl.* **35**, 95-102.

Traub-Dargatz, J.L.; Ralston, S.; Bennett, D.; and Collins, J. (1985) Outbreak of EVA at CSU-VTH *J. Equine Vet. Sci.* **5**, 168.

Trent, D.W., and Grant, J.A. (1980) A comparison of new world alpha-viruses in the western equine encephalitis complex by immunochemical and oligonucleotide fingerprinting techniques. *J. Gen. Virol.* **47**, 261-82.

Trent, D.W.; Grant, J.A.; Rosen, L.; and Monath, T.P. (1983) Genetic variation among dengue 2 viruses of different geographic origin. *Virology* **128**, 271-84.

Van der Zeijst, B.A.M.; Horzinek, M.C.; and Moening, V. (1975) The genome of equine arteritis virus. *Virology* **68**, 418-25.

Westaway, E.G.; Brinton, M.A.; Gaidamovich, S.Y.; Horzinek, M.C.; Igarashi, A.; Kaariainen, L.; Lvov, D.K.; Porterfield, J.S.; Russell, P.K.; and Trent, D.W. (1985) Togaviridae. *Intervirology* **24**, 125-39.

Young, J.F.; Taussig, R.; Aaronson, R.P.; and Palese, P. (1981) Advantages and limitations of the oligonucleotide mapping technique for analysis of viral RNAs. In *The Replication of Negative Strand Viruses*, pp. 209-15. Elsevier North Holland, New York.

Response of Vaccinated and Non-Vaccinated Mares to Artificial Insemination with Semen from Stallions Persistently Infected with Equine Arteritis Virus

William H. McCollum, Peter J. Timoney, A. Wayne Roberts, Judy E. Willard, and Gene D. Carswell

SUMMARY

Twenty horses were used to study the pathogenesis of the TWH and TB-SS strains of equine arteritis virus (EAV), including the protection afforded by vaccination. Ten mares, seven vaccinated and three nonvaccinated, were inseminated with semen from a Tennessee Walking Horse stallion infected with the TWH strain. Eight seronegative mares were used as contacts to monitor possible transmission of infection from the mares exposed venereally. Six mares, three vaccinates and three nonvaccinates, were inseminated with semen from a Thoroughbred stallion infected with the TB-SS strain.

The TWH and TB-SS strains of EAV produced a rather mild disease in susceptible seronegative mares. Signs of disease did not develop in vaccinated mares after insemination, but all mares became infected, as evidenced by the isolation of virus for a brief period from the nasopharynx and buffy coat and by an elevated antibody response.

Virus was present in the nasopharynx and blood of nonvaccinated mares in much greater quantities and for longer periods of time than in the vaccinated mares. In vaccinated mares exposed venereally to the TWH strain of EAV, the quantity of virus shed nasally was detectable in cell cultures for only one to three days. Similar observations were made in vaccinated and nonvaccinated mares inseminated with semen containing the TB-SS strains of EAV.

Infection was readily transmitted to a susceptible contact mare from nonvaccinated mares after insemination.

Infection developed in only one of the seven seronegative mares held in close contact with vaccinated mares challenge-exposed by the venereal route to the TWH strain of EAV. This indicated that the small quantity of virus eliminated by vaccinated mares was insufficient to establish infection in most instances, or that it was effectively diluted by the environment.

The use of the vaccine is advisable in mares when a carrier horse, or "viral shedder," is known to exist.

McCollum, Timoney, Roberts: Department of Veterinary Science, University of Kentucky, Lexington, Kentucky 40546. Willard, Carswell: Morehead State University, Morehead, Kentucky 40351. Published as paper No. 87-4-176 with approval of the Director of the Kentucky Agricultural Experiment Station; supported by a grant from the Grayson Foundation, Inc.

INTRODUCTION

The carrier horse, especially the stallion, is probably the major factor in the dissemination of equine viral arteritis and the perpetuation of the causative virus (Pottie 1888; Clark 1892; Bergman 1913; Schofield 1937; McCollum et al. 1971; Timoney 1985; Timoney et al. 1986, 1987). Many of the measures currently in force in Kentucky to control this infection in the wake of the 1984 epizootic are designed to protect both stallions and the mares to which they are bred (Kentucky Department of Agriculture 1986). As part of an ongoing study to elucidate further the "carrier state" in the stallion persistently infected with EAV, the pathogenesis of selected strains of EAV isolated from carrier stallions was investigated in mares exposed by the venereal route. In conjunction with this, the efficacy of the commercial vaccine Arvac was evaluated in mares challenged venereally with the selected strains of EAV within three weeks of vaccination.

This study was designed to investigate the pathogenesis of two strains of EAV (TWH and TB-SS), and the immunity that mares developed against virus challenge by the venereal route after inoculation with the commercial vaccine.

MATERIALS AND METHODS

Horses. Of the 20 crossbred mares seronegative to EAV in the study, Nos. 123, 124, 125, 128, 129, 135, 136, 137, 138, and P1 were two to three years old, and Nos. 58, 60, 61, 64, 66, 68, 69, 70, 71, and 72 were older. Of the 20 mares, Nos. 123, 129, 136, and 137 were used on two different occasions, as they did not become infected or undergo seroconversion during the initial experiment.

Vaccine. Arvac (Fort Dodge Laboratories, Fort Dodge, Iowa) was administered according to instructions.

Carrier stallions, semen collection, and insemination. The two stallions in the study, a 14-year-old Tennessee Walking Horse (TWH) and a nine-year-old Thoroughbred, were both persistently infected with EAV. Certain mares bred to the TWH stallion in September 1985 confirmed the stallion to be a "semen shedder" of EAV. Since then, virus has been recovered reglarly from semen in cell culture. Semen was collected from this stallion using a phantom mare and a

Table 1. TWH strain of EAV: Clinical responses and virus isolations from mares after insemination with semen from a persistently infected stallion

Mare No.	Days of thermal response (max. C°)	Days of virus isolation: Nasopharynx	Buffy coat	Cervix	Signs of arteritis
		Nonvaccinated			
69	2-8 (39.7)	4-8	2,4-7	2-5	Mild
124	4-9 (39.2)	4-10	3-9	4-8	Mild
128	3-10 (39.2)	4-8	3-10	6-7	Mild
		Vaccinated			
58	4,5 (39.2)	5,6	4	Not done	None
60	4-6 (38.9)	7,9	5,6	Not done	None
61	4-7 (38.6)	6,7	4	Not done	None
64	4,5 (38.4)	4,5,6	4	Not done	None
66	3,4 (39.1)	5,6,7	3,4	Not done	None
68	3,4,6,7 (39.6)	4,5	3,4	Not done	None
72	4,5 (39.0)	4,5,10	4,5	Not done	None

modified Colorado-type artificial vagina fitted with a plastic liner and a filter-equipped plastic bottle. The spermatozoa were counted using a calibrated spectrophotometer. The semen was immediately placed on ice and transported to the farm where the mares were located. The mares were artificially inseminated using a 21-inch dairy-type plastic insemination pipette and a 10/25-ml syringe. Each mare was inseminated twice on alternate days, each time receiving 5×10^8 spermatozoa.

The TB-SS stallion was first confirmed as a long-term carrier of EAV in May 1985, in a testing program that the Kentucky State Department of Agriculture mandated for the Thoroughbred stallion population in the state. Since then, EAV has been isolated regularly from the semen of this stallion. The procedures for collecting and inseminating the semen of this stallion were the same as for the TWH stallion.

Experimental design. Two similar studies were conducted, one utilizing the TWH strain of EAV and the second the TB-SS strain. In the TWH study, seven mares were vaccinated with Arvac: Nos. 58, 60, 61, 64, 66, 68, and 72. Eighteen or 19 days later, these mares and three nonvaccinated mares, Nos. 69, 124 and 128, were inseminated with semen from the TWH stallion. Three days after initial insemination, the mares were paired with seronegative mares in the following manner: No. 58 (135), 60 (125), 61 (136), 64 (129), 66 (123), 68 (137), 72 (P1), and Nos. 124 and 128 with No. 138. Mare 69 did not have a seronegative contact. With one exception, all pairings were in box stalls (12 ft × 12 ft). Rectal temperatures and signs of disease were recorded twice daily for 14 days. Nasopharyngeal swabs and buffy coat samples were obtained from the inseminated mares for 14 days and from the contact mares on days when they were febrile. Cervical swabs were obtained from the vaccinated mares, but not routinely. Aliquots of these specimens were inoculated into 25-cm^2 flasks of the RK-13 rabbit kidney cell line for recovery of virus. Serum neutralizing (SN) antibody titers were determined on pre- and postvaccination and postinsemination serum samples. Procedures for the propagation and maintenance of cell cultures, for collecting specimens, isolating and assaying EAV, and quantitating serum neutralizing antibodies have been described previously (McCollum 1970; McCollum et al. 1971).

In the case of the TB-SS strain of EAV, three mares, Nos. 70, 71, and 129, were inseminated three weeks after vaccination, along with nonvaccinated mares Nos. 123, 136, and 137. Procedures to monitor for clinical signs of disease and to collect and process specimens were the same as those described for the TWH study.

RESULTS

Clinical responses and recovery of virus from nasopharynx, buffy coat, and cervix. All the vaccinated mares remained afebrile and asymptomatic throughout the 18 to 21 days before insemination. Responses of the mares to cervical insemination with raw semen from stallion TWH are summarized in Table 1. Four of the vaccinated mares were febrile for two days; two for three days; and one for four days. The maximum temperatures ranged from 38.4°C to 39.6°C. There were no other signs of disease. The nonvaccinated mares were febrile for six to eight days, with maximum temperatures ranging from 39.2°C to 39.7°C. Mild signs of pinkeye, inappetence, and nasal discharge developed in these mares. Virus was recovered from the nasopharynx of four vaccinated mares for two days and from the other three mares for three days. Virus was recovered from the nasopharynx of nonvaccinated mares for five to seven days. Virus was recovered from buffy coats of vaccinated mares for one to two days, and for five to eight days from corresponding samples of nonvaccinated mares. Cervical swabs obtained from nonvaccinated mares contained virus for two to five days.

Table 2. TB-SS strain of EAV: Clinical responses and virus isolations from mares after insemination with semen from a persistently infected stallion

Mare no.	Days of thermal response (max. C°)	Days of virus isolation			Signs of arteritis
		Nasopharynx	Buffy coat	Cervix	
		Nonvaccinated			
123	1-9 (39.6)	4-10	3-13	7	Mild
136	1-9 (39.0)	2-10	3-13	1-7	Mild
137	2-9 (39.9)	2-10	2-13	3-6	Mild
		Vaccinated			
70	3 (39.3)	3-6	2-8	1-6	None
71	2-4 (39.1)	5-7	3-8	3-6	None
129	2-3 (39.0)	4-7	2-8	1-4	None

Results for mares inseminated with raw semen from stallion TB-SS were similar (Table 2). The nonvaccinated mares developed mild signs of arteritis and were febrile for eight to nine days, the maximum temperatures ranging from 39.0°C to 39.9°C. Virus was present in the nasopharynx for seven to nine days, in the buffy coats for 10 to 11 days, and on the cervix for one to seven days. Although otherwise asymptomatic, vaccinated mares were slightly febrile for one to three days, the maximum temperatures ranging from 39.0°C to 39.3°C. Virus was isolated from the buffy coats for six to seven days and from cervical swabs for four to six days.

Estimation of quantity of virus in nasopharynx. The three nonvaccinated mares inseminated with semen from the TWH stallion commenced nasal shedding of the virus on the fourth day, with the quantity of virus present in the nasopharynx ranging from 70 to 480 plaque-forming units (PFU) per milliliter of nasal swab extract (Table 3). The amount of virus was maximum on the sixth day after insemination, ranging from 1500 to >2000 PFU/ml of nasal swab extract. Virus was not detected in the nasal tract 11 to 14 days after insemination. Swabs from vaccinated horses yielded much smaller quantities of virus for two to three days. The maximum quantity of virus detected was 16 PFU/ml of swab extract on day four from Mare 68. All other values were 8 PFU/ml or less.

Nonvaccinated Mares 123, 136, and 137, inseminated with semen collected from the TB-SS stallion, commenced shedding virus from the second through the fourth day after first insemination and continued to shed through the tenth or eleventh day (Table 4). The quantity of virus peaked on the sixth day, ranging from 500 to 10,000 PFU/ml of swab extract. Vaccinated mares 70, 71, and 129 commenced shedding virus on the third to the fifth day and continued to shed for three to four more days. Maximum concentrations of virus—30 PFU (Mare 129) and 52 PFU (Mare 71)—occurred on the sixth day after insemination. The concentration of virus present on the remaining days was 10 PFU or less.

Table 3. Quantitation of TWH strain of EAV in nasopharynx of mares after cervical insemination with semen from a stallion persistently infected with TWH strain

Mare no.	Days after insemination; PFU[a]/ml of nasal swab extract								
	1-3	4	5	6	7	8	9	10	11-14
				Nonvaccinated					
69	0	280	2000	>2000	>2000	100	0	0	0
124	0	480	600	1500	1000	10	2	2	0
128	0	70	1100	1500	650	10	0	0	0
				Vaccinated					
58	0	0	6	2	0	0	0	0	0
60	0	0	0	0	2	0	2	0	0
61	0	0	0	8	2	0	0	0	0
64	0	2	2	0[b]	0	0	0	0	0
66	0	0	6	0[b]	2	0	0	0	0
68	0	0[b]	16	0	2	0	0	0	0
72	0	2	2	0	0	0	0	2	0

[a] PFU = plaque-forming units.
[b] Virus recovered on 2nd passage.

Thermal, serologic and clinical response of seronegative mares in contact with inseminated mares. Six of the seven seronegative mares in contact with vaccinated mares venereally exposed to the TWH strain of EAV did not become febrile, develop signs of disease, or undergo seroconversion (Table 5). Contact mare No. 125, however, became slightly febrile for four days, and after four weeks had an SN titer of 1:256. EAV was isolated from the nasopharynx and buffy coat. Mare 138, in contact with nonvaccinated mares Nos. 124 and 128, had a titer of 1:256 four weeks after the latter mares had been inseminated, but this mare did not develop signs of arteritis.

Serological responses to insemination. The nonvaccinated mares had serum-neutralizing titers which were inconclusive one week after insemination with semen from the TWH stallion (Table 6). These titers rose to 1:256 to ≥1:512 after four weeks. Vaccinated horses had titers ranging from 1:4 to 1:16 at the time of insemination, 18-19 days after vaccination. One week later the titers had increased to 1:256 to ≤1:512,

Table 4. Quantitation of TB-SS strain of EAV in nasopharynx of mares after cervical insemination with semen from a persistently infected stallion

Mare no.	Days after insemination; PFU[a]/ml of nasal swab extract													
	1	2	3	4	5	6	7	8	9	10	11	12	13	14
	Nonvaccinated													
123	0	0	0	25	250	500	500	10	10	5	0	0	0	0
136	0	30	100	500	2500	5000	2500	100	60	10	0	0	0	0
137	0	20	500	2500	2500	10,000	2500	100	100	20	2	0	0	0
	Vaccinated													
70	0	0	3	3	5	1	0	0	0	0	0	0	0	0
71	0	0	0	0	4	52	2	0	0	0	0	0	0	0
129	0	0	0	10	3	30	1	0	0	0	0	0	0	0

[a] PFU = plaque-forming units.

Table 5. TWH strain of EAV: Clinical and serologic response of seronegative mares in contact with mares inseminated with semen from a persistently infected stallion

Control mare no. (contact mare, inseminated)	Days of thermal response (Max. C°)	Serum-neutralizing titers: Precontact	Serum-neutralizing titers: 4 weeks after contact	Signs of arteritis
		Nonvaccinated contact mares		
138 (124, 128)	ND[a]	Negative	1:256	None
		Vaccinated contact mares		
135 (58)	None (38.3)	Negative	Negative	None
125[b] (60)	12-15 (38.6)	Negative	1:256	None
136 (61)	None (38.3)	Negative	Negative	None
129 (64)	None (38.3)	Negative	Negative	None
123 (66)	None (38.4)	Negative	Negative	None
137 (68)	None (38.3)	Negative	Negative	None
P1 (72)	None (38.4)	Negative	Negative	None

[a] ND = not done.
[b] EAV was isolated from nasopharyngeal swabs on Days 9 through 14 after being placed in contact with Mare 60.

Table 6. TWH strain of EAV: Serologic responses of mares to cervical insemination with semen from a persistently infected stallion

Mare no.	Serum-neutralizing titers: Before vaccination	Before insemination (18-19 days postvac.)	Weeks after insemination: 1	Weeks after insemination: 4
		Nonvaccinated		
69		Negative	Inconclusive	≥1:512
124		Negative	Inconclusive	1:512
128		Negative	Inconclusive	1:256
		Vaccinated		
58	Negative	1:4	≥1:512	≥1:512
60	Negative	1:16	1:512	256
61	Negative	ND[a]	1:256	256
64	Negative	1:8	≥1:512	≥1:512
66	Negative	1:8	1:512	1:512
68	Negative	1:8	1:512	1:256
72	Negative	1:16	1:512	1:512

[a] ND = not done.

Table 7. TB-SS strain of EAV: Serological responses of mares to cervical insemination with semen from a persistently infected stallion

Mare no.	Serum-neutralizing titers			
	Before vaccination	Before insemination (18-19 days postvac.)	Weeks after insemination 1	4
		Nonvaccinated		
123		Negative	1:4	1:128
136		Negative	Inconclusive	1:32
137		Negative	1:4	1:256
		Vaccinated		
70	Negative	1:64	1:256	≥1:512
71	Negative	1:128	1:128	≥1:512
129	Negative	1:32	1:128	≥1:512

and were relatively unchanged when retested four weeks after insemination.

One nonvaccinated mare, No. 136, exposed to semen from the TB-SS stallion, had an inconclusive SN titer after one week, which increased to 1:32 after four weeks (Table 7). The other two nonvaccinated mares developed titers of 1:4 after one week, increasing to 1:128 to 1:256 after four weeks. Vaccinated mares had titers ranging from 1:32 to 1:128 at the time of insemination, which was carried out 21 days postvaccination. The titers ranged from 1:128 to 1:256 after one week and ≤1:512 four weeks after insemination.

DISCUSSION

The TWH and TB-SS strains of EAV produced a comparatively mild disease in nonvaccinated seronegative mares. Nasal discharge, a slight degree of pinkeye, and slight depression for one or two days were the maximum signs of disease that developed. Nevertheless, such strains of EAV are considered abortigenic, and due precautions should be taken to prevent EAV infection. Vaccination protected against development of clinical signs of disease but did not prevent the mares from becoming infected. However, the duration of shedding and the quantity of virus present in the nasopharynx and blood were much less in vaccinated mares than in the nonvaccinated controls. In fact, the quantity of virus shed nasally by nonvaccinated mares was 100 to 1,000 times more than the maximum amount demonstrated in the nasopharynx of vaccinated mares.

The question remains as to what quantity of virus is necessary to establish infection and under what circumstances. In this study, the possibility of lateral spread or contact transmission of the infection from inseminated vaccinated mares to seronegative contact mares was maximized by boxing the pairs in close quarters one or two days after the second insemination. In only one instance was EAV transmitted by vaccinated mares to the nonvaccinated contacts. Although only one mare was used as a contact control with nonvaccinated mares, infection was readily transmitted to it. It is probably fair to assume that if the study had matched each nonvaccinated mare with a seronegative contact mare, all such contacts would have acquired the infection. Therefore, the vaccine used could be considered to have moderated the infection caused by this strain of virus by reducing nasal shedding to a level that greatly reduced the possibility of transmission to susceptible horses in normal contact with the vaccinates. Revaccination with Arvac greatly enhances the immunity to EVA and should be considered as part of any control program (Timoney et al. 1987). In emergencies when timing is critical, an alternative is vaccines that are less attenuated and that elicit more protection (Doll et al. 1957; McCollum 1970).

REFERENCES

Bergman, A.M. (1913) Beitrage zur Kenntnis der Virustrager bei Rotlaufseuche, Influenza erysipelatosa, des Pferdes. *Z. Infekt. Kr.* **13**, 161-74.

Clark, J. (1892) Transmission of pink-eye from apparently healthy stallions to mares. *J. Comp. Path.* **5**, 261-64.

Doll, E.R.; Bryans, J.T.; McCollum, W.H.; and Crowe, M.E.W. (1957) Isolation of a filterable agent causing arteritis of horses and abortion by mares. Its differentiation from the equine abortion (influenza) virus. *Cornell Vet.* **47**, 3-41.

Kentucky Department of Agriculture (1986) Restrictive equine viral arteritis. Administrative Regulation 301, *KAR* **20**, 180 (Nov. 16, 1986).

McCollum, W.H. (1970) Vaccination for equine viral arteritis. In *Equine Infectious Diseases*, Vol. 2, pp. 143-51. Karger, Basel.

McCollum, W.H., and Bryans, J.T. (1972) Serological identification of infection by equine arteritis virus in horses of several countries. *Proc. 3d Int. Conf. Equine Infect. Dis.*, pp. 256-63.

McCollum, W.H.; Prickett, M.E.; and Bryans, J.T. (1971) Temporal distribution of equine arteritis virus in respiratory mucosa, tissues and body fluids of horses infected by inhalation. *Res. Vet. Sci.* **2**, 459-64.

Pottie, A. (1888) The propagation of influenza from stallions to mares. *J. Comp. Path.* **1**, 37-38.

Schofield, F.W. (1937) A report of two outbreaks of equine influenza due to virus carriers (stallions). Annual report, Department of Agriculture, Ontario.

Timoney, P.J. (1985) Clinical, virological and epidemiological features of the 1984 outbreak of equine viral arteritis in the Thoroughbred population in Kentucky, USA. *Proc. Grayson Found. Intl. Conf. Thoroughbred Breeders* Orgs on EVA, pp. 24-33.

Timoney, P.J.; McCollum, W.H.; Roberts, A.W.; and Murphy, T.W. (1986) Demonstration of the carrier state in naturally acquired equine arteritis virus infection of the stallion. *Res. Vet. Sci.* **41**, 279-80.

Timoney, P.J.; McCollum, W.H.; Murphy, T.W.; Roberts, A.W.; Willard, J.G.; and Carswell, C.D. (1987) The carrier state in equine arteritis virus infection in the stallion with specific emphasis on the venereal mode of virus transmission. *J. Reprod. Fert. Suppl.* **35**, pp. 95-102.

Safety Evaluation of a Commercial Modified Live Equine Arteritis Virus Vaccine for Use in Stallions

Peter J. Timoney, Norman W. Umphenour, and William H. McCollum

SUMMARY

The safety of a modified live equine arteritis virus (EAV) vaccine for stallions was assessed under experimental conditions. No clinical sequelae of either a local or systemic nature and no significant hematologic or blood biochemical changes were detected in any of the 16 stallions that were vaccinated. With the exception of a 17-23% reduction in the percentage of sperm with normal morphology two to three weeks after vaccination, no significant effects on semen quality were observed. Although vaccine virus was isolated sporadically from the blood and nasopharynx of some of the stallions, it could not be recovered from urine or semen. Serum neutralizing antibody titers to EAV developed in all of the vaccinated stallions within 5 to 8 days, but by Day 42 had decreased to undetectable levels in 25% of the group. None of the vaccinated stallions transmitted EAV infection either to in-contact controls or to mares to which they were bred after vaccination. The results of the study confirm the safety of this modified live EAV vaccine for use in stallions.

INTRODUCTION

With the isolation of equine arteritis virus (EAV) during an epizootic of abortion on a Standardbred farm in Bucyrus, Ohio, in 1953 (Doll et al. 1957), equine viral arteritis (EVA) was first identified as a separate disease of the horse. Before that, the etiology of EVA had often been confused with that of equine influenza and rhinopneumonitis. Severity of the disease is variable, with many cases being subclinical in nature. It is characterized clinically by fever, anorexia, depression, limb and ventral edema, leucopenia, rhinitis, conjunctivitis, skin rash, and abortion in pregnant mares.

Equids are the only natural hosts of the causative virus (McCollum 1970), which belongs to the family Togaviridae, genus *Arterivirus* (Westaway *et al.*, 1985). The virus is readily transmitted by the respiratory and venereal routes, and to a lesser extent by indirect contact with contaminated fomites during the acute phase of the infection (McCollum, Prickett & Bryans 1971; McCollum & Swerczek 1978; Timoney & McCollum 1985). Transmission by persistently infected carrier stallions occurs primarily by the venereal route (Timoney et al. 1987b). Immunity following natural EAV infection is both solid and long-lasting and would appear to persist for several years (McCollum 1969; Gerber et al. 1978).

In spite of the apparent worldwide distribution of EAV (Timoney & McCollum 1985), recorded outbreaks or epizootics of the disease have been limited and sporadic (Timoney & McCollum 1987). The epizootic of EVA in Kentucky in 1984 marked the first occasion this disease had been reported in the Thoroughbred population of North America (Timoney 1985). There is ample serologic evidence to indicate that the preponderance of acute infections are subclinical, not only in the United States (McCollum & Bryans 1973; Timoney & McCollum, unpublished data), but also in a variety of other countries (Akashi, Konishi & Ogata 1976; Gerber et al. 1978; Konishi et al. 1975; Matumoto, Shimizu & Ishizaki 1965; Moraillon & Moraillon 1978).

Occurrences of EVA were infrequently reported in the scientific literature before 1984, despite the widespread distribution of the causal virus. Prior to the 1984 epizootic in Kentucky, virtually no organized attempts were made to prevent and control this disease, at either the national or international level. Although an experimental modified live vaccine had been developed against EVA almost 20 years earlier (Doll et al. 1968; McCollum 1969), few saw the need for a commercial vaccine. The 1984 epizootic, however, reawakened awareness of the abortifacient potential of EAV. Even more important, it provided the first indication that a relatively high percentage of stallions become chronic carriers and remain constant semen shedders following infection with the virus (Timoney & McCollum 1985). The timing was right for commercial production of an experimental EAV vaccine that had been developed previously by attenuation of the prototype Bucyrus strain of the virus, following serial passage in primary cultures of equine kidney, rabbit kidney, and a diploid equine dermal cell line (McCollum 1981; Harry & McCollum 1981). Although a number of experimental modified live EAV vaccines have been shown to be both safe and effective (Doll et al. 1968; McCollum 1969; Harry & McCollum 1981; McCollum 1981; Fukunaga et al. 1982; McCollum 1986; McCollum et al. 1987), the safety of these vaccines for use in stallions has not been investigated. Such information is a prerequisite if a control program for EVA is to be based on vaccination of a breeding stallion population.

The present study was undertaken to evaluate the safety for

Timoney, McCollum: Department of Veterinary Science, Gluck Equine Research Center, University of Kentucky, Lexington, Kentucky 40546. Umphenour: Gainesway Farm, Lexington, Kentucky 40511. Published as paper No. 86-4-307 by permission of the Dean and Director, College of Agriculture and Kentucky Agricultural Experiment Station.

stallions of a modified live EAV vaccine (Arvac; Fort Dodge Laboratories, Fort Dodge, Iowa). Specific objectives were to investigate the potential for local or systemic reaction in stallions; effects on hematologic and blood chemical parameters and on semen quality; shedding of vaccine virus in the nasopharynx, semen, or urine or its circulation in the blood; and transmission of the virus by vaccinated stallions, either venereally or by aerosol transmission.

MATERIALS AND METHODS

Horses. *Stallions.* Sexually mature stallions, seronegative for antibodies to EAV, were obtained from a commercial vendor. The majority had been used previously for breeding to nurse mares or as teaser stallions. They comprised Thoroughbred (6), Quarter Horse (3), Appaloosa (2), Belgian (1), Tennessee Walking Horse (1), pony (1), and crossbred (6). The ages ranged from two to more than 12 years and, excluding three who exceeded 12 years, the mean age was 7.2 years.

Mares. Mares for test breeding to the vaccinated stallions were obtained from a commercial vendor and confirmed seronegative for antibodies to EAV. With the exception of a number of crossbred animals, they were either Thoroughbred or Quarter Horse mares.

Vaccine. The commercial modified live EAV vaccine used was ARVAC, of passage history HK-131/RK-111/ECID-24. It was administered by the intramuscular route in accordance with the manufacturer's recommendations, using the same lot of vaccine throughout. After vaccination, an aliquot of vaccine was titrated in monolayer cultures (25 cm^2 flasks) of RK-13 cells (ATCC. ccl-37) and found to have an infectivity titre of 1.9×10^7 plaque-forming units (PFU)/ml.

Experimental design. This study was conducted over a six-to-seven-week period extending from late December to early February of the following year. A total of 19 stallions were individually maintained in adjoining stalls extending the length of each side of a barn; 16 were vaccinated against EVA and three were kept as in-contact controls. Pre- and postvaccination testing of each stallion comprised: (*a*) clinical examination for evidence of any local or systemic reaction; (*b*) determination of various hematologic and blood biochemical parameters; (*c*) semen evaluation based on sperm motility, density, and morphology; (*d*) attempted virus isolation from nasopharynx, buffy coat, serum, urine, and semen; (*e*) determination of the serum neutralizing antibody response to EAV; and (*f*) attempted venereal transmission of vaccine virus to two groups of test mares bred on Days 14-17 and 28-31, respectively, after vaccination. Two additional mares were included as in-contact stall and paddock controls.

Experimental procedures. *Clinical examination.* Each stallion was clinically examined and the rectal temperature recorded twice daily at 7:00 A.M. and at 3:00 P.M. for five days before and 14 days after vaccination. Special attention was paid to the possibility of undesirable local reactions at the site of vaccination.

Hematology. A comprehensive hematologic profile was undertaken daily on each stallion from three days before vaccination to Day 17 after. The statistics included total white cell count (WBC), total red cell count (RBC), packed cell volume (PCV), hemoglobin, mean corpuscular volume (MCV), mean corpuscular hemoglobin (MCH), and mean corpuscular hemoglobin concentration (MCHC). Determinations were carried out on a Profile 750 cell counter (Mallinckrodt, Inc., Bohemia, New York).

Blood biochemistry. An extensive range of blood biochemical parameters was examined on each stallion over a period from two days before vaccination to three weeks after (Days 2, 4, 6, 8, 10, 12, 13, and 21). Determinations of glucose, calcium, phosphorus, total bilirubin, creatine phosphokinase (CPK), lactic dehydrogenase (LDH), aspartate aminotransferase (AST), AST, alkaline phosphatase, urea nitrogen, creatinine, and albumin were carried out using a Gemstar chemistry analyzer (Electro-Nucleonics, Inc., Fairfield, N.J.); sodium and potassium using a Corning Model 480 flame photometer (Corning Medical, Medfield, Massachusetts); chloride and bicarbonate using an Oxford Model 600 titration system (Oxford Laboratories, Inc., Foster City, Calif.); and total serum protein using a refractometer (American Optical, Buffalo, N.Y.). Globulin levels were calculated by deducting respective albumin concentrations from those for total serum protein.

Semen evaluation. Semen evaluations were attempted on the day of vaccination and after that, on Days 3, 7, 10, 14-17, and 21. For a number of reasons, mainly difficulties with some stallions in breeding artifically and the time of semen collection in relation to the breeding season, possible changes in semen quality could not be monitored for a significant number of the stallions throughout the sampling period.

Semen was collected using a closed-ended artifical vagina (modified Colorado-type) and a teaser mare. When it was not feasible to obtain a semen collection by this means, as between Days 14 and 17, when the stallions were bred to the first group of test mares, dismount samples were collected at time of breeding. No antiseptics or disinfectants were used in washing the external genitalia of the stallions before collection.

Semen evaluations determined gel volume, gel-free seminal volume, percent progressive sperm motility, sperm concentration, and percent sperm with normal morphology. An aliquot of semen (approximately 2-5 ml) was refrigerated on freezer packs immediately after collection and transported to the laboratory for virus isolation.

Motility estimates were performed on wet mounts of semen as described by Neu and Timoney (1988). On occasion, the excessively cold weather prevailing at the time caused temperature shock of semen samples. With the exception of an initial few specimens for which sperm concentration was calculated using a Neubauer hemocytometer (American Optical, Buffalo, N.Y.) after the method of Neu and Timoney (1988), sperm densities were determined on gel-free semen samples using a Model 340 digital spectrophotometer (Sequoia-Turner, Mountain View, Calif.) at a wavelength of 550 nm. No attempt was made to correct for the number of sperm present in the gel fraction of the semen. Morphologic assessment of sperm was performed on smears of semen stained with eosin-nigrosin and examined using oil immersion at 1000 ×.

Virus isolation. Virus isolation was attempted from the following specimens collected from each stallion after vaccination: (*a*) nasopharyngeal swabs, buffy coat cells, and serum on Days 1-17, 21, and 28; (*b*) urine on Days 3, 7, 10, 14, 21, and 28; and (*c*) semen on Days 3, 7, 10, 14-17, 21, and 28-31. Following collection, all samples were refrigerated on freezer packs for transport to the laboratory, where they were either processed immediately or frozen at −80°C and tested at a later date. The procedures used to collect and attempt virus isolation from nasopharyngeal swabs, buffy coat cells, serum, and semen were similar to those of Timoney and colleagues (1987b). Virus isolation was attempted in monolayer cultures (25 cm^2 flasks) of RK-13 cells. Midstream urine samples were collected in sterile containers following intravenous administration of 150 mg furosemide (Butler Co., Columbus, Ohio). These were concentrated by overnight dialysis at 4°C against an 8% solution of polyethylene glycol (MW 15,000-20,000) using dialysis sacks (Sigma, St. Louis, Mo.) with retention capability for proteins of greater than 2,000 molecular weight. Concentrated urine samples were harvested aseptically and inoculated undiluted and diluted 1:10 into cell culture.

The identity of isolants of EAV was confirmed in a one-way plaque-reduction assay using horse antiserum prepared against the Bucyrus strain of the virus.

Serology. The serum neutralizing antibody response to EAV was monitored in each stallion before vaccination and on Days 1-14, 17, 21, 28, and 42 after vaccination. Antibody titers to EAV were determined by a microneutralization test in RK-13 cells in the presence of guinea pig complement (Miles Scientific, Naperville, Ill.).

Test breeding. Two groups of eight mares each were test-bred to the vaccinated stallions, the first group during Days 14-17 after vaccination and the second group during Days 28-31. Mares were synchronised in estrous with estradiol cypionate (Upjohn, Kalamazoo, Mich.) and alfa prostol (Hoffman La Roche, Nutley, N.J.) Each mare was assigned to two stallions and bred by natural service to those stallions once a day for

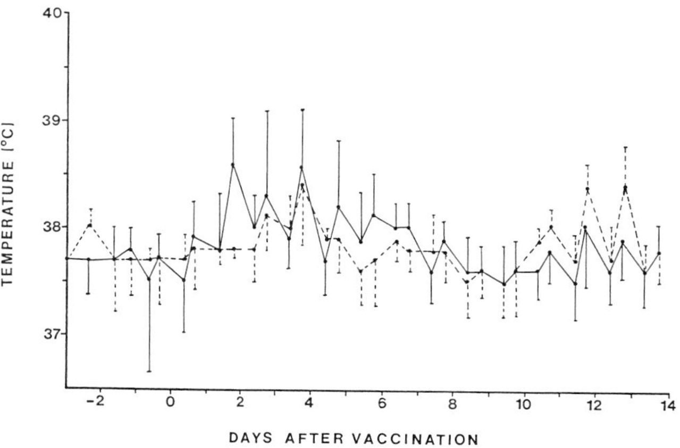

Fig. 1. Diurnal temperatures of stallions after vaccination with a modified live equine arteritis virus vaccine (Arvac). Temperature expressed as mean values ±1 standard deviation: *solid lines*, vaccinates ($N = 16$); *dashed lines*, controls ($N = 3$).

four consecutive days, for a total of eight matings per mare. All mares, including the two in-contact controls, were monitored for clinical evidence of infection and for seroconversion for EAV on Days 7, 14, 21, and 28 after breeding.

Statistical analysis. The Student's t-test was used to analyze the data on WBC counts, sperm motility, concentration, and morphology. In all cases, only differences with a probability of $P < 0.05$ were considered significant.

RESULTS

Clinical observations. None of the stallions exhibited any overt clinical signs of illness following vaccination. Febrile responses, if present, were mild, generally not exceeding 39.2° C. They occurred principally during the first three days after the stallions were vaccinated (Fig. 1). Only three stallions (Nos. 4, 14, and 17) developed temperatures in excess of 39.2° C, the maximum temperature recorded being 40.2° C in stallion No. 4 on the second day. Febrile responses were transient, lasting only 24 hr in most cases, and two to five days for the others (Nos. 2, 4, 7, and 14). No adverse local reactions were observed at the site of inoculation in any of the stallions after vaccination.

Hematologic responses. No major alterations were detected in the range of hematologic parameters investigated following vaccination. No statistically significant differences were demonstrated between pre- and postvaccination red cell values (total RBC, PCV, hemoglobin, MCV, MCH, and MCHC) for any of the stallions. Although there was a slight elevation in the mean PCV of the vaccinated stallions between Days 2 and 7 after vaccination, an equivalent rise occurred concomitantly in the corresponding values of the control animals (Fig. 2).

The first week after vaccination marked a minor decrease

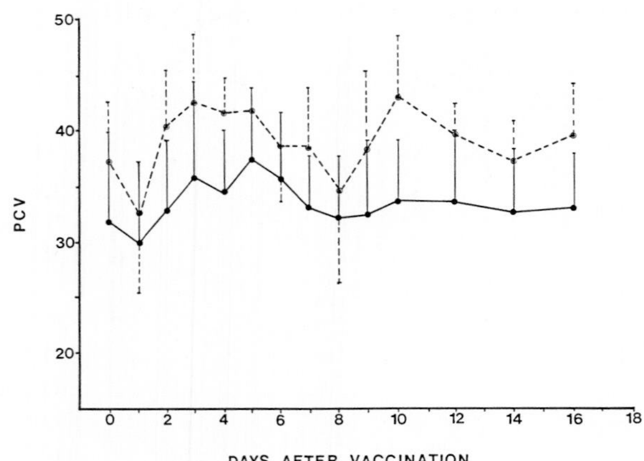

Fig. 2. Packed red cell volume in stallions after vaccination with a modified live equine arteritis virus vaccine (Arvac). Packed cell volume expressed as mean values ±1 standard deviation: *solid lines*, vaccinates ($N = 16$); *dashed lines*, controls ($N = 3$).

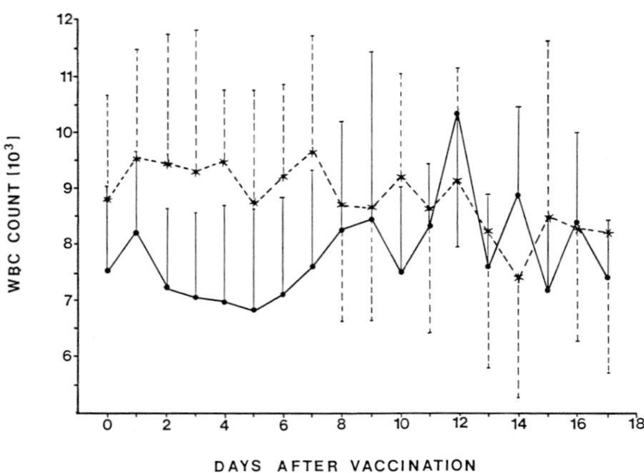

Fig. 3. Total leucocyte count in stallions after vaccination with a modified live equine arteritis virus vaccine (Arvac). Leucocyte count expressed as mean values ±1 standard deviation: *solid lines*, vaccinates ($N = 16$); controls ($N = 3$).

in the mean total WBC count of the vaccinated stallions (Fig. 3). The depression in mean WBC count was short-lived and differences between pre- and postvaccination values were significant only on Days 4 ($P<0.05$) and 5 ($P<0.01$) after vaccination. This leucopenia was followed by an even more transient leucocytosis lasting approximately 48 hr, which occurred on Days 11 ($P<0.001$) and 12 ($P<0.01$).

Blood biochemical responses. Although some variation was in observed pre- and postvaccination values, no significant differences were demonstrated in the blood biochemical parameters.

Changes in semen quality. The quality of semen from the stallions before and after vaccination was evaluated primarily on the basis of sperm motility, concentration, and morphology. Due to difficulties in getting many of the stallions to breed artificially, mean values were based on data derived from a total of eight animals. With the exception of values obtained on Days 3 and 7 postvaccination, no significant changes were observed in the percentage of progressive sperm motility in the vaccinated stallions (Table 1). Since ambient temperature was well below freezing on both days, the drop in percent motility that occurred may have been due to temperature shock of some semen samples.

While there was a certain amount of variation in the mean sperm concentration of the stallions after vaccination (Table 2), the changes seen were not significant. The percentage of sperm with normal morphology in the semen of vaccinated stallions decreased gradually over a two- to three-week period, from a mean of 75% at time of vaccination to a minimum of 57.6% on Day 17, increasing slightly to 59.6% four days later (Table 3; Fig. 4). Mean values for three of the last four collection days were significantly lower (Day 15, $P<0.01$; Days 17 and 21, $P<0.001$) than at the start of the experiment.

Virologic responses. Multiplication of vaccine virus was detected sporadically in a number of the vaccinated stallions. Virus was recovered most frequently from buffy coat cultures, with 12 stallions yielding virus, three of which were also positive on nasopharyngeal culture (Table 4). The vaccine strain of EAV was not found in the buffy coat of stallions for one to seven days (mean 3.1 days) after vaccination. The duration of circulating virus detectable in cell culture varied from 1-21 days, with the majority of stallions remaining positive for an average of 6.7 days. The quantity of EAV detected in buffy coat cultures was very low: 1-22 PFU of virus. Concentrations of virus reached a maximum between Days 4 and 7 after vaccination in all but two stallions. In those two, values peaked within 48 hr of vaccination.

Vaccine virus was recovered from the nasopharynx of four vaccinated stallions (Table 4). It was not found in the nasal tract for three to four days (mean 3.5 days) after vaccination. Duration of virus shedding ranged from three to seven days, with an average of five days. The amount of vaccine virus present in nasopharyngeal swabs was low (4-80 PFU/ml), with maximal concentrations between Days 3 and 6 after vaccination.

The vaccine strain of EAV was not recovered from any of the urine ($N = 91$) or semen ($N = 148$) samples collected following vaccination.

One of the in-contact control stallions (No. 10) yielded another RNA virus, differing from EAV in physicochemical characteristics and in the absence of neutralization by antiserum to the reference Bucyrus strain of EAV. The virus was isolated from the nasopharynx (Days 9-13) and urine (Days 7, 14, 21, and 28) of the control. The same virus was also isolated on multiple occasions from the urine of six of the vaccinated stallions, in two animals on every sampling occasion. One of the latter two stallions (No. 3) was retained, killed 62 days after vaccination, and necropsied. A wide range of tissues were sampled for attempted virus isolation

Table 1. Percent sperm motility in semen from stallions after vaccination with a modified live equine arteritis virus vaccine

	Percent normal motility, days after vaccination								
Stallion no.	0 (AV)[a]	3 (AV)	7 (AV)	10 (AV)	14 (Dis)[b]	15 (Dis)	16 (Dis)	17 (Dis)	21 (AV)
1	ND[c]	ND	ND	ND	35	35	ND	0	ND
2	65	60	15	70	80	50	50	0	75
3	ND	ND	ND	ND	70	55	50	40	ND
4	ND	ND	ND	ND	55	45	60	0	ND
5	65	10	50	65	75	55	30	0	50
6	75	80	0	65	40	35	35	75	70
7	ND	ND	ND	ND	30	40	50	50	ND
8	ND	ND	ND	ND	35	60	25	05	ND
9	60	40	25	25	65	70	65	55	40
12	25	45	5	65	20	55	70	65	75
13	60	50	20	60	65	65	65	15	80
14	45	20	5	55	25	45	65	50	55
15	40	5	0	55	70	45	75	65	55
17	15	20	40	55	ND	ND	ND	ND	ND
18	ND	ND	ND	ND	50	65	25	30	ND
20	ND	ND	ND	ND	35	55	50	50	ND
Mean ($N=8$):	54.4	38.7	15*	57.5	55	52.5	56.9	40.6	62.5
Standard deviation:	±16.3	±25.7	±16.9	±14.1	±23.3	±11.3	±16.7	±30.8	±14.4

Note: Vaccine used was Arvac. [a] AV = Semen collected using an artificial vagina. [b] Dis = Dismount semen sample. [c] Not done. * $P<0.001$.

(selected thoracic and abdominal lymphatic glands, lung, liver, spleen, kidney, ureters, and bladder), as well as bodily fluids (peritoneal, pleural, and pericardial). Whereas EAV was not detected in any of the bodily fluids or clarified 10% tissue suspensions, the RNA virus unrelated to EAV was isolated from the urine but not from any other site.

Serologic findings. Serum neutralizing antibody titers to EAV developed in all of the vaccinated stallions within five to eight days (Table 5). Peak titers of 1:16-1:128 were attained by Days 10-14, with the maximal mean titer of 1:46 occurring on Day 14 after vaccination. Antibody levels subsequently dropped off rapidly, and at six weeks four of the group had become seronegative and the remainder carried titers ranging from 1:4 to 1:64 (mean, 1:11.2).

Transmission findings. None of the vaccinated stallions transmitted EAV infection either to the in-contact controls or to the mares to which they were bred. Both test mares and controls remained seronegative for antibodies to EAV for the duration of the study.

DISCUSSION

Under the conditions of this experimental study, the modified live EAV vaccine Arvac was found to be safe for use in stallions. With the exception of a slight febrile response, no adverse clinical sequelae, either local or systemic, developed in any of the vaccinated stallions. This is consistent with the findings of previous studies on experimental EAV vaccines,

Table 2. Sperm concentration in semen from stallions after vaccination with a modified live equine arteritis virus vaccine

	Number of sperm/ml (10^6), days after vaccination						
Stallion no.	0 (AV)[a]	3 (AV)	7 (AV)	10 (AV)	14 (Dis)[b]	17 (Dis)	21 (AV)
1	ND[c]	ND	ND	ND	550	ND	ND
2	613	451	280	844	ND	ND	505
3	ND	ND	ND	ND	ND	ND	ND
4	ND	ND	ND	ND	ND	ND	ND
5	592	511	680	355	ND	ND	228
6	479	162	15	350	ND	ND	105
7	ND	ND	ND	ND	ND	ND	ND
8	ND	ND	ND	ND	ND	ND	ND
9	146	78	359	170	ND	ND	58
12	143	157	215	260	ND	ND	220
13	80	183	70	68	ND	ND	145
14	82	74	33	132	ND	ND	108
15	169	73	114	54	ND	ND	158
17	ND	ND	ND	ND	ND	ND	ND
18	ND	ND	ND	ND	ND	ND	ND
20	ND	ND	ND	ND	ND	ND	ND
Mean ($N=8$)	288	211.1	220.7	279.1			190.9
Standard deviation:	±231.6	±172.8	±222.1	±256.1			±139.4

Note: Vaccine used was Arvac.
[a] AV = semen collected using an artificial vagina.
[b] Dis = dismount semen sample.
[c] Not done.

Table 3. Percent sperm with normal morphology in semen from stallions after vaccination with a modified live equine arteritis virus vaccine

	Percent normal sperm, days after vaccination								
Stallion no.	0 (AV)[a]	3 (AV)	7 (AV)	10 (AV)	14 (Dis)[b]	15 (Dis)	16 (Dis)	17 (Dis)	21 (AV)
1	ND[c]	ND	ND	ND	37	35	40	36	ND
2	71	46	63	59	36	48	66	50	60
3	ND	ND	ND	ND	84	80	84	84	ND
4	ND	ND	ND	ND	69	52	44	48	ND
5	50	57	78	65	49	46	58	ND	50
6	76	88	80	78	80	75	80	ND	63
7	ND	ND	ND	ND	62	68	71	ND	ND
8	ND	ND	ND	ND	50	48	41	ND	ND
9	82	71	50	63	59	59	63	ND	65
12	73	77	63	68	81	75	69	ND	54
13	88	72	80	75	69	65	63	65	69
14	76	76	74	69	45	57	68	50	48
15	84	86	75	76	78	69	57	65	68
17	ND	ND	ND	ND	52	57	59	55	ND
18	ND	ND	ND	ND	66	63	45	30	ND
20	ND	ND	ND	ND	54	55	52	50	ND
Mean ($N=8$):	75	71.6	70.4	69.1	62.1	61.7*	65.5	57.5**	59.6**
Standard deviation:	±11.6	±14.1	±10.7	±6.75	±17.5	±11.2	±7.27	±8.66	±8.09

Note: Vaccine used was Arvac.
[a] AV = semen collected using an artifical vagina. [b] Dis = dismount semen sample. [c] Not done. * $P < 0.01$. ** $P < 0.001$.

all of which confirm that a mild fever of short duration is the only clinical response observed following intramuscular inoculation with modified virus (Doll et al. 1968; McCollum 1969; Harry & McCollum 1981; McCollum 1981; Fukunaga et al. 1982; McCollum 1986; McKinnon et al. 1986).

Although vaccination was not associated with major hematologic changes in the stallions, a slight leucopenia of several days' duration did occur. Similar observations were made by Doll and colleagues (1968), McCollum (1969, 1981), Fukunaga and colleagues (1982) and McKinnon and colleagues (1986), all of whom reported a decrease in WBC counts after injection with EAV of differing passage levels in cell culture, the leucopenia appearing within two to three days of vaccination and lasting three to five days. The transient leucocytosis that supervened a few days after the leucopenia in the present study has not been recorded previously. Although it may have resulted from an intercurrent infection in the vaccinated stallions, there was no similar finding in the in-contact controls. The WBC counts recorded in the former group were significantly greater than prevacccination values and are hardly likely to represent normal biological variation.

The absence of significant alteration in the wide range of blood biochemical parameters investigated, and of any overt clinical signs of systemic dysfunction, attests to the safety of this vaccine following parenteral administration.

Evaluation of semen quality in the stallions, though limited by failure to obtain collections from 50% of the group prior to vaccination, provided no evidence of any resultant adverse changes, in either progressive sperm motility or sperm concentration. McKinnon and colleagues (1986), in a similar study, reported no alteration in percent sperm motility in ejaculates from stallions collected on Days 11 and 25 after vaccination. In contrast to these findings with respect to the vaccine strain of EAV, Neu and Timoney (1988) demonstrated significant decreases of six to seven weeks' duration, both in sperm motility and concentration, in stallions experimentally infected with an unmodified strain of this virus isolated during the 1984 epizootic of EVA in Kentucky (Timoney 1985). The reduction in percentage of sperm with normal morphology observed in the present study was unex-

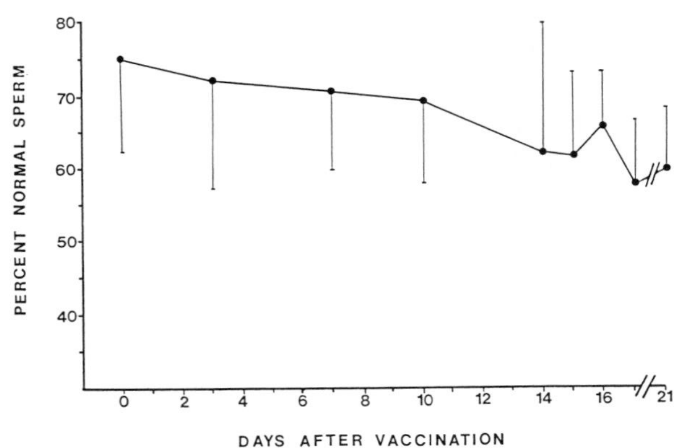

Fig. 4. Percentage of sperm with normal morphology in semen from stallions after vaccination with a modified live equine arteritis virus vaccine (Arvac). Percent sperm expressed as mean values ($N = 8$) ±1 standard deviation.

Table 4. Virus isolation from buffy coat samples and nasopharyngeal swabs from stallions after vaccination with a modifed live equine arteritis virus vaccine

Stallion no.	Virus isolation[a], days after vaccination											
	1	2	3	4	5	6	7	8-10	11	12-17	21	28
1	0	0	0	0	0	0	0	0	0	0	0	0
2	0	3	6(16)[b]	0(22)	7(44)	0(80)	0(6)	0	0	0	0	0
3	0	0	0	5	8	3	17	0	0	0	0	0
4	0	0	0	20	18	14	5	0	1	0	1	0
5	0	0	0	0	3	0	0	0	0	0	0	0
6	0	0	0	0	6	0	5	0	0	0	0	0
7	0	0	0	0	0	0	0	0	0	0	0	0
8	0	0	0	0	2	0	6	0	0	0	0	0
9	1	0	0	3(24)	2	1(4)	0	0	0	0	0	0
12	0	1	0	19	3	0	0	0	0	0	0	0
13	0	0	0	0	0	0	1	0	0	0	0	0
14	3	0	0	0	0	0	0	0	0	0	0	0
15	22	16	0	5	0	0	0	0	0	0	0	0
17	0	0	0	0	0	0	0	0	0	0	0	0
18	10	16	0(10)	5	0	1	0	0	0	0	0	0
20	0	0	0	0(4)	0	0	0	0	0	0	0	0

Note: Vaccine used was Arvac.

[a] Virus isolation attempted in monolayer cultures of RK-13 cells; infectivity expressed in plaque-forming units (PFU).

[b] Nasopharyngeal isolation in parentheses, expressed in PFU/ml of nasal swab extract.

Table 5. Serum neutralizing antibody response in stallions after vaccination with a modified live equine arteritis virus vaccine

Stallion no.	SN titer, days after vaccination											
	0-4	5	6	7	8	10	12	14	17	21	28	42
1	0	0	0	0	4	16	32	64	64	64	16	4
2	0	4[a]	4	8	16	16	32	32	32	32	16	16
3	0	4	4	4	4	16	32	64	64	64	16	16
4	0	0	4	16	16	32	64	64	64	64	64	64
5	0	4	4	4	8	8	32	32	32	32	16	4
6	0	0	4	8	8	8	16	32	32	32	16	8
7	0	4	4	4	4	4	8	32	32	32	16	8
8	0	0	0	4	4	8	8	16	16	16	16	16
9	0	4	4	16	16	32	32	32	32	32	16	8
12	0	0	4	8	16	8	8	32	32	32	16	4
13	0	0	0	8	8	8	8	16	16	16	16	0
14	0	0	4	8	16	16	16	32	16	16	8	0
15	0	4	4	8	16	16	32	32	32	32	16	16
17	0	0	0	0	4	4	16	64	64	32	16	0
18	0	4	8	32	32	32	64	128	128	64	32	8
20	0	4	4	16	8	32	64	64	64	64	16	0
Mean ($N = 16$):		2	3.25	9	11.2	16	28	46	45	39	19.5	11.2
Standard deviation:		±2.07	±2.18	±7.93	±7.62	±10.4	±20.2	±27.9	±28.7	±18.4	±12.7	±15.5

Note: Vaccine used was Arvac.

[a] Reciprocal of SN antibody titre; neutralizing antibodies detected using a microneutralization assay in RK-13 cells.

pected. From an initial value of 75%, the mean number of normal sperm progressively decreased over the term of the study, falling as low as 23.3% on Day 17 after vaccination. It appeared, however, that the percentage of sperm with normal morphology was returning to prevaccination values at the time of final semen collection, three weeks after the stallions were vaccinated. In a study of experimental infection of stallions with an unmodified strain of EAV, Neu and Timoney (1988) reported a highly significant decrease ($P<0.001$) in the percentage of normal sperm, accompanied by an increase in sperm with abnormal morphology. Morphologic changes appeared during the first week after inoculation, and the percentage of normal sperm declined to a low of 14.8% during Week 7 and remained significantly depressed for 20 weeks after virus challenge. They considered these changes to have resulted from the combined thermal effects of elevated body temperature and scrotal edema on spermatogenesis and did not regard them as virus-specific in nature. The decrease in percentage of sperm with normal morphology observed in the present study, while far less dramatic, requires further investigation, since none of the vaccinated stallions exhibited any major elevations in body temperature nor any evidence of scrotal edema. Although no attempt was made to investigate the possible effects of EAV vaccination on fertility, subsequent studies over a two-year period have failed to demonstrate any detrimental effect on stallion fertility following extensive use of the vaccine in the Thoroughbred stallion population in Kentucky (Timoney et al. 1987a).

Vaccination of stallions with Arvac was associated with recovery of the virus from over 75% of the group, two-thirds of which were positive for virus only on buffy coat culture. These findings contrast with those of Doll and colleagues (1968), who failed to demonstrate virus in nasopharyngeal secretions following intramuscular inoculation with an experimental live EAV vaccine. McKinnon and colleagues (1986), in a similar study with Arvac, also were unsuccessful in isolating vaccine virus from a total of 64 buffy coat and 32 semen samples from a group of 16 vaccinated stallions. In an earlier report on the pathologic features in horses inoculated intramuscularly with modified EAV of passage history HK-131/RK-80/EC1D-10, McCollum (1981) recovered virus from cervical lymph nodes in every animal up to Day 8 after vaccination but made no isolation from nasal swab or serum samples. Fukunaga and colleagues (1982), in a subsequent study with a modified strain of EAV of unspecified passage history, isolated virus from four out of nine horses. The virus was isolated transiently from nasal and rectal swabs and buffy coat cultures from two of the horses, and relatively continuously from the buffy coat of the two others—in one animal up to Day 32 postinoculation. In the present study, virus was recovered for a maximum of 21 days after vaccination, also from a buffy coat culture.

The absence of detectable EAV in urine and semen of the stallions in this study is consistent with the finding of McKinnon and colleagues (1986), who, based on a more limited sampling protocol, failed to isolate virus from the semen of a similar group of vaccinated stallions. Vaccine virus has, however, been demonstrated previously in urine up to postvaccination Day 6 (McCollum 1981). The identity and significance of the other RNA virus clearly distinguishable from EAV, recovered principally from the urine of the vaccinated stallions, is under current investigation.

In the present study, although a modified strain of EAV multiplied in the majority of the vaccinated stallions, virus shedding was restricted to the nasopharyngeal route and was limited to 25% of the group. Lateral transmission of vaccine virus from vaccinated to susceptible in-contacts was not demonstrated in any instance and was considered unlikely to occur in view of the very small quantity of virus detected in nasopharyngeal secretions. McCollum and colleagues (1987), in a study of the responses of vaccinated and nonvaccinated mares to insemination with semen infected with EAV, reached a similar conclusion with respect to the amount of field virus that vaccinated mares shed nasally after challenge.

Whereas all the stallions in the present study responded serologically to EAV after vaccination, peak neutralizing antibody titers were variable and did not exceed a mean of 1:46. The responses were characterized by a rapid fall-off in antibody titers, with 25% of the group reverting to seronegativity within six weeks of vaccination. Fukunaga and colleagues (1982) and McKinnon and collegaues (1986) reported similar serological findings in their respective vaccination studies. Subsequent field studies have confirmed that revaccination with Arvac results in an excellent anamnestic response, with development of high antibody titers to EAV that are maintained relatively undiminished for at least nine to 12 months (Timoney, McCollum, Umphenour, and Roberts, unpublished data). In light of these findings, revaccination with Arvac should be considered integral to any control program that uses the currently available vaccine.

Failure to achieve transmission of EAV infection to either group of test mares corroborated the negative virus isolation attempts from semen and urine. There was no evidence that vaccine virus was shed venereally by any of the stallions after vaccination. These results are similar to those of McKinnon and colleagues (1986) in an independent study with Arvac, who failed to demonstrate seroconversion to EAV in mares bred to stallions between Days 10 and 25 after the latter were vaccinated.

The findings of the present study confirm the safety of this modified live EAV vaccine for use in stallions. While no attempt was made to evaluate the efficacy of the vaccine, it was apparent from the serologic data that the level and duration of protection it afforded would be considerably enhanced by revaccination. Subsequent field studies have attested to the safety of this vaccine (Timoney et al. 1987a); mandatory vaccination of the Thoroughbred stallion population constitutes the basis of the current successful program to control EVA in Kentucky.

ACKNOWLEDGMENTS

We thank Drs. B. Kincaid, S. Neu, M. Osborne, and K. Shiner; Ms. J. Gerstenblatt, Ms. M. Meyer, and Ms. J. O'Neill; Messrs. T. Johnson, A. Roberts, and K. Whittaker, who participated in this study; also Mr. J. Taylor, Dr. J. Hendricks and the Kentucky State veterinarian, Dr. R. Hail. This work was largely supported by Gainesway Farm, Lexington, Kentucky.

REFERENCES

Akaski, H.; Konishi, S.; and Ogata, M. (1976) Studies on equine viral arteritis. II. A serological survey of equine viral arteritis in horses imported in 1973/74. *Jpn. J. Vet. Sci.* **38,** 71-73.

Doll, E.R.; Bryans, J.T.; McCollum, W.H.; and Crowe, M.E.W. (1957) Isolation of a filterable agent causing arteritis of horses and abortion of mares. Its differentiation from the equine abortion (influenza) virus. *Cornell Vet.* **47,** 3-41.

Doll, E.R.; Bryans, J.T.; Wilson, J.C,; and McCollum, W.H. (1968) Immunisation against equine viral arteritis using modified live virus propagated in cell cultures of rabbit kidney. *Cornell Vet.* **48,** 497-524.

Fukunaga, Y.; Wada, R.; Hirasawa, K.; Kamada, M.; Kumanomido, T.; and Akiyama, Y. (1982) Effect of the modified Bucyrus strain of equine arteritis virus experimentally inoculated into horses. *Bull. Equine Res. Inst.* **19,** 97-101.

Gerber, H.; Steck, F.; Hofer, B.; Walther, L.; and Friedli, U. (1978) Clinical and serological investigations on equine viral arteritis. *Proc. 4th Int. Conf. Equine Infect. Dis.*, pp. 461-65.

Harry, T.O., and McCollum, W.H. (1981) Stability of viability and immunising potency of lyophilised, modified equine arteritis live-virus vaccine. *Am. J. Vet. Res.* **42,** 1501-5.

Konishi, S.; Akashi, H.; Sentsui, A.; and Ogata, M. (1975) Characterisation of the virus and trial survey on antibody with Vero cell culture. *Jpn. J. Vet. Sci.* **37,** 259-67.

McCollum, W.H. (1969) Development of a modified virus strain and vaccine for equine viral arteritis. *J. Am. Vet. Med. Assoc.* **155,** 318-22.

———. (1970) Vaccination for equine viral arteritis. Proc. 2d *Int. Conf. Equine Infect. Dis.*, pp. 143-51.

———. (1981) Pathologic features of horses given avirulent equine arteritis virus intramuscularly. *Am. J. Vet. Res.* **42,** 1218-20.

———. (1986) Responses of horses vaccinated with avirulent modified-live equine arteritis virus propagated in the E. Derm (NBL-6) cell line to nasal inoculation with virulent virus. *Am. J. Vet. Res.* **47,** 1931-34.

McCollum, W.H., and Bryans, J.T. (1973) Serological identification of infection by equine arteritis virus in horses of several countries. *Proc. 3d Int. Conf. Equine Infect. Dis.*, pp. 256-62.

McCollum, W.H., and Swerczek, T.W. (1978) Studies of an epizootic of equine viral arteritis in racehorses. *J. Equine Med. Surg.* **2,** 293-99.

McCollum, W.H.; Prickett, M.E.; and Bryans, J.T. (1971) Temporal distribution of equine arteritis virus in respiratory mucosa, tissues and body fluids of horses infected by inhalation. *Res. Vet. Sci.* **2,** 459-64.

McCollum, W.H.; Timoney, P.J.; Roberts, A.W.; Willard, J.E.; and Carswell, G.D. (1987) Response of vaccinated and non-vaccinated mares to artificial insemination with semen from stallions persistently infected with equine arteritis virus. *Proc. 5th Int. Conf. Equine Infect. Dis.* In press.

McKinnon, A.O.; Colbern, G.C.; Collins, J.K.; Bowen, R.A.; Voss, J.L.; and Umphenour, N.W. (1986) Vaccination of stallions with modified live equine viral arteritis virus. *J. Equine Vet. Sci.* **6,** 66-69.

Matumoto, M.; Shimizu, T.; and Ishizaki, R. (1965) Constat anticorps contre le virus de l'arterite equine dans le serum de juments indiennes. *C. R. Soc. Biol.* **159,** 1262-64.

Moraillon, A.; and Moraillon, R. (1978) Results of an epidemiological investigation on viral arteritis in France and some other European and African countries. *Ann. Rech. Vet.* **9,** 43-54.

Neu, S.M., and Timoney, P.J. (1988) Changes in semen quality in stallions experimentally infected with equine arteritis virus. *Am. J. Vet. Res.* Submitted for publication.

Timoney, P.J. (1985) Clinical, virological and epidemiological features of the 1984 outbreak of equine viral arteritis in the Thoroughbred population in Kentucky, USA. *Proc. Grayson Found. Int. Conf. of Thoroughbred Breeders Organizations on EVA.* pp. 24-33.

Timoney, P.J., and McCollum, W.H. (1985) The epidemiology of equine viral arteritis. *Proc. 31st Ann. Conv. Am. Assoc. Equine Practnr.*, pp. 545-51.

———. (1987) Equine viral arteritis. *Canad. Vet. J.* **28,** 693-95.

Timoney P.J.; McCollum, W.H.; Roberts, A.W.; and McDonald, M.J. (1987a) Equine viral arteritis status of Kentucky for 1985. *J. Am. Vet. Med. Assoc.* **191,** 36-39.

Timoney, P.J.; McCollum, W.H.; Murphy, T.W.; Roberts, A.W.; Willard, J.G.; and Carswell, G.D. (1987b) The carrier state in equine arteritis virus infection in the stallion with specific emphasis on the venereal mode of virus transmission. *J. Reprod. Fert. Suppl.* **35,** 95-102.

Westaway, E.G.; Brinton, M.A.; Gaidamovich, S. Y., Horzinek, M.C.; Igarashi, A.; Kaariainen, L.; Lvov, D.K.; Porterfield, J.S. Russell, P.K.; and Trent, D.W. (1985) Togaviridae. *Intervirology* **24,** 125-39.

Shedding and Maintenance of *Streptococcus equi* in Typical and Atypical Strangles

John F. Timoney

SUMMARY

A spontaneous outbreak of atypical strangles in a group of yearling ponies was investigated with respect to nasal shedding of *Streptococcus equi,* serum antibodies to M protein of the causative strain, and molecular characteristics of the M protein. Localization and nasal shedding studies were also performed on ponies inoculated with a virulent isolate of *S. equi*.

Nasal shedding of *S. equi* by the atypically affected ponies was observed for at least three to four weeks, and in one pony it persisted for some six weeks. Evidence was obtained, moreover, that the atypically affected ponies maintained the infection for at least eight months and were the source of the severe, typical form of strangles in foals with which they were later comingled. Serum antibody to the M protein of *S. equi* was present in all the ponies when signs of the infection were first observed, suggesting that specific immunity was of significance in the atypical disease expression. Supporting this observation, the M protein of an isolate from the outbreak was found to be identical to M proteins on isolates from typical strangles.

In experimentally inoculated ponies, *S. equi* was localized in the soft palate and tonsillar area when sampled an hour after inoculation. It reappeared in this area when systemic signs of disease became evident. Nasal shedding began after a latent period of four to seven days. Two out of three ponies in which nasal shedding had ceased still carried the organism at necropsy, three to four weeks later.

INTRODUCTION

Strangles is still one of the most frequently encountered infectious diseases of the horse despite the widespread use of bacterin and M protein extract vaccines. The causative agent, the group C streptococcus *S. equi,* is an obligate parasite of Equidae and survives only briefly in the environment unless protected in moist discharges. Interepizootic maintenance of the organism has not been well explained other than by survival in herds that have experienced cases of strangles. The organism commonly disappears from herds of horses, and even from geographic regions, following epizootics of strangles, and in only one instance has a prolonged carrier state been documented (George et al. 1983). When infection is introduced into a herd or stables free of the disease, the usual agent is an animal that is incubating the disease. In some instances, however, the disease breaks out in stables that have had no recent arrivals and no known contact with infected horses.

S. equi infection has three clinical forms—typical, atypical (catarrhal), and malignant, or bastard, strangles (Todd 1910). The atypical, catarrhal form of strangles is characterized by a slight purulent nasal discharge, cough, occasional slight fever of short duration, and abscessation of lymph nodes in a small proportion of cases. The signs are much milder than in the typical disease, a severe illness with high fever, dysphagia, pharyngitis, marked lymphadenitis, and a heavy mucopurulent nasal discharge. The atypical disease has been described in England (Mahaffey 1962), Australia (Woolcock 1975), Canada (Prescott et al. 1982) and Ireland (Timoney, Timoney & Strickland 1984) in association with a matt colony form of the organism. However, in the Irish study both mucoid and matt colony forms were isolated from atypically affected animals, suggesting that the matt colonial phenotype was not an essential prerequisite of the atypical disease.

Matt strains have been shown to be lysogenized with one of two related bacteriophage that encode hyaluronidase, which breaks down the hyaluronic capsule (Spanier & Timoney 1977; Timoney, Timoney & Strickland 1984). The loss of the capsule possibly renders the organism more susceptible to phagocytosis and therefore less virulent. Other observations, however, including those of Todd (1910), who noted that atypical strangles was more common in older animals experiencing a secondary infection, suggest that the immune status of the animal is important in the atypical expression.

MATERIAL AND METHODS

S. equi strains. A heavily encapsulated strain of *S. equi* (CF32) obtained from the abscess of a horse infected during an epizootic of typical strangles in New York State in 1981 was used in the experimental studies. Cultures were grown overnight at 37°C in Todd Hewitt broth (THB) with 0.1% yeast extract added. Organisms were stored in THB at −70°C. Other mucoid virulent strains used for immunoblot comparisons had been isolated in the United States and Europe from strangles outbreaks during the period 1976 to 1986.

Department of Microbiology, Immunology and Parasitology, New York State College of Veterinary Medicine, Cornell University, Ithaca, New York 14853.

Opsonic antibody. Opsonic antibody was estimated as described by Timoney and Eggers (1985). All assays were performed in triplicate. Blood for the test was obtained from a pony raised in isolation, never exposed to *S. equi*. The negative control serum was obtained from a similar pony. The positive control serum came from a horse with chronic *S. equi* pleuritis.

Intranasal inoculation of experimental ponies. Four yearling ponies raised in isolation in the experimental pony herd at Cornell University were used for the experimental pathogenesis studies. The ponies, housed individually, were inoculated by the intranasal insufflation of an overnight culture of CF32 suspended in 3 ml of Todd Hewitt broth. Culture was administered by means of a nasal atomizer (Model No. 251; DeVilbiss Co., Somerset, Pa.). The number of organisms administered was 5×10^8 cfu for ponies in which experimental strangles was produced for study of long-term shedding, and 5×10^9 cfu for ponies used to study the distribution of *S. equi* during the early phase of infection.

Nasal and pharyngeal cultures. Cultures from the nasal mucosa, about 5 inches from the external meatus, were taken by Culturette swabs (Marion Scientific, Kansas City, Mo.). The swabs were plated on Colombia agar (CNA) within an hour of collection and incubated at 37°C for 18 hr. Swabs were similarly taken at necropsy from the cheeks, tongue, hard palate, ventral and dorsal soft palate, tonsils, retronares, and entrance to the guttural pouch. Mucus from the soft palate and retronares was also cultured by placing 50-µl aliquots directly on CNA. Samples (1.0 g) of soft palate mucosa, tonsil, submandibular and retropharyngeal lymph nodes, and posterior nares mucosa were collected within 15 min of euthanasia and homogenized in 3-ml sterile saline in Tenbroeck grinders. One-milliliter aliquots of the homogenate were cultured in triplicate by the pour plate method in CNA. Beta hemolytic colonies were identified by inoculation into lactose, ribose, sorbitol, and trehalose.

Immunoblotting. Acid extracts of *S. equi* strains were prepared by the technique of Lancefield (1928) at a pH of 2.5. The polypeptide fragments released by the host acid treatment were separated by sodium dodecyl sulphate polyacrylamide gel electrophoresis (SDS-PAGE, 10%), electrophoretically transferred to cellulose nitrate, and then immunoblotted with horse serum (Timoney & Trachman 1985).

Elisa. *S. equi* M protein was harvested by acid extraction of cells from an 18-hr culture in Todd Hewitt broth and purified by affinity chromatography (Timoney & Trachman 1985). Enzyme-linked immunosorbent assay (ELISA) plates, polystyrene with 96 wells, were coated with M protein (1.0 µg/well) in a moist chamber at 37°C for 3 hr and washed four times in BSAPBST solution, containing 0.1 M PBS, 0.05% Tween 20, and 1% BSA. After drying, the wells were blocked by adding to each well 50 µl of 0.1 M PBS containing 0.05 Tween 20, 3% BSA, and 1% normal rabbit serum. The following day, blocking solution was removed and the wells were washed three times in BSAPBST. Sera were heat-inactivated at 56°C for 40 min and then diluted 1:80 in BSAPBST. Aliquots in triplicate of the serum dilution were added to the coated wells, incubated for 1 hr at 37°C in a moist chamber, and washed five times. Peroxidase conjugated rabbit antihorse IgG (Cappel, Malvern, Pa.), diluted 1:1000 in BSAPBST, was added in aliquots of 100 µl to each well and incubated for 1 hr at 37°C. The plates were then washed five times in BSAPBST before addition of 50-µl aliquots of O-phenylenediamine substrate.

The color reaction was stopped after 5 min. by adding 50 µl of 2.5-M sulfuric acid. The wells were read at an O.D. of 490 nm in a Minireader II (Dynatech, Alexandria, VA.), following blanking against a normal, nonimmune serum control. This serum and a positive control serum were the same as used in assay of opsonic antibody.

RESULTS

Atypical strangles outbreak. An atypical strangles outbreak occurred spontaneously in a herd of 14 yearling ponies in a nutrition experiment on the MB farm at Cornell University. The ponies, raised on another farm at the university, had no known previous exposure to *S. equi*, by either vaccination or infection. On November 14, 1982, during routine blood sampling, three ponies in an adjoining lot were noted to be slightly depressed and to have purulent nasal discharges. When nasal swabs were collected from the three and plated on CNA, they yielded growths of mucoid *S. equi*.

On January 6, 1983, the 14 ponies, which appeared clinically normal, were moved about 3 miles to the E barn at the Cornell Equine Research Park. On February 18, all the ponies except Pony 16 were noted to have slight purulent nasal discharges and to be coughing. Three ponies, 49, 47, and 17, had small, submandibular abscesses. Nasal swabs were collected from all 14 ponies and blood samples taken on February 18 and again on March 8 and 31. Pus from abscesses was also collected for culture on CNA.

A mucoid *S. equi* (ERP) was isolated from nasal swabs of eight ponies and from each submandibular abscess (Table 1). On March 8, nasal discharges were still evident in some of the ponies. *S. equi* was isolated from nasal swabs of six animals, of which two had no evident nasal discharge at the time of sampling. Another, Pony 16, had a submandibular abscess from which *S. equi* was isolated. On March 31, nasal discharges were still evident in seven ponies, but *S. equi* was isolated from a nasal swab of only one (Pony 17). Serum antibody titers to the M protein of *S. equi* were measured by ELISA and opsonic assay (Table 2). The reactivities of acute and convalescent sera from five representative ponies are shown in Figure 1. The ponies were not subsequently

Table 1. Clinical and bacteriologic findings in a group of 14 yearling ponies affected with atypical strangles

Pony No.	Februrary 18			March 8			March 31	
	Nasal Discharge	*S. equi*	Abscess[a]	Nasal discharge	*S. equi*	Abscess[a]	Nasal discharge	*S. equi*
02	+	+			+		+	
16		+		+	+	+M	+	
17	+	+	+R				+	+
18	+	+		+	+		+	
20	+				+		+	
46	+							
47	+	+	+M	+	+		+	
48	+							
49	+	+	+M	+				
50	+							
51	+	+		+	+			
53	+	+						
54	+							
55	+						+	

[a] M = mandibular lymph node; R = retropharyngeal lymph node.

sampled. On July 10, 1983, the group of 14 ponies was moved to SD farm some miles away and mingled with a group of seven pony mares and foals, which had been held in isolation since foaling some two to four months previously.

During the next five weeks all the foals developed acute, severe strangles, with high temperatures, submandibular and retropharyngeal abscesses, and purulent nasal discharges. A mucoid *S. equi* was isolated from abscesses and nasal swabs of these foals.

Experimentally infected ponies. The numbers of *S. equi* detected on nasal swabs from inoculated ponies were not closely correlated with the appearance and extent of nasal discharges, which became evident in Ponies 67 and 68 on Day 7 and in Ponies 69 and 70 on Day 4 after inoculation. Cultural studies of the distribution of *S. equi* in the nasopharynx of the experimentally inoculated ponies revealed large numbers of the organism on the soft palate and adjacent tonsillar tissue an hour after inoculation (Table 3). The organism was not found in significant numbers elsewhere in the nasopharynx. In Pony 249, *S. equi* was found in only small numbers on the soft palate after 48 hr, but in greater numbers in the submandibular lymph node. In Pony 247, killed at five days, the organism had again appeared in large numbers on the soft palate and tonsil and in the retropharyngeal lymph nodes. By this time the animal was febrile and had a neutrophilia.

Nasal shedding of *S. equi* was highly variable from inoculated ponies that subsequently developed clinically severe strangles (Table 4). During a latent period of four to seven days after inoculation, *S. equi* was virtually absent from nasal swabs. The onset of severe clinical signs followed, including high fever, neutrophilia, anorexia, depression, dysphagia, coughing, and nasal discharge. Pony 69 died of *S. equi* pneumonia and pleuritis on Day 12. Large numbers of *S. equi* appeared on nasal swabs of Pony 67 on Day 12 and heavy shedding continued during the next nine days. For the next 14 days, only small numbers of organisms were present. Pony 68 shed heavily from Day 18 through 21 then only lightly for the next two days. Shedding by Pony 70 was very intermittent and light, but extended over a period of 31 days. All ponies had ceased to shed by Day 52. At necropsy of Pony 67 on Day 69, a small abscess was found in a medial retropharyngeal lymph node, from which a pure culture of *S. equi* was isolated. *S. equi* was not isolated from any site at necropsy of Pony 68 on Day 64, but was recovered from the tonsillar and palatine tissue of Pony 70 at necropsy on Day 76.

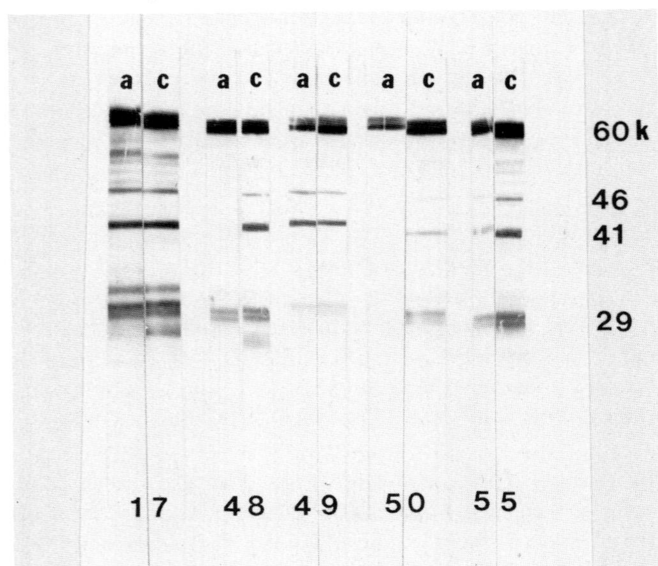

Fig. 1. Reactions of acute (*a*) and convalescent (*c*) sera of atypically affected ponies with acid-extracted protein of *S. equi*. Proteins were separated by SDS-PAGE, electrophoretically transferred to strips of nitrocellulose, and immunoblotted. Molecular weights of the most reactive bands are shown at right.

Table 2. Acute and convalescent serum antibody to M protein of *S. equi* in yearling ponies affected with atypical strangles

Pony no.	Elisa[a] February 18	Elisa[a] March 31	Opsonic antibody[b] February 18	Opsonic antibody[b] March 31
02	0.49	0.65	0.76	0.12
16	0.36	0.70	0.64	0.48
17	0.36	0.54	0.80	0.01
18	0.50	0.63	0.76	0.20
20	0.30	0.40	1.08	0.36
46	0.38	0.37	0.88	0.76
47	0.21	0.59	0.40	0.08
48	0.20	0.42	1.00	0.08
49	0.54	0.70	1.32	0.12
50	0.33	0.38	0.76	0.40
51	0.40	0.26	0.84	2.00
53	0.56	0.65	2.16	0.12
54	0.30	0.42	1.24	0.04
55	0.65	0.61	0.52	0.04
Negative control	0.02		1.00	
Positive control	0.56		0.01	

Note: Each value is the mean of three replications.

[a] Each test was run in triplicate and blanked against the negative control serum.

[b] Estimated by dividing the mean of the three test values by the negative control value.

Table 3. Distribution of *S. equi* in equine nasopharynx following intranasal inoculation of 9 x 10^9 colony-forming units

	Length of time after inoculation			
	1 hr		2 days	5 days
	Pony WM	Pony BM	Pony 249	Pony 247
Tonsil	+ + +	+ + +		+
Dorsal soft palate	+ + +	+ + +		+ + +
Ventral soft palate	+ + +	+ + +	+	+ + +
Cheek				
Hard palate				
Posterior nares	+	+		+
Mandibular lymph node	+		+ + +	
Retropharyngeal lymph node				+ + +

Note: + = 1 to 5 colonies; + + + = many colonies.

DISCUSSION

The prolonged character of the atypical strangles outbreak, and the occurrence of typical strangles in in-contact foals four months after the return of clinical normality for the atypically affected ponies, strongly suggest that *S. equi* can be maintained in groups of horses for very extended periods. The clinical signs noted in February and March were mild and similar to those described in cases of atypical or catarrhal strangles (Todd 1910; Mahaffey 1962). Moreover, Todd stated that in older horses or those having secondary attacks, the disease usually took the atypical, catarrhal form, and such cases were often the origin of clinically severe strangles in young horses.

Inherent in these epizootiologically significant observations is the implication that host immunity modifies expression of the disease. The ELISA results from sera collected on February 18 support this hypothesis. Serum antibody to the M protein of *S. equi* was present in varying amounts in all the ponies, suggesting that exposure to *S. equi* had occurred some time before. Serum opsonic activity against *S. equi* was low at this time, but had increased greatly in nine out of 14 ponies by March 31. The lack of correlation between ELISA and opsonic antibody activity is explained by the fact that opsonic antibodies are formed later than antibodies against other more immunodominant epitopes on streptococcal M proteins (Lancefield 1959; Timoney & Eggers 1985). Some horses at no time produce detectable opsonic responses, although capable of responding to other epitopes on the M protein (Timoney & Eggers 1985).

Immunoblotting of acid-extracted *S. equi* M protein fragments from sera of five representative ponies in the acute stage (February 18) and the convalescent stage (March 31) further supports the conclusion that the ponies were already making antibody responses to *S. equi* on February 18, when nasal discharges were first noted. Ponies 17, 49, and 55 had antibody reactivity to the 29-, 41-, and 46-kilodalton fragments of the M protein on February 18. Ponies 48 and 50 had much less antibody on this date, but gave strong reactions on March 31.

Ponies 48, 54, and 55, which were culturally negative for *S. equi* throughout the observation period, developed strong serum opsonic activity. It is probable that nasopharyngeal infection of those ponies had ceased before February 18. The nasopharyngeal infection of Pony 17 continued despite the presence of strong serum opsonic activity on March 31. Although unproven, local nasopharyngeal antibody reponses in this animal may have been inadequate (Galán & Timoney 1985). The persistence of purulent nasal discharge from ponies that were culturally negative for *S. equi* suggests that other infectious agents were present. A mucoid *S. zooepidemicus* strain was detected in large numbers in all of the nasopharyngeal swabs that were negative for *S. equi* and in some of the swabs that were positive. The effect of this infection or that of respiratory viruses on local nasopharyngeal immune responses to *S. equi* is unknown, but could be significant in nasopharyngeal persistence of *S. equi*.

Alterations in the infectious agent are a well-established source of variation in the disease expressed. In the case of *S. equi*, matt colony forms of the organism have been associated with a clinically mild, atypical form of strangles (Mahaffey 1962; Woolcock 1975; Prescott et al. 1982). Matt colony forms are due to phage-encoded hyaluronidase that is expressed when the colony is 10 to 12 hr old (Spanier & Timoney 1977; Timoney, Pesante, & Ernst 1982). During an atypical strangles outbreak in Ireland, both colony types were

Table 4. Nasal shedding of *S. equi* following experimental nasal inoculation

Pony no.	Days[a] after inoculation																						
	2	4	7	8	9	11	12	13	14	15	16	17	18	19	20	21	22	23	27	30	35	42	45
67					+R[b]	+	+ + +	+ + +	+ + +	+ + +	+ + +	+	+ + +	+	+ + +	+ + +	+	+	+	+	+	+	+
68	+		+	+		+	+		M[c]	+	R		+ + +	+ + +	+ + +	+ + +	+	+					
69		+	+	+ +	+ +	+ +	Died																
70			+	+					+M			+	+	+	+						+		

Note: + = 1 to 5 colonies; $\substack{+\\+}$ 5 to 20 colonies; $\substack{+\\+\\+}$ many colonies.

[a] = Ponies were swabbed daily until Day 52 after inoculation.
[b] M = mandibular lymph node abscess.
[c] R = retropharyngeal lymph node abscess.

present in strains from affected animals (Timoney et al. 1984). Matt and mucoid colony forms were isolated both from animals with nasal discharges alone and from more severely affected animals, suggesting that the matt colony condition was not critical in the atypical character of the disease. Moreover, both the amount of M protein and the acid-extracted polypeptide fragments of matt colony forms were similar to those of typical mucoid strains. *S. equi* isolated from the Cornell outbreak were uniformly heavily mucoid and carried an M protein identical in polypeptide fragment profile to *S. equi* strains isolated from typical strangles in the United States and Europe. It is, of course, possible that the loss of disease-producing capability may involve other as-yet-unrecognized virulence factors of *S. equi* that are unrelated to M protein or encapsulation. However, the outbreak of severe strangles in foals following comingling with ponies that had harbored the atypical disease suggests that host factors rather than bacterial influences are of importance in atypical disease expression.

Although adherence of *S. equi* to equine tongue, cheek, and nasal epithelial cells has been observed in vitro by Srivastava and Barnum (1983), the data from the experimentally infected ponies suggests that adhesion to these sites is not important in the living animal. It is more likely that the epithelium of the soft palate and tonsillar area is the site of initial localization and penetration of the organism, as well as subsequent maintenance. This conclusion is supported by studies on porcine strangles caused by the group E streptococcus *S. porcinus* that have clearly demonstrated the tonsil to be the portal of entry of the invading organism (Gosser & Olson 1973). The isolation of *S. equi* from the submandibular lymph node of Pony WM suggests that penetration this far from the tonsil can occur within an hour of inoculation. Although clinical signs were absent and no nasal shedding was detected six weeks after experimental infection, the organism persisted beyond this time, as detected at necropsy. Although unproven in this study, shedding of the organism by such latently infected animals could be a source of infection for in-contact susceptible animals.

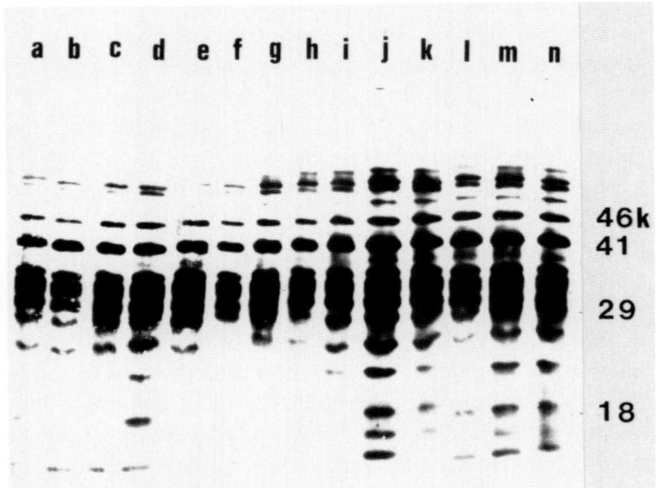

Fig. 2. SDS-PAGE and immunoblot analysis of acid-extracted M proteins of *S. equi* isolates from typical and atypical strangles; blot was developed with rabbit antiserum to *S. Equi* M protein. Isolates: *a*, Boldmani (Ireland, 1983); *b*, CF32 (New York, 1980); *c*, Battisti (Ohio, 1980); *d*, F43 (U.S. vaccine strain); *e*, Crafty Red (New York, 1982); *f*, Vi331 (Sweden); *g*, Melody (New York, 1983); *h*, 22 (Ireland, 1983); *i*, ERP (New York, 1982); *j*, Sprinkle Misty (New York, 1981); *k*, Headache (New York, 1983); *l*, e23 (New York, 1975); *m*, Lady M (Ireland, 1983); *n*, Top Sun (New Jersey, 1975). The extracts on tracks *i* and *m* were from isolates from outbreaks of atypical strangles.

Earlier writers on strangles, including Todd (1910), emphasize that infection can break out in stables where there have been no recent arrivals and no known contact with infected horses. In addition, Todd very insightfully stated his conviction that "*S. equi* remains in the glands and follicles of the nasal mucous membrane of some recovered horses for a considerable time after recovery." The first convincing bacteriological evidence supporting this was provided by George and others (1983), who described nasopharyngeal carriage of *S. equi* in a mare that persisted for 11 months with minimal clinical signs. Our data on both the atypical and typical forms of the disease substantiate and extend the observations of these workers on the role of recovered, clinically normal animals in maintenance of *S. equi*. Moreover, these findings point to the need for further detailed study of the interaction of *S. equi* with the equine nasopharynx, to explain the protective effect of local antibody in convalescent or intranasally immunized animals (Galán & Timoney 1985; Timoney & Galán 1985).

ACKNOWLEDGMENTS

The assistance of Jorge Galán, Jennifer Schroeder, and Clarence Marquis during the course of these studies is gratefully acknowledged.

REFERENCES

Galán, J.E., and Timoney, J.F. (1985) Mucosal nasopharyngeal immune responses of horses to protein antigens of *Streptococcus equi*. *Infect. Immun.* **47,** 623-28.

George, S.Y.; Reif, J.S.; Schideler, R.K.; Small, C.J.; Ellis, R.P.; Snyder, S.P.; and McChesney, A.E. (1983) Identification of carriers of *Streptococcus equi* in a naturally infected herd. *J. Am. Vet. Med. Assoc.* **183,** 80-84.

Gosser, H.S., and Olson, L.D. (1973) Chronologic development of streptococci lymphadenitis in swine. *Am. J. Vet. Res.* **34,** 77-82.

Lancefield, R.C. (1928) The antigenic complex of *Streptococcus haemolyticus*. I. Demonstration of a type-specific substance in extracts of *Streptococcus haemolyticus*. *J. Exp. Med.* **47,** 91-103.

———. (1959) Persistence of type-specific antibodies in man following infection with group A streptococci. *J. Exp. Med.* **110,** 272-92.

Mahaffey, L.W. (1962) Respiratory conditions in horses. *Vet. Rec.* **74,** 1295-1311.

Prescott, J.F.; Srivastava, S.K.; de Ganes, R.; and Barnum, D.A. (1982) A mild form of strangles caused by an atypical *Streptococcus equi*. *J. Am. Vet. Med. Assoc.* **180,** 293-94.

Spanier, J., and Timoney, J.F. (1977) Bacteriophages of *Streptococcus equi*. *J. Gen. Virol.* **35,** 369-75.

Srivastava, S.K., and Barnum, D.A. (1983) Adherence of *S. equi* on tongue, cheek, and nasal epithelial cells of ponies. *Vet. micro* 8:493-504.

Timoney, J.F., and Eggers, D. (1985) Serum bactericidal responses to *Streptococcus equi* of horses following infection or vaccination. *Equine Vet. J.* **17,** 306-10.

Timoney, J.F., and Galán, J.E. (1985) The protective response of the horse to an avirulent strain of *Streptococcus equi*. In *Recent advances in steptococci and streptococcal diseases*, pp. 294-95. Eds. Y. Kimura, S. Kotani, and Y. Shiokawa. Reedbooks, Bracknell, Berkshire.

Timoney, J.F., and Trachman, J. (1985) The immunologically reactive proteins of *Streptococcus equi*. *Infect. Immun.* **48,** 20-34.

Timoney, J.F.; Pesante, L.; and Ernst, C. (1982) Hyaluronidase associated with a temperate bacteriophage of *Streptococcus equi*. In *Microbiology*—1982, pp. 145-46. Ed. D. Schlessinger. American Society for Microbiology, Washington, D.C.

Timoney, J.F.; Timoney, P.J.; and Strickland, K.L. (1984) Lysogeny and the immunologically reactive proteins of *Streptococcus equi*. *Vet. Rec.* **115,** 148-49.

Todd, A.G. (1910) Strangles. *J. Comp. Pathol. Ther.* **23,** 212-29.

Woolcock, J.B. (1975) Studies in atypical *Streptococcus equi*. *Res. Vet. Sci.* **19,** 115-119.

Expression and Localization of the *Streptococcus equi* M Protein in *Escherichia coli* and *Salmonella typhimurium*

Jorge E. Galán, John F. Timoney, and Roy Curtiss III

SUMMARY

Avirulent mutants of *Salmonella typhimurium* Δ*cya* Δ*crp* carrying a plasmid with the M protein gene of *Streptococcus equi* were constructed. The M protein gene was expressed at high levels in both *S. typhimurium* and *Escherichia coli*. The majority of the *Strep. equi* M protein localized to the periplasmic space in both organisms, although M protein activity was detected in other cell fractions. These constructs will provide a better means of stimulating a protective mucosal immune response to strangles.

INTRODUCTION

An important virulence factor of *Strep. equi* is the M protein, a surface structure with antiphagocytic activity (Bazeley 1942 & 1943; Bazeley et al. 1949; Erickson & Norcross 1975; Woolcock 1974). We have demonstrated that protection against strangles correlates with the presence of mucosal nasopharyngeal antibodies against two polypeptide fragments of acid-extracted M protein of *Strep. equi*. These fragments are different in size from the one carrying the determinants that induce the production of serum bactericidal antibodies (Galán & Timoney 1985b; Galán, Timoney & Lengemann 1986; Timoney, Timoney & Strickland 1984; Timoney & Eggers 1985; Timoney & Trachman 1985). Although available vaccines can stimulate serum bactericidal antibodies, they do not give a high level of protection, probably because of failure to stimulate a local immune response in the upper respiratory tract (Timoney & Eggers 1985). The use of nonreplicating antigens to stimulate mucosal immune responses has been hampered by a lack of adjuvants that effectively induce secretory immunity (Genco, Linzer & Evans 1983; Taubman et al. 1983). Live replicating antigens are known to stimulate mucosal immune responses better, partly because they tend to persist longer (Ganguly & Waldman 1980). An avirulent strain of *Strep. equi*, Cornell 709-27, has been successfully used to immunize horses against strangles (Timoney & Galán 1985) and is effective in inducing a protective mucosal immune response. It is not safe, however, when given in large doses to foals of less than four months.

Galán, Curtiss: Department of Biology, Washington University, Saint Louis, Missouri 63130. Timoney: New York State College of Veterinary Medicine, Cornell University, Ithaca, New York 14853.

Recombinant DNA technology has provided several new approaches toward the development of safer and more efficacious vaccines. One approach is the use of avirulent strains of *S. typhimurium* carrying heterologous antigens that can be presented as bivalent oral vaccines (Clements et al. 1986; Curtiss et al. 1986; Curtiss et al. 1988a; Curtiss et al. 1988b; Dougan, Hormaeche & Maskell 1987; Formal et al. 1981; Stevenson & Manning 1985). Following oral administration, *S. typhimurium* invades and proliferates in the gut-associated lymphoid tissue (GALT) (Carter & Collins 1974). Antigen delivered into the GALT leads to an immune response at other mucosal sites (Bienstock et al. 1978; Cebra et al. 1976). Several investigators have made use of avirulent strains of *S. typhimurium* to deliver into the GALT heterologous antigens encoded for by cloned recombinant genes to induce a generalized secretory immune response to the recombinant virulence antigens (Clements et al. 1986; Curtiss et al. 1986; Curtiss et al. 1988a; Stevenson & Manning 1985). Several avirulent mutants of *S. typhimurium* have been used, including *aroA* deletion (Δ) mutants (Hoiseth & Stocker 1981), Δ*galE* (Germanier & Furer 1975; Hone et al. 1987; and Δ*asd* (Curtiss et al. 1987b). There have been recent descriptions of the use of *S. typhimurium* strains lacking adenylate cyclase and the cyclic AMP receptor protein (CRP) due to deletion mutations in the *cya* and *crp* genes, respectively (Curtiss & Kelly 1987 Curtiss et al. 1988a).

We recently cloned and expressed in *E. coli* the entire structural M protein gene of *Strep. equi* (Galán & Timoney 1987a, b). The recombinant protein appears in SDS-polyacrylamide gels as three closely spaced bands with molecular weights of 58,000, 53,000 and 50,000, similar to the native *Strep. equi* M protein. We have initiated studies toward the development of *S. typhimurium* Δ*cya* Δ*crp* strains carrying the structural gene for the *Strep. equi* M protein as a means of stimulating a generalized secretory immune response against the M protein.

MATERIALS AND METHODS

Bacterial strains, bacteriophage, plasmid, and growth conditions. *E. coli* strain Y1089 lysogenic for lambda gt11/SEM7 carrying the *Strep. equi* M protein gene (Galán & Timoney 1987b) and the *E. coli* HB101 strain have been described (Maniatis & Fritsch 1982). The other organisms are described as follows: *S. typhimurium* strains χ 4062

Δ*cya* Δ*crp*, cured of the virulence plasmid pStSR100, and χ 4064 Δ*cya* Δ*crp*, containing the virulence plasmid pStSR100 (Curtiss & Kelly 1987); *S. typhimurium* χ 3477 (*hsdL6*, *hsdSA29*), a recombination-deficient, modification-proficient strain (S. A. Tinge & R. Curtiss III, unpublished); *S. typhimurium* Δ*aroA* strain SL3261 (Hoiseth & Stocker 1981); *Strep. equi* strain CF32 (Galán & Timoney 1985b); plasmid vectors pWM401 (Wirth & Clewell 1987); pREG153, a gift from R. E. Gill (University of Colorado); and pCVD305, a gift from J. Kaper (University of Maryland School of Medicine). *E. coli* and *S. typhimurium* strains were grown on L broth or luria agar. *Strep. equi* strain CF32 was grown on Todd Hewitt broth. When appropriate, antibiotics were used at the following concentrations: ampicillin 100 μg/ml, tetracycline 10 μg/ml.

DNA manipulations. Plasmid DNA was isolated by the method of Birnboin (1983), and bacteriophage λgt11/SEM7 DNA by the method of Ivanov and colleagues (1985). Restriction endonuclease digestions, DNA ligations, and Klenow fill-in reactions were done with commercially available enzymes (Bethesda Research Laboratories, Gaithersburg, Md.; International Biotechnology Inc., New Haven, Conn.). Transformation of *E. coli* and *S. typhimurium* was performed as described by Humphreys and colleagues (1979). To overcome the restriction barriers, plasmid DNA isolated from *E. coli* strains was routinely transformed into *S. typhimurium* strain χ 3477, and plasmid DNA isolated from this strain was used to transform *S. typhimurium* strains χ 4062, χ 4064, and SL3261.

Construction of plasmid vector pYA2204. The plasmid vector pYA2204 was constructed as follows. The cosmid vector pREG153 is an IncW low-copy-number plasmid that encodes for ampicillin resistance and has the λ *cos* site on a BglII fragment. The unique BamHI and EcoRI sites of pREG153 were eliminated by restriction endonuclease digestion, Klenow fill-in, and religation. The lacZ multiple cloning site of m13 mp8 obtained in a BglII fragment from pCVD305 was ligated to BglII digested pREG153. Lactose$^+$ transformants were screened for loss of the *cos* site and the presence of a single multiple-cloning site by restriction analysis.

Colony immunoblot. Colony immunoblot was done according to modifications of procedures described by Heleman and colleagues (1983). Overnight colonies were lifted from agar plates onto nitrocellulose filters and immediately lysed by exposing them to chloroform vapors for 15 min at 37°C. Filters were washed in NET buffer (50 mM Tris, 150 mM NaCl, 5 mM EDTA, 0.25% gelatin [w/v], 0.05% Triton × 100 [w/v]; pH 7.4) for 2 hr (Galán & Timoney 1985b).

Cell fractionation of *E. coli* and *S. typhimurium*. Cell fractionation of *E. coli* and *S. typhimurium* was done as described by Schnaitman (1981), with some modifications. Cells were grown overnight at 37°C in 100 ml of L broth and collected by centrifugation at 7,000 g. The culture supernatant, designated fraction A, was processed as described below, and the cell pellet was washed once with 150 mM NaCI, resuspended in 5 ml of PBS (phosphate-buffered saline, pH 7.4) and disrupted in a cell homogenizer (B. Braun, Melsungen AG, West Germany). The cell lysate was then centrifuged at 5,000 g for 10 minutes, and the cell-free supernatant was centrifuged at 100,000 g for 1 hr. The supernatant containing cytoplasmic and periplasmic proteins was designated fraction B. The pellet was resuspended in 2% sarcosyl in PBS and centrifuged at 100,000 g for 1 hr. Supernatant enriched for cytoplasmic membranes was designated fraction D, and pellet enriched for outer membranes was resuspended in 0.1% SDS and designated fraction C.

A separate experiment to separate cytoplasmic from periplasmic fractions was based on the procedures described by Dobrogosz (1981). Cells were grown overnight in 50 ml of L broth, washed once with 150 mM NaCl, resuspended in 5 ml of 30 mM Tris (pH 7.4), 3 mM EDTA, and 25% sucrose (w/v), and incubated at 25°C for 10 min while shaking. Cells were spun down at 13,000 g, pellet resuspended in ice-cold 0.5 mM MgCl, and centrifuged at 13,000 g for 15 min. The supernatant was designated periplasmic fraction. The pellet was resuspended in PBS, cells disrupted in a cell homogenizer, and centrifuged at 100,000 g for 1 hr. The supernatant was designated cytoplasmic fraction.

Table 1. Distribution of the *S. equi* M protein in *S. typhimurium* and *E. coli* cell fractions

Fraction	*S. typhimurium* (%)	*E. coli* (%)
Culture supernatant	6	5
Outer membrane	6	5
Periplasmic space	77	80
Cytoplasmic membrane	4	4
Cytoplasm	7	6

Culture supernatant. Culture supernatants of *E. coli* and *S. typhimurium* were saturated to 50% ammonium sulfate and incubated at 4°C overnight with stirring. Precipitated proteins were recovered by centrifugation at 12,000 g for 20 min, resuspended in PBS, and extensively dialyzed against several volumes of the same buffer.

E. coli and S. typhimurium whole-cell lysates. Cells from 500 μl of cultures of *E. coli* or *S. typhimurium* standing overnight were collected by centrifugation at 12,000 g for 1 min, resuspended in 50 μl of Laemmli loading buffer (Laemmli 1970), boiled for 5 min and centrifuged again at 12,000 g for 1 min. Usually 1 to 2 μl of the whole-cell lysates were loaded on SDS-PAGE gels for further analysis. *E. coli* strain Y1089 (λgt11/SEM7) lysates were prepared as described elsewhere (Galán & Timoney 1987b).

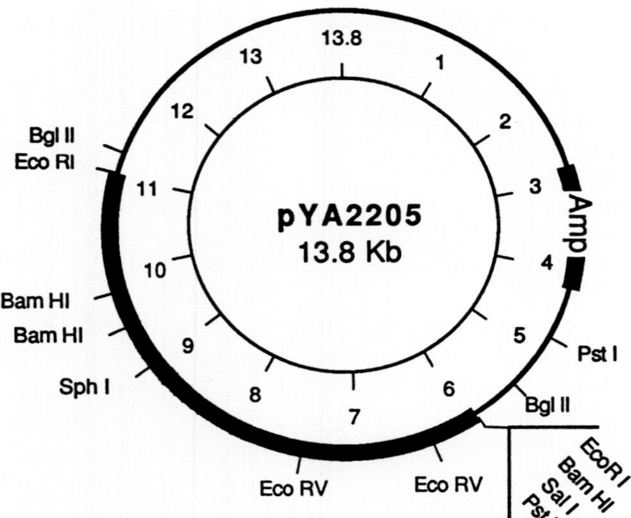

Fig. 1. Restriction endonuclease site map of pYA2205. *Heavy line*, 5.1-kb *Strep. equi* insert DNA.

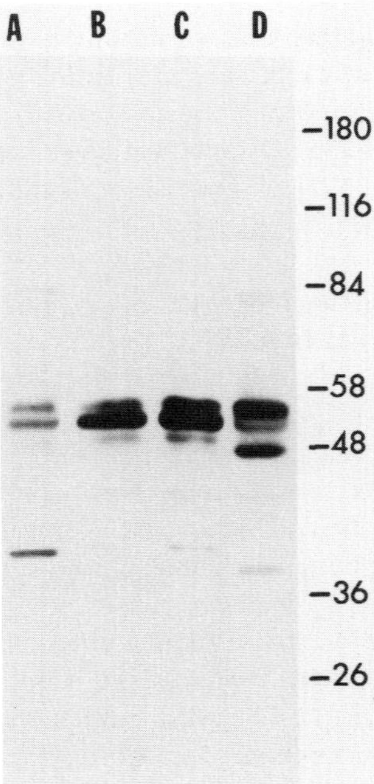

Fig. 2. SDS-PAGE and immunoblot analysis of whole cell lysates from Δ*aroA S. typhimurium* SL 3261 (*Lane A*), Δ*cya* Δ*crp S. typhimurium* χ 4062 (*Lane B*) and χ 4064 (*Lane C*), and *E. coli* χ 6060 containing the plasmid pYA2205 that carries the *Strep. equi* M protein gene. Blot was developed with *Strep. equi* M protein antiserum. Numbers at right represent positions of molecular weight standards.

Native *S. equi* M protein. Native *Strep. equi* M protein was obtained from strain CF32 (Galán & Timoney 1987b).

***Strep. equi* M protein antiserum.** *Strep. equi* M protein antiserum was prepared (Timoney & Trachman 1985). To eliminate cross-reactive antibodies, the serum was extensively adsorbed with *E. coli* and *S. typhimurium* extracts (Galán and Timoney 1987b).

SDS-PAGE and Western blotting. SDS-PAGE and Western blot analysis was performed as described (Galán and Timoney 1985b; Towbin, Staehelin & Gordon 1979).

RESULTS

Subcloning of *Strep equi* M protein gene. Lambda gt11/SEM7 carries the entire M protein gene in a 5.1-kb fragment. The *Strep. equi* M protein gene is not fused to the lacZ gene of λgt11 and is expressed from its own promoter (Galán & Timoney 1987b). Lambda gt11/SEM7 DNA was digested with EcoRl, and the 5.1-kb fragment containing the *Strep. equi* M protein gene was isolated from agarose gels (Langridge, Langridge & Berquist 1980). Subcloning of the *Strep. equi* M protein gene into large-copy-number plasmids such as pBR322 or pUC18 was not successful, presumably because the high level of the *Strep. equi* M protein gene product is harmful for the bacterial host. Subcloning into the shuttle vector pWM401 yielded the plasmid pJEG34, which stably expressed the M protein gene in *E. coli* strain HB101. Expression of the M protein in this plasmid, though, was extremely unstable following introduction into *S. typhimurium* strains χ 3477, χ 4062, χ 4064, and SL 3261 and DNA rearrangements, resulting in inactivation of the M protein gene after overnight growth in the presence of the

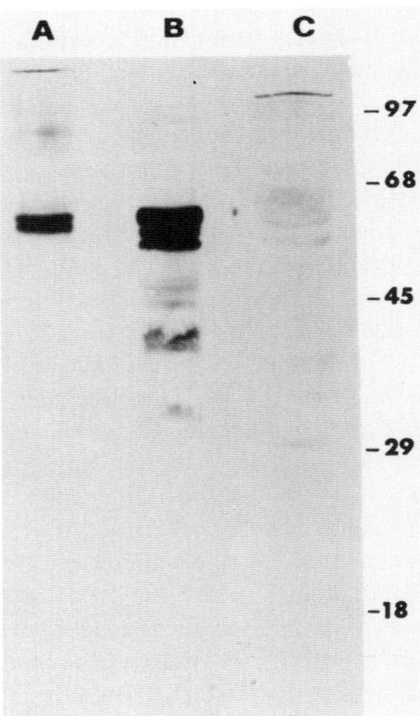

Fig. 3. SDS-PAGE and immunoblot analysis of native *Strep. equi* M protein (*Lane A*) and a lysate of *E. coli* Y1089 (λgt11/SEM7) containing *Strep. equi* M protein gene (*Lane B*). *Lane C* is a lysate of *E. coli* Y1089 (λgt11) as a negative control. Numbers at right represent positions of the molecular weight standards. Blot was developed with *Strep. equi* M protein antiserum.

antibiotic selection marker. Subcloning of the M protein gene into the low-copy-number plasmid pYA2204 yielded plasmid pYA2205. This plasmid stably expressed the *Strep. equi* M protein gene in *E. coli* and *S. typhimurium* strains when grown in the presence of the antibiotic selection marker (Fig. 1).

Expression of the *Strep. equi* M protein gene in *E. coli* and *S. typhimurium*. pYA2205 was introduced into *E. coli* strain χ 6060, and *S. typhimurium* strains χ 4062, χ 4064, and SL3261 by transformation. A western blot analysis of whole-cell lysates from the different strains using *Strep. equi* M protein antiserum is shown in Figure 2. The *Strep. equi* M protein was efficiently expressed in all the strains tested, as demonstrated by the presence of closely spaced bands with molecular weights ranging from 50,000 to 58,000. This molecular weight distribution is characteristic of the native *Strep. equi* M protein as well as the recombinant protein expressed in λgt11/SEM7 (Fig. 3) (Galán & Timoney 1987a, b). Since equal amounts of protein were loaded in each track, it is evident that Δ*cya* Δ*crp S. typhimurium* strains expressed the M protein gene at higher levels than *E. coli* or Δ*aroA S. typhimurium* strain SL 3261. In addition, it is apparent that the *Strep. equi* M protein was less degraded in Δ*cya* Δ*crp S. typhimurium* strains than in *E. coli* or Δ*aroA S. typhimurium* strain SL3261, since a higher intensity of the smaller molecular weight bands was observed in the latter two strains.

Localization of the *Strep. equi* M protein *E. coli* and *S. typhimurium*. To more accurately determine the distribution of the *Strep. equi* M protein among the different *E. coli* and *S. typhimurium* cell fractions, amounts of each fraction were loaded on polyacrylamide gels to obtain bands of approximately equal intensity in Western blots reacted with the *Strep. equi* M protein antiserum. The percentage of M protein in each fraction was then established by considering the total volume of each fraction and the amount loaded. The quantitative distribution of the *Strep. equi* M protein in the different cell fractions was very similar in *E. coli* and *S. typhimurium* (Table 1). Figures 4 and 5 show the Western blot analysis of cell fractions of Δ*cya* Δ*crp S. typhimurium* strain χ 4062 *E. coli* strain χ 6060. Although most of the M protein reactivity (approximately 80%) was associated with fraction B, composed of periplasm and cytoplasm, M protein reactivity was also detected in fractions A (culture supernatant), C (outer membranes), and D (cytoplasmic membranes). A separate experiment conducted to differentiate cytoplasmic from periplasmic fractions determined that most of the M protein was localized in the periplasm with little activity present in the cytoplasmic fraction (data not shown). From Figures 4 and 5, it is evident that some forms of the M protein selectively localize to specific compartments of the *E. coli* and *S. typhimurium* cells. The 50,000 M protein polypeptide copurified with the outer membrane fraction of *S. typhimurium* was barely detectable in either of the other

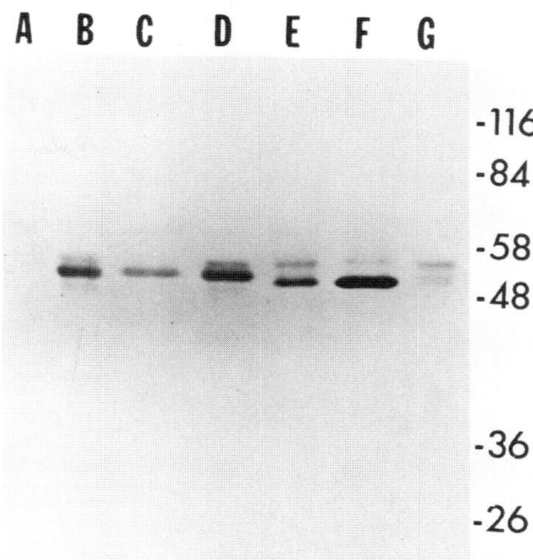

Fig. 4. SDS-PAGE and immunoblot analysis of different cell fractions of Δ*cya* Δ*crp S. typhimurium* χ 4062 containing the plasmid pYA2205 that carries *S. equi* M protein gene: *Lane C*, culture supernatant; *Lane D*, periplasm and cytoplasm; *Lane E*, cytoplasmic and outer membranes; *Lane F*, outer membranes; *Lane G*, cytoplasmic membranes. Controls: *Lane A*, whole cell lysate of *S. typhimurium* χ 4062 containing the plasmid vector pYA2204 (negative control); *Lane B*, whole cell lysate of *S. typhimurium* χ 4062 containing the plasmid pYA2205 (positive control). Blot was developed with *Strep. equi* M protein antiserum. Numbers at right represent positions of molecular weight standards.

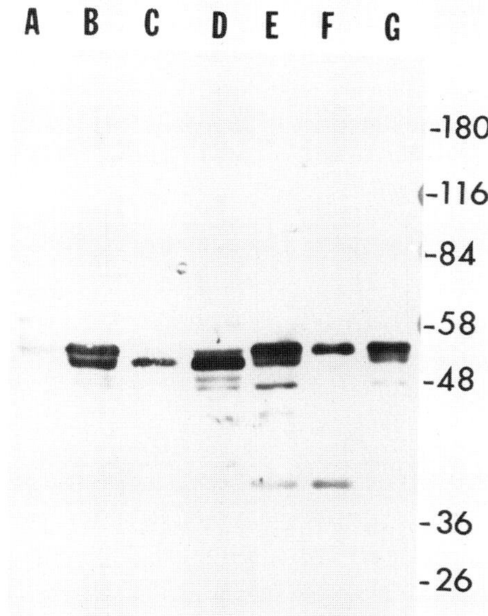

Fig. 5. SDS-PAGE and immunoblot analysis of cell fractions of *E. coli* χ 6060 containing the plasmid pYA2205 that carries *Strep. equi* M protein: *Lane C*, culture supernatant; *Lane D*, periplasm and cytoplasm; *Lane E*, cytoplasmic and outer membranes; *Lane F*, outer membranes; *Lane G*, cytoplasmic membranes. Controls: *Lane A*, whole lysate from *E. coli* containing the plasmid vector pYA2204 (negative control); *Lane B*, whole lysate of *E. coli* χ 6060 containing the plasmid pYA2205 that carries the *Strep. equi* M protein gene (positive control). Blot was developed with *Strep. equi* M protein antiserum. Numbers at right represent positions of molecular weight standards.

fractions. In contrast, the 58,000 polypeptide was localized in the outer membrane of *E. coli*, and very little of the lower molecular weight forms of the M protein were detected in that fraction. In culture supernatants of *E. coli* and *S. typhimurium*, only the 53,000 polypeptide was present.

DISCUSSION

The tropism of *S. typhimurium* for Peyer's patches (Carter & Collins 1974) makes avirulent derivatives of this organism possible vehicles to deliver foreign antigens into the GALT to elicit a generalized secretory immune response at other mucosal sites, provided that the mutations involved to render them avirulent do not interfere with tissue tropism. *S. typhimurium* Δ*cya* Δ*crp* strains are avirulent for mice and confer protective immunity against subsequent challenge with high doses of wild-type virulent *S. typhimurium* (Curtiss & Kelly 1987; Curtiss et al. 1988a). The relative avirulence of the Δ*cya* Δ*crp* mutants has been enhanced by curing them of the 100-kb virulence plasmid pStSR100 without impairing immunogenicity or tissue tropism (Gulig & Curtiss 1987). Unlike some other avirulent strains of *Salmonella*, virulence of *cya crp* strains cannot be restored by dietary or host components (Hoiseth & Stocker, 1981). The location of the *cya* and *crp* genes in the chromosome (11 minutes apart) (Sanderson & Roth 1983), increases the safety of these avirulent mutants because reversion to virulence requires restoration of both genes to the wild type, a very unlikely event given the distance between them. Since the tissue tropism of *cya crp* mutants is not affected, they are suitable vehicles to deliver foreign antigens into the GALT (Curtiss & Kelly 1987). We have now constructed Δ*cya* Δ*crp S. typhimurium* carrying the *Strep. equi* M protein gene. The gene, although present in a low-copy-number plasmid vector, is expressed to high levels as shown in the Western blot analysis of Figure 2. Expression was higher in the Δ*cya* Δ*crp S. typhimurium* with or without the pStSR100 virulence plasmid than in *E. coli* or Δ*aroA S. typhimurium* strain SL3261. No explanation for this phenomenon is yet available, although it does not seem to be peculiar to the *Strep. equi* M protein gene since similar results have been obtained with the *Streptococcus sobrinus* surface protein antigen A gene (Curtiss et al. 1988a). In Δ*cya* Δ*crp* mutants there was less degradation of the recombinant M protein than in Δ*aro* mutants or *E. coli*, as shown by the lower intensity of the smaller molecular weight bands (Fig. 2).

The cell fractionation analysis indicates that the majority of the *Strep. equi* M protein localizes to the periplasmic space of *S. typhimurium* and *E. coli* (Table 1), although M protein reactivity was readily apparent in other cell fractions. The type 6 M protein of *Streptococcus pyogenes* expressed in *E. coli* has also been found to localize in the periplasmic space (Fischetti et al. 1984).

As shown in Figure 3, *Strep. equi* M protein is expressed in λgt11/SEM7 as three closely spaced bands with molecular weights of 50,000, 53,000 and 58,000. Some other smaller molecular weight bands are also present, presumably degradation products since they are much less apparent in fresh preparations. The native M protein of *S. equi* is most often seen as two closely spaced bands of molecular weight similar to that of the higher two bands of *E. coli* M protein. Some forms of the M protein seem to selectively copurify with particular fractions of *E. coli* or *S. typhimurium* cells. The 50,000 molecular weight polypeptide seems to preferentially copurify with the outer membrane fraction of *S. typhimurium*, while the 58,000 form of the M protein will copurify with the same fraction of *E. coli*. Stability problems were encountered in the expression of *Strep. equi* M protein when the M protein gene was cloned in vectors of high copy number. If indeed some forms of the M protein are associated with the outer membrane of *E. coli* and *S. typhimurium*, it is likely that that association may alter the outer membrane of these organisms, which could account for the lack of stability observed in those vectors. Conceivably, the deletion of part of the amino terminal region of the M protein gene could prevent that interaction and allow for the expression of the *Strep. equi* M protein gene at higher levels in those hosts. A similar approach has been successfully taken with the *S. sobrinus* surface protein antigen A gene, allowing high expression of that protein in *E. coli* and *S. typhimurium* with no apparent harmful effects to the host.

Low levels of *Strep. equi* M protein were detected in culture supernatants of *E. coli* and *S. typhimurium*. The presence of M protein in culture supernatants is probably not due to active secretion but rather to "leakage" or passive release after cell death. It is interesting that only the 53,000 form of the M protein was present in culture supernatant preparations of both *S. typhimurium* and *E. coli*. Fischetti and colleagues (1984) did not find *S. pyogenes* M protein serotype 6 in culture supernatants of *E. coli* carrying the M protein serotype 6 gene. Although M protein is not commonly found in culture supernatants of *S. pyogenes*, it is readily detectable in culture supernatants of *Strep. equi* as a single band with a molecular weight of 53,000 (Timoney & Trachman 1985).

We have previously demonstrated the involvement of *Strep. equi* M protein in the pathogenesis of purpura hemorrhagica (Galán & Timoney 1985a). Epitope mapping of the M protein gene is now in progress to dissect the protective determinants from those involved in the development of purpura hemorrhagica. The ultimate goal is to construct a safer bivalent *Salmonella* vaccine, one that induces a protective immune response against strangles without increasing the risk of purpura hemorrhagica.

In conclusion, we have constructed avirulent strains of *S. typhimurium* carrying the entire structural *Strep. equi* M protein gene in a low-copy plasmid vector. Immunization studies to evaluate the protective ability and safety of these constructs are in progress.

REFERENCES

Bazeley, P.L. (1942) Studies with equine streptococci. 4. Cross-immunity to *S. equi*. *Aust. Vet. J.* **19**, 189-94.

———. (1943) Studies with equine streptococci. 5. Some relations between virulence of *S. equi* and immune response in the host. *Aust. Vet. J.* **19**, 62-85.

Bazeley, P.L.; Baldwin, S.; Dickson, H.; and Thayer, J.R. (1949) The keeping qualities of strangles vaccine. *Aust. Vet. J.* **25**, 130-33.

Bienstock, J.; McDermott, M.; Befus, D.; and O'Neill, M. 1978. A common mucosal immunologic system involving the bronchus, breast, and bowel. *Adv. Exp. Med. Biol.* **107**, 53-59.

Birnboim, H.C. (1983) A rapid alkaline extraction method for the isolation of plasmid DNA. *Meth. Enzymol.* **100**, 243-55.

Carter, P.B., and Collins, F.M. (1974) The route of enteric infection in normal mice. *J. Exp. Med.* **139**, 1189-1203.

Cebra, J.J.; Gearhart, P.J.; Kamat, R.; Robertson, S.M.; and Tseng, T. (1976) Origin and differentiation of lymphocytes involved in the secretory IgA response. *Cold Spring Harbor Symp. Quant. Biol.* **41**, 201-15.

Clements, J.D.; Lyon, F.L.; Lowe, K.L.; Farrand, A.L.; and El-Morshidy, S. (1986) Oral immunization of mice with attenuated *Salmonella enteritidis* containing a recombinant plasmid which encodes for the production of the B subunit of heat-labile *E. coli* enterotoxin. *Infect. Immun.* **53**, 685-92.

Curtiss, R., III, and Kelly, S.M. (1987) *Salmonella typhimurium* deletion mutants lacking adenylate cyclase and cyclic AMP receptor protein are avirulent and immunogenic. *Infect. Immun.* **55**, 3035-43.

Curtiss, R., III; Goldschmidt, R.; Pastian, R.; Lyons, M.; Michalek, S.M.; and Mestecky, J. (1986) Cloning virulence determinants from *Streptococcus mutans* and the use of recombinant clones to construct bivalent oral vaccine strains to confer protective immunity against *S. mutans*-induced dental caries. In *Molecular Microbiology and Immunobiology of* Streptococcus mutans, pp. 173-80. Eds. S. Hamada, S.M. Michalek, H. Kiyono, L. Menaker, and J. R. McGhee. Elsevier, Amsterdam.

Curtiss, R., III; Goldschmidt, R.; Kelly, S.M.; and Fletchall, N. (1988a) Avirulent *Salmonella typhimurium* Δcya Δcrp oral vaccine strains expressing a streptococcal colonization and virulence antigen. *Vaccine*, **6**, 155-60.

Curtiss, R., III; Goldschmidt, R.; Kelly, S.M.; Lyons, M.; Michalek, S.; Pastian, R.; and Stein, S. (1988b) Construction and testing of live bivalent vaccine strains for oral immunization against *Streptococcus mutans*-induced dental caries. *Proc. 10th Intl. Convoc. on Immunology*, pp. 261-71.

Dobrogosz, W.J. (1981) Enzymatic activity. In *Manual of Methods for General Bacteriology*, p. 367. ASM, Washington, D.C.

Dougan, G.C.; Hormaeche, E.; and Maskell, D.J. (1987). Live oral *Salmonella* vaccines: potential use of attenuated strains as carriers of heterologous antigens to the immune system. *Parasite Immunol.* **9**, 151-60.

Erickson, E.D., and Norcross, N.L. (1975) The cell surface antigens of *Streptococcus equi*. *Can. J. Comp. Med.* **39**, 110-15.

Fischetti, V.A.; Jones, K.F.; Manjula, B.N.; and Scott, J.R. (1984) Streptococcal M 6 protein expressed in *Escherichia coli*: localization, purification and comparison with streptococcal-derived M protein. *J. Exp. Med.* **159**, 1083-95.

Formal, S.B.; Baron, L.S.; Kopecko, D.J.; Powell, C.; and Life, C.A. (1981) Construction of a potential bivalent vaccine strain: introduction of *Shigella sonnei* form I antigen genes into the *galE Salmonella typhy* Ty21a typhoid vaccine strain. *Infect. Immun.* **34**, 746-50.

Galán, J.E., and Timoney, J.F. (1985a) Immune complexes in purpura hemorrhagica of the horse contain IgA and M antigen of *Streptococcus equi*. *J. Immunol.* **135**, 3134-37.

———. (1985b) Mucosal nasopharyngeal immune response of horses to protein antigens of *Streptococcus equi*. *Infect. Immun.* **47**, 623-28.

———. (1987a) Molecular and genetic analysis of the M protein of *Streptococcus equi*. In *Streptococcal Genetics*, pp. 181-84. Eds. J.J. Ferretti and R. Curtis III. ASM, Washington, D.C.

———. (1987b) Molecular analysis of the M protein of *Streptococcus equi* and cloning and expression of the M protein gene in *Escherichia coli*. *Infect. Immun.* **55**, 3181-87.

Galán J.E.; Timoney, J.F., and Lengemann, F.W. (1986). Passive transfer of mucosal antibody to *Streptococcus equi* in the foal. *Infect. Immun.* **54**, 202-6.

Ganguly, R., and Waldman, R. (1980) Local immunity and local immune responses. *Prog. Allergy* **27**, 1-68.

Genco, R.J.; Linzer, R.; and Evans, R.T. (1983) Effect of adjuvants on oral administered antigens. *Ann. N.Y. Acad. Sci.* **409**, 650-68.

Germanier, R., and Furer, E. (1975) Isolation and characterization of *galE* mutant Ty21a of *Salmonella typhi*: a candidate strain for live, oral typhoid vaccine. *J. Infect. Dis.* **131**, 553-58.

Gulig, P.A., and Curtiss, R. III. (1987) Plasmid associated virulence of *Salmonella typhimurium*. *Infect. Immun.* **55**, 2891-2901.

Heleman, D.M.; Feramisco, J.R.; Fiddes, J.C.; Thomas, G.P.; and Hughes, S.H. (1983) Identification of clones that encode chicken tropomyosin by direct immunological screening of a cDNA expression library. *Proc. Natl. Acad. Sci. USA*, **80**, 31-35.

Hoiseth, S.K., and Stocker, B.A.D. (1981) Aromatic-dependent *Salmonella typhimurium* are nonvirulent and effective as live vaccines. *Nature* **291**, 238-39.

Hone, D.; Morona, R., Attridge, S.; and Hackett, J. (1987) Construction of defined *galE* mutants of *Salmonella* for use as vaccines. *J. Infect. Dis.* **156**, 167-74.

Humphreys, G.O.; Weston, A.; Brown, M.G.M.; and Saunders, J.R. (1979) *Transformation 1978*, pp. 254-79. Ed. S. W. Glover, and L. O. Butler. Costworld Press, Oxford.

Ivanov, I., and Gigova, L. (1985) Isolation of lambda DNA by hydroxylapatite chromatography. *Analyt. Biochem.* **146**, 389-92.

Laemmli, U.K. (1970) Cleavage of structural proteins during the assembly of the head of bacteriophage T4. *Nature* (London) **227**, 680-85.

Landgridge, J.; Landgridge, P.; and Bergquist, P.L. (1980) Extraction of nucleic acids from agarose gels. *Analyt. Biochem.* **103**, 264-71.

Lennox, E.S. (1955) Transduction of linked genetic characters of the host by bacteriophage P1. *Virology* **1**, 190-206.

Maniatis, T., and Fritsch, E.F. (1982) *Molecular cloning, a laboratory manual*. Ed. J. Sambrook. Cold Spring Harbor Laboratory, Cold Spring Harbor, N.Y.

Moore, B.O., and Bryans, J.T. (1970) Type specific antigenicity of group C streptococci from disease of the horse. *Proc. 2d Int. Conf. on Equine Infect. Dis.*, pp. 231-38.

Sanderson, K.E., and Roth, J.R. (1983) Linkage map of *Salmonella typhimurium*, 6th ed. *Microb. Rev.* **47**, 410-53.

Schnaitman, C.A. (1981) Cell fractionation. In *Manual of Methods for General Bacteriology, 60*. ASM, Washington, D.C.

Stevenson, G., and Manning, P.A. (1985) Galactose epimeraseless (*galE*) mutant G30 of *Salmonella typhimurium* is a good potential live oral vaccine carrier for fimbrial antigens. *FEMS Microbiol. Letters* **28**, 317-21.

Taubman, M.A.; Ebersole, J.L.; Smith, D.J.; and Stack, W. (1983) Adjuvants for secretory immune responses. *Ann. N.Y. Acad. Sci.* **409**, 637-49.

Timoney, J.F., and Eggers, D. (1985) Serum bactericidal responses to *Streptococcus equi* of horses following infection or vaccination. *Equine Vet. J.* **17**, 306-10.

Timoney, J.F., and Galán, J.E. (1985) The protective response of the horse to an avirulent strain of *Streptococcus equi*. In *Recent advances in streptococci and streptococcal diseases*, pp. 294-95. Eds. Y. Kimura, S. Kotami, and Y. Shiokawa. Reedbooks, Bracknell, Berkshire.

Timoney, J.F., and Trachman, J. (1985) Immunologically reactive proteins of *Streptococcus equi*. *Infect. Immun.* **48**, 29-34.

Timoney, J.F.; Timoney, P.J.; and Strickland, K.C. (1984) Lysogeny and the immunologically reactive proteins of Streptococcus equi. *Vet. Rec.* **115**, 148-49.

Towbin, H.; Staehelin, T.; and Gordon, J. (1979) Electrophoretic transfer of proteins from polyacrilamide gels to nitrocellulose membranes sheets. *Proc. Natl. Acad. Sci. USA* **76**, 4350-54.

Weisz-Carrington, P.; Roux, M.E.; McWilliams, M.; Phillip-Quagliata, J.M.; and Lamm, M.E. (1979) Organ and isotype distribution of plasma cells producing specific antibody after oral immunization: evidence for a generalized secretory immune system. *J. Immunol.* **123**, 1705-8.

Wirth, R.; An, F.; Clewell, D.B. (1987) Highly efficient cloning system for *Streptococcus faecalis*: protoplast transformation, shuttlevectors, and applications. In *Streptococcal genetics*, pp. 25-27. Ed. J. J. Ferretti and R. Curtiss III. ASM, Washington, D.C.

Woolcock, J.B. (1974) Purification and antigenicity of an M-like protein of *Streptococcus equi*. *Infect. Immun.* **10**, 116-22.

Evidence for *Streptococcus pneumoniae* as a Cause of Respiratory Disease in Young Thoroughbred Horses in Training

Mary E. Mackintosh, Susan T. Grant, and Michael H. Burrell

SUMMARY

Many young Thoroughbreds in racing stables experience episodes of respiratory disease of uncertain etiology during training. In a collaborative project, the possible causes were investigated in a group of two- and three-year-olds in training in one yard in Newmarket. Virology, bacteriology, hematology, and cytology were evaluated, together with a clinical assessment including endoscopy, for each horse over a period of one to two years. Bacteria recovered from tracheal washes were enumerated and identified. The host's response to the potential pathogen *Streptococcus pneumoniae* was considered in light of the results in the other disciplines. *S. pneumoniae* was cultured and identified by conventional methods. Strains were confirmed as capsule type 3 by immunofluorescent techniques, and antibodies to *S. pneumoniae* type 3 were estimated by indirect immunofluorescence. In the study, *S. pneumoniae* was isolated from horses with clinical signs of a respiratory infection that could not be attributed to a virus. Such horses had a rising titer of 1:64 to 1:512 to *S. pneumoniae* type 3 over a period of two to four weeks following onset of clinical signs.

Results of the virological study suggest that episodes of bacterial infection may be preceded by a clinical or subclinical virus infection. *S. pneumoniae* was usually present in a mixed bacterial infection although it was not necessarily the predominant organism. *S. pneumoniae* was isolated from horses in full training that showed no clinical signs of respiratory infection but had low antibody titers, ranging from 1:2 to 1:64.

These results indicate that *S. pneumoniae* is a causative agent of respiratory infection and that it can be carried asymptomatically, serving as a reservoir of infection.

INTRODUCTION

S. pneumoniae has long been recognized as a serious human respiratory pathogen. It is still an important cause of pneumonia, meningitis, and septicemia, although it is often carried asymptomatically in children and young adults (Lockley & Wise 1984). The isolation of *S. pneumoniae* from the horse has recently been reported (Benson & Sweeney 1984; Burrell, Mackintosh & Taylor 1986). This report describes the results of bacteriology and serology on a group of young Thoroughbred (TB) horses in training over a period of one or two flat racing seasons.

Animal Health Trust, Bacteriology Unit, Lanwades Park, Kennett, Newmarket, Suffolk CB87PN, England. Burrell: 10 Evesham Road, Reigate, Surrey RH29DF, England.

MATERIALS AND METHODS

A total of 26 young TB horses from one training yard in Newmarket were sampled at monthly intervals for six to 18 months as part of a multidisciplinary investigation of respiratory disease. At the beginning of the study, 16 horses were randomly selected: 11 two-year-olds and five three-year-olds. At the end of the first season, all of the older and five of the younger horses left the yard and were replaced. In the second season, nine two-year-olds and one three-year-old were added to the six that had been two-year-olds the previous season, giving a total of seven three-year-olds. These 26 horses were monitored for clinical signs of respiratory disease, and at monthly intervals serum samples were collected. At four- to six-week intervals the horses were examined with an endoscope and tracheal washings were collected for virological, bacteriological, and cytological examinations. Any horse that developed clinical signs of respiratory disease was investigated by endoscopy and tracheal washing, and an acute-phase serum sample was taken.

Endoscopy and tracheal washings. Endoscopic examination was always carried out after exercise. No clinical restraint or local anaesthetic was used, the horse being restrained by a bridle and twitch. A 1.8-meter human colonoscope (Olympus) was introduced via the ventral nasal meatus into the nasal pharynx and guided through the laryngeal additus and into the tracheal lumen. It was then passed down the length of the trachea until the carina could be seen. A sterile plastic catheter plugged with sterile agar was passed via the biopsy channel to the level of the carina. Thirty milliliters of sterile phosphate-buffered saline (PBS) was directed from a 50-ml syringe through the catheter into both main stream bronchi. The fluid drained cranially to the level of the thoracic inlet, where it pooled and was aspirated back into the syringe. The sample was divided into three aliquots after thorough mixing, and the one for bacteriology was dispensed into a sterile bijou. On the passage down the trachea, the amount of exudate visible was graded on a scale of 0-3, with 3 being a profuse amount, as previously described (Burrell et al. 1985).

Table 1. Bacteria isolated from tracheal washes of young Thoroughbred horses in training

Aerobes	Anaerobes
Potential pathogens	
S. zooepidemicus	Peptostreptococcus spp.
S. pneumoniae	Fusobacterium spp.
B. bronchiseptica	
P. pneumotropica	
P. haemolytica	
Uncertain significance	
Staphylococcus spp.	B. fragilis
S. equisimilis	B. oralis
S. milleri	B. melaninogenicus
α Streptococcus spp.	Peptococcus spp.
P. multocida	Clostridium spp.
Ps. aeruginosa	Cl. perfringens
Ps. maltophila	Veillonella spp.
Ps. pickettii	
M. phenylpyruvica	
M. nonliquefaciens	
E. coli	
A. lwoffii	
E. agglomerans	
Alcaligens spp.	
Bacillus spp.	
Corynebacterium spp.	
Streptococcus (CO_2 dependent)	
Transient	
Ps. acidovorans	
Ps. cepacia	
Ps. diminuta	
Ps. paucimobilis	
Actinobacillus spp.	
M. urethralis	
S. rubidaea	
F. multivarium	
Vibrio spp.	

Bacteriology. A 2-mm loopful of each sample of tracheal washing was inoculated onto each of two plates of Wilkins-Chilgren 5% horse blood agar. One plate was incubated microaerophilically and the other anaerobically. All plates were incubated at 37°C, those for microaerophilic culture for 24 hr and those for anaerobic culture for 48 hr.

To estimate number of viable bacteria present in each sample of tracheal washing, a 0.1-ml sample was mixed with an equal volume of a mucolitic agent, and the mixture allowed to stand for 15 min at 37°C with occasional gentle agitation. Serial 100-fold dilutions were made in anaerobic broth (Lab M). Each dilution was inoculated onto a Wilkins-Chilgren agar containing 5% horse blood agar by means of a calibrated 10-µl loop. The plates were incubated microaerophilically at 37°C for 24 hr. The colonies derived from those dilutions that gave the largest number of single colonies were counted and the results expressed as the number of colony-forming units per milliliter (cfu/ml) of the original sample. No correction was made for the difference between the 30-ml sterile PBS used for the wash and the volume actually recovered by aspiration. The bacteria isolated were identified by conventional tests (Cowan & Steel 1974; Willis 1977). All strains of *S. pneumoniae* isolated were capsule-typed.

Serum antibody levels to *S. pneumoniae* capsule type 3 were determined by indirect immunofluorescence. The antigen used was an *S. pneumoniae* isolated from an equine tracheal washing that had been typed as capsule type 3 by the Central Public Health Laboratory, Colindale, England. It was inoculated into brain-heart infusion broth (Oxoid Limited, Basingstoke, England) containing 5% sterile pig serum, which was incubated aerobically for 18 hr and then centrifuged at 3,000 rpm for 10 min. The pellet was washed twice in sterile PBS, pH 7.3, resuspended in PBS, and vortex-mixed to give a suspension of $10^{8\text{-}9}$ cfu/ml. Using a standard loop, 2 µl of suspension was placed on each of the 15 wells of a multitest slide (Flow Laboratories Limited, Irvine, UK). The slides were allowed to dry, fixed in acetone for 10 min, and stores at -20°C. Before use the slides were allowed to equilibrate to room temperature and then dried.

Indirect immunofluorescence. Each serum was initially tested at doubling dilutions in sterile PBS. Dilutions of sera were pipetted onto the appropriate well in 10-µl aliquots and incubated in a moist chamber for 30 min at 37°C. The slide wells were individually washed with distilled water, then washed twice with PBS over a period of 15 min. The slide was then dried. Onto each well was pipetted 10 ml of fluoracine-labeled antihorse immunoglobulin (Wellcome Diagnostics, Dartford, England), at the working dilution of 1:60 in PBS. After incubation in a moist chamber at 37°C for 30 min, the slide was rinsed and washed as previously described before being dried and mounted in buffered glycerol saline (90% glycerol, 10% sterile PBS).

Positive and negative antisera were run with each test. The negative control was gnotobiotic horse serum with Wellcome antihorse fluoracine conjugate. The positive control was bactopneumococcus antisera type 3 (Difco Laboratory, Detroit, Mich.) raised in a rabbit with Wellcome fluoracine-labeled antirabbit. The fluorescence was a solid unbroken halo around a dark centre. The fluorescence was graded under four categories.

RESULTS

No bacteria were isolated from 62 (18%) of the 338 tracheal washings taken during the study. The number of aerobic bacteria isolated ranged from 0 to $10^{7\text{-}8}$ cfu/ml. Most cultures contained two to nine different bacterial species. Thirty-one aerobic and nine obligate anaerobic species identified were grouped as potential pathogens, bacteria of uncertain significance, and nonsignificant or transient organisms. These groupings were based on clinical history and endoscopic

Table 2. Incidence of clinical infection, seroconversion, and isolation of *S. pneumoniae* among young Thoroughbred horses in training

Horse No.	Clinical signs[a]	Sero conversion	Maximum antibody titer detected	*S. pneumoniae* isolated: No. samples	*S. pneumoniae* isolated: No. positive
		Clinical and subclinical infections			
1	C	+	1:256	9	2
2	C	+	1:128	15	2
3	C	+	1:512	7	3
4	C	+	1:256	18	2
5	C	+	1:64	2	2
6	C	+	1:128	8	6[b]
7	Sub.	+	1:64	14	7[b]
8	Sub.	+	1:256	8	4[b]
9	Sub.	+	1:128	8	7[b]
10	Sub.	+	1:64	10	1
11	Sub.	+	1:128	11	3
		Uninfected and carriers			
12	None	−	1:32	17	13[b]
13	None	−	1:64	7	5[b]
14	None	−	1:64	10	6[b]
15	None	−	1:32	11	1
16	None	−	1:32	6	1
17	None	−	1:32	5	0
18	None	−	1:64	11	0
19	None	−	1:64	6	0
20	None	−	1:32	8	0
21	None	−	1:32	12	3
22	None	−	1:32	11	0
23	None	−	1:64	8	0
24	None	−	1:64	15	0
25	None	−	1:128	9	1
26	None	−	1:64	5	0

[a] At time of seroconversion: C = clinical infection; Sub. = subclinical infection.
[b] Persistent carrier.

examination of the horse, bacterial enumeration and pathogenicity in the horse or other species, and cytological examination of the tracheal washings. The principal organisms considered to be involved in respiratory disease episodes were *Streptococcus zooepidemicus*, *S. pneumoniae*, *Bordetella bronchiseptica*, *Pasteurella pneumotropica*, *P. haemolytica*, Peptostreptococcus spp., and Fusobacterium spp. (Table 1).

S. pneumoniae was isolated on one or more occasions from 18 of the 26 horses, including four or more consecutive monthly samples from seven horses. The seven were considered to be persistent carriers. All isolates were capsule type 3.

All 26 horses had detectable serum antibody levels to *S. pneumoniae* type 3, with titers ranging from 1:4 to 1:512 (Table 2). A seroconversion of fourfold increase in antibody titer from consecutive samples occurred in 14 horses. During the course of the study, 16 horses showed clinical symptoms of respiratory disease. *S. pneumoniae* was isolated with an associated seroconversion at the time of the episode from six horses, all two-year-olds. In only one episode was *S. pneumoniae* isolated in pure culture. In the other five it was present in a mixed culture, with *S. zooepidimicus* occurring most frequently. In one case *B. bronchiseptica* was also present. The antibody titers to *S. pneumoniae* in these six cases were raised to 1:256 except for one animal that received antibiotic therapy. In this case the titer was 1:64 when treatment was initiated, and no further rise was observed.

Five horses seroconverted with no clinical signs of infection, and two of them became persistent carriers after seroconversion. Twelve horses did not seroconvert during the study. *S. pneumoniae* was not recovered on any occasion from eight of them, and on no more than two occasions from the remaining four, in low numbers and mixed cultures in all cases.

Of the seven horses found to be persistent carriers, six were first identified as such when two-year-olds. One of them carried for its entire two- and three-year-old seasons with no evidence of clinical or subclinical infection or seroconversion; two of them were carriers between February and August; two were still carrying in November, when they left the study; and the remaining two-year-old, clinically infected in March, was a carrier until treated in June. The seventh horse was identified as a persistent carrier when it joined the study as a three-year-old and continued to carry for the season until November.

DISCUSSION

The bacteria most frequently isolated in association with respiratory disease episodes were *S. zooepidemicus, S. pneumoniae, B. bronchiseptica, P. haemolytica,* Peptostreptococcus spp., and Fusobacterium spp. The importance of *S. zooepidemicus* has been recognized for many years (Knight & Hietala 1978; Whitwell & Greet 1984), and during the present study it was frequently isolated from the respiratory tract of both sick and healthy horses.

The isolation of *S. pneumoniae* from 19 of the 26 horses in this study suggests that it is not a rare occurrence. Culturally, *S. pneumoniae* may be considered fastidious, with media and cultural conditions critical for isolation (Burrell, Mackintosh & Taylor 1986). Although it is classed as an aerobe, recovery is often superior under obligate anaerobic conditions and since certain other bacteria are less well adapted, *S. pneumoniae* is easier to identify.

Although serology is routinely used to diagnose viral respiratory disease, its use for assessing bacterial disease in the horse is very limited and has not previously been reported for *S. pneumoniae*. In humans, where serology is used extensively to diagnose bacterial infections (Kerttula 1987; Austrian 1984), 83 capsule types of *S. pneumoniae* have been identified, based on specific antigenicity of the polysaccharide capsule. All *S. pneumoniae* isolated in this study were capsule type 3, which in humans has long been recognized as a particularly pathogenic strain, associated with a higher mortality than other types of pneumococcal infections (Austrian & Gold 1964).

The carrier state of *S. pneumoniae* provides a potential reservoir of infection (Austrian 1984; Gray et al. 1981), both for new animals coming into the yard and as an endogenous source. Secondary bacterial infection has long been recognized as a major complication of acute respiratory viral disease in humans (Jakab 1982; Austrian 1984). Results from this study suggest that *S. pneumoniae* infections may follow upon clinical or subclinical virus infections. Seroconversions to equid herpes virus-1 and equine rhinovirus tended to occur in November and December, but *S. pneumoniae* was first isolated in January, while seroconversions occurred in four of the six horses in March. The time span between the two episodes is longer than would be expected from human experience. The lapse may represent a gradual buildup of bacterial numbers prior to infection and seroconversion, or bacterial infection may be secondary to other viral agents or factors such as stress caused by race training. In a study of human pneumonia, *S. pneumoniae* was identified as the most common etiological agent, and 58% of viral pneumonia cases showed evidence of mixed infection with bacteria (Kerttula et al. 1987). Antibiotic treatment of *S. pneumoniae* in humans alleviates clinical symptoms but may not affect carriage (Hendley et al. 1975). The etiology of respiratory disease in horses is complex, involving both viruses and bacteria, and *S. pneumoniae* should be considered an important component. The serological results from this study strongly suggest that a titer greater than 1:64 indicates exposure to *S. pneumoniae* antigen. Demonstration of a fourfold increase in titer, or an elevated titer (>1:64) associated with a cough or signs of respiratory distress, may be considered indicative of infection in young TB horses.

REFERENCES

Austrian, R. (1984) Pneumococcal infections. In *Bacterial Vaccines*, pp. 257-88. Ed. R. Germaier. Academic Press, New York.

Austrian, R., and Gold, J. (1964) Pneumococcal bacteremia with especial reference to bacteremic pneumococcal pneumoniae. *Ann. Intern. Med.* **60**, 759-76.

Benson, C.E., and Sweeney, C.R. (1984) Isolation of *Streptococcus pneumoniae* type 3 from equine species. *J. Clin. Microbiol.* **20**, 1028-30.

Burrell, M.H.; Mackintosh, M.E.; Whitwell, K.E.; Mumford, J.A.; and Rossdale, P.D. (1985) A two year study of respiratory disease in a Newmarket stable: Some preliminary observations. *Proc. Soc. Vet. Epidemiol. & Prev. Med.* (Reading), pp. 74-83.

Burrell, M.H.; Mackintosh, M.E.; and Taylor, C.E.D. (1986) Isolation of *Streptococcus pneumoniae* from the respiratory tract of horses. *Equine Vet. J.* **18**, 183-86.

Cowan, S.T., and Steel, K.J. (1974) *Manual for the Identification of Medical Bacteria*, 2d ed. Cambridge University Press.

Hendley, J.O.; Sande, M.A.; Stewart, P.M.; and Gwaltney, J.M. (1975) Spread of *Streptococcus pneumoniae* in families. I. Carriage rates and distribution of Types. *J. Infect. Dis.* **132**, 55-61.

Jakab, G.J. (1982) Viral bacterial interaction in pulmonary infections. *Adv. Vet. Sci. Comp. Med.* **26**, 155-71.

Kerttula, Y.; Leinonen, M.; Koskela, M. and Makela, P.H. (1987) The aetiology of pneumonia. Application of bacterial serology and basic laboratory methods. *J. Infection* **14**, 12-20.

Knight, H.D., and Hietala, S. (1978) Transtracheal aspiration revisted. *Proc. Ann. Sci. Meet. Am. Coll. Vet. Internal Med.*, pp. 120-31.

Lockley, M.R., and Wise, R. (1984) Pneumococcal infections. *Br. Med. J.* **288**, 1179-80.

Whitwell, K.E., and Greet, T.R.C. (1984) Collection and evaluation of tracheobronchial washes in the horse. *Equine Vet. J.* **16**, 499-508.

Willis, A.T. (1977) *Anerobic Bacteriology*. Butterworths, London.

Influenza

Origin of the A/equine/Johannesburg/86(H3N8) Virus: Antigenic and Genetic Analyses of Equine-2 Influenza A Hemagglutinins

Yoshihiro Kawaoka, William J. Bean, and Robert G. Webster

SUMMARY

A severe influenza outbreak occurred among horses in South Africa during 1986 and 1987. The causative agent was identified as an equine-2 influenza A virus [A/equine/Johannesburg/86(H3N8)]. Antigenic analyses of the hemagglutinin (HA) with ferret antisera and monoclonal antibodies showed that the virus is similar to other recent equine-2 influenza A viruses. The nucleotide sequence information on the HA genes of A/equine/Johannesburg/86 and other equine-2 influenza A viruses, together with the epidemiological data, clearly demonstrated that the virus was derived from an equine-2 influenza A virus that had been circulating among horses in the United States during 1986-87. The epidemiological information suggests that the unusual severity of the influenza outbreak in South Africa was due to lack of immunity in the horse population rather than to genetic changes in the virus.

INTRODUCTION

Despite extensive vaccination, equine influenza outbreaks occur every year in many countries. It is unusual for the virus to be introduced into a country where an influenza epidemic has not been experienced, as the majority of the equine population worldwide has been exposed to the disease. The South African population, however, escaped an epidemic until December 1986, when an outbreak occurred there that was unusually severe, resulting in the death of some animals. The causative agent was identified as an equine-2 influenza A virus, which epidemiological studies suggested had been introduced by horses imported from the United States. Possible reasons for the severity of the outbreak include a highly virulent virus or the lack of immunity among a susceptible population.

The object of the study was to determine the origin of the virus and to explain the severity of the outbreak.

MATERIALS AND METHODS

A/equine/Johannesburg/86(H3N8) was obtained from Dr. Jenny Mumford (Animal Health Trust); A/equine/Kentucky/2/87(H3N8) from James Wilson (University of Kentucky); and the other equine-2 influenza A viruses from the repository of St. Jude Children's Research Hospital. First or second egg passages of field isolates were used whenever possible. Viruses were grown in 11-day-old embryonated hens' eggs and purified by differential sedimentation through 25-70% sucrose gradients in a Beckman Sw28 rotor. Virion RNA was isolated by treatment of purified virus with proteinase K and sodium dodecyl sulfate, followed by extraction with phenol:chloroform (1:1) as described by Bean, Sriram, and Webster (1980).

Department of Virology and Molecular Biology, St. Jude Children's Research Hospital, 211 North Lauderdale, P.O. Box 318, Memphis, Tennessee 38101.

Cloning of hemagglutinin (HA) gene. Full-length cDNA was prepared by reverse transcription of virion RNA using the methods of Huddleston and Brownlee (1982). A 12-base synthetic primer complementary to the 3′ terminus of the negative-strand RNA was phosphorylated with T4 polynucleotide kinase and then used to prime reverse transcription of total virion RNA in the presence of [α^{32}P]dATP. Second-strand DNA synthesis was carried out using a phosphorylated 13-base synthetic primer complementary to the 3′ end of the cDNA and Klenow fragment of *Escherichia coli* DNA polymerase I.

Full-length double-stranded copies of Segment 4 were blunt-end ligated into the *PvuII* site of pATX153 obtained from C. Naeve (St. Jude Children's Research Hospital). Transformants were screened by a modification of the Grunstein and Hogness (1975) colony hybridization method (Rothstein et al. 1979) using a ^{32}P-labeled "short copy" cDNA probe to identify positive colonies.

Nucleic acid sequencing. Nucleotide sequencing of the cloned HA genes was performed by the method of Zagursky and colleagues (1987) using alkali-denatured DNA template. Oligonucleotide primers complementary to the virion HA gene segment were synthesized on a Model 380A synthesizer (Applied Biosystems, Foster City, Calif.) by the solid-phase phosphoramidite method. The reaction products were resolved on 6% polyacrylamide-7 *M* urea thin gels containing a 1.0 to 4× TBE (90 m*M* Tris-borate, pH 8.0, 1 m*M* EDTA) gradient (Biggin, Gibson & Hong 1983).

Serological tests. HA titrations and hemagglutination inhibition (HI) tests were done in microtiter plates (Palmer et al. 1975) with ferret antisera and monoclonal antibodies to the HA of equine-2 influenza A virus obtained from Judy Appleton (Cornell University).

Table 1. Antigenic comparisons of equine-2 influenza A viruses

Virus	HI titers[a] (× 10) with ferret antisera to: A/equine/Miami/63	A/equine/Uruguay/63	A/equine/Kentucky/76	A/equine/Fontainebleau/79
A/equine/Miami/1/63	>128	2	1	1
A/equine/Uruguay/1/63	>128	128	128	16
A/equine/Romania/1/80	4	4	8	8
A/equine/Santiago/85	8	8	>128	>128
A/equine/Tennessee/86	>128	128	>128	>128
A/equine/Johannesburg/86	16	32	>128	>128

[a] Hemagglutinin inhibition titer is expressed as the reciprocal of the highest antibody dilution inhibiting 4 hemagglutinating units of virus.

Table 2. Antigenic comparisions of equine-2 influenza A viruses using monoclonal antibodies

Virus	HI titers[a] (× 100) with MAb to A/equine/Miami/1/63: Monoclone 2/1	Monoclone 3/1	Monoclone 4/1
A/equine/Miami/1/63	4	1	>128
A/equine/Uruguay/1/63	8	<1	4
A/equine/Romania/1/80	<1	<1	1
A/equine/Santiago/85	<1	<1	1
A/equine/Tennessee/86	2	1	4
A/equine/Johannesburg/86	<1	<1	1

[a] Hemagglutination inhibition titer is expressed as the reciprocal of the highest antibody dilution inhibiting 4 hemagglutinating units of virus.

Table 3. Nucleotide differences in HA gene between A/equine/Johannesburg/86 and other equine-2 influenza A viruses

Other virus	No. of nucleotide differences
A/equine/Uruguay/1/63	102
A/equine/Miami/1/63[a]	110
A/equine/Tokyo/71	138
A/equine/Algeria/72	136
A/equine/Newmarket/76	47
A/equine/Fontainebleau/79	68
A/equine/Romania/1/80	38
A/equine/Santiago/85	28
A/equine/Tennessee/86	2
A/equine/Kentucky/86	10
A/equine/Kentucky/2/87	5

[a] The nucleotide sequences of A/equine/Miami/1/63 and A/equine/Fontainebleau/79 viruses were obtained from Daniels and colleagues (1985).

RESULTS

Antigenic analysis of HA molecule with ferret sera. The antigenicity of the HA molecule of A/equine/Johannesburg/86 was compared with that of other equine-2 influenza A viruses by means of ferret antisera (Table 1). A/equine/Johannesburg/86 virus was antigenically quite different from early equine-2 influenza A viruses such as A/equine/Miami/1/63 and A/equine/Uruguay/1/63. The recent equine-2 influenza A viruses, including Johannesburg/86, are similar to each other in reactivity, but they can be differentiated with ferret sera. Analyses with ferret sera also showed that there are antigenic differences in the index isolates of equine-2 influenza A viruses (e.g., Miami/1/63 and Uruguay 1/63).

Antigenic analyses of HA molecule with monoclonal antibodies. The antigenicity of the equine-2 influenza A HA molecules was further examined with monoclonal antibodies to A/equine/Miami/1/63 virus (Table 2). The A/equine/Johannesburg/86 HA could be differentiated from other equine-2 influenza A viruses, similar to the results with the ferret antisera. Antigenically different equine-2 influenza A viruses cocirculate, and antigenic variation was observed between the viruses isolated during 1963.

Nucleotide sequence analysis of HA genes. The nucleotide sequence of the HA genes of A/equine/Johannesburg/86 and other equine-2 influenza A viruses was compared to provide information on the origin of the Johannesburg/86 virus. The number of nucleotide differences increases in parallel with the length of time between the isolation of Johannesburg/86 and the isolation of other equine-2 influenza A viruses (Table 3).

There were only two nucleotide differences between the HA genes of A/equine/Johannesburg/86 and A/equine/Tennessee/86 viruses, and there were fewer than 10 nucleotide differences between A/equine/Johannesburg/86 and equine-2 influenza A viruses isolated during 1986-87 in the United States.

One of the nucleotide substitutions detected between Johannesburg/86 and Tennessee/86 viruses resulted in an amino acid change at Residue 263. The other nucleotide change was silent. Although Residue 263 is located on the globular head of HA molecules in the three-dimensional structure (Wilson, Skehel & Wiley 1981), it is not in the antigenic sites. This amino acid substitution may cause conformational changes that would explain the antigenic differences between the two viruses.

Comparison of amino acid sequence at cleavage site. Cleavage of the HA molecule of influenza virus is a prerequisite for viral infectivity. In avian influenza viruses, vir-

Table 4. Amino acid sequence at cleavage site of hemagglutinin

							HA1	HA2
Virulent avian influenza A virus	Gln	Arg	Lys	Arg	Lys	Lys	Arg	Gly
Avirulent avian influenza A virus	Gln	—	—	Arg	Glu	Thr	Arg	Gly
Equine influenza A virus	Glu	—	—	Lys	Glu	Ile	Arg	Gly

Note: Underscore indicates basic amino acids.

Table 5. Amino acid sequence in receptor binding pocket of hemagglutinin

	Residue site				
Source of hemagglutinin	224	225	226	227	228
Human influenza A virus (H3)[a]	Arg	Gly	Leu	Ser	Ser
Avian influenza A virus (H3)[a]	Arg	Gly	Gln	Pro	Gly
Equine influenza A virus (H3)	Arg	Gly	Gln	Ser	Gly

[a] Fang and colleagues (1981).

ulence is correlated with cleavage of the HA and with plaque formation in tissue cultures in the absence of additional trypsin. A series of basic amino acids at the cleavage site of the virulent influenza virus is important for cleavage activation of the molecule (Bosch et al. 1981; Kawaoka & Webster 1988). When we examined the amino acid sequence at the cleavage site of the A/equine/Johannesburg/86 HA, we found that it contained only one basic amino acid in this region of the molecule, similar to other equine-2 influenza A viruses (Table 4).

Comparison of receptor binding site. The HA molecule is responsible for viral attachment to cell-surface receptors. The differences in receptor specificity and in the amino acid sequence around the receptor binding site of the HA have been shown among influenza viruses isolated from various species of animals. The alteration of receptor specificity could result in differences in the host range and virulence of the virus. We, therefore, compared the amino acids around the receptor binding pocket of the HA of A/equine/Johannesburg/86 and other equine-2 influenza A viruses (Table 5). Although variations were detected among influenza viruses isolated from other species of animals, Johannesburg/86 virus had the same amino acid sequence at the receptor binding site as other equine-2 influenza A viruses.

DISCUSSION

Antigenic analyses of the influenza virus isolated from horses in South Africa indicated that A/equine/Johannesburg/86 virus is related to other equine-2 influenza A viruses but can be discriminated from equine-2 influenza A viruses circulating in North America in 1986 and 1987. Comparison of the nucleotide sequence of the HA genes demonstrated that A/equine/Johannesburg/86 virus is very similar to recent equine-2 influenza A viruses isolated in the United States, especially A/equine/Tennessee/86. The two nucleotide variations and the single amino acid difference between Johannesburg/86 and Tennessee/86 indicate that the HAs on these viruses are very closely related.

This information, together with epidemiological evidence, strongly suggests that A/equine/Johannesburg/86 virus was derived from an equine-2 influenza A virus circulating in the United States.

Influenza infection among horses in the United States in recent years has not been very severe, being limited to fever, a frequent cough, and nasal discharge, and mortality is very rare. Although we examined only the HA gene, comparison of the nucleotide sequence clearly showed the A/equine/Johannesburg/86 virus is closely related to A/equine/Tennessee/86 virus. The single amino acid substitution detected between Johannesburg/86 and Tennessee/86 viruses occurred in the globular head, and no changes were detected in regions of the HA associated with virulence. Although we cannot exclude the possibility that mutation(s) in other genes may have been responsible for the severity of the South African outbreak, we think that this is unlikely, for the HA is a key gene product in determining virulence. A/equine/Tennessee/86 virus was isolated from a young horse that had been vaccinated twice with inactivated influenza vaccine, at three and four months before natural infection occurred. This suggests that influenza vaccination does not prevent horses from becoming infected but may modify the severity of disease.

The difference in the immune status between the horse population of the United States and that of South Africa may be the reason why the influenza outbreak in South Africa was so severe.

ACKNOWLEDGMENTS

This work was supported by U.S. Public Health Research Contract AI 52586 from the National Institute of Allergy and Infectious Diseases; Cancer Center Support (CORE) Grant CA 21765; and American Lebanese Syrian Associated Charities. The authors thank Dr. Clayton W. Naeve for preparation of the oligonucleotide primers. Daniel Channell, Scott Krauss, James Watkins, and Laura Whitworth provided excellent technical assistance, and we thank Glenith D. White for typing the manuscript.

REFERENCES

Bean, W.J.; Sriram, G.; and Webster, R.G. (1980) Electrophoretic analysis of iodine-labeled influenza virus RNA segments. *Anal. Biochem.* **102**, 228-32.

Biggin, M.D.; Gibson, T.J.; and Hong, G.F. (1983) Buffer gradient gels and ^{35}S-label as an aid to rapid DNA sequence determination. *Proc. Natl. Acad. Sci. USA* **80**, 3963-65.

Bosch, F.X.; Garten, W.; Klenk, H.D.; and Rott, R. (1981) Proteolytic cleavage of influenza virus hemagglutinins: Primary structure of the connecting peptide between HA1 and HA2 determines proteolytic cleavability and pathogenicity of avian influenza viruses. *Virology* **113**, 725-35.

Daniels, R.S.; Skehel, J.J.; and Wiley, D.C. (1985) Amino acid sequences of haemagglutinins of influenza viruses of the H3 subtype isolated from horses. *J. Gen. Virol.* **66**, 457-64.

Fang, R.; Min Jou, W.; Huylebroeck, D.; Devos, R.; and Fiers, W. (1981) Complete structure of A/duck/Ukraine/63 influenza hemagglutinin gene: Animal virus as progenitor of human H3 Hong Kong 1968 influenza hemagglutinin. *Cell* **25**, 315-23.

Grunstein, M., and Hogness, D. (1975) Colony hybridization: A method for the isolation of cloned cDNAs that contain a specific gene. *Proc. Natl. Acad. Sci. USA* **723**, 3961-65.

Huddleston, J.A., and Brownlee, G.G. (1982) The sequence of the nucleoprotein gene of human influenza A virus strain, A/NT/60/68. *Nucl. Acids Res.* **10**, 1029-37.

Kawaoka, Y., and Webster, R.G. (1988) Sequence requirements for cleavage activation of influenza virus hemagglutinin expressed in mammalian cells. *Proc. Natl. Acad. Sci. USA*. In press.

Palmer, D.F.; Coleman, M.T.; Dowdle, W.R.; and Schild, G.C. (1975) Advanced laboratory techniques for influenza diagnosis. In *Immunology Series No. 6*, pp. 51-52. U.S. Department of Health, Education, and Welfare.

Rothstein, R.J.; Call, L.F.; Babl, C.P.; Norang, S.A.; and Wu, R. (1979) Synthetic adaptors for cloning DNA. In *Methods in Enzymology*, Vol. 69, pp. 101-10. Ed. A. San Pietro. Academic Press, New York.

Wilson, I.A.; Skehel, J.J.; and Wiley, D.C. (1981) Structure of the hemagglutinin membrane glycoprotein of influenza virus at 3 Å resolution. *Nature* **289**, 366-73.

Zagursky, R.; Baumeister, K.; Lomax, N.; and Berman, M. Dideoxy DNA sequencing directly from plasmid DNA using reverse transcriptase. In *Gene Analysis Techniques*, Vol. 2. In press.

Hemagglutinin Gene Sequencing Studies of Equine-1 Influenza A Viruses

C.A. Gibson, Rodney S. Daniels, J.W. McCauley, and Geoffrey C. Schild

SUMMARY

This study was undertaken to investigate, at the molecular level, the apparently low degree of antigenic drift in equine-1 influenza A(H7N7) strains as demonstrated by serological analyses. The sequences of the hemagglutinin (HA) genes (the HA1 portions) of 10 influenza viruses isolated between 1956 and 1977 were determined using an oligonucleotide primer extension method in the presence of dideoxynucleotides. Genetically and antigenically, the viruses can be divided into two groups covering the periods 1956-63 and 1964-77. Within those groups, low levels of antigenic drift are observed, but between them a major drift is apparent. Potential antigenic sites are identified by aligning the equine H7HA protein sequence with that of the prototype human influenza virus H3HA, the three-dimensional structure of which is known. Two models for the occurrence of the two groups in the equine-1 influenza A population are discussed.

INTRODUCTION

Equine-1 influenza A virus containing hemagglutinin (HA) of the Heq-1 subtype was first isolated from horses in 1956 (Sovinova et al. 1958). The virus was reclassified in 1980 as equine-1 influenza A(H7N7) on the basis of reactions with hyperimmune sera prepared against other members of this subtype of avian origin (WHO 1980).

Since 1956, antigenically related viruses have caused outbreaks of equine influenza worldwide, the last viral isolate being reported for 1978 (Tumova 1980), although serology suggests that the subtype is still circulating (R.G. Webster, personal communication). In relatively limited studies, with few viral isolates and immune sera, only minor antigenic drift of the HA has been reported (Powell et al. 1974; Burrows & Denyer 1982). This contrasts with results obtained for influenza of the H3 subtype isolated from humans (Webster & Laver 1980) and horses (Hinshaw et al. 1983).

Our extensive study of equine-1 influenza A viruses supports the concept of a low level of antigenic drift of this influenza subtype in this species. This is confirmed by the amino acid sequences, deduced from the nucleotide sequence of virus RNAs, of HAs of 10 virus isolates representative of the pandemic period 1956-77. The sequence of the prototype equine H7 HA derived from A/equine/Prague/1/56(H7N7) is compared with the published sequences of H7 HAs of avian origin [A/FPV/Rostock/34(H7N7); Porter et al. 1979] and seal origin [A/seal/Massachusetts/1/80(H7N7); Naeve & Webster 1983] and the antigenicity of the equine-1 influenza A virus is discussed in terms of the structure of the HA of the prototype human influenza A(H3N2) virus (Wilson, Skehel & Wiley 1981).

Gibson, Daniels, Schild: National Institute for Biological Standards and Control, Virology Division, Blanche Lane, South Mimms, Potters Bar, Herts EN6 3QG, England. McCauley: Institute for Animal Disease Research, Pirbright, Woking, Surrey GU24 ONF, England. Present address, Daniels: National Institute for Medical Research, Virology Division, The Ridgeway, Mill Hill, London NW7 1AA, England.

MATERIALS AND METHODS

The following 16 equine-1 influenza A(H7N7) viruses were used: A/Prague/1/56, A/Cambridge/1/63, A/Detroit/1/64, A/Connaught Detroit 1/64 (a vaccine manufacturer's seed stock), A/Lexington/1/66, A/Switzerland/125/72, A/Switzerland/137/72, A/London/899/73, A/London/905/73, A/London/1416/73, A/Cambridge/1/73, A/Sao Paulo/1/76, A/Uruguay/1/76, A/Newmarket/1/77, A/Argentina/1/77, and A/Santiago/1/77. The viruses are maintained in the reference collection of the National Institute for Biological Standards and Control. All were grown in 10-day-old embryonated hens' eggs and purified, and RNA was extracted (Hay et al. 1977).

Hemagglutination inhibition (HI) tests were carried out (WHO technical report series 1953) using 0.7% turkey erythrocytes, allantoic fluids containing infectious virus, and either postinfection ferret antisera or postvaccination (A/Prague/56) pony sera.

Nucleotide sequences were determined using the dideoxynucleotide chain-terminating procedure of Sanger and colleagues (1977) and 5′ -^{32}P-labeled oligodeoxynucleotide primers of reverse transcription (Daniels et al. 1983). All primers were made on an Applied Biosystems 381A DNA-synthesizer and corresponded to bases 5-AAAGCAGGGGA-15, 151-GTTGTCAATGCA-162, 412-ATGGGATTCAC-422, 585-CTGGGGAATCCACCA-599, 877-TGTGAAGGTGAATG-890 of the A/Prague/56 sequence (Fig. 1).

RESULTS

To examine the antigenic relatedness of equine-1 influenza A viruses associated with outbreaks of disease, a range of viruses from Europe and the Americas were studied in HI tests (Table 1). Eleven of 16 ferret sera gave higher titers with

Table 1. Hemagglutination inhibition tests—comparison of equine-1 influenza A virus isolates

Anti-serum	Virus strain Pr 56	C 63	D 64	CD 64	LE 66	S125 72	S137 72	L899 73	L905 73	L1416 73	C 73	SP 76	Ur 76	NM 77	Arg 77	Sant 77
Postinfection ferret sera																
Pr/56	5120	5120	1016	1280	905	1613	640	1280	905	1280	640	905	905	905	302	905
C/63	160	226	160	127	160	25	80	80	80	127	57	57	80	80	57	113
D/64	320	320	508	403	320	403	160	453	226	160	160	160	320	320	160	320
CD/64	113	113	127	202	80	113	113	113	113	160	113	113	226	160	80	80
LE/66	1200	1613	1280	1016	806	806	806	2032	1280	806	806	1016	1613	1613	640	1280
S137/72	640	905	50	1016	640	640	640	905	905	640	640	320	640	640	453	905
L889/73	57	57	80	63	80	40	60	40	40	40	28	20	80	28	20	80
L905/73	90	1280	1016	2032	1810	1280	1810	1810	2560	1280	905	1280	1280	1810	640	1810
L1416/73	3620	2560	3225	4064	1810	2560	3620	>5120	3620	2560	2560	1280	2560	3620	2560	2560
Ur/76	905	905	1016	1280	905	905	905	905	905	1280	453	905	905	1810	905	1810
NM/77	905	1280	2560	2560	2560	1280	1810	2560	1810	3225	1280	1810	2560	3620	1810	2560
Arg/77	1280	905	1016	1280	1280	640	905	905	905	1016	905	640	905	905	1810	1810
Sant/77	1280	905	640	905	905	640	320	640	905	403	640	320	320	320	640	1810
Postvaccination pony sera																
20/5	5120	3225	4063	4063	2560	5120	—	—	—	4063	1613	2560	—	2560	—	—
30/5	1613	4063	4063	2560	1613	1613	—	—	—	3225	4063	2560	—	4063	—	—
20/4	40	80	80	80	80	127	—	—	—	80	40	60	—	80	—	—

Notes: Homologous titers are underlined. All titers (reciprocal) are expressed as the geometric means of at least three independent assays. For complete names of virus strains, see *Materials and Methods* section.

homologous virus than with heterologous viruses, but in general, all sera were reactive with all viruses. The most striking difference in titer was observed for the A/Prague/56-infected ferrets. Their sera distinguished the two early viruses (A/Prague/56 and A/Cambridge/63) from the rest of the group. This distinction was not supported by the results obtained wih postvaccination pony sera. A range of responses to the immunogen was seen in individual ponies, and all gave sera broadly reactive to heterologous viruses with higher titer in some cases. To further investigate this high degree of antigenic relatedness, 10 of the viruses were selected for HA gene sequencing studies, on the basis of their high growth potential in hens' eggs and differences in their HAs suggested by migration differences on sodium dodecylsulphate–polyacrylamide gel electrophoresis (SDS-PAGE) (results not shown).

Figure 1 shows the nucleotide sequence of the A/Prague/56 HA gene (mRNA sense) covering the 5′ noncoding region and the coding regions for the signal peptide, HA1, and the polybasic connecting peptide—a total of 1,068 bases. The noncoding region is assumed to be 21 bases long due to the conservation of this region between A/FPV/Rostock/34 (Porter et al. 1979) and A/seal/Massachusetts/1/80, (Naeve & Webster, 1983), the sequences of which were determined from full-length cDNA clones; the specificity of primer 5 AAAGCAGGGGA 15 in the present study suggests nucleotide sequence is conserved over this region. All three H7 HA genes contain 54 nucleotides (Nos. 22-75) encoding the highly hydrophobic signal peptides, which show homologies of 66.7% (A/FPV/34→A/Prague/56), 57.4% (A/FPV/34→A/seal/80), and 55.6% (A/Prague/56→A/seal/80) at the nucleotide level (Table 2). The HA1 coding region of A/FPV/Rostock/34 is 957 nucleotides long (Porter et al. 1979). The A/Prague/56 and A/seal/80 sequences align well over this region to give homologies of 77.3% (A/FPV/34→A/Prague/56), 74.4% (A/FPV/34→A/seal/80), and 71.7% (A/Prague/56→A/seal/80), but 3 and 24 nucleotide extensions are present in the respective HA gene sequences of A/seal/80 and A/Prague/56 (Table 2). The connecting peptide coding regions are 3, 12, and 15 nucleotides long for A/seal/80, A/Prague/56 and A/FPV/34, respectively, encoding basic amino acids prior to a conserved sequence of 30 nucleotides (data not shown) encoding the first 10 amino acids of HA2. Overall the coding sequences are 1,026, 1,047 and 1,017 nucleotides long and indicate gene base compositions rich in T (33.9%, 35.9%, and 32.2%) and low in G (20.1%, 19.6%, and 20.9%) for A/FPV/34, A/Prague/56 and A/seal/80 respectively. Between A/Prague/56 and A/Detroit/64, there are 57 nucleotide differences—2, 54, and 1 in the signal peptide, HA1, and connecting peptide coding regions, respectively (Fig. 1). For HA1 this represents 5.5% variation and a nucleotide substitution rate of 0.69%/year.

The deduced amino acid sequence of A/Prague/56 HA signal peptide, HA1, and connecting peptide are shown in Fig. 2. The signal peptides of all H7 viruses are 18 amino acids long and show relatively low homology (50% A/FPV/34→A/Prague/56, 50% A/FPV/34→A/seal/80, 33.3% A/Prague/56→A/seal/80; Table 2). The HA1 of A/FPV/Rostock/34 is known to be 319 amino acids long with a Lys at its carboxy-terminus (Porter et al. 1979), whilst the A/seal/80

Fig. 1. Nucleotide sequence of A/equine/Prague/56 hemagglutinin (HA1).

The initiation codon is at positions 22 to 24, the HA1 reading frame starts at nucleotide 76 and terminates at 1056, thereafter nucleotides encoding the connecting peptide are shown.
X Nucleotides not determined in the present study.

```
                                                         10                  20
          A/Equine/Detroit/64
          A /Equine/Prague/56           x x x x x x x x x x x x x x x x x x x A

                 30                  40                  50                  60
A A T G A A C A C T C A A A T T C T A A T A T T A G C C A C T T C G G C A T T C

                 70                  80                  90                 100
C       G
T T C T A T G T A C G T G C A G A T A A A A T C T G C C T A G G A C A T C A T G

                110                 120                 130                 140
              C
C T G T G T C T A A T G G A A C C A A A G T A G A C A C C C T T A C T G A A A A

                150                 160                 170                 180
G
A G G A A T A G A A G T T G T C A A T G C A A C A G A A A C A G T T G A A C A A

                190                 200                 210                 220
  A                   C                                   G                   A
A C A A A C A T C C C T A A G A T C T G C T C A A A A G G A A A A C A G A C T G

                230                 240                 250                 260
                                                                A
T T G A C C T T G G T C A A T G T G G A T T A C T A G G G A C C G T T A T T G G

                270                 280                 290                 300
      C                 C
T C C T C C C C A A T G T G A C C A A T T T C T T G A A T T C T C T G C T A A T

                310                 320                 330                 340
            A         G           A
T T A A T A G T T G A A A G A A G G G A A G G T A A T G A C A T T T G T T A T C

                350                 360                 370                 380
                            G                                   C
C A G G C A A A T T T G A C A A T G A A G A A A C A T T G A G A A A A A T A C T

                390                 400                 410                 420
                                                A
C A G A A A A T C C G G A G G A A T T A A A A A G G A G A A T A T G G G A T T C

                430                 440                 450                 460
A C A T A T A C C G G A G T G A G A A C C A A T G G A G A G A C T A G C G C A T

                470                 480                 490                 500
                                                              A
G T A G A A G G T C A A G A T C T T C C T T T T A T G C A G A G A T G A A A T G

                510                 520                 530                 540
      C               A                           G T       C
G C T T C T A T C C A G C A C A G A C A A T G G G A C A T T T C C A C A A A T G

                550                 560                 570                 580
          A                                       G     A G
A C A A A G T C C T A C A A G A A C A C T A A G A A G G T A C C A G C T C T G A

                590                 600                 610                 620
                                                              C G
T A A T C T G G G G A A T C C A C C A C T C A G G A T C A A C T A C T G A A C A

                630                 640                 650                 660
                  G                       A           G
G A C T A G A T T A T A T G G A A G T G G G A A T A A A T T G A T A A C A G T T

                670                 680                 690                 700
          T                                             C
T G G A G C T C C A A A T A C C A A C A A T C T T T T G T C C C A A A T C C T G

                710                 720                 730                 740
              G                 A           C
G A C C A A G A C C G C A A A T G A A T G G T C A A T C A G G A A G A A T T G A

                750                 760                 770                 780
        T                       T                                           A
C T T T C A C T G G C T G A T G C T A G A T C C C A A T G A T A C T G T C A C T
```

Fig. 1. (continued)

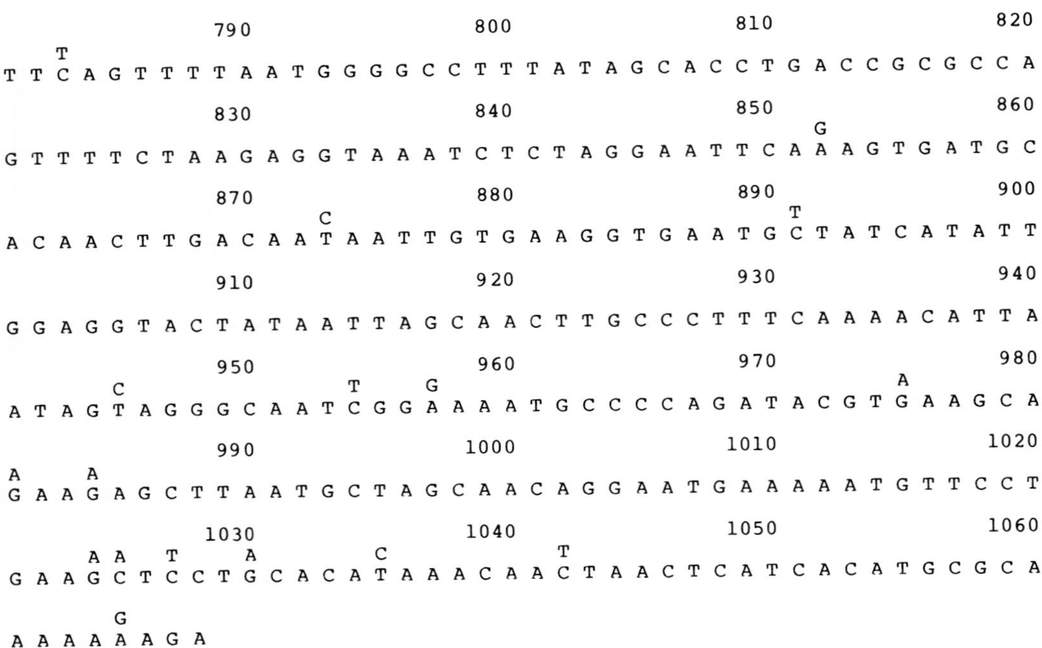

molecule may contain an additional Thr at its carboxy-terminus (Naeve & Webster 1983). In the A/Prague/56 sequence, the terminal Lys is substituted by Ala and the polypeptide is probably extended by 8 amino acids (His-Lys-Gln-Leu-Thr-His-His-Met). If, for comparison purposes (Table 2), the potential carboxy-terminal extensions of HA1 are disregarded, the H7HA1s show high homologies of 84.0% (A/FPV/34→A/Prague/56), 84.6% (A/FPV/34→A/seal/80), and 79.9% (A/Prague/56→A/seal/80). HA1 of A/FPV/Rostock/34 contains five glycosylation sites (Keil et al. 1985) at positions 22, 38, 133, 160, and 240 (Fig. 2) and four of these are present in A/Prague/56 (22, 38, 160, 240) and A/seal/80 (22, 38, 133, 240). The connecting peptide of A/FPV/34 contains five predominantly basic amino acids; four of these are conserved in the A/Prague/56 sequence whilst A/seal/80 has a single Arg at this site. In protein sequence, A/Detroit/64 differs from A/Prague/56 at 20 sites—two in the signal peptide and 18 in HA1—which represents 5.5% variation and an amino acid substitution rate of 0.69%/year for HA1 (Fig. 2).

A/Cambridge/63 is closely related to A/Prague/56, having only six nucleotide differences (373A→C, 527C→T, 584T→C, 696T→C, 717G→C, 949G→A) in the HA1 coding position, five of which result in amino acid substitutions. Nucleotide substitutions 584 and 949, resulting in amino acid changes (numbered according to the alignment shown in Fig. 2) at 179 (Ile→Thr) and 301 (Ala→Thr), are unique to A/Cambridge/63, whilst the substitutions at 373 and 717 producing amino acid changes 110 (Lys→Gln) and 23 (Met

Table 2. Sequence homologies between hemagglutinins of H7 influenza viruses of avian, equine, and seal origin

		Nucleotide sequence homology			
		A/equine/ Prague/56	A/equine/ Detroit/64	A/FPV/ Rostock/34	A/seal Massachusetts/80
	A/equine/ Prague/56	—	a96.3	66.7	55.6
		—	b94.6	77.3	71.7
Amino acid sequence homology	A/equine/ Detroit/64	88.9	—	66.7	53.7
		94.4	—	79.1	71.7
	A/FPV/ Rostock/34	50.0	50.0	—	57.4
		84.0	84.6	—	74.4
	A/seal Massachusetts/80	33.3	33.3	50.0	—
		79.9	79.6	84.6	—

Note: For each virus comparison, homologies are shown for: (a) signal peptide domains (54 nucleotides and 18 amino acids) and (b) HA1 domains (957 nucleotides and 319 amino acids).

Fig. 2. Amino Acid sequence of A/equine/Prague/56 hemagglutinin (HA1).

All sequences are compared with that of A/equine/Prague/56. The sequences are aligned to maximise homology with X31, the 3-dimensional structure of which is known (Wilson et al. 1981). Numbers refer to the X31 sequence. (*) No amino acid present in that particular sequence. Potential glycosylation sites are underlined.

```
                                                          -15       -10       -5
A/Aichi/1/68 (X31)                                      K   I   A L S Y I F C L A L G * *
A/Equine/Detroit/64                                                           L C
A/Equine/Prague/56                                    M N T Q I L I L A T S A F F Y V R A

                    10                  20                  30                  40
Q D L P G N D N S T A T L                   P _____ L   K   I   D D Q           _____
* * * * * * * * * * D K I C L G H H A V S N G T K V D T L T E K G I E V V N A T

                    50                  60                  70                  80
  L   Q S S S T G         N N P H R I L   G I D   T   I D A L L   D   H     V   Q
          K                           I                     I
E T V E Q T N I P K I C S K G K Q T V D L G Q C G L L G T V I G P P Q C D Q F L

                    90                  100                 110                 120
N E T W D   F       S K A F S N     Y D V P D Y A S     S L V A S     T L E F
              I                               D         Q
E F S A N L I V E R R E G N D I C Y P G K F D N E E T L R K I L R K S G G I K K

                    130                 140                 150                 160
I T E       W T     T Q     G S N     K   G P G   G   F S R L N     T K   G S T
                                            *                             N
E N M G F T Y T G V R T N G E T S A C R R S * R S S F Y A E M K W L L S S T D N

                    170                 180                 190
* * Y   V L N V T M P   N D N F D K   Y             P S T N Q       S     V Q A
  V                           R E                           A
G T F P Q M T K S Y K N T K K V P A L I I W G I H H S G S T T E Q T R L Y G S G

200                 210                 220                 230
S G R V     S T R R S     T I I     I   S     W V R   L   S     S I Y   T I V K
                            A                   I                   Y
N K L I T V W S S K Y Q Q S F V P N P G P R P Q M N G Q S G R I D F H W L M L D

240                 250                 260                 270
  G   V L V I N S     N L       R G Y F K M   T       S I M R       * P I D T
          N                                  *
P N D T V T F S F N G A F I A P D R A S F L R * G K S L G I Q S D A Q L D N N C

  280                 290                 300                 310
I S     I T P N   S     P N D K       V   K I T Y   A     K       N T   K

E G E C Y H I G G T I I S N L P F Q N I N S R A I G K C P R Y V K Q K S L M L A

  320                 328
      R               K Q T * * * * * * * * *     * * *
                      N S T
T G M K N V P E A P A H K Q L T H H M     R K K R
```

→Ile) are present in later viruses. The change at position 527 causing amino acid substitution 160^{++} (Thr→Ile) is notable in that it results in the loss of a potential glycosylation site, which is also absent from all the later viruses due to the substitution 160^{++} Thr→Val (Fig. 2). Another potential glycosylation site is lost from the A/London/1416/73 HA1 due to amino acid substitution at position 24 (Thr→Ile), whilst A/Detroit/64, A/Connaught Detroit/64, and A/Newmarket/77 contain an additional glycosylation site due to substitution at 244 (Thr→Asn; Table 3). In addition, all viruses isolated in 1964 and later contain a potential glycosylation site as a result of a tripeptide substitution at residues 326-328 (Ala-Pro-Ala→Asn-Ser-Thr; Fig. 2).

Table 3 summarizes the differences between the HAs of A/Detroit/64 and seven other equine-1 influenza A viruses isolated between 1964 and 1977. For the region encoding the signal peptide, HA1, and connecting peptide, no nucleotide insertions or deletions were observed. Of the 1,047 nucleotides sequenced for each gene, only 42 positions (4.0%) showed nucleotide substitutions in at least one HA. Only 17 of these substitutions resulted in amino acid changes, at one position in the signal peptide and at 16 positions in HA1.

The relatedness of the later group of viruses (1964-77) is shown by the strong conservation of 49 nucleotide substitutions (two in the signal peptide and 47 in HA1 coding regions; Fig. 1), with viruses only occasionally showing reversion to A/Prague/56 sequence, e.g. A/Newmarket/77 at nucleotides 566, 612, and 717 (Table 3). Additional conserved nucleotide substitutions were first apparent in A/Lexington/66 (positions 254 and 325) and A/Switzerland/125/72 (positions 50, 645, 777, 858, 948, 1002, and 1041). This conservation is reflected in the amino acid sequences. Relative to A/Prague/56, all viruses isolated since 1964 have the same amino acid substitutions at positions −5 and −4 of the signal peptide and 46, 59, 88, 110, 157, 160^{++}, 173, 174, 189, 214, 223, 233, 326, 327, and 328 of HA1 (Fig. 2); only two virus HAs show reversion to A/Prague/56 sequence: A/London/1416/73 at position 110 and

Table 3. Differences between hemagglutinins of A/Detroit/64 and later equine-1 influenza A virus isolates

Nucleotide no. and base in A/Detroit/64		Base substitutions in later viruses							Amino acid substitutions compared with A/Detroit/64[a]		
		CD 64	LE 66	S125 72	L1416 73	C 73	SP 76	NM 77			
33	A	–	–	–	–	–	–	G	–15	Q	
50	C	–	–	T	T	T	T	T	–9	T-I	
95	A	–	G	–	–	–	–	–	7	H-R	(17)
102	T	C	–	–	–	–	–	–	9	A	
104	T	C	–	–	–	–	–	–	10	V-A	(20)
		–	A	–	–	–	–	–		V-E	
108	C	–	T	T	T	T	T	T	11	S	
116	C	–	–	–	T	–	–	–	14	T-I	(24)
153	T	–	–	–	–	–	–	C	26	V	
254	T	–	C	C	C	C	C	C	60	I-T	(70)
321	A	–	–	–	–	–	G	–	82	E	
325	A	–	G	G	G	G	G	G	84	N-D	(94)
330	C	–	–	–	–	–	–	T	85	D	
355	G	–	A	A	A	A	A	A	94	D-N	(104)
373	C	–	–	–	A	–	–	–	100	Q-K	(110)
405	A	–	G	G	G	G	G	G	110	K	
459	A	C	–	C	C	C	C	C	128	A	
510	C	–	–	–	–	–	–	T	145	S	
524	G	A	–	–	–	–	–	–	150	G-E	(160+)
566	G	–	–	–	–	–	–	A	164	R-K	(173)
579	G	–	–	–	A	A	–	–	168	L	
612	C	–	–	–	–	–	–	T	179	T	
615	T	–	–	–	–	–	C	–	180	A	
626	G	–	–	A	–	–	–	–	184	R-K	(193)
639	T	–	–	–	–	C	–	–	188	S	
643	A	–	–	G	–	–	–	–	190	N-D	(199)
645	T	–	–	C	C	C	C	C		N	
652	A	–	–	–	–	–	G	–	193	I-V	(202)
680	A	–	–	–	–	–	G	–	202	Q-R	(211)
696	T	–	–	C	C	C	C	C	207	N	
711	G	–	–	–	–	–	T	–	212	P	
717	A	–	–	–	–	–	–	G	214	I-M	(223)
777	C	–	–	T	T	T	T	T	234	V	
779	A	–	C	C	C	C	C	–	235	N-T	(244)
783	T	–	–	C	C	C	C	C	236	F	
850	C	–	–	A	–	–	–	–	259	Q-K	(269)
858	T	–	–	C	C	C	C	C	261	D	
909	T	–	–	–	–	–	–	C	278	T	
948	G	–	–	A	A	A	A	A	291	R	
975	A	–	–	–	–	–	G	–	300	V	
1002	A	–	–	C	C	C	C	C	309	T	
1041	A	–	–	G	G	G	G	G	322	Q	
1065	G	–	A	A	A	A	A	A	3	K	

Note: Base substitutions occurring in signal peptide, HA1, and connecting peptide coding regions are shown

[a] Numbers in brackets refer to equivalent positions of amino acids in the H3 (x31) HA1 structure.

A/Newmarket/77 at positions 173 and 223 (Table 3). Other conserved substitutions are apparent from 1966 (A/Lexington) at positions 70 and 94 and from 1972 (A/Switzerland/125) at position −9 (Table 3).

Nonconserved nucleotide substitutions occur at 19 positions in the HA1 coding regions of viruses isolated during 1964-77, resulting in amino acid substitutions that are virus-specific at 11 sites (Table 3). Both 1964 virus isolates have amino acid substitutions at positions 104 (Asn→Asp) and 244 (Thr→Asn), which are not conserved in later viruses.

The A/Connaught Detroit/64 strain has unique substitutions at positions 20 (Val→Ala) and 160 + (Gly→Glu). The other viruses have nonconserved changes, at positions 17 (His →Arg) and 20 (Val→Glu) for A/Lexington/66; 193 (Arg →Lys), 199 (Asn→Asp), and 269 (Gln→Lys) for A/Switzerland/125/72; 24 (Thr→Ile) for A/London/1416/73; 202 (Ile→Val) and 211 (Gln→Arg) for A/Sao Paulo/76; and 244 (Thr→Asn) for A/Newmarket 77.

DISCUSSION

From the data presented here, equine-1 influenza A viruses can be divided into two antigenic groups based on the time scales 1956-63 and 1964-77. Rates of amino acid substitutions in HA1 can be calculated to 0.214%/year and 0.412%/year for the early and late groups, whilst the rates of silent mutation are 0.014%/year and 0.169%/year, respectively. Generally, the figures agree well with estimates made for antigenically drifted equine-2 influenza A viruses in horses and are considerably lower than the rate of variation of human influenza A(H3N2) (Daniels, Skehel & Wiley 1985). The mutation rate between A/Prague/56 and A/Cambridge/63 may not be representative as it is based on only two sequences; additional isolates over this time period were not available. However, with the increase in transport of horses between countries in more recent years, the number of virus replication cycles may have increasd, thereby producing the higher rate seen in the later (1964-77) virus group.

It seems unlikely that the major antigenic drift during 1963-64 was due to some unidentified mutagenic force. A more likely explanation is that the 1964 viruses represent a minor variant in the equine-1 influenza A pool, which through mutation gained an infectious advantage over the viruses that predominated during 1956-63. Alternatively, the 1964 viruses may reflect the introduction of a highly related virus from another species, possibly avian (Webster et al. 1980). The high degree of nucleotide and amino acid homologies between A/FPV/Rostock/34, A/Prague/56, and A/seal/80 predicts strongly an ancestral relationship, but the timing of possible interspecies transmission cannot be predicted from the present study. However, an ongoing epidemiological study of avian H7 isolates involving extensive sequencing of the HA genes has not yielded a single virus with carboxy-terminal extension of HA1, which is characteristic of equine-1 influenza A viruses. In addition, the HA sequence homologies of A/Detroit/64 to A/Prague/56 are considerably higher than to A/FPV/Rostock/34 or A/seal/80, which suggests an equine virus progenitor of A/Detroit/64. Further to this, attempts to generate equine-avian H7 recombinants in the laboratory have proved unsuccessful and the equine-1 influenza A viruses are not pathogenic in chickens (J.W. McCauley, unpublished observations). These observations suggest that interspecies transmission was not the cause of the appearance of the 1964 viruses.

If generation of a more infectious virus was responsible for

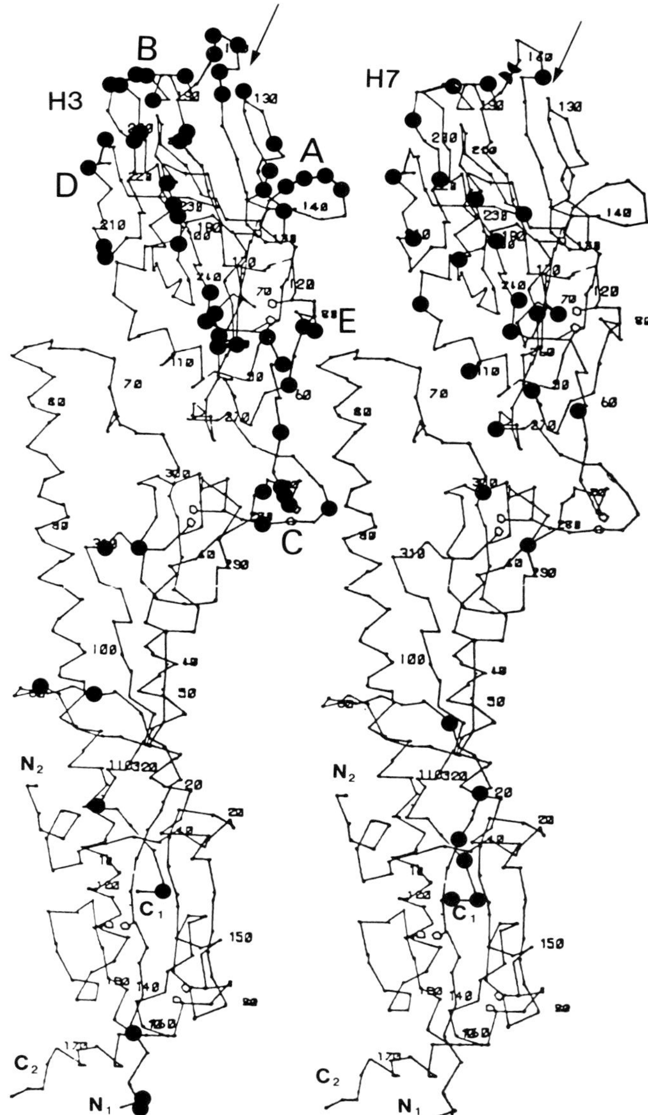

Fig. 3. Location of amino acid substitutions in equine-1 influenza A HA1 on the human influenza A H3HA three-dimensional structure.

The α-carbon tracing of the structure of human influenza A virus H3HA (Wilson, Skehel and Wiley 1981) is shown with changes in HA1 that occurred during 1968-83 for H3 viruses isolated from humans (*left*; R. Daniels, unpublished data) and 1956-77 for equine-1 influenza A viruses isolated from horses (*right*). Amino-termini of HA1 (N_1) and HA2 (N_2), carboxy-termini of HA1 (C_1) and HA2 (C_2), and the location of five antigenic sites (A-E) suggested for the prototype human H3 virus (Wiley, Wilson and Skehel 1981) are shown. Arrows indicate location of receptor binding site. On H7 diagram (*right*), the two adjacent semicircles at top indicate an insertion of two amino acids (160 +, 160 + +) compared to the H3 structure, both of which have been substituted in at least one virus (*Fig. 2; Table 3*), but the invariant eight amino acid carboxy-terminal extension of HA1 (*Fig. 2*) is not shown.

the 1964 epizootic, the HA may be the gene product at issue, considering its roles in receptor binding and membrane fusion, which initiate infection. Of 12 amino acid substitutions that first occur in the HA1 of viruses isolated in 1964, all are present in all the later viruses. To investigate the possible roles of these amino acids in modifying infectivity, the equine HA1 sequences were aligned with those of the human influenza A(H3N2) virus A/Aichi/1/68 (Fig. 2, Table 3). For all sequences, the nine Cysteines important in maintaining the three-dimensional structure of HA are conserved, as are residues 98 (Tyr), 153 (Trp), 183 (His), 190 (Glu), and 194 (Leu), which are important for the receptor binding function of the protein (Wilson et al. 1981). In addition, all the equine-1 influenza A HA1s have Gln at residue 226, which is associated with an α-2:3 sialic acid binding specificity (Rogers et al. 1983), the known specificity of equine-1 and -2 influenza A viruses isolated from horses (Rogers & Paulson 1983). These considerations suggest a strong structure-function relationship in HA that is conserved between the influenza subtypes.

Figure 3 shows a plot, on the H3HA three-dimensional structure, of all the amino acid substitutions in equine H7HA1s for 1956-77 and compares it with a similar plot for human H3N2 viruses over the period 1968-83. Five antigenic sites were proposed, A→E, on the H3HA (Wiley, Wilson & Skehel 1981); of these, only sites B, D, and E are evident in the equine H7HA, although the high cross-reactive titers in HI-tests (Table 1) suggest that animals have antibody responses to more conserved domains of HA. Only three of the 12 amino acid substitutions totally conserved in viruses isolated since 1964 occur in the vicinity of the receptor binding pocket: residues 189 (Thr→Ala), 160^{++} (Thr→Val), and 157 (Ser→Asn) on the H3HA structure. The substitution at 160^{++} results in the loss of a potential glycosylation site, which was also lost from A/Cambridge/63 due to a similar substitution (160^{++} Thr→Ile). All these amino acid substitutions result from single nucleotide changes, and one or more of them may be involved in modifying the receptor binding properties of the equine-1 influenza A viruses. Toward the carboxy-terminus of HA1 is a highly conserved tripeptide substitution (326-328 Ala-Pro-Ala→Asn-Ser-Thr), which results in the introduction of a potential glycosylation site. This tripeptide substitution required changes at four nucleotide sites, an event that may have required multiple replication cycles over eight years (1956-64). In the three-dimensional structure, this would be close to the amino-terminus of HA2. Amino acid substitutions in this vicinity have been shown to alter the fusion properties of HA of the human H3 and avian H7 subtypes (Daniels, et al. 1985). In the avian H5 subtype, the loss of a potential glycosylation site from amino acid 21 (H3 numbering system) of HA1 (which in the three dimensional structure is close to the amino-terminus of HA2 and residues 326-328 of HA1), has been associated with the acquisition of virulence (Webster, Kawaoka & Bean 1986). Further sequencing studies are required to test whether the occurrence of two groups of equine-1 influenza A viruses in horses resulted from either interspecies transmission or the intraspecies generation of viruses by point mutations with an infectious advantage over A/Prague/56. In particular, such studies would focus on viruses from the 1956-63 period, together with characterization of the receptor binding and fusion properties of the HA.

ACKNOWLEDGMENTS

We thank F. Burki, A. Kendal, J. Mumford, R.G. Webster, and M. Weiss for supplying viruses included in the NIBSC reference collection and are grateful to P. Young and S. Prime for their assistance in preparing this manuscript. This work was supported by research grants from the Horserace Betting Levy Board (VETRS/88-CAG) and NIAID (A120591-GCS).

REFERENCES

Burrows, R., and Denyer, M. (1982) Antigenic properties of some equine influenza viruses. *Arch. Virol.* **73**, 15-24.

Daniels, R.S.; Douglas, A.R.; Skehel, J.J.; and Wiley, D.C. (1983) Analyses of the antigenicity of influenza hemagglutinin at the pH optimum for virus-mediated membrane fusion. *J. Gen. Virol.* **64**, 1657-62.

Daniels, R.S.; Downie, J.C.; Hay, A.J.; Knossow, M.; Skehel, J.J.; Wang, M.L.; and Wiley, D.C. (1985) Fusion mutants of the influenza virus hemagglutinin glycoprotein. *Cell* **40**, 431-39.

Daniels, R.S.; Skehel, J.J.; and Wiley, D.C. (1985) Amino acid sequences of hemagglutinins of influenza viruses of the H3 subtype isolated from horses. *J. Gen. Virol.* **66**, 457-64.

Hay, A.J.; Lomniczi, B.; Bellamy, A.R.; and Skehel, J.J. (1977) Transcription of the influenza virus genome. *Virology* **83**, 337-55.

Hinshaw, V.S.; Naeve, C.W.; Webster, R.G.; Douglas, A.; Skehel, J.J.; and Bryans, J. (1983) Analysis of antigenic variation in equine-2 influenza A viruses. *Bull. Wld Hlth Org.* **61**, 153-58.

Keil, W.; Geyer, R.; Dabrowski, J.; Dabrowski, V.; Niemarin, H.; Stirm, S.; and Klenk, H.D. (1985) Carbohydrates of influenza virus. Structural elucidation of the individual glycans of the FPV hemagglutinin by two-dimensional 'H n.m.r. and methylation analysis. *EMBO. J.* **4**, 2711-20.

Naeve, C.W., and Webster, R.G. (1983) Sequence of the hemagglutinin gene from influenza virus A/Seal/Mass/1/80. *Virology* **129**, 298-308.

Porter, A.G.; Barber, C.; Carey, N.H.; Hallewell, R.A.; Threlfall, G.; and Emtage, J.S. (1979) Complete nucleotide sequence of an influenza virus hemagglutinin gene from cloned DNA. *Nature* **282**, 471-77.

Powell, D.G.; Thompson, G.R.; Spooner, P.; Plowright, W.; Burrows, R.; and Schild, G.C. (1974) The outbreak of equine influenza in England, April/May 1973. *Vet. Rec.* **94**, 282-87.

Rogers, G.N., and Paulson, J.C. (1983) Receptor determinants of human and animal influenza virus isolates: differences in receptor specificity of the H3 hemagglutinin based on species of origin. *Virology* **127**, 361-73.

Rogers, G.N.; Paulson, J.C.; Daniels, R.S.; Skehel, J.J.; and Wiley,

D.C. (1983) Single amino acid substitutions in the influenza hemagglutinin change the specificity of receptor binding. *Nature* **304**, 76-78.

Sanger, F.; Nicklen, S.; and Coulson, A.R. (1977) DNA sequencing with chain-terminating inhibitors. *Proc. Natl. Acad. Sci. USA.* **74**, 5463-67.

Sovinova, O.; Tumova, B.; Pouska, F.; and Nemec, J. (1958) Isolation of a virus causing respiratory diseases in horses. *Acta. Virol* **1**, 52-61.

Tumova, B. (1980) Equine influenza—a segment in influenza virus ecology. *Comp. Immun. Microbiol. Infect. Dis.* **3**, 45-59.

Webster, R.G., and Laver, W.G. (1980) Determination of the number of non-overlapping antigenic areas on Hong Kong (H3N2) influenza virus hemagglutinin with monoclonal antibodies and the selection of variants with potential epidemiological significance. *Virology* **104**, 139-48.

Webster, R.G.; Hinshaw, V.S.; Bean, W.J.; and Sriram, G. (1980) Influenza transmission between species. *Phil. Trans. R. Soc. Lond.* **B288**, 439-47.

Webster, R.G.; Kawaoka, Y.; and Bean, W.J. (1986) Molecular changes in A/Chicken/Pennsylvania/83 (H5N2) influenza virus associated with acquisition of virulence. *Virology* **149**, 165-73.

Wiley, D.C.; Wilson, I.A.; and Skehel, J.J. (1981) Structural identification of the antibody-binding sites of Hong Kong influenza hemagglutinin and their involvement in antigenic variation. *Nature* **289**, 373-78.

Wilson, I.A.; Skehel, J.J.; and Wiley, D.C. (1981) Structure of the hemagglutinin membrane glycoprotein of influenza virus at 3A resolution. *Nature* **289**, 366-73.

World Health Organisation (1980) A revision of the system of nomenclature for influenza viruses (Memorandum). *Bull. Wld Hlth Org.* **58**, 585-91.

World Health Organisation Expert Committee (1953) Influenza: first report. WHO Technical Report Series No. 64.

The Influence of the Host Cell on the Antigenic Properties of Equine-2 Influenza A Viruses

R. Frank Cook, Jennifer A. Mumford, A. Douglas, and John M. Wood

SUMMARY

Three equine-2 influenza A viruses were isolated in eggs and in Madin-Darby canine kidney (MDCK) cells. These cell and egg isolates were compared in terms of their reactivity against postinfection and postvaccination equine sera and against monoclonal antibodies (MAbs), as measured by hemagglutination inhibition (HI) tests, enzyme-linked immunosorbent assay (ELISA), antibody-capture ELISA, and radioisotopic antiglobulin binding assay (RABA).

ELISA detected MAbs that were egg virus–specific. Egg-grown virus produced significantly smaller plaques on MDCK cells than did MDCK-grown virus, indicating biological as well as antigenic differences.

HI reactions with postinfection sera, postvaccination sera, and MAbs indicated that early-passage cell-grown virus was significantly more sensitive as an antigen than its egg-grown counterpart. Disruption of the viral membrane with Tween 80–ether increased the reactivity in HI tests of both cell- and egg-grown viruses, suggesting that HI results were not due to an egg-derived inhibition of hemagglutination. Despite differences in HI, the binding of equine sera and MAbs was found to be equivalent in solid-phase binding essays.

INTRODUCTION

Equine influenza A viruses are routinely isolated and propagated in embryonated hens' eggs prior to antigenic characterization. Evidence exists that cultivation of influenza viruses in eggs results in selection of variants that may differ significantly from the viruses that replicate and produce disease in vivo. Burnet and Bull (1943) reported biological modification of influenza viruses on adaption to growth in eggs. More recently monoclonal antibodies have been produced that are capable of differentiating between human influenza B virus that is egg-isolated and the same virus isolated in mammalian (MDCK) cells (Schild et al. 1983; Robertson et al. 1985). Furthermore, sera from unvaccinated children and young adults exhibit a significantly greater reactivity in HI tests with influenza B mammalian cell isolates than with equivalent egg isolates (Schild et al. 1983). This suggests that isolation in mammalian cells, compared with conventional isolation in eggs, produces a virus population with a closer antigenic resemblance—at least in the hemagglutinin (HA) molecule—to naturally occurring influenza B viruses. Nucleotide sequence analysis of the hemagglutinin gene of cell and egg influenza B viruses has suggested that antigenic differences result from the absence in egg isolates of a specific glycosylation site at the distal tip of the HA molecule adjacent to the cell receptor binding site (Robertson et al. 1985). Examples of antigenic variation between egg and mammalian cell isolates have also been discovered in human influenza A viruses (J.M. Wood, unpublished data).

Since the host cell can select antigenic variants, speculation arises as to whether egg-grown influenza viruses are the most appropriate for epidemiological studies, diagnostic reagents, and vaccines.

This report concerns the primary isolation of equine-2 influenza A viruses in mammalian cell cultures and embryonated hens' eggs, which are characterized antigenically using monoclonal antibodies and polyclonal anisera.

Cook, Mumford: Equine Virology Unit, Animal Health Trust, Lanwades Park, Kennett, Newmarket, Suffolk CB8 7PN, England. Douglas: National Institute for Medical Research, Mill Hill, London NW7 1AA, England. Wood: National Institute for Biological Standards and Control, South Mimms, Potters Bar, Hertfordshire EN6 3QG, England.

MATERIALS AND METHODS

Virus isolate N79 [A/equine/Newmarket/79(H3N8)] was isolated from a sick horse in Newmarket during an outbreak of influenza in 1979. Virus isolates 3247 and 3248 [A/equine/Pau/3247-3248/83(H3N8)] were obtained from two horses at the training center in Pau, France, during an epidemic of influenza in 1983.

Influenza A viruses were isolated by inoculation of nasopharyngeal swab material into the allantoic cavity of 11-day-old fertile hens' eggs or by inoculation onto monolayers of MDCK cells. MDCK cells were maintained in bovine serum–free 199 medium (Flow Laboratories, Scotland) containing 1.25 µg/ml trypsin (3.4.21.4 BDH Chemicals Ltd., Poole, England). Following harvesting of infected allantoic and tissue culture fluids, the viruses were serotyped using polyclonal rabbit and ferret antisera, confirming them to be equine-2 influenza A viruses.

Monoclonal antibodies. MAbs to equine-2 influenza viruses and human influenza A (H3N2)viruses were prepared using established protocols (Kohler & Milstein 1975; Web-

Table 1. HI titers of sera from nonvaccinated horses against egg and MDCK equine-2 influenza A isolates

Serum	3247		3248		N79	
	MDCK	Egg	MDCK	Egg	MDCK	Egg
France 1983						
3244	16	<.8	32/64	<.8	ND	ND
3249	8	<.8	32	<.8	ND	ND
Brentwood 1979						
5102	ND	ND	ND	ND	16	<.8
5103	ND	ND	ND	ND	16	<.8
5114	ND	ND	512	32	512	64
5260	ND	ND	ND	ND	256	64
5262	16/32	<.8	16	<.8	64	<.8
5263	128	8	64	8	ND	ND
5264	16	<.8	8	<.8	32	<.8
5266	64	8	64	8	128	16
5275	ND	ND	512	64	512	128
5277	ND	ND	128	<.8	64/128[a]	8
Iraq 1984						
4	ND	ND	64	<.8	64	<.8
19	ND	ND	128	<.8	128	16
34	ND	ND	ND	ND	16	<.8
35	ND	ND	128	8	64/128[a]	16
412	16	<.8	32	<.8	ND	ND
417	16	<.8	64	<.8	ND	ND
420	16	<.8	128	<.8	ND	ND

Note: ND = not determined. [a] = end point between the dilutions quoted.

ster & Berton 1981; Campbell 1984). Ascites fluids were prepared in Balb/c mice (Hoogenraad, Helman & Hoogenraad 1983).

Hemagglutination inhibition test. HI tests were performed in microtiter plates using standard methods with chicken erythrocytes (Wood et al. 1983). Tween 80–ether treatment of influenza viruses was as described by Berlin and colleagues (1963) and John and Fulginiti (1966). Egg and MDCK isolates were used at passage level 2 unless otherwise stated. The dosage of each antigen was 4 hemagglutination units.

Purification of equine influenza A viruses. Viruses were collected from tissue culture medium or from allantoic fluid by centrifugation (50,000 × g for 3 hr at 4°C) and purified by centrifugation (45,000 × g for 12 hr at 20°C) in 25-50% w/v sucrose gradients (in 50 mM Tris/HC1; 100 mM NaC1, pH7.4).

ELISA and antibody-capture indirect ELISA. Monoclonal antibodies diluted in phosphate-buffered saline (PBS) containing 0.05% Tween 20 and 1% bovine serum albumin (Fraction V) were added to polystyrene 96-well plates (Becton Dickinson, Oxnard, Calif.). The plates were coated, using $NaHCO_3/Na_2CO_3$, pH9.6, with purified influenza A virus derived from growth in eggs or MDCK cells following incubation for 2 hr at 4°C. Plates were washed five times in PBS plus 0.05% Tween 20 and incubated with a peroxidase conjugated rabbit antiserum to mouse immunoglobulins (DAKO, Denmark) for 2 hr at 4°C. After five further washings, final incubation was done with O-phenylenediamine substrate (0.37 mM O-phenylenediamine, 50 mM sodium citrate, 150 mM sodium phosphate containing 50µl/H_2O_2 per 100 ml) for 30-60 minutes at room temperature. All assays were carried out in triplicate and recorded as mean values corrected for substrate background absorbance.

In antibody-capture indirect ELISA, purified influenza A viruses were added to 96-well plates (Becton Dickinson). Plates were coated, using $NaHCO_3/Na_2CO_3$, pH9.6), with a polyclonal rabbit antiserum to A/equine/Kentucky/81 and were incubated for 12 hr at 4°C. Subsequent steps were as described above.

Radioisotopic antiglobulin binding assay. RABA was performed essentially as described by Hannant, Donaldson, and Bolton (1985). Postinfection equine sera (diluted 1:100) was added to Removawells (Dynatech Laboratories, Billingshurst, England), coated with purified influenza A viruses derived from eggs or MDCK cells, and incubated for 2 hr at 37°C. After washing in PBS + 0.05% Tween 20 + 1% bovine serum albumin, wells were incubated for 2 hr at 37°C with a rabbit antiserum to equine IgG_{ab} (J. Kent, Animal Health Trust). Final incubation used iodine-125 labeled protein A (Amersham International, Amersham, England) at 10^5 counts per minute (CPM) per well. Results were expressed as bound CPM after subtracting, as a control, the CPM bound using equine-2 influenza A seronegative equine sera from a gnotobiotic foal.

RESULTS

The reactivity of the virus isolates was tested in ELISA against a panel of 28 hemagglutinin-specific MAbs raised against a variety of human influenza A (H3N2) isolates, mainly egg-grown. ELISA plates were coated with gradient-purified egg and cell isolates on the basis of equivalent hemagglutination units, which corresponded to equivalent concentrations of total protein. In each ELISA test the reactivity of two MAbs (3G9, 10G6), directed aganst the influenza group A antigen nucleoprotein (Cook, Sinclair & Mumford 1987), were tested as a marker of the relative amounts of egg and MDCK antigens bound to the solid phase. The majority (78%) of the human influenza A MAbs did not react in ELISA, reflecting antigenic divergence between human influenza A (H3N2) and equine-2 influenza A viruses. However, three MAbs (x31/H19; E864 HC/5; NIB/8/HC/89) were identified as cross-reactive between egg and MDCK equine-2 influenza A isolates; more important, three others (W1C/114/5; MRC11/H1; NIB/8/HC/68) were found to be egg isolate–specific. Unfortunately, the egg isolate–specific

Table 2. HI antibody titers of postvaccination equine sera

	N79		A/equine/ Miami/63	A/equine/ Newmarket/79
	MDCK	Egg	T80-ether	T80-ether
Ponies				
76	32/64	8	64	ND
79	16	<.8	32	ND
80	64	8	64	ND
83	16	<.8	32/64	ND
91	64	8/16	32/64	ND
92	64	8	64	ND
Horses in training				
64506	128	16	512	512
64507	512	32	512	512
64544	256	16	256	512
64515	512	128	1024	1024
64516	16	<.8	32	16
64517	64	16	256	128
64519	1024	256	1024	1024
64525	64	8	128	64

Note: ND = not determined

MAbs did not inhibit the hemagglutination reaction of equine-2 influenza A viruses.

A difference in plaque size was rated between egg and MDCK isolates grown on MDCK cells. The egg N79 isolate produced small (<0.5 mm) plaques, whereas the MDCK isolate produced plaques approximately 2.0 mm in size.

Using postinfection equine sera, HI titers in sera were greater when tested with MDCK isolates than with egg isolates (Table 1). Sera from horses that had been vaccinated with inactivated egg-grown influenza A virus were examined for any preferential reaction with egg-isolated virus over MDCK-isolated virus in the HI test. Sera were obtained from six ponies with no known history of natural infection that had been vaccinated at an interval of four weeks with two doses of 15 μg HA egg-grown A/equine/Newmarket/79 virus. The sera reacted preferentially in the HI test with MDCK-isolated N79 virus as compared with egg-isolated N79 (Table 2). Similar results were obtained with sera from eight Thoroughbred horses in training, with no known history of natural infection, that had also been regularly immunized with inactivated egg-grown equine influenza A vaccine virus (Table 2).

A panel of equine-2 influenza A–specific MAbs were also found to have significantly greater HI reactivity against the N79 MDCK isolates (Table 3). Although MAb 4E2 was raised against N79 MDCK-isolated virus, M63 and F79 were prepared against egg-isolated and egg-grown A/equine/Miami/63 and A/equine/Fontainebleau/79. Identical reactivities in HI tests were also obtained with egg and MDCK isolates of 3248. The stability of enhanced reactivity in HI tests of MDCK-isolated equine-2 influenza A viruses was tested by passage in MDCK cells at low multiplicity of infection (1 plaque-forming unit per 1000 cells) to minimize the risks of generating defective interfering particles. By passage level 6 (p6) there was a significant drop in HI titer against a panel of postinfection equine sera, to approximately the same level as egg-isolated virus (Table 3). Similar results were obtained with a panel of equine-2 influenza A–specific MAbs. Only with MAb 4E2 was there no signifcant drop in

Table 3. Effects of passage level on HI antibody titer of MDCK-isolated equine-2 influenza A N79 virus

	MDCK					Egg	T80-Ether MDCK	T80-Ether MDCK
	p2	p3	p4	p5	p6	p3	p2	p6
Monoclonal antibody								
4E2[a]	800	ND	ND	ND	1,600	50	1,600	800
F/79[b] H1	>32,000	ND	ND	ND	<.25	100	>32,000	400
H2	4,000	ND	ND	ND	25	200	>32,000	400
H3	2,000	ND	ND	ND	<.25	400	1,600	200
H4	800	ND	ND	ND	<.25	100	3,200	50
M/63[c] H1	16,000	ND	ND	ND	400	3,200	>32,000	3,200
H2	2,000	ND	ND	ND	50	200	>32,000	3,200
H3	4,000	ND	ND	ND	800	400	16,000	3,200
Sera postinfection								
5260	1024	512	512	128	256	64	ND	ND
5262	64	32	16	<.8	<.8	<.8	>1024	256
5263	256	256	64/128	32	32	ND	ND	ND
5264	64/128	64	16	<.8	ND	<.8	>1024	256
5266	256	128	128	64	64	32	>1024	>1024
5279	128/256	128	64/128	64	64	ND	ND	ND

Note: ND = not determined

[a] 4E2 = N79 MDCK isolate A/equine/Newmarket/79.

F/79 = egg isolate A/equine/Fontainebleau/79.

M/63 = egg isolate A/equine/Miami/63.

Table 4. Effect on HI antibody titer of Tween 80–ether treatment of egg and MDCK N79 isolates

		N79 MDCK		N79 egg	
		Untreated	T80-ether	Untreated	T80-ether
Postinfection serum		128	>1024	<.8	256
Postvaccination serum		256	>1024	32	512
MAb					
4E2[a]		800	1600	50	100
F/79[b]	H1	>32,000	>32,000	100	800
	H2	4000	>32,000	200	3,200
	H3	2000	16,000	200	1,600
	H4	800	3,200	100	400
M/63[c]	H1	16,000	>32,000	3,200	3,200
	H2	2,000	>32,000	200	3,200
	H4	4,000	16,000	400	3,200

Note: starting dilutions: equine sera, 1:8; with MAbs, 1:25
[a] 4E2 = N79 MDCK isolate A/equine/Newmarket/79.
[b] F/79 = egg isolate A/equine/Fontainebleau/79.
[c] M/63 = egg isolate A/equine/Miami/63.

HI titer. The reduction in HI titer between MDCK p2 and MDCK p6 N79 virus was also present after Tween 80-ether treatment (Table 3).

The influence of Tween 80 and ether on the two methods of virus isolation was also examined. The sensitivity of non-disrupted MDCK N79 virus in HI tests was similar to that of the Tween 80–ether treated egg-derived antigens A/equine/Miami/63 and A/equine/Newmarket/79 used routinely in this laboratory (Table 2). Tween 80–ether treatment significantly increased the sensitivity of both MDCK and egg isolates of N79 virus with postinfection and postvaccination equine sera (Table 4). Similar results were obtained with a panel of equine-2 influenza A–specific MAbs. Tween 80–ether treatment significantly increased the HI sensitivity of epitopes F/79 H1 (N79 egg isolate); F/79 H2, H3, and H4; M/63 H2 and H4 (N79 egg and MDCK isolates). However, epitopes 4E2 (N79 MDCK and egg isolates) and M/63 H1 (N79 egg isolate) were not significantly enhanced by Tween 80–ether treatment, indicating that such treatment did not affect all the epitopes.

Solid-phase binding assays determined the amount of HI antibody bound to the hemagglutinin of MDCK isolates compared with egg isolates. Binding of HI antibody in postinfection equine sera was measured using RABA. Remova-wells were coated with gradient-purified MDCK or egg N79 isolates on the basis of equivalent hemagglutination units (HAU), corresponding to equivalent amount of total protein. Under conditions where antigen concentration was not limiting, all the postinfection sera tested were bound in equivalent amounts by both types of isolate (Table 5).

Postinfection equine sera contain antibodies to other influenza proteins besides hemagglutinin, which in solid-phase assays obscure the results of HI tests. This does not occur in

Table 5. Binding of postinfection sera from nonvaccinated horses to egg and MDCK isolates of N79

	RABA, counts per minute	
Serum	N79 egg	N79 MDCK
France 1983		
3244	2995 ± 48	2859 ± 286
3247	2077 ± 145	1913 ± 53
Brentwood 1979		
5262	12,486 ± 125	11,908 ± 952
5264	12,902 ± 387	12,992 ± 1170
5266	21,736 ± 869	17,134 ± 788
5269	6,724 ± 403	7,168 ± 322
5279	20,467 ± 409	19,560 ± 782
Iraq 1984		
1	11,030 ± 77	10,389 ± 415
2	5,644 ± 282	6,008 ± ,240
3	8,326 ± 250	7,666 ± 230
4	10,619 ± 152	9,400 ± 282
5	8,813 ± 126	7,555 ± 340
6	9,603 ± 768	9,199 ± 46
7	8,120 ± 384	7,996 ± 719
8	7,672 ± 97	7,395 ± 369
15	7,888 ± 223	7,215 ± 404

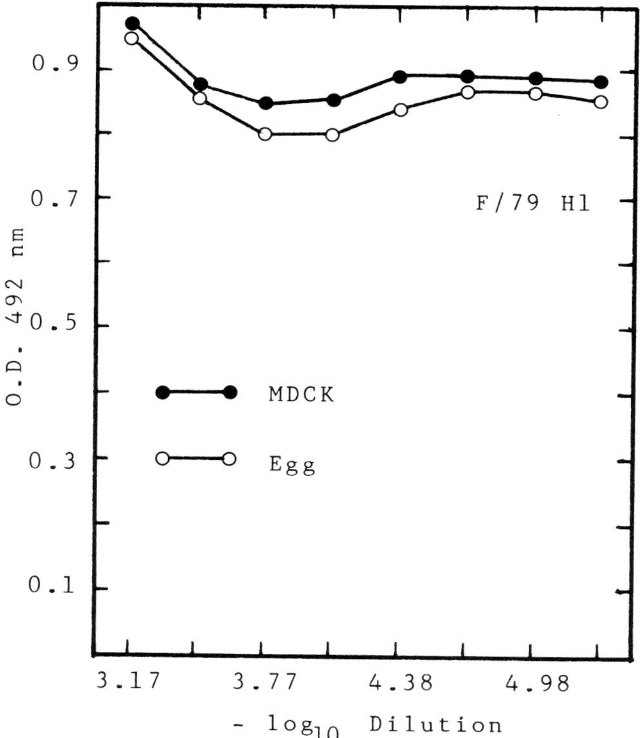

Fig. 1. Binding of hemagglutinin-specific equine-2 influenza A MAbs to egg and MDCK isolates of N79, measured by ELISA. Mean optical density (O.D. 492 nm) values of MAb prepared against egg-grown A/equine/Fontainebleau/79 (F/79 H1) bound to egg and MDCK isolates of N79. MAbs were diluted from 1:1500 to 1:192,000 in twofold steps. Only approximate $\log_{10}$ values are shown.

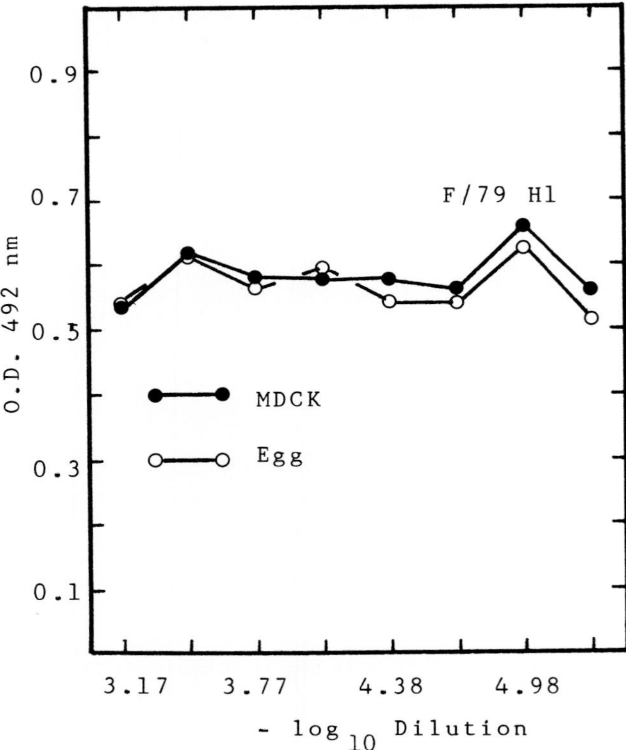

Fig. 2. Binding of hemagglutinin-specific equine-2 influenza A MAbs to egg and MDCK isolates of N79, measured by antibody-capture ELISA. Mean optical density (O.D. 492 nm) values of MAbs bound to egg and MDCK isolates of N79 bound to the solid phase via a polyclonal rabbit antiserum raised against A/equine/Kentucky/81. MAb prepared against egg-grown A/equine/Fontainebleau/79 (F/79 H1). MAbs were diluted from 1:1500 to 1:192,000 in twofold steps. Only approximate $\log_{10}$ values are shown.

solid-phase assays using hemagglutinin-specific MAbs. The binding of MAb F/79 H1 (A/equine/Fontainebleau/79) to the egg and MDCK isolates of N79 as measured by ELISA is shown in Figure 1. Similar results were observed using MAb F/79 H2, H3, and H4 (A/equine/Fontainebleau/79) and MAb M/63 H1 and H4 (A/equine/Miami/63).

Conditions were not limiting in terms of the concentrations of antigen (based on equivalent HAU/total protein) and of rabbit antimouse immunoglobulin peroxidase conjugate. Similar amounts of each MAb were bound by both antigens over a dilution range of 1:1500 to 1:192,000. MAb 4E2 did not react in ELISA with equine-2 influenza A antigen directly bound to the solid phase, but did react with antigen immobilized via specific equine-2 influenza A antibody. Direct coating of equine-2 influenza A antigen for ELISA or radioimmune assay therefore results in the loss of at least one epitope, suggesting possible conformational changes that affect the binding of other MAbs. This was tested by measuring amounts of the MAb F/79 H1-H4, M63/H4, and 4E2 bound to egg and MDCK N79 antigens in an antibody-capture ELISA. As with the standard ELISA, similar amounts of each MAb were bound by both antigens. Figure 2 presents the results of one of these assays using egg-grown MAb, F/79 H1.

Purification of the hemagglutinin molecule did not alter the reactivity of MDCK and egg isolates in the HI test. MDCK N79 gradient-purified virus produced an enhanced HI response to a variety of equine-2 influenza A MAbs as compared with egg-isolated N79 virus (Table 6).

Table 6. HI antibody titers of gradient-purified egg and MDCK isolates of N79

Monoclonal antibody		N79 MDCK	N79 egg
F79[a]	H2	≥3200	200
	H3	≥3200	200
	H4	800	100
M/63[b]	H4	≥3200	800

[a] F/79 = egg isolate A/equine/Fontainebleau/79.
[b] M/63 = egg isolate A/equine/Miami/63.

DISCUSSION

Evidence has been presented that isolation of equine-2 influenza A viruses in embryonated eggs produces virus that differs antigenically and perhaps biologically, as well as differing in HI reactivity, from equine-2 influenza A virus isolated in MDCK cells from the same clinical sample. Antigenic differences were demonstrated by the identification of three MAbs to the hemagglutinin H3 that were egg virus–specific. Whether these MAbs react against the same or different epitopes remains to be determined. However, as with human influenza B viruses (Schild, et al. 1983; Robertson et al. 1985), MAb data provides good evidence for host cell selection of antigenic variants in equine-2 influenza A viruses.

Host selection for biological differences may be indicated, based on the demonstration that egg-isolated equine-2 influenza A viruses produced smaller plaque variants than equivalent MDCK isolates when grown in MDCK cells. Similar differences have not been reported in egg and MDCK isolated human influenza B viruses (Robertson et al. 1985).

HI results using postinfection sera and postvaccination sera from egg-derived vaccines to MAbs raised against egg-grown equine-2 influenza A viruses demonstrated that MDCK-isolated virus was a more sensitive HI antigen than its egg-grown counterpart. Early-passage MDCK equine-2 influenza A isolates were almost equivalent in sensitivity to standard Tween 80–ether treated antigens, suggesting that such isolates may be of value in epidemiological studies. Although Tween 80–ether disruption of equine-2 influenza A viruses increases the absolute value detected by the HI test (Berlin et al. 1963), it reduces the specificity-obscuring differences generated by antigenic drift. Nondisrupted early-passage MDCK isolates would not be affected in this manner.

Early-passage MDCK equine-2 influenza A antigens were equivalent in sensitivity to standard Tween 80–ether treated egg-isolated antigens, suggesting the existence of an egg-specific hemagglutination inhibitor that required Tween 80–ether treatment for its removal. However, this did not appear likely since Tween 80–ether treatment increased the sensitivity of both egg and MDCK isolates to postinfection and postvaccination equine sera.

The use of MAbs in the HI test provided information on the effects of Tween 80–ether treatment on individual epitopes. Two classes of epitope were recognized in both egg and MDCK isolates. The first, defined by MAbs F/79 H1-H4 and M/63 H2 and H4, stimulated a significant HI increase following Tween 80–ether treatment, whereas the second, defined by MAbs 4E2 and possibly M63 H1, exerted no effect. In the first class of epitopes MDCK isolates retained their enhanced HI reactivity whereas egg isolates were stimulated only to the level found in nondisrupted MDCK-isolated virus. The results indicate that, in terms of absolute values for the detection of antibodies to equine-2 influenza A viruses, the sensitivity of HI tests may be significantly enhanced by the use of early-passage Tween 80–ether treated MDCK-isolated antigens instead of conventional egg-isolated antigens.

The relative performance of egg and MDCK isolates in HI tests could not be explained by detectable differences in antibody binding to the hemagglutinin of each isolate, as measured by solid-phase binding assays. With postinfection equine sera, differences in antibody binding to hemagglutinin could have been masked by binding to other influenza proteins, but this would not have been the case with hemagglutinin-specific MAbs. Using MAbs, the differences in HI titer were not mirrored by differences in antibody binding. These results did not stem from changes in the hemagglutinin molecule that may have been induced by purification, since significant differences in HI titer were observed with the gradient-purified egg and MDCK isolates. Differences in HI reactivity may have arisen from small changes in antibody binding that were not detected under the assay conditions, or the origin may have been conformational in nature, such that less antibody was required to inhibit hemagglutination reactions in MDCK isolates than in egg isolates.

Whatever the mechanism, the enhanced reactivity in HI tests of MDCK isolates was unstable following passage in the homologous system. By passage 6 in MDCK cells, there was a significant reduction in HI titer using postinfection equine sera to all the MAbs tested except 4E2. It would thus appear that equine-2 influenza A viruses undergo comparatively rapid adaptation to growth in MDCK cells. Similar adaptation of MDCK cells has not been observed in influenza B viruses (Schild et al. 1983; Robertson et al. 1985).

Studies are now in progress to determine the structural basis for the antigenic and biological differences between early-passage egg and MDCK isolates of equine-2 influenza A viruses.

ACKNOWLEDGMENTS

The authors are grateful to Dr. D. Hannant for helpful discussions and to Mrs. D. R. Burkett for secretarial assistance. This work was supported by the Animal Health Trust and the Horserace Betting Levy Board.

REFERENCES

Berlin, B.S.; McQueen, J.L.; Minuse, E.; and Davenport, F.M. (1963) A method of increasing the sensitivity of the hemagglutination inhibition test with equine influenza virus. *Virology* **21**, 665-66.

Burnet, F.M., and Bull, D.R. (1943) Changes in influenza virus associated with adaptation to passage in chick embryos. *Aust. J. Exp. Biol. Med. Sci.* **21**, 55-69.

Campbell, A.M. (1984) Monoclonal antibody technology. In *Laboratory Techniques in Biochemistry and Biology*, Vol. 13. Eds. R.H. Burdon and P.H. van Knippenberg. Elsevier, Amsterdam.

Cook, R.F.; Sinclair, R.; and Mumford, J.A. (1987) Detection of influenza nucleoprotein antigen in nasal secretions from horses infected with A/equine/influenza (H3N8) viruses. Submitted for publication.

Hannant, D.; Donaldson, K.; and Bolton, R.E. (1985) Immunomodulatory effects of mineral dust. 1. Effects of intraperitoneal dust inoculation on splenic lymphocyte function and humoral immune responses *in vivo*. *J. Clin. Lab. Immunol.* **16**, 81-85.

Hoogenraad, H.; Helman, T.; and Hoogenraad, J. (1983) The effect of pre-infection of mice with pristane on ascites tumour formation and monoclonal antibody production. *J. Immunol. Meth.* **61**, 317-20.

John, T.J., and Fulginiti, V.A. (1966) Parainfluenza 2 virus. Increase in hemagglutinin titre on treatment with tween-80 and ether. *Proc. Soc. Exp. Biol. Med.* **212**, 109-11.

Kohler, G., and Milstein, C. (1975) Continuous cultures of fused cells secreting antibody of predefined specificity. *Nature*, **256**, 495-96.

Robertson, J.W.; Naeve, C.W.; Webster, R.G.; Bootman, J.S.; Newman, R.; and Schild, S.G. (1985) Alternations in the hemagglutinin associated with adaptation of influenza B virus to growth in eggs. *Virology* **143**, 166-74.

Schild, G.C.; Oxford, J.S.; de Jong, J.C.; and Webster, R.G. (1983) Evidence for host-cell selection of influenza virus antigenic variants. *Nature* **303**, 706-9.

Webster, R.G., and Berton, M.T. (1981) Analysis of antigenic drift in the hemagglutinin molecule of influenza B virus with monoclonal antibodies. *J. Gen. Virol.* **54**, 243-51.

Wood, J.M.; Mumford, J.A.; Folkers, C.; Scott, A.M.; and Schild, G.C. (1983) Studies with inactivated equine influenza vaccine. 1. Serological responses of ponies to graded doses of vaccine. *J. Hyg., Camb.* **90**, 371-84.

Nasopharyngeal, Tracheobronchial, and Systemic Immune Responses to Vaccination and Aerosol Infection with Equine-2 Influenza A Virus (H3N8)

Duncan Hannant, D.M. Jessett, T. O'Neill, B. Sundqvist, and Jennifer A. Mumford

SUMMARY

The immune responses to vaccination and experimental infection with equine-2 influenza A virus were studied in ponies. Clinical influenza was induced by exposing ponies to standardized doses of infectious virus by nebulized aerosol. Subunit vaccines were injected intramuscularly in the form of immune stimulating complexes (ISCOMs). Virus-specific antibodies (IgG_{ab}, IgM, IgA) in the serum, nasopharynx, and trachea were measured by radioisotopic antiglobulin binding assays. Cytotoxic lymphocyte activity of peripheral blood mononuclear cells was measured by a 3-hr radioactive chromium release assay using autologous and allogeneic combinations of effectors and virus-infected target cells.

Virus-specific antibody was detected in the serum and respiratory tract by Day 7 after primary infection of native ponies. High levels of antibody, a typical anamnestic response, were detected in both these sites on Day 4 on rechallenge with the same virus. Virus-specific IgG_{ab} in the nasopharynx and trachea did not show the features of long duration seen with serum antibody of this isotype. Systemic vaccination with ISCOMs resulted in a significant but transitory IgG_{ab} antibody response in the trachea, whereas antibody production in the nasopharynx was delayed and appeared to be accumulatory on boosting. Genetically restricted cytotoxic lymphocyte activity was demonstrated in virus-infected ponies. However, the identity of the effector cell in vivo is still the subject of some controversy because effector cells that function across a histocompatibility barrier have also been identified in such animals.

INTRODUCTION

Recent studies on equine influenza have shown important differences between immunity induced by infection and the effects of vaccination with inactivated antigens. For example, a close relationship between immunity and the level of circulating antibody to hemagglutinin has been established in horses vaccinated with inactivated whole virus vaccines (Mumford et al. 1983, 1987). On the other hand, even low levels of serum antibody have been effective in protecting against rechallenge in ponies that had been infected as long as 62 weeks previously (Hannant, Mumford & Jessett 1988). Clearly, the protective immune mechanisms that operate following infection with equine influenza differ in some respects from those induced by inactivated vaccines.

The contribution of local (respiratory tract) antibody to protection from challenge with equine influenza is poorly understood, although studies have shown that nasopharyngeal antibody may be detected (Rouse & Ditchfield 1970; Kumanomido & Akiyama 1975). Its importance may be inferred from human studies (Murphy et al. 1973; Johnson et al. 1985, 1986), which indicated that prechallenge nasal IgA was associated with protection. Local antibody memory, as defined by anamnestic responses, has been demonstrated in the upper respiratory tract of humans after rechallenge of primed individuals (Callard 1979). The potential of cell-mediated immune mechanisms in protection against and recovery from equine influenza may be predicted by analogy with the extensive studies of humans and rodents (Askonas, McMichael & Webster 1982; Ada & Jones 1986).

As the primary site for equine influenza virus replication is the respiratory tract, this study examines the serum and local (nasopharyngeal and tracheal) antibody responses to primary and secondary infections, and compares them with the local responses stimulated by systemic immunization with ISCOM-based vaccines. At least two types of antigen-specific cell-mediated immune responses are represented by cytotoxic effector cells that are both restricted and non-restricted genetically.

MATERIALS AND METHODS

Challenge virus. The equine influenza A virus used for aerosol infection of naive or previously infected ponies was the second egg passage of A/equine/Newmarket/D55/79 (H3N8) recovered from the nasopharynx of an unvaccinated pony.

Infection protocol. Welsh Mountain yearling ponies, seronegative for equine-2 influenza A viruses, were infected by exposure to an aerosol generated from 20 ml of allantoic fluid containing a total of $10^{7.9}$ EID_{50} of the challenge virus using a Model 65 nebulizer (De Vilbiss, Somerset, Pa.) as described by Mumford and colleagues (1987).

Vaccination. Ponies were immunized intramuscularly with A/equine/Solvalla/79(H3N8) virus antigens in the form of

Hannant, Jessett, O'Neill, Mumford: Equine Virology Unit, Animal Health Trust, Lanwades Park, Newmarket, Suffolk CB8 7PN, England. Sundqvist: National Veterinary Institute, Uppsala, Sweden.

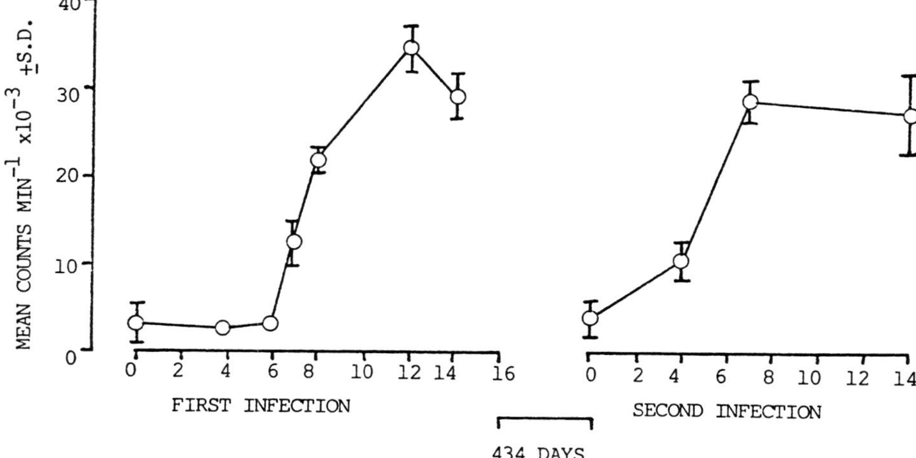

Fig. 1. Development of virus-specific IgG_{ab} measured by RABA in sera of ponies after first and second infection with A/equine/Newmarket/79. Results are means ±SD of six ponies. Interval between first and second infections = 450 days.

ISCOMs prepared by the method of Morein and colleagues (1984). The vaccine was standardized at 15 μg hemagglutinin (HA) per dose by the single radial diffusion technique (Wood et al. 1983).

Nasal and tracheal wash samples. Nasal washes were collected by flushing the nasopharynx with approximately 100 ml of sterile PBS using a flexible polythene tubing attached to a large syringe. Tracheal washes were collected with a bronchoendoscope (Burrell, Mackintosh & Taylor 1986). Nasal and tracheal washes were stored on ice and frozen at −20°C after the addition of 0.02% NaN_3. Before antibody measurements were carried out, samples were concentrated approximately tenfold by dialysis against Aquacide (Calbiochem).

Antibody measurement. All samples were assayed by a radioisotopic antiglobulin binding assay (RABA) (Hannant et al. 1987). The variable and unknown dilution of nasal and tracheal washes was controlled by expressing antibody measurements in terms of micrograms of equine serum albumin (ESA) in the samples. ESA was measured by an inhibition radioimmunoassay using reagents prepared in this laboratory.

Equine peripheral blood mononuclear cells (PBMCs). Whole blood was collected in heparinized tubes (Vacutainer, Becton Dickinson, Meylan, France) and diluted 1:1 with 0.85% NaCl before PBMCs were isolated by Ficoll-Hypaque (Pharmacia, Hounslow, England) centrifugation (Hudson & Hay 1976). Washed PBMCs were used as virus-infected targets and as effector cells for cytotoxic assays. Target cells were infected with A/equine/Miami/63(H3N8) in serum-free RPMI1640 medium (Gibco, Paisley, UK) (McMichael & Askonas 1978) before radiolabeling with ^{51}Cr. Induction culture of cytotoxic effector cells was carried out for five days at 37°C, 5% CO_2 in complete RPMI1640 which contained 10% fetal calf serum (Gibco), 10^{-5}M 2-mercaptoethanol (Sigma, St. Louis, Mo.) and influenza A/equine/Newmarket/79(H3N8) antigen. Virus-infected ^{51}Cr labeled target cells were plated at 2×10^4 cells 100 μl^{-1} well^{-1} in round-bottomed 96-well microplates (Nunc, Roskild, Denmark) Effector cells (100 μl) were added at killer:target ratios ranging from 100:1 to 25:1. Percentage cytotoxicity was calculated using the standard formula (McMichael & Askonas 1978).

RESULTS

Serum antibody responses to primary and secondary infections. Ponies seronegative to equine-2 influenza viruses were infected with A/equine/Newmarket/79 and rechallenged 15 months later. The development of virus-specific serum IgG_{ab} antibody as measured by RABA is shown in Figure 1. There was an initial increase in antibody levels at Day 7 postinfection ($P<0.01$), and antibody levels continued to rise over the next six days. RABA-defined antibody declined to prechallenge levels over the period of approximately 15 months When the ponies were rechallenged with the same virus at 450 days, there was evidence of anamnestic response, in that all ponies showed a secondary antibody response by Day 4 ($P<0.01$; Fig. 1).

Confirming the long duration of virus-specific IgG_{ab} isotype after primary infection, the initial rise in antibody in a group of three ponies was maintained until a second challenge 62 days later (Fig. 2). There was no evidence of a significant further increase in antibody at Day 4 after rechallenge but increases in levels were detected at eight days. The high levels of circulating IgG_{ab} were maintained until at least 32 days after the second challenge.

Primary and secondary responses of other antibody isotypes were studied only in the ponies that were rechallenged at 62 days. Virus-specific IgM antibody development in these ponies is summarized in Figure 3, which shows that the rise of IgM on primary infection had declined by about 50% at the time of rechallenge. The secondary rise in IgM antibody after rechallenge was not anamnestic and was also of relatively short duration, showing a marked decline by 32 days after

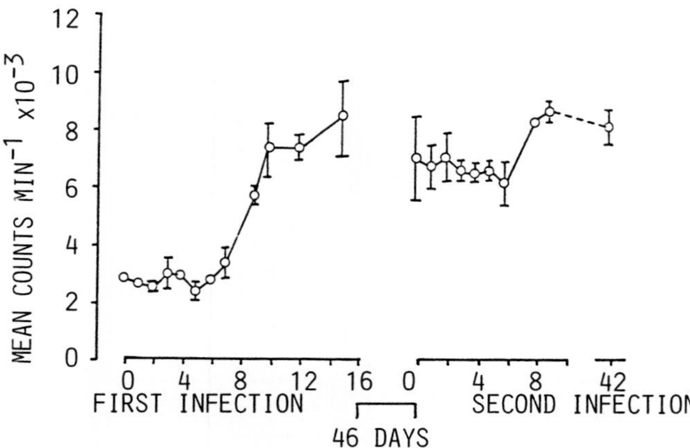

Fig. 2. Development of virus-specific IgG_{ab} measured by RABA in sera of ponies after first and second infection with A/equine/Newmarket/79. Results are means ±SD of three ponies. Interval between first and second infections = 62 days.

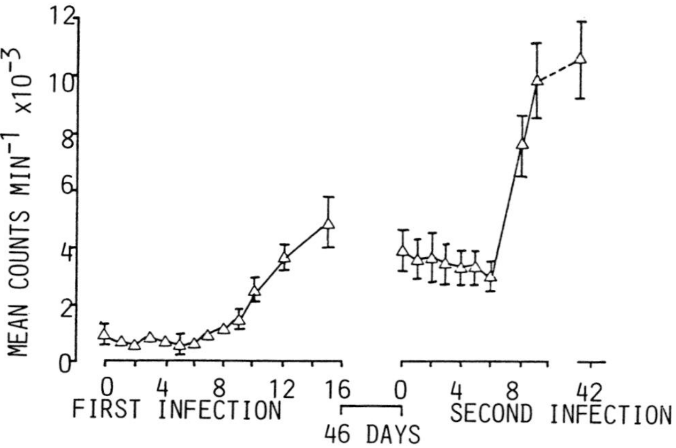

Fig. 4. Development of virus-specific IgA measured by RABA in sera of ponies. (*For details, see Fig. 2.*)

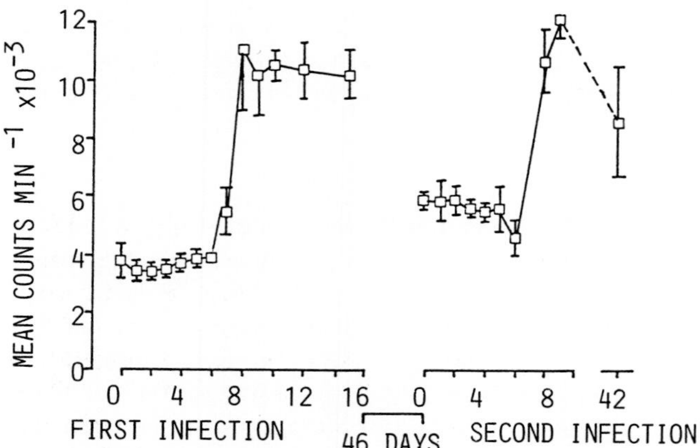

Fig. 3. Development of virus-specific IgM measured by RABA in sera of ponies. (*For details, see Fig. 2.*)

second infection. In contrast to the kinetics of IgM development, serum antibody of the IgA isotype rose much more slowly after first infection and had declined by approximately 20% at the time of rechallenge (Fig. 4). There was a stronger and more rapid response in serum IgA on rechallenge, and the high levels were maintained until at least 42 days after second infection.

Nasopharyngeal and tracheobronchial antibody responses to primary and secondary infections. Virus-specific nasopharyngeal antibody to equine-2 influenza A was measured in nasal washes by means of RABA. To correct for variable sample dilution and serum transudation, antibody measurements are presented in terms of ESA content. The kinetics of virus-specific nasopharyngeal IgG_{ab} production after first infection (Fig. 5) appeared to be similar to that of serum IgG_{ab} in first infections (Figs. 1 and 2). However, there was a marked decline in nasal wash antibody by 62 days, and when rechallenged a typical secondary antibody response was detected by Day 4 (Fig. 6). The anamnestic response to rechallenge detected in the nasopharynx was confirmed by the kinetics of virus-specific antibody in tracheal wash samples from the same animals (Fig. 6).

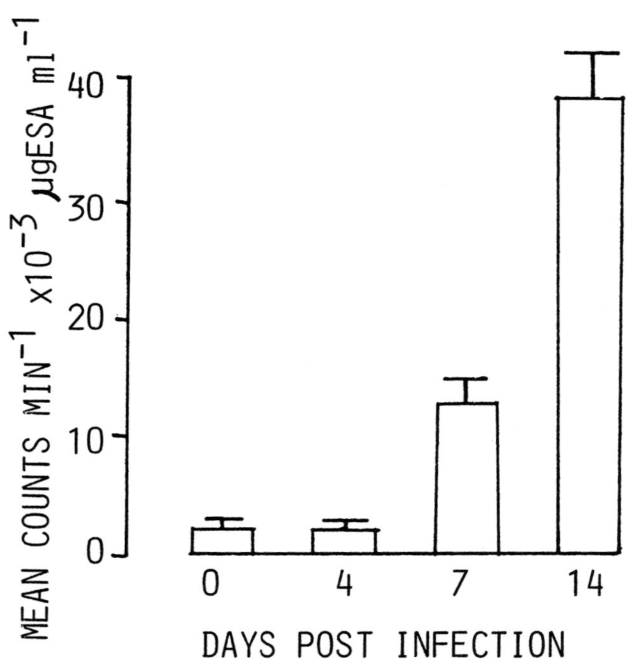

Fig. 5. Virus-specific IgG_{ab} measured by RABA in nasal washes of naive ponies (n = 3) after infection with A/equine/Newmarket/79.

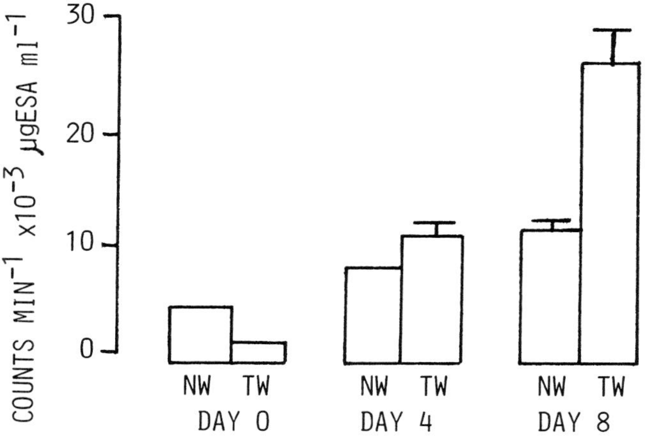

Fig. 6. Virus-specific IgG_{ab} measured by RABA in nasal washes (NW) and tracheal washes (TW) of ponies rechallenged with A/equine/Newmarket/79 62 days after first infection.

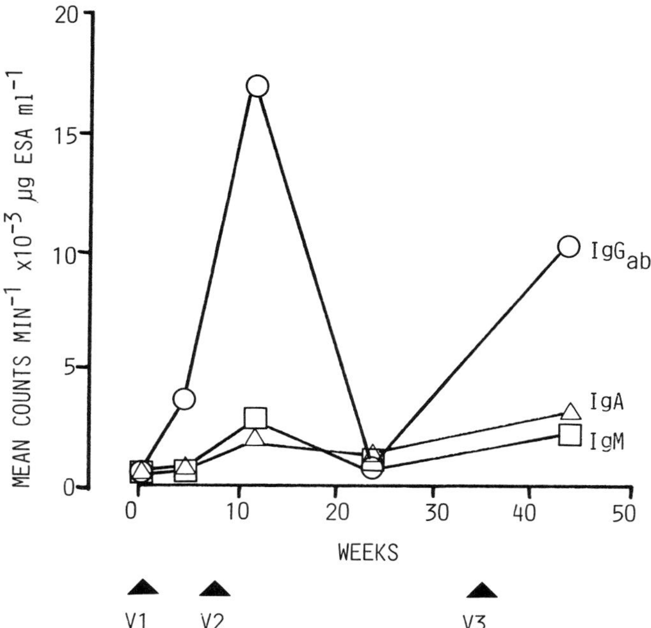

Fig. 7. Development of virus-specific IgG_{ab}, IgM, and IgA measured by RABA in trachea of ponies after ISCOM vaccination. Vaccination dates indicated by arrows.

Nasopharyngeal and tracheal antibody responses to ISCOM vaccination. The development of virus-specific IgG_{ab}, IgM, and IgA in the upper respiratory tract of ponies undergoing ISCOM vaccination is shown in Figures 7 and 8. Four ponies were inoculated with 15-μg dose $^{-1}$HA A/equine/Solvalla/79(H3N8) in the form of ISCOMs, and nasal and tracheal wash samples were collected over a period of 45 weeks. Virus-specific antibody as measured by RABA is

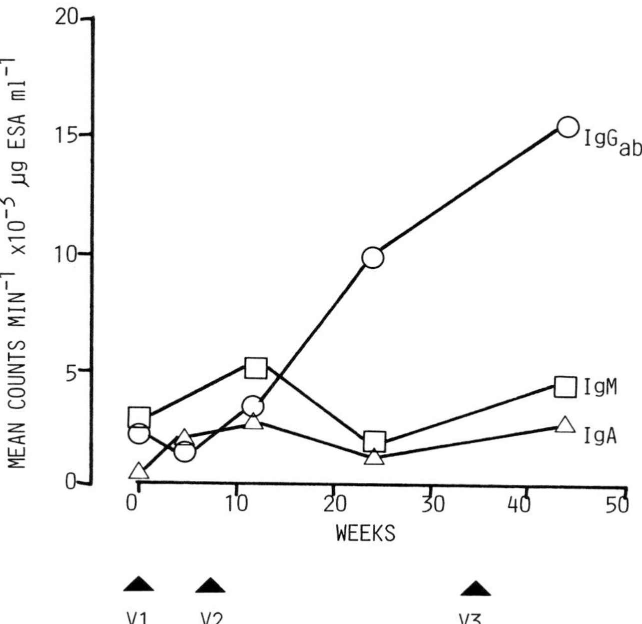

Fig. 8. Development of virus-specific IgG_{ab}, IgM, and IgA measured by RABA in nasopharynx of ponies after ISCOM vaccination.

presented in terms of ESA content; each point represents the mean of four ponies, and each sample was analyzed in triplicate. Standard deviations did not exceed 15%. Reactivity to egg allantoic fluid antigens was negligible in nasal and tracheal wash samples. During development of virus-specific antibody in tracheal washes, there was a rapid rise in IgG_{ab}, which declined by about 25 weeks after the initial course of two doses of vaccine (Fig. 7). The rises in virus-specific IgA and IgM were not so marked. On boosting (V3) at 35 weeks, there was a further significant rise in IgG_{ab}, but again the IgA and IgM responses were not of the same order. In marked contrast, nasopharyngeal antibody at 12 weeks showed a transient rise in virus-specific IgM (Fig. 8), followed by development of high levels of IgG_{ab} at 25 weeks. Unfortunately, no samples were available between 25 weeks and the third vaccination at 35 weeks to show whether nasopharyngeal IgG_{ab} declined over this period. However, after boosting (V3) there was a further rise in IgG_{ab}, whereas the IgA and IgM responses were not remarkable.

Virus antigen expression on infected equine PBMCs in vitro. Equine PBMCs were infected with influenza in vitro, and development of cell-surface virus antigens was detected by the binding of a monospecific xenogeneic polyclonal antiserum to equine-2 influenza A virus as revealed by uptake of radiolabeled Protein A. The kinetics of virus antigen expression on equine PBMCs is shown in Figure 9. Antigen was first detected about 1.5 hr after infection, increasing over the following 48 hr. Cell viability was approximately 75%

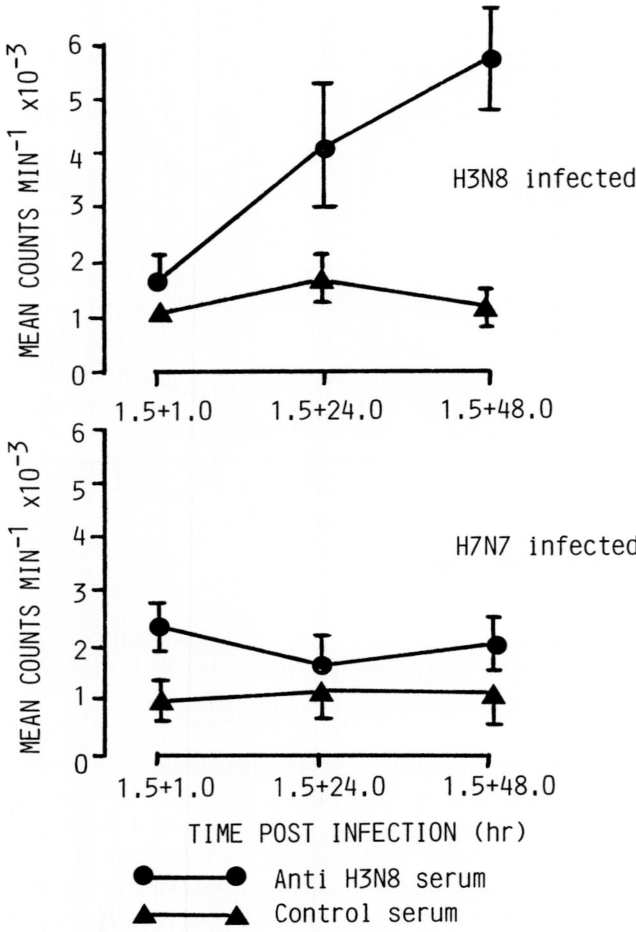

Fig. 9. Expression of A/equine/Newmarket/79 antigen on in vitro-infected equine peripheral blood mononuclear cells.

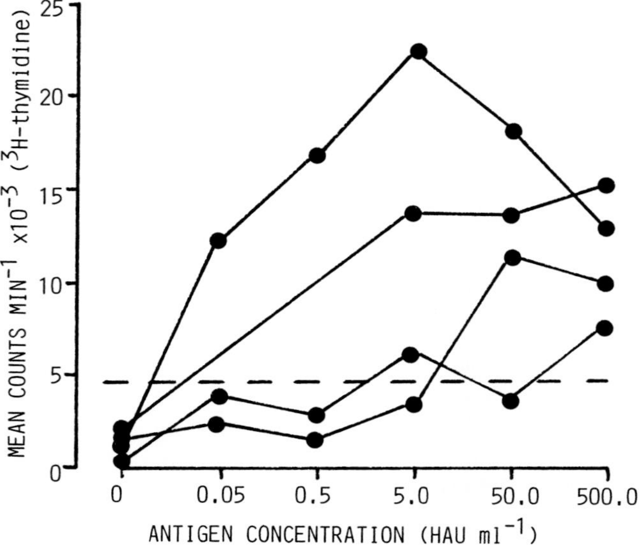

Fig. 10. Lymphocyte proliferation responses to equine-2 influenza A; lymphocytes were taken from four ponies 14 days after infection with A/equine/Newmarket/79.

(trypan blue exclusion) at 24 hr. This experiment confirmed the suitability of in vitro–infected PBMCs as targets for cytotoxicity studies.

Generation of virus-specific T-lymphocytes in ponies after influenza infection. Specific lymphocyte reactivity to influenza virus antigens was assessed by proliferation assays using PBMCs prepared from four ponies 14 days after infection. PBMCs were cultured for five days in the presence of varying amounts of equine-2 influenza A virus antigens, and specific T-cell proliferation was assessed by uptake of radiolabeled nucleic acid precursor ^{3}H-thymidine (Amersham International, Amersham, UK) (Fig. 10). These experiments showed that specifically sensitized T-lymphocytes were present in ponies 14 days after infection with influenza. The proliferation was considered to be a property of T-cells because no antibody was detected in the culture supernatants using a sensitive radioimmunoassay (data not shown).

Cytotoxic activity of equine lymphocytes for virus-infected targets. Autologous and allogeneic combinations of effector cells with uninfected and virus-infected target cells were studied using a 3-hr ^{51}Cr release assay for cytotoxicity. If culture conditions were optimized for the production of large numbers of in vitro–induced cytotoxic cells, their cytotoxic activity was not genetically restricted. Thus, cytotoxicity was demonstrated in allogeneic combinations of effector and target cells (Fig. 11) only if the target cells were expressing virus antigens. The obvious interpretation was that cytotoxic effector cell populations contained large numbers of natural killer cells. Monocyte/macrophage-mediated cytotoxicity was considered unlikely because of the short time of the assay (3 hr). Moreover, the very limited killing of noninfected target cells suggested that nutrient depletion by macrophages was not a feature of this cytotoxic system. Attempted purification of T-lymphocytes from other effector cells by nylon wool adherence failed to reveal genetic restriction of cytotoxic effector cells (data not shown).

To control for possible activators of natural killer cells in vitro, experiments were carried out to modify the induction process for cytotoxic effector cells. These studies, in combination with modifications of the cytotoxic assay itself, showed that genetically restricted cytotoxicity could be revealed (unpublished data). Table 1 shows the results of a typical assay for genetically restricted cytotoxic T-lymphocyte activity in equine-2 influenza A–infected target cells. The most effective modifications of the induction culture for cytotoxic lymphocytes were small numbers of cells and low concentrations of equine interleukin-2 (IL-2) made in this laboratory.

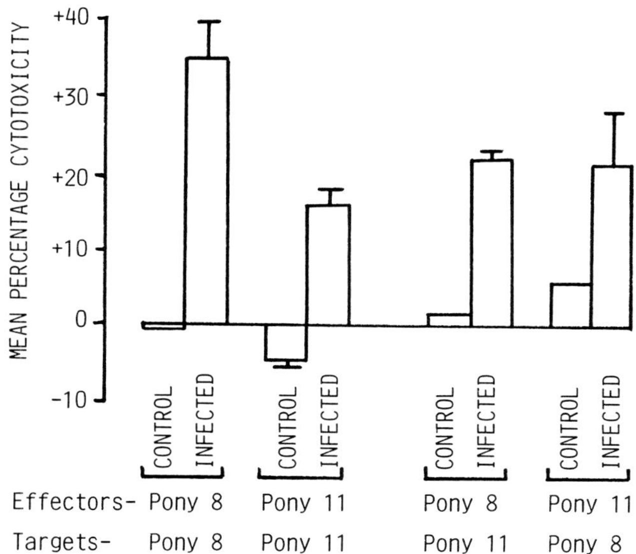

Fig. 11. Cell-mediated cytotoxicity of in vitro-induced lymphocytes after infection with A/equine/Newmarket/79.

DISCUSSION

The results presented in this paper extend our recent studies on the duration of antibody stimulated by infection with A/equine/Newmarket/79 virus (Hannant et al. 1988). The specificity of the RABA-defined isotype responses has yet to be ascribed to individual viral antigens, and the kinetics of virus-specific serum IgM and IgA in primary and secondary infections suggest that the consequences of antigenic stimulation by infectious virus are complex. It is therefore not yet possible to attribute functional significance to these responses in terms of protection from challenge. However, the present study highlights some of the immune mechanisms stimulated by infection that may be important for effective immunoprophylaxis.

The long duration of virus-specific serum IgG_{ab} was notable after infection with equine-2 influenza A virus, whereas serum IgM responses were short-lived after both primary and secondary infections. The latter response, similar to the duration of antibody to HA as measured by the SRH test (Hannant et al. 1988), served to emphasize the differences in antigen specificity as revealed by single radial hemolysis (SRH) and RABA. It is not known whether the transient IgM response during first and second infections showed specificity similar to that of the antibodies defined by SRH, although equine IgM would function in a test based on complement-mediated lysis such as SRH (McGuire, Crawford & Henson 1973). The development of virus-specific serum IgA on first infection was not so rapid as for IgG_{ab} and IgM. Circulating IgA did not show a major decline over the 62-day period before second challenge. There was a more rapid rise in serum IgA on rechallenge and the high levels of antibody that resulted were of long duration. Therefore, second infection with

Table 1. Genetic restriction of cytotoxic lymphocytes for equine influenza–infected target cells

Pony no.	Killer:Target ratio	% Cytotoxicity[a]	
		Autologous	Allogeneic
A	100:1	27.4	8.9
A	50:1	15.1	7.9
B	100:1	32.2	10.0

[a] Calculated as described by McMichael and Askonas (1978).

equine-2 influenza A virus caused antigenic stimulation sufficient to generate secondary increases in serum IgA and IgM in the presence of high levels of circulating IgG_{ab}.

Previous studies have shown that ponies were protected from rechallenge by nebulized aerosol of equine-2 influenza A virus over this time period (Hannant et al. 1988). Clinical protection was defined as absence of pyrexia, dyspnoea, and cough. However, some virus replication occurred in experiments, similar to those summarized in Figures 3 and 4, with occasional low levels of virus recovery (Hannant et al. 1988). Seroconversions did not occur in ponies exposed to inactivated virus of the same antigenic mass used for nebulized aerosol infection with live virus (D. Hannant and J.A. Mumford, unpublished).

The high levels of IgM stimulated by first infection had declined within 50 days, which suggests that measurement of virus-specific IgM by RABA may be useful in detecting recent or multiple infections where levels of serum IgG_{ab} are already high.

Unlike serum IgG_{ab}, antibody detected in the nasopharynx and trachea was relatively short-lived after infection with equine-2 influenza A virus. By 62 days after first infection, virus-specific IgG_{ab} in the upper respiratory tract had declined to prechallenge levels. When rechallenged, local antibody memory was demonstrated by an anamnestic response. Although the kinetics of antibody production in the nasopharynx and serum were similar, local virus-specific IgG_{ab} was not long-lasting. The short duration is at odds with the suggestion that nasal wash IgG was transudated from serum in human influenza infections (Wagner et al. 1987).

Further evidence to support local antibody production in the nasopharynx and trachea after equine-2 influenza A infection was obtained by applying the formulas described by Stockley and Burnett (1980) to the antibody measurements in this study. In randomly selected samples, the proportion of locally produced antibody in the upper respiratory tract varied from 15% to 60% (data not shown). However, in gauging the degree of local antibody production during an inflammatory response after influenza infection, estimates are liable to error unless it is possible to measure components of the antibody molecules that are unique to nasopharyngeal and tracheal secretions. Studies are thus in progress to measure secretory IgA in the upper respiratory tract of horses, based on two site assays specific for secretory component and alpha chain of immunoglobulin.

Systemic vaccination with influenza ISCOMs revealed a significant but transitory rise in virus-specific IgG_{ab} in the trachea, lasting about 25 weeks, whereas the antibody response in the nasopharynx was more delayed and appeared to be accumulative. Again, the predominant antibody isotype detected in the upper respiratory tract was IgG_{ab}, although some increases in IgM and IgA were also observed. If a transient tracheal antibody response is a common feature of systemic vaccination, it may be sufficient to prevent a challenge infection by the aerosol route where virus replication in the tracheal epithelium is a common finding (R.F. Cook, personal communication).

The essential reagents for the demonstration of virus-specific T-lymphocyte cytotoxicity in horses have been developed—namely, target cells expressing large amounts of virus antigens and in vitro–induced virus-specific T-lymphocytes. The genetic restriction phenomenon, typical of cytotoxic T-cell activity (Zinkernagel & Doherty 1974), proved difficult to demonstrate with equine cellular reagents in vitro, and only after the cytotoxic cell induction phase and the assay conditions were modified was genetic restriction observed.

It is probable that more than one type of cytotoxic effector cell is operative in the control of equine influenza infection and recovery from disease. However, in the absence of equine lymphocyte surface phenotype markers, it is only possible to describe effector cells on the basis of functional activity. Therefore, despite the identification of genetically restricted T-cells and cytotoxic cells that function across a histocompatibility barrier in horses, the identity of effector cells in the respiratory tract remains to be established.

The demonstration of cytotoxic effector cells of at least two functional types using different culture methods is not without precedent. Recent studies have suggested that genetically restricted cytotoxic T-cells represent a differentiation step in the development of nonrestricted cytotoxic cells of "promiscuous" target specificity (Brooks, Holscher & Urdal 1985; Havele, Bleackley & Paetkau 1986). Cloned cytotoxic T-cells have been shown to expand their target cell range from autologous to xenogeneic cells, displaying features consistent with natural killer cells (Brooks & Holscher 1987). The changes in target cell specificity were induced by exposure of cloned T-cells to lymphokines in vitro, such as interferon and IL-2. These studies have some parallels with the results presented here, where large amounts of IL-2 favored the development of large numbers of cytotoxic cells in vitro that were genetically nonrestricted.

Studies are in progress on the in vitro requirements for cytotoxic lymphocyte generation, to identify the target antigens recognized by cytotoxic effector cells. The rationale behind this approach is that only if such antigens are incorporated into subunit vaccines will cell-mediated immune mechanisms be stimulated by immunoprophylaxis.

ACKNOWLEDGMENTS

This study was supported by the Horserace Betting Levy Board and the Animal Health Trust. We thank Mr. H. Sawyer and his staff for excellent management of the pony herd, Mr. M. Price for technical assistance, and Mrs. Denise Burkett for preparation of the manuscript. The antiglobulin reagent to equine IgG_{ab} was kindly donated by Miss J. Kent.

REFERENCES

Ada, G.L., and Jones, P.D. (1986) The immune response to influenza infection. *Curr. Top. Microbiol. Immunol.* **128**, 1-54.

Askonas, B.A.; McMichael, A.J.; and Webster, R.G. (1982) The immune response to influenza viruses and the problem of protection against infection. In *Basic and Applied Influenza Research*, pp. 157-88. Ed. P.A.S. Beare. C.R.C. Press, Boca Raton.

Brooks, C.G., and Holscher, M. (1987) Cell surface molecules involved in NK reconition by cloned cytotoxic T lymphocytes. *J. Immunol.* **138**, 1331-37.

Brooks, C.G.; Holscher, M.; and Urdal, D. (1985) Natural killer activity in cloned cytotoxic T lymphocytes: regulation by interleukin 2, interferon and specific antigen. *J. Immunol.* **135**, 1145-52.

Burrell, M.H.; Mackintosh, M.E.; and Taylor, C.E.D. (1986) Isolation of *Streptococcus pneumoniae* from the respiratory tract of horses. *Equine Vet. J.* **18**, 183-86.

Callard, R.E. (1979) Specific *in vitro* antibody response to influenza virus by human blood lymphocytes. *Nature* **282**, 734-36.

Hannant, D.; Mumford, J.A.; and Jessett, D.M. (1988) Duration of circulating antibody and immunity following infection with equine influenza virus. *Vet. Rec.* **122**, 125-28.

Havele, C.; Bleackley, R.C.; and Paetkau, V. (1986) Conversion of specific to nonspecific cytotoxic T lymphocytes. *J. Immunol.* **137**, 1448-54.

Hudson, L., and Hay, F.C. (1976) *Practical Immunology*. Blackwell Scientific Publications, Oxford.

Johnson, P.R.; Feldman, S.; Thompson, J.M.; Mahoney, J.D.; and Wright, P.F. (1985) Comparison of long-term systemic and secretory antibody responses in children given live, attenuated, or inactivated influenza A vaccine. *J. Med. Virol.* **17**, 325-35.

———. (1986) Immunity to influenza A virus infection in young children : a comparison of natural infection, live cold-adapted vaccine, and inactivated vaccine. *J. Infect. Dis.* **154**, 121-27.

Kumanomido, T., and Akiyama, Y. (1975) Immuno-effect of serum and nasal antibody against experimental inoculation with influenza A-Equi-2 virus. *Exp. Rep. Equine Hlth Lab.* **12**, 44-52.

McGuire, T.C.; Crawford, T.B.; and Henson, J.B. (1973) The isolation, characterization and functional properties of equine immunoglobulin classes and subclasses. *Proc. 3d Int. Conf. Equine Infect. Dis.*, pp. 364-381.

McMichael, A.J., and Askonas, B.A. (1978) Influenza virus-specific cytotoxic T cells in man; induction and properties of the cytotoxic cell. *Eur. J. Immunol.* **8**, 705-11.

Morein, B.; Sundqvist, B.; Hoglund, S.; Dalsgaard, K.; and Osterhaus, A. (1984) ISCOM, a novel structure for antigenic presentation of membrane proteins from enveloped viruses. *Nature* **308**, 457-60.

Mumford, J.A.; Wood, J.M.; Scott, A.M.; Folkers, C.; and Schild,

G.C. (1983) Studies with inactivated equine influenza vaccines. 2. Protection against experimental infection with influenza virus A/equine/Newmarket/79 (H3N8). *J. Hyg., Camb.* **90**, 385-95.

Mumford, J.A.; Hannant, D.; Jessett, D.M.; and Scott, A.M. (1987) Experimental infection of ponies with equine influenza (H3N8) virus by intranasal inoculation or exposure to aerosols. *Equine Vet. J.* In press.

Murphy, B.R.; Chalub, E.G.; Nusinoff, S.R.; Kasel, J.; and Chanock, R.M. (1973) Temperature-sensitive mutants of influenza virus. III. Further characterization of the *ts*-1[E] influenza A recombinant (H3N2) virus in man. *J. Infect. Dis.* **128**, 479-87.

Rouse, B.T., and Ditchfield, W.J.B. (1970) The response of ponies to *Myxovirus influenzae* A-Equi-2. III. The protective effect of serum and nasal antibody against experimental challenge. *Res. Vet. Sci.* **11**, 503-7.

Stockley, R.A., and Burnett, D. (1980) Local IgA production in patients with chronic bronchitis : effect of acute respiratory infection. *Thorax* **35**, 202-6.

Wagner, D.K.; Clements, M.L.; Reiner, C.B.; Snyder, M.; Nelson, D.L.; and Murphy, B.R. (1987) Analysis of immunoglobulin G antibody responses after administration of live and inactivated influenza A vaccine indicates that nasal wash immunoglobulin G is a transudate from serum. *J. Clin. Microbiol.* **25**, 559-62.

Wood, J.M.; Schild, G.C.; Folkers, C.; Mumford, J.A.; and Newman, R.W. (1983) Standardization of inactivated equine influenza vaccines by single-radial immunodiffusion. *J. Biol. Stand.* **11**, 133-36.

Zinkernagel, R.M., and Doherty, P.C. (1974) Restriction of *in vitro* T cell mediated cytotoxicity in lymphocytic choriomeningitis within a syngeneic or semiallogeneic system. *Nature* **248**, 701-2.

Single Radial Immunodiffusion Potency Tests for Inactivated Equine Influenza Vaccines

John M. Wood, Jennifer A. Mumford, Una Dunleavy, Valerie Seagroatt, Robert W. Newman, Denise Thornton, and Geoffrey C. Schild

SUMMARY

The potency of equine vaccines is conventionally assessed by hemagglutination or immunogenicity tests in small animals and horses, which can be time-consuming, and the results may vary. There is a need for a reliable in vitro assay of equine influenza vaccine hemagglutinin (HA) antigen, the major protective antigen of influenza virus. The single radial immunodiffusion (SRD) test, developed several years ago to measure human influenza virus HA, is now the internationally accepted standard for human influenza vaccine. We have prepared freeze-dried SRD reagents (calibrated antigen and specific anti-HA serum) for A/equine/Prague/56(H7N7), A/equine/Miami/63(H3N8) and A/equine/Kentucky/81(H3N8) viruses. Results from a recent equine SRD collaborative study involving 13 laboratories from seven countries indicate that the test is highly reproducible (geometric coefficient of variation <7%) and sensitive enough to measure HA antigen content of conventional equine vaccines. Clinical trials of A/equine/Miami/63 vaccine in ponies demonstrated an excellent correlation between SRD-detectable vaccine HA concentration and postvaccination antibody responses.

INTRODUCTION

Despite widespread use of inactivated equine influenza vaccine, outbreaks of influenza can cause serious problems, especially in Thoroughbred training stables. Efforts to improve vaccine efficacy focus on standardization of vaccine potency, which calls for reliable in vitro assay of equine influenza vaccine hemagglutinin, the major protective viral antigen. The SRD test for the measurement of human influenza virus HA provides a more reliable estimate of vaccine potency than hemagglutination tests (Ennis et al. 1977). SRD techniques are applicable in testing equine influenza vaccine potency (Wood et al. 1983a), and SRD potency estimates correlate well with vaccine immunogenicity (Wood et al. 1983b).

We have prepared freeze-dried SRD reagents for A/equine/Prague/56(H7N7), A/equine/Miami/63(H3N8), and A/equine/Kentucky/1/81(H3N8) viruses and have examined the A/equine/Prague/56(H7N7) reagents in an international collaborative study. Results demonstrate that protection against equine influenza correlates well with vaccine SRD potency.

Wood, Dunleavy, Newman, Schild: National Institute for Biological Standards and Control, Blanche Lane, South Mimms, Potters Bar, Herts EN6 3QG, England. Mumford: Equine Virology Unit, Animal Health Trust, Lanwades Park, Kennett, Newmarket, Suffolk CB8 7DW, England. Seagroatt: Unit of Clinical Epidemiology, Oxford Record Linkage Study, Oxford Regional Health Authority, Old Road, Headington, Oxford OX3 7LF, England. Thornton: Central Veterinary Laboratory, New Haw, Weybridge, Surrey KT15 3NB, England.

MATERIALS AND METHODS

Viruses. The strains A/equine/Miami/63(H3N8) and A/equine/Prague/56(H7N7) used for laboratory virus preparations came from the stocks of the National Institute for Biological Standards and Control (NIBSC). The A/equine/Kentucky/1/81(H3N8) strain was obtained from J. Skehel, National Institute for Medical Research (NIMR), London. Viruses were grown on embryonated hens' eggs and purified as described by Oxford and colleagues (1981). The A/equine/Miami/63 virus for infecting ponies, obtained at the sixth egg passage level (Skehel, NIMR), was passaged twice in ponies and once more in eggs.

Vaccines. Beta-propiolactone A/equine/Miami/63 whole virus aqueous vaccine (Duphar, Weesp, Holland) was standardized by SRD to contain 1, 5, 15, or 50 μg HA per dose.

SDS-PAGE. Virus proteins were analyed by the sodium dodecylsulphate polyacrylamide gel (SDS-PAGE) system of Laemmli (1970), modified by Oxford and colleagues (1981). After staining with Coomassie blue, gels were scanned with a Vitatron densitometer, and peak areas of the tracings were quantified using a Kontron MOP digiplan apparatus.

Immunoblotting. PAGE bands were identified by immunoblotting (Thorpe et al. 1987), using sheep or goat antisera to HA and rabbit antisera to nucleoprotein and matrix protein.

Protein assay. Protein content of virus preparations was measured in acid-hydrolyzed samples by O-phthalaldehyde (OPA) fluorometric assay (Benson & Hare 1975; Phelan et al. 1980), using bovine plasma albumen (Armour Pharmaceutical, Eastbourne, UK) as standard.

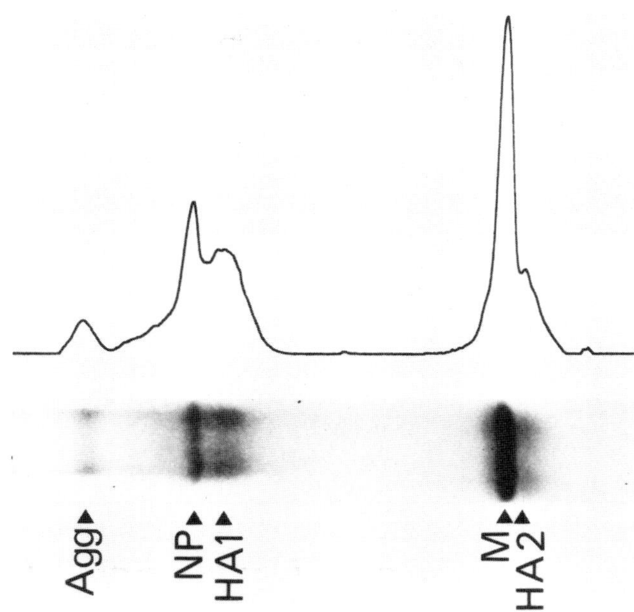

Fig. 1. PAGE separation and densitometer tracings of A/equine/Miami/63 virus structural proteins. Hemagglutinin was resolved into HA1 and HA2, which can be seen as shoulders on peaks of the nucleoprotein (NP) and matrix protein (M), respectively. A high-molecular-weight band was identified by immunoblotting as an aggregate of HA, NP, and M.

SRD reagents. Specific goat antisera to purified HA of A/equine/Prague/56 HA (GH13, 84/673) and A/equine/Miami/63 HA (GH15, 84/677) were produced as described by Wood and colleagues (1983a). Sheep antiserum to A/equine/Kentucky/1/81 HA (S64, 85/516) was produced by intramuscular injection of one dose of 150 µg of purified HA (Brand & Skehel 1972) with Freunds' complete adjuvant (FCA), followed two weeks later by two further doses of 75 µg HA with FCA. Serum was collected five weeks after the initial immunization. Reference virus antigens were prepared from formalin-inactivated whole virus vaccine (Duphar B.V., Holland, and Behringwerke A.G., West Germany). Antiserum and antigens were freeze-dried in 1-ml amounts according to NIBSC procedures (Campbell 1974).

SRD test. Antiserum and antigen reagents were used to assay vaccines by SRD as described by Wood and colleagues (1977), except that Zwittergent 3-14 detergent (1% w/v final concentration; Calbiochem-Behring, La Jolla, Calif.) was used to disrupt virus particles.

SRD collaborative study. The study involved 15 laboratories from seven countries; preliminary data are presented from 13 of the laboratories. Two freeze-dried preparations of formalin-inactivated A/equine/Prague/56 virus (85/557 and 85/530) were distributed as test vaccines to the participants, along with A/equine/Prague/56 reference antigen 85/553 and antiserum reagent 84/673. Participants were required to assay vaccines by SRD on three separate occasions and to submit data for analysis to NIBSC. Data were analyzed by the slope ratio method (Finney 1978), relating zone diameter^2 to antigen dilution. The data were tested by analysis of variance, including tests for nonlinearity and deviation from common intercept. Vaccine potency was expressed as a percentage of the reference antigen 85/553. The overall variability of the estimates was expressed as the geometric coefficient of variation (GCV) (Kirkwood 1979).

Clinical trial. Welsh Mountain pony yearlings, seronegative for A/equine/Miami/63 by single radial hemolysis (SRH) test (Oxford et al. 1979), were divided into four groups of eight each. Each group received two doses of vaccine containing 1, 5, 15, or 50 µg HA at four-week intervals, and four ponies from each group received a third dose 10 weeks later. Sera were taken at two- to four-week intervals and tested for antibody to influenza HA by SRH test. All vaccinated ponies and six unvaccinated ponies were challenged intranasally with A/equine/Miami/63 ($10^{8\cdot7}$ egg infectious dose 50), 13½ weeks after the second dose and 3½ weeks after the third dose of vaccine. Serum samples, rectal temperatures, and nasopharyngeal swabs for virus isolation were dealt with as described by Mumford and colleagues (1983).

RESULTS

Calibration of SRD reference antigens. The PAGE separation of structural proteins of purified A/equine/Miami/63 virus is illustrated in Figure 1. Under the reducing conditions of the gel, the HA protein was resolved into HA1 and HA2 polypeptides. The nucleoprotein (NP) and matrix protein (M) migrated as densely staining bands corresponding to proteins of molecular weight 65 and 25 kilodaltons, respectively (Skehel & Schild 1971). The neuraminidase and polymerase proteins could not be resolved in the gels, but this had little quantitative importance, as these proteins normally contribute less than 10% of the total influenza virus protein (Oxford, Corcoran & Hugentobler 1981). One band of high molecular weight was identified by immunoblotting as an aggregate of HA, NP, and M proteins.

The optical density of each band was calculated from the area under the densitometric peaks (Fig. 1). When two peaks were incompletely separated (as for NP and HA1), they were divided by a line drawn at right angles to the baseline, intersecting the point where the shoulder met the main peak. In this manner the areas under the two peaks could be quantified separately. The proportion of HA present in the virus preparations was calculated as follows: (1) the percentage protein in each PAGE band was estimated from the areas under the optical density tracings. (2) The amount of HA in the high "molecular weight aggregate" was estimated on the assumption that the percentage HA in the aggregate would be the same as the value obtained in (1). (3) The percentage HA

Table 1. Calibration of reference antigens

Virus strain	%HA protein (± stand. dev.)	Reference antigen	HA concentration in reference antigen[a] (µg/ml)
A/equine/ Miami/63	37.2 (2.5)[b]	87/510	27
A/equine/ Kentucky/1/81	39.2 (2.5)[c]	85/520	28
A/equine/ Prague/56	32.3 (4.5)[c]	85/553	110

[a] Based on SRD tests of calibrated laboratory virus and freeze-dried reference antigen.
[b] Mean of PAGE gels of 5 purified virus preparations.
[c] Mean of PAGE gels of 4 purified virus preparations.

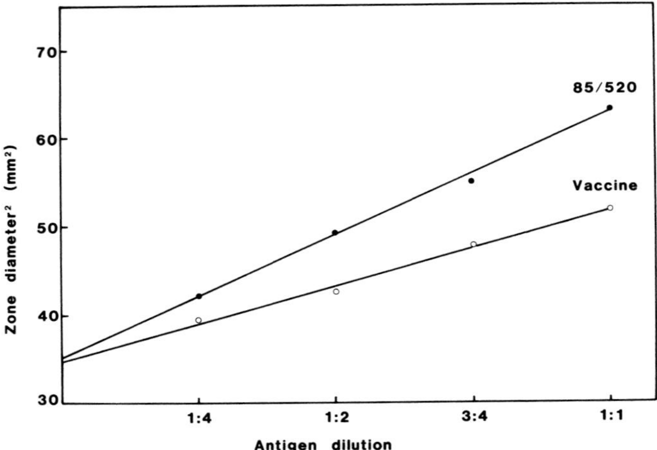

Fig. 3. SRD potency test of an aqueous A/equine/Kentucky/1/81 vaccine. Dilutions of Zwittergent 3-14 detergent–treated (1% w/v final concentration) vaccine and reference A/equine/Kentucky/1/81 antigen (85/520, 24 µg HA/ml) were tested on SRD plates containing homologous antiserum reagent 85/516. By comparing the graphs of SRD zone diameter² against antigen dilution for vaccine and reference antigen, it was possible to calculate the vaccine potency (15 µg HA/ml).

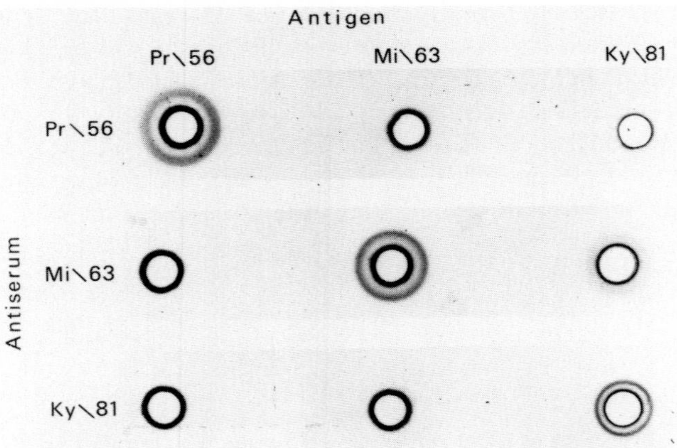

Fig. 2. Specificity of equine SRD test. Reference antigens for A/equine/Prague/56 (85/553), A/equine/Miami/63 (87/510) and A/equine/Kentucky/1/81 (85/520) were tested on SRD plates containing antisera to the three strains (antiserum reagents 84/673, 84/677, and 85/516, respectively). A/equine/Prague/56 and A/equine/Miami/63 antigens reacted only with homologous antisera, whereas the A/equine/Kentucky/1/81 antigen gave intense zones with homologous antiserum, weak zones with antiserum to A/equine/Miami/63, and no reaction with antiserum to A/equine/Prague/56.

in the virus preparation including the aggregate was estimated by combining the HA values from (1) and (2).

PAGE tracings were derived in a similar manner for the A/equine/Prague/56 and A/equine/Kentucky/1/81 viruses. The relative amounts of HA were calculated from the tracings of the three equine viruses (Table 1). The values were used to calculate the amount of HA in laboratory-purified virus of known protein content. The freeze-dried reference antigens were then assigned potency values based upon SRD comparisons with the laboratory-purified virus (Table 1).

SRD specificity. The reference antigens gave clearly visible diffusion zones on SRD plates incorporating the corresponding antiserum reagent (Fig. 2). There was no SRD reaction of the A/equine/Prague/56 antigen (85/553) on plates containing antiserum to equine-2 influenza A virus (reagents 84/677 or 85/516) and similarly the equine-2 influenza A antigens (87/510 and 85/520) did not react on plates containing antiserum to A/equine/Prague/56 (84/673). However, there was some antigenic cross-reactivity between the two equine-2 influenza A viruses, as the A/equine/Kentucky/1/81 antigen reacted weakly with the A/equine/Miami/63 antiserum (Fig. 2).

SRD vaccine potency test. In a representative analysis of SRD data (Fig. 3), an aqueous A/equine/Kentucky/1/81 vaccine was tested on plates containing homologous antiserum (reagent 85/516) and compared with 85/520 reference antigen. Based on a graph of diffusion zone diameter² against antigen dilution, the dose response slope of the vaccine was compared with that of the calibrated reference antigen. The vaccine in this comparison contained 15 µg HA/ml, which is equivalent to the potency of conventional equine influenza vaccines (Wood et al. 1983a). Similar SRD data were obtained for vaccines containing A/equine/Prague/56 and A/equine/Miami/63 antigens using the appropriate SRD reagents.

Collaborative study. The 13 laboratories participating in the study contributed data from 39 assays, of which only five were judged to be statistically invalid. The potency estimates from the individual assays (expressed as ratios to 85/553 potency) are illustrated in Figure 4. There was good agreement between potency estimates with the exception of those from Laboratory 8 for vaccine 85/557, which were among

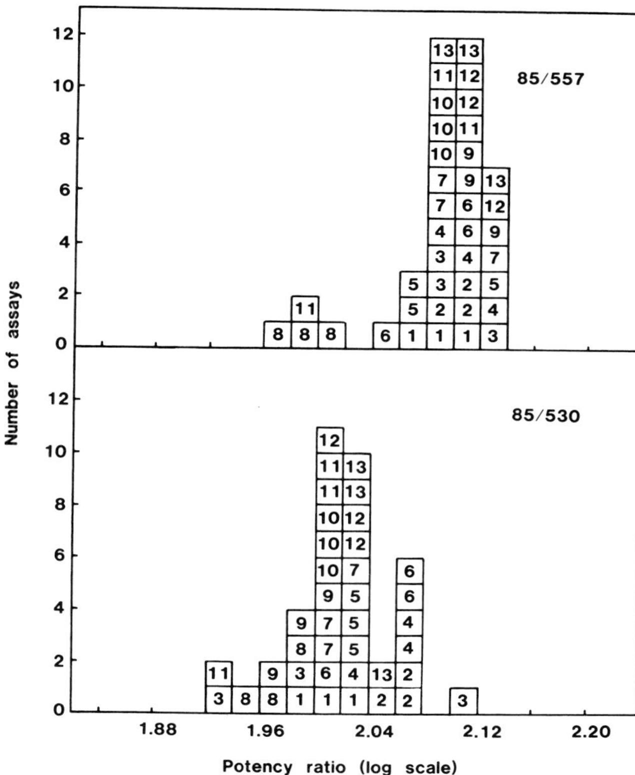

Fig. 4. Frequency distributions of SRD potency estimates from the collaborative study. Potency estimates of vaccines 85/557 and 85/530 are expressed as ratios to the activity of reference antigen 85/553. Each box represents the result from one assay; numbers in boxes refer to the laboratory code.

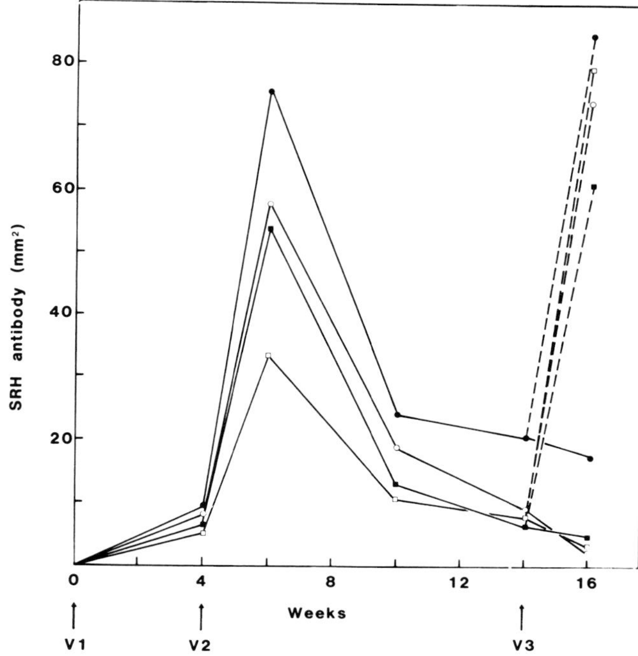

Fig. 5. Postvaccination SRH responses of seronegative yearling ponies to A/equine/Miami/63 virus. Four weeks after the first A/equine/Miami/63 vaccine dose (V_1), ponies were given a second dose (V_2); 10 weeks later, half the ponies were given a third dose (V_3, dashed lines). Responses to vaccines: *open squares*, 1 μg HA per dose; *solid squares*, 5 μg; *open circles*, 15 μg; *solid circles*, 50 μg.

those judged to be statistically invalid. The geometric coefficient of variation for all potency estimates of 85/557 was 8.0%; for 85/530 the GCV was 7.2%. When the variability was examined by analysis of variance, it was found to be significant ($P<0.01$) for 85/557 and marginally significant ($P<0.05$) for 85/530. When results from Laboratory 8 were excluded, the GCVs were 3.3% and 6.4%, respectively, and the variability was no longer significant.

Clinical studies. Figure 5 illustrates the SRH antibody responses following the first (V_1), second (V_2), and third (V_3) doses of vaccine containing 1, 5, 15, and 50 μg HA/dose. Weak antibody responses were observed after one dose; they were greatly elevated after the second dose, but fell rapidly within six weeks of boosting. The antibody responses were vaccine dose–related after the first and second doses. After the third dose, antibody responses were in general higher than those stimulated by the second dose, but were no longer dose-related.

In the same study, ponies were subsequently challenged with A/equine/Miami/63 virus (Mumford et al. unpublished data) and it was demonstrated that all ponies with prechallenge SRH antibody of >74 mm² were completely protected.

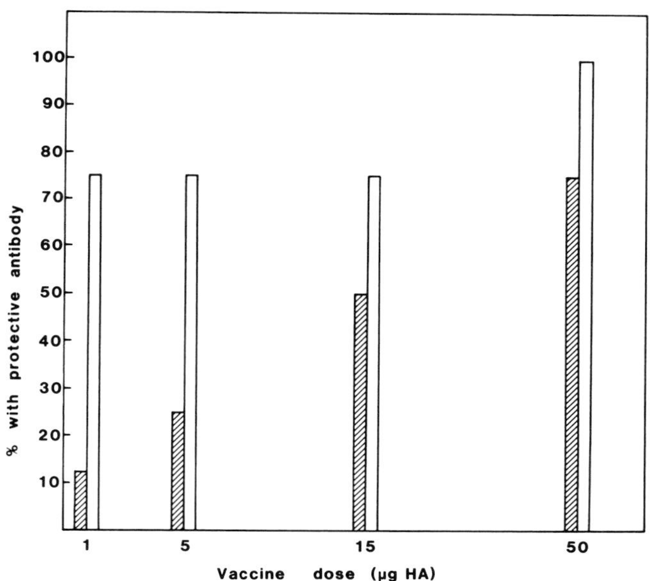

Fig. 6. Correlation between vaccine SRD potency and incidence of postvaccination protective antibody (SRH≥74 mm²) after two vaccine doses (shaded bars) and three vaccine doses (open bars). Protective level of antibody was calculated from challenge studies in which vaccinated ponies were infected intranasally with A/equine/Miami/63 virus.

After two doses of vaccine there was a clear correlation between SRD-detectable vaccine potency and incidence of protective antibody (Fig. 6). After three vaccine doses, >70% of ponies developed protective antibody at all vaccine concentrations.

DISCUSSION

After preparing freeze-dried reagents (calibrated antigen and specific antiserum) for A/equine/Miami/63, A/equine/Kentucky/1/81 and A/equine/Prague/56 virus strains, we demonstrated their suitability for SRD potency tests of equine influenza vaccine. Because the antisera are influenza subtype–specific, each component of a bivalent vaccine containing equine-1 and -2 influenza A virus can be assayed independently. However, the antigenic homology between A/equine/Miami/63 and A/equine/Kentucky/1/81 viruses is sufficient for cross-reactivity in the SRD test. Thus, in mixtures of the two equine-2 influenza A viruses, it would not be possible to assay each strain separately.

The collaborative study has demonstrated the reproducibility (GCV < 7%) of the SRD technique for equine influenza vaccines, as was demonstrated in earlier studies of SRD with human influenza vaccines (Wood et al. 1981) and rabies vaccines (Ferguson, Seagroatt & Schild 1984).

We have also demonstrated that SRD potency values are clinically relevant to the protective efficacy of equine influenza vaccines. Our studies showed that more than three doses of aqueous vaccine of conventional potency (15 μg HA per dose; Wood et al. 1983a) would be required to stimulate protective levels of antibody in all ponies. However, adjuvanted vaccines make it possible to achieve protective levels of antibody with fewer doses of vaccine (Wood et al. 1983b; J. Mumford, unpublished observations).

One difficulty with the use of SRD for equine influenza vaccines is that many contain adjuvants, which often interfere with antigen diffusion. In SRD tests, the result is low potency estimates. Such interference can be avoided by using SRD before addition of adjuvant and then standardizing final vaccine potency based upon predetermined clinical trial data.

In conclusion, we have demonstrated that it is now possible to achieve international standardization of equine influenza vaccines by the use of the simple and reliable SRD test. One problem, however, is the variety of strains incorporated in the various commercial equine influenza vaccines, since antigenic homology between reference and test antigens is important in the SRD test (Ferguson et al. 1987; Mayner & Needy 1987; Wood et al., unpublished observations). At the present time several vaccines contain strains other than A/equine/Miami/63, A/equine/Kentucky/1/81, or A/equine/Prague/56. It would not be realistic to produce SRD reagents for all vaccine strains, but one possible solution would be to follow the strategy adopted by the World Health Organization for human influenza vaccines. Current epidemiological data are the basis for what the WHO recommends each year for human influenza vaccine strain composition, and SRD reagents are then made for each strain included in vaccines. It may now be appropriate to review the equine influenza strains circulating worldwide and to attempt international vaccine standardization.

ACKNOWLEDGMENTS

We are grateful to Dr. Peter Phillips, Risha Yetts, and Cae Neville for assistance in preparing the SRD reagents; to Gillian Harrison for assistance in the clinical study; to all the participants in the collaborative study; and to Sandra Prime for typing the manuscript. Financial assistance was gratefully received from the Horserace Betting Levy Board and the Animal Health Trust.

REFERENCES

Benson, J.R., and Hare, P.E. (1975) O-phthalaldehyde: fluorogenic detection of primary amines in the picomole range. Comparison with fluorescamine and ninhydrin. *Proc. Natl. Acad. Sci. USA* **72**, 619-22.

Brand, C.M., and Skehel, J.J. (1972) Crystalline antigen from the influenza virus envelope. *Nature New Biol.* **238**, 145-47.

Campbell, P.J. (1974) International biological standards and reference preparations II. Procedures used for the production of biological standards and reference preparations. *J. Biol. Stand.* **2**, 259-67.

Ennis, F.A.; Mayner, R.E.; Barry, D.W.; Manischewitz, J.E.; Dunlap, R.C.; Verbonitz, M.W.; Bozeman, F.M.; and Schild, G.C. (1977) Correlation of laboratory studies with clinical responses to A/New Jersey influenza vaccines. *J. Infect. Dis.* **136**, 5397-5406.

Ferguson, M.; Seagroatt, V.; and Schild, G.C. (1984) A collaborative study on the use of single radial immunodiffusion for the assay of rabies virus glycoprotein. *J. Biol. Stand.* **12**, 283-94.

Ferguson, M.; Wachmann, B.; Needy, C.F.; and Fitzgerald, E.A. (1987) The effect of strain differences on the assay of rabies virus glycoprotein by single radial immunodiffusion. *J. Biol. Stand.* **15**, 73-77.

Finney, D.T. (1978) *Statistical Method in Biological Assay*, 3d ed. Griffin, London.

Kirkwood, T.B.L. (1979) Geometric means and measures of dispersion. *Biometrics* **35**, 908-9.

Laemmli, U.K. (1970) Cleavage of structural proteins during the assembly of the head of bacteriophage T4. *Nature* **227**, 680-85.

Mayner, R.E., and Needy, C.F. (1987) Evaluation of the single radial-immunodiffusion assay for measuring the glycoprotein content of rabies vaccines. *J. Biol. Stand.* **15**, 1-10.

Mumford, J.; Wood, J.M.; Scott, A.M.; Folkers, C.; and Schild, G.C. (1983) Studies with inactivated equine influenza vaccine 2. Protection against experimental infection with influenza virus A/equine/Newmarket/79 (H3N8). *J. Hyg., Camb.* **90**, 385-95.

Oxford, J.S.; Corcoran, T.; and Hugentobler, A.L. (1981) Quantitative analysis of the protein composition of influenza A and B viruses using high resolution SDS polyacrylamide gels. *J. Biol. Stand.* **9**, 483-91.

Oxford, J.S.; Schild, G.C.; Potter, C.W.; and Jennings, R. (1979) The specificity of the anti-hemagglutinin antibody response induced in man by inactivated influenza vaccines and by natural infection. *J. Hyg., Camb.* **82**, 51-61.

Phelan, M.A.; Mayner, R.E.; Bucher, D.J.; and Ennis, F.A. (1980) Purification of influenza virus glycoproteins for the preparation and standardization of immunological potency testing reagents. *J. Biol. Stand.* **8**, 233-42.

Skehel, J.J., and Schild, G.C. (1971) The polypeptide composition of influenza A viruses. *Virology* **44**, 396-408.

Thorpe, R.; Brasher, M.D.R.; Bird, C.R.; Garrett, A.J.; Jacobs, J.P.; Minor, P.D.; and Schild, G.C. (1987). An improved immunoblotting procedure for the detection of antibodies against HIV. *J. Virol. Meth.* **16**, 87-96.

Wood, J.M.; Schild, G.C.; Newman, R.W.; Seagroatt, V. (1977) An improved single-radial-immunodiffusion technique for the assay of influenza hemagglutinin antigen. Application for potency determinations of inactivated whole virus and subunit vaccines. *J. Biol. Stand.* **5**, 237-47.

Wood, J.M.; Seagroatt, V.; Schild, G.C.; Mayner, R.E.; Ennis, F.A. (1981) International collaborative study of single-radial-immunodiffusion and immunoelectrophoresis techniques for the assay of hemagglutinin antigen of influenza virus. *J. Biol. Stand.* **9**, 317-30.

Wood, J.M.; Schild, G.C.; Folkers, C.; Mumford, F.; and Newman, R.W. (1983a). The standardization of inactivated equine influenza vaccines by single-radial-immunodiffusion. *J. Biol. Stand.* **11**, 133-36.

Wood, J.M.; Mumford, J.; Folkers, C.; Scott, A.M.; and Schild, G.C. (1983b). Studies with inactivated equine influenza vaccine 1. Serological responses of ponies to graded doses of vaccine. *J. Hyg., Camb.* **90**, 371-84.

Generation of Vaccinia Virus–Equine Influenza A Virus Recombinants and Their Use as Immunogens in Horses

Beverly Dale, Rhonda Brown, Jean M. Kloss, Barbara Cordell, Bobby O. Moore, and Tilahun Yilma

SUMMARY

Protective serotype-specific immunity to influenza virus infection in horses is presumably due primarily to the appropriate host responses to the two surface glycoproteins of the virus, especially the hemagglutinin. Complete cDNA clones of the hemagglutinin and neuraminidase genes of equine-1 and -2 influenza A viruses were isolated. Four separate vaccinia virus recombinants were generated, each bearing a hemagglutinin or neuraminidase gene. Each recombinant was shown to express a native-appearing equine influenza A protein as judged by migration in SDS-PAGE gels and immunoreactivity with antisera raised against wild-type equine influenza A virus. In addition, the neuraminidase recombinants expressed functional enzyme as measured by a sialic acid cleavage assay. The four recombinants of vaccinia virus and equine influenza A virus (vac-EIV) were used separately and in various combinations to immunize horses. The animals responded in a serotype-specific fashion as assayed by hemagglutination inhibition, single radial hemolysis, and serum neutralization assays. The availability of the vac-EIV recombinants will allow dissection of the host immune response by analyzing the impact of specific antihemagglutinin and antineuraminidase responses.

INTRODUCTION

It has recently been suggested that influenza virus is the most comprehensively studied infectious agent in terms of understanding the components of a host protective immune response (Ada & Jones 1986). With the advent of molecular cloning and sequencing techniques, X-ray crystallographic methods, and monoclonal antibody technology, the influenza virion has been dissected to the point of indicating how individual proteins—in fact, subunits of proteins—affect the induction of protective immune responses. Most studies so far have addressed the immune response to human influenza viruses in humans or in animal models such as mice, hamsters, and ferrets. The results have shown the host immune response to be exceedingly complex, including a long-established role for neutralizing antibody and major involvement of cell-mediated immunity (Mitchell, McMichael & Lamb 1985; Ada & Jones 1986).

One might argue that conclusions drawn from studies of host immunity to human influenza virus can be readily extended to influenza viruses that cause disease in other species such as the horse. This argument is supported by the conservation seen in the structure (although not necessarily the sequence) of the genes and proteins from all viruses in the A group. Another justification is the similarity of the disease syndromes in heterologous species. However, while all influenza A viruses are quite similar, the animals that these viruses infect are quite different, and in many cases the understanding of these species' immune response mechanisms is primitive at best. While many aspects of human and murine response to human influenza A viruses can be extrapolated to the equine disease, ultimately a study of equine viruses in the equine host is necessary.

In this paper we describe the generation of four recombinant vaccinia viruses that express surface glycoproteins encoded by genes isolated from the two currently circulating equine-1 and -2 influenza A viruses. These recombinant viruses (vac-EIVs), which express either a hemagglutinin (HA) or a neuraminidase (NA) of a single serotype, were administered singly or in combination to horses, and the resultant immune sera was analyzed by conventional means for anti-influenza virus activity. Now that the equine influenza A virus can be separated into individual antigenic components that are presented to the host animal as a part of a replicating infectious agent (vac-EIV), accuracy should improve in dissecting the equine immune response to equine viruses. In addition, the vac-EIVs themselves may be studied for their potential as protective immunogens in the horse.

MATERIALS AND METHODS

Cells. Madin Darby canine kidney (MDCK) cells, human 143 tk^- cells and CV-1 cells were grown in Eagle's medium (EMEM) supplemented with 10% fetal bovine serum.

Viruses. Vaccinia virus (Wyeth strain) was isolated from a vial of Wyeth smallpox vaccine and amplified on CV-1 cells. Influenza virus A/equine/Prague/56(H7N7) (Fort Dodge

Dale, Brown, Kloss, Cordell: California Biotechnology Inc., 2450 Bayshore Parkway, Mountain View, California 94043. Moore: Fort Dodge Laboratories, Fort Dodge, Iowa 50501. Yilma: University of California at Davis, Davis, California 95616.

Laboratories, Fort Dodge, Iowa) was the twenty-second egg passage of a strain originally designated A/equine-1/Prague and confirmed by the U.S. Animal Influenza Viral Reference Center (World Health Organization). Influenza virus A/equine/Kentucky/81(H3N8) (Fort Dodge Laboratories) was the third fertile egg passage of seed virus obtained from R.G. Webster.

Insertion of influenza genes into Vaccinia virus plasmid vectors. The derivation of full-length cDNA clones of the HA and NA genes of two equine influenza A serotypes is described elsewhere (Dale et al. 1986; Dale & Cordell 1986). The influenza viruses used for the cDNA cloning were obtained from Dorothy Holmes (Cornell University). The equine-1 influenza A virus, originally isolated from an infected horse in Florida in 1973, was passed in four isolation ponies at Cornell University before being propagated in MDCK cells. The virus is designated A/Cornell/16/74 (H7N7). The equine-2 influenza A virus, designated A/Kentucky/1/81(H3N8), was originally obtained as an allantoic fluid preparation from Virginia Hinshaw at St. Jude Children's Research Hospital, Memphis Tennessee. It was subsequently passed in MDCK cells.

The full-length cDNAs encoding the H7(equine-1), H3 (equine-2), N7(equine-1), and N8(equine-2) proteins were inserted individually into the vaccinia virus plasmid insertion vector pGS20 (Mackett, Smith & Moss 1984) provided by B. Moss. In each case the cDNAs were modified at the 5′ end either by naturally occurring restriction sites or by insertion of such sites by in vitro mutagenesis. Similar manipulations were performed at the 3′ end of each gene (Dale and Cordell 1986).

Transient expression assay. pGS20 plasmid vectors bearing equine influenza A cDNAs were analyzed for the ability to produce authentic equine influenza A antigens by the method of Cochran, Mackett, and Moss (1985). CV-1 cells grown on 60-mm dishes were infected with wild-type vaccinia virus at a multiplicity of infection (m.o.i.) of 30 plaque-forming units (PFU)/cell. After a 30-min adsorption period at 37°C, cells were transfected with 10 µg of $CaCl_2$-precipitated plasmid insertion vector DNA in HEPES buffer (140 mM NaCl, 5 mM KCl, 1 mM Na_2HPO_4, 0.1% dextrose, and 20 mM N-2-hydroxyethylpiperazine-N-2-ethanesulfonic acid (HEPES), pH adjusted to 7.05). After an incubation period of 30 min at 25°C, the monolayer was overlayed with EMEM containing 8% fetal calf serum and the dishes incubated at 37°C until 8-18 hr postinfection. Cells were labeled with 150 µCi of ^{35}S methionine in medium lacking this amino acid for 4 hr and then lysed in 0.5% Nonidet P-40. Radioimmunoprecipitation (RIP) of the labeled cell lysates was carried out with rabbit hyperimmune serum. In the case of the 10C serum, rabbits were immunized with three doses of 10^8 PFU of sucrose-gradient purified wild-type equine-1 influenza A—A/Cornell/16/74(H7N7)—initially with complete Freund's adjuvant and then boosted with incomplete Freund's adjuvant. In the case of the 11B serum, rabbits were immunized with three injections of a commercially available inactivated equine-1 and 2 influenza A vaccine. RIPs were subsequently analyzed by sodium dodecyl sulphate–polyacrylamide gel electrophoresis (SDS-PAGE) and autoradiography.

Generation of vac-EIV recombinant viruses. pGS20 insertion vectors (Fig. 1) were utilized to generate vac-EIV recombinant viruses (Mackett et al 1984). Briefly, CV-1 cells were infected with wild-type vaccinia virus at an m.o.i. of 0.05 PFU/cell. Two hours postinfection, the viral inoculum was aspirated and calcium phosphate precipitated DNA (5-10 µg pGS20 derivative and 1-2 µg purified wild-type vaccinia virus DNA) was added. Forty-eight hours postinfection, the cells were harvested and thimidine kinase (tk^-)–recombinant virus was selected by plaque-purifying on 143 cells in the presence of 25 µg/ml of BUdR in the agar overlay. BUdR-resistant plaques (tk^-) were replaqued twice and small stocks grown on CV-1 cells. The presence of equine influenza A–specific coding sequences was confirmed by DNA-DNA dot blot hybridization or RIP of infected cell lysates (Dale & Cordell 1984). Vac-EIV recombinants were amplified on CV-1 cells. Crude stocks (not cell-free) were prepared and titered on CV-1 cells yielding 5×10^7 to 5×10^8 PFU/ml. Viral stocks used in the horse immunizations were grown on HeLa cells and had titers of 10^9 to 4×10^9 PFU/ml.

Immunization with recombinant vaccinia viruses. Horses were housed in pairs in a large animal P3 facility inspected and approved by the Animal and Plant Health Inspection Service of the U.S. Department of Agriculture. All animals were seronegative at the beginning of the immunization regimen except J.T.; for this horse, the preexisting equine-2 influenza A titer persisted throughout the study. Horses were first bled for negative control sera, then were given 0.5 ml of Rompun i.v. (Haver, Shawnee, Kans.) as a sedative. Hair was removed with clippers from an area approximately 6×6 inches on the side of the neck. The horses were vaccinated at four locations with 0.5 ml of the appropriate virus inoculum per location. The vaccination was administered intradermally followed by scarification with a needle until exudation of blood occurred.

Sera were collected for antibody studies at various times before and after primary and secondary immunization. Sera were tested for antibodies by serum neutralization (SN), hemagglutination inhibition (HI), and single radial hemolysis (SRH) assays.

Serum neutralization assay. Horse sera were heat-inactivated at 56°C for 30 min. Serial twofold dilutions of each serum were performed in a 96-well V-bottom microtiter plate using 0.2% bovine serum albumin (BSA) in PBS as the diluent. An equal volume of the test virus (100 $TCID_{50}$) was

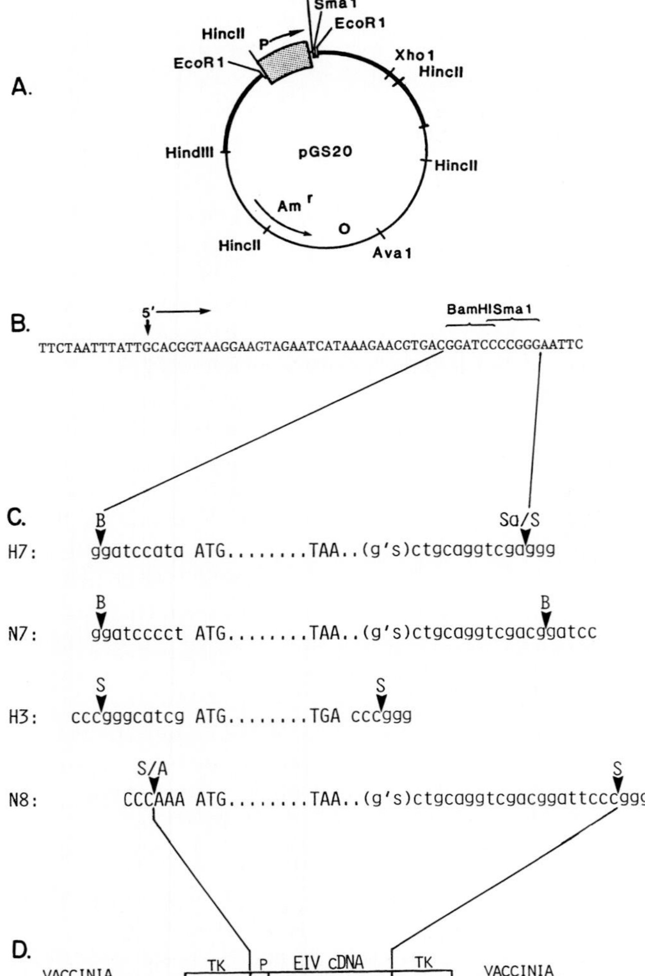

Fig. 1. A. Schematic representation of plasmid insertion vector pGS20: *solid line*, pBR328 bacterial plasmid sequences; *heavy solid line*, vaccinia virus tk gene sequences; *stippled box*, vaccinia 7.5-kdal promoter sequences, with arrow indicating direction of transcription. B. Nucleotide sequence of the transcriptional start site (5′) in the 7.5-kd promoter and the relative positions of the unique cloning sites in pGS20. C. Nucleotide sequence surrounding equine influenza A cDNA coding regions (ATG . . . TAA or TGA represents cDNA sequence) *B* = BamHI; *Sa* = SalI; *S* = SmaI; *A* = AhaIII. D. Schematic representation of heterologous gene insertion in vaccinia genome.

added to each well, mixed, and incubated at room temperature for 1 hr. Following the neutralization period, the serum-virus mixtures were added to monolayers of MDCK cells grown in 96-well flat-bottom microtiter plates. The virus was allowed to adsorb for 1 hr at 37°C; the cells were then refed with serum-free EMEM containing 2μg/ml trypsin. At 48-72 hr postinfection, the monolayers were stained with 1% crystal violet in 50% ethanol. The serum neutralization and point titer was defined as the last well in which the monolayer was 100% protected.

Hemagglutination inhibition assay. Horse sera were treated by the trypsin-periodate method (Moore & Whalen 1987), to remove nonspecific inhibitors of hemagglutinin, followed by a further adsorption with chicken red blood cells (CRBC). Serial twofold dilutions of each serum were prepared in U-bottom microtiter plates using 0.01 M PBS as the diluent. An equal volume of test virus containing 4 HA units was then added to each well and incubated for 30 min at room temperature. After the incubation period, an equal volume of a 0.5% CRBC suspension was added and allowed to settle at room temperature until the CRBC control wells formed a negative pattern. The last dilution showing complete inhibition of hemagglutination was considered the end point.

Single radial hemolysis assay. An 8% solution of sheep red blood cells (SRBC) was mixed with clarified whole virus and then with an equal volume of a 1/400 dilution of 2.25 M $CrCl_3$ (Moore and Whalen 1987). The virus-sensitized SRBCs were then sedimented, washed, and resuspended again to an 8% solution. At that point, 0.9 ml of sensitized SRBC was added to 7.8 ml of agarose at 42°C, followed by addition of 0.3 ml of undiluted guinea pig complement. The mixture was poured into plastic dishes and allowed to harden. Holes 3 mm in diameter were punched in the agarose and filled with 10 μl of the appropriate heat-inactivated test serum. The plates were incubated for 20 hr in a moist chamber at 35°C. The antibody titers are expressed as the area (mm^2) of hemolysis surrounding each test well. The area is calculated from the mean diameter of the hemolysis zone.

RESULTS

Expression of equine influenza A–specific proteins by vac-EIV recombinant viruses. It is now well known that vacccinia virus has the genetic capacity to integrate heterologous genes into nonessential regions of the vaccinia genome (Panicali & Paoletti 1982; Mackett et al. 1982). These genes are stably maintained and faithfully expressed when the vaccinia recombinants are used to infect susceptible cell monolayers or experimental animals. Genes that encode a number of viral glycoproteins, including the human influenza virus HA, have been incorporated into vaccinia genomes to investigate how the independent expression of individual antigens affects the host immune response to the pathogen as a whole (Smith, Murphy & Moss 1983; Smith, Mackett & Moss 1983; Paoletti et al. 1984; Wiktor et al. 1984; Mackett, et al. 1985; Cranage et al 1986; Olmsted et al. 1986).

Vaccinia virus recombinants bearing individual equine influenza virus genes encoding the HA and NA proteins were generated by the methods of Mackett and colleagues (1984). These methods require preparation of plasmid insertion vectors that will satisfy vaccinia transcriptional requirements and facilitate introduction of the foreign gene into the vaccinia genome. Certain features of the plasmid insertion vector pGS20 (Fig. 1A) facilitate generation of such recombinants. Two unique restriction sites, BamHI and SmaI, which allow the insertion of heterologous cDNAs or genes 3′ to the 7.5-kilodalton (kdal.) promoter of vaccinia virus. Figure 1B denotes the position of the unique cloning sites relative to the 5′ transcriptional start site of the promoter. The promoter-cDNA sequences are then flanked by an interrupted vaccinia thymidine kinase gene that serves two functions: (1) it allows for the homologous recombination of the tk-promoter-cDNA-tk cassette into the native vaccinia tk gene during cell culture infection, and (2) the loss of tk function in a vaccinia virus receiving such a cassette is useful in recombinant selection—that is, the generation of tk^- viruses that survive and plaque when grown on tk^- cells in the presence of the nucleotide analog, bromodeoxyuridine. Figure 1C illustrates the exact nucleotide sequences surrounding the equine influenza cDNA coding regions (ATG . . . TAA or TGA) in the four pGS20 insertion plasmids used to generate vaccinia recombinants. In the original cDNA cloning of these genes (Dale & Cordell 1986), each cDNA was flanked by 5′ and 3′ poly C or G tracts. For each cDNA, the 5′ C/Gs were removed prior to insertion into pGS20 and subsequent generation of recombinant viruses. The 3′ C/Gs were removed only from the H3 cDNA. Figure 1D illustrates schematically the final arrangement of the plasmid insertion sequence in a vaccinia genome after recombination through the tk region.

The vaccinia plasmid insertion vectors were assayed for appropriate expression of the heterologous cDNA insert prior to generation of recombinant viruses (Fig. 2). Each plasmid was transfected into a monolayer of CV-1 cells previously infected with wild-type vaccinia virus (supplying necessary transcriptional elements), labeled with ^{35}S methionine, and analyzed by RIP and SDS-PAGE. In each case, infection by a wild-type equine-1 influenza A virus (A/Cornell/16/74) or equine-2 influenza A virus (A/Kentucky/1/81) was analyzed in a similar fashion, to compare recombinant-expressed protein with native influenza virus protein. A pGS20 plasmid vector containing no equine influenza A–cDNA insert constituted the negative control. The two antisera used for the RIP were raised in rabbits, but with different immunogens.

The pGS20-N7, -N8, and -H3 plasmids used in the transient assays are the same plasmids used to generate vac-EIV recombinants (Fig. 1). The pGS20-H7g construct includes a moderately long poly G tract 5′ to the ATG of the H7 coding region. It has been suggested that any length of nontranslated nucleotides placed between the transcription start site and the ATG of the inserted heterologous gene (Fig. 1B) may reduce expression, particularly if the untranslated stretch is C/G rich. The pGS20-H7p construct lacks the 5′ poly C/G tract but contains, 3′ to the H7 coding region, 2.7 kilobase of pUC bacterial plasmid sequences. The pGS20-H7 construct used to generate the recombinant virus possesses the 5′ end of the H7p plasmid but lacks the bacterial sequences.

The equine-1 influenza A cDNAs (N7 and H7) contained in pGS20 generated native-appearing NA and HA proteins

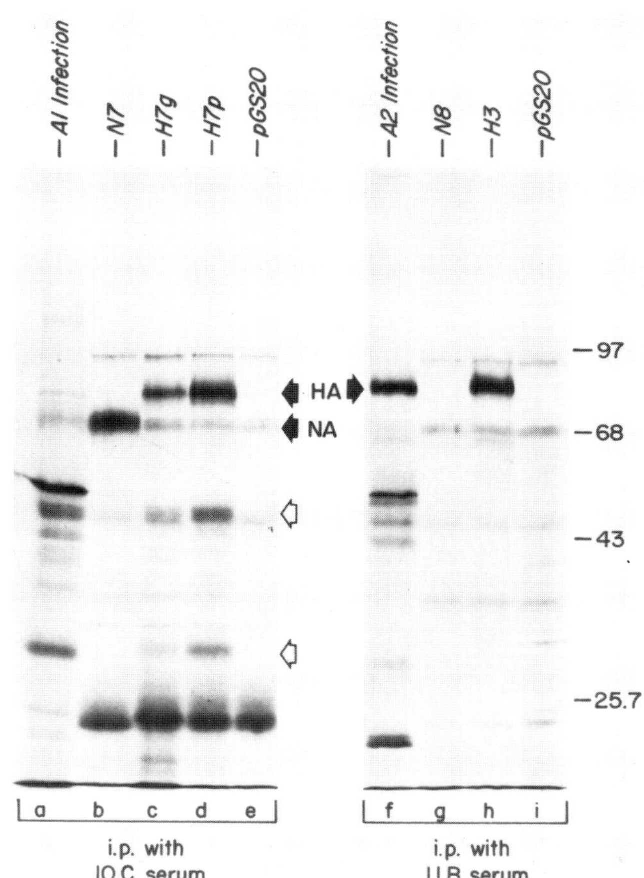

Fig. 2. Radioimmunoprecipitation of equine influenza A–specific polypeptides synthesized by wild-type equine influenza A or pGS20–equine influenza A plasmid transfected and vaccinia virus infected CV-1 cells: *Lanes a* and *f*, cells infected with equine-1(A1) and equine-2(A2) influenza A virus; *Lanes b, c, d, e, g, h, i*, pGS20 plasmid transfected and vaccinia virus infected cells (*Lanes e* and *i*, cells transfected with a pGS20 plasmid carrying no insert). The equine influenza A cDNA contained in each pGS20 plasmid is indicated above each lane.

that were specifically immunoprecipitable by 10C antisera (Fig. 2, Lanes b, c, d). The NA protein expressed by pGS20-N7 comigrates at a molecular weight of about 65 kdal. with a protein in the equine-influenza A infected cell lysate (Lane a). Immunoreactive protein expressed by both pGS20-H7 constructs comigrates with a faint band at 80 kdal and with more intense bands at 50 kdal and 30 kdal in the equine-1 influenza A–infected cell lysates. The lower molecular weight proteins may include the HA1 and HA2 molecules of processed HA, suggesting that recombinant vaccinia H7 is processed similarly to wild-type equine-influenza A, H7 although perhaps not as completely. The reduced amount of HA, HA1, and HA2 in the pGS20-H7g lysate when compared with the pGS20-H7p lysate may indicate that 5′ poly C/Gs do indeed interfere with efficient expression of heterologous cDNAs.

Table 1. Serum neutralization titers in immunized horses

Weeks after first immunization	Immunogen (horse): VSV (Lola) Equine-1	VSV (Lola) Equine-2	H3, H7, N7, N8 (Fanny) Equine-1	H3, H7, N7, N8 (Fanny) Equine-2	H3, H7 (Leo) Equine-1	H3, H7 (Leo) Equine-2	N7, N8 (Howard) Equine-1	N7, N8 (Howard) Equine-2
0	<20	40	<20	40	<20	40	<20	40
1	<20	40	160	160	1280	640	20	40
3	<20	40	160	320	2560	2560	160	80
4	<20	40	160	320	1280	640	160	80
(Second immunization)								
5	<20	40	160	>2560	960	640	160	160
6	<20	40	80	1280	320	640	80	80
8	<20	40	80	640	320	320	80	80
12	<20	40	160	320	160	320	160	40
18	<20	ND[a]	80	ND	160	ND	80	ND

Weeks after first immunization	H3 (Q.D.) Equine-1	H3 (Q.D.) Equine-2	H7 (J.T.) Equine-1	H7 (J.T.) Equine-2	H3, H7 (Tiger) Equine-1	H3, H7 (Tiger) Equine-2	Equicine[b] (Calm Storm) Equine-1	Equicine[b] (Calm Storm) Equine-2
0	<20	40	<20	80	<20	40	<20	40
1	<20	160	40	80	80	160	320	1280
3	<20	640	160	80	320	1280	>2560	640
4	<20	640	160	80	160	1280	2560	1280
5	ND	ND	ND	ND	ND	ND	ND	ND
(Second immunization)								
6	<20	2560	>2560	160	640	>2560	>2560	>2560

Notes: Equine-1 test virus = A/equine/Cornell/16/74. Equine-2 test virus = A/equine/Kentucky/1/81.
[a] ND = test not done.
[b] Manufactured by Haver, Shawnee, Kans.

The pGS20-H3 plasmid generated an 80-kd immunoreactive protein (Lane h) with no readily discernible cleavage products. Indeed, in the equine-2 influenza A–infected cell lysates, the majority of the HA protein remains uncleaved (Lane f). There is no obvious immunoreactive band in the RIPs of the pGS20-N8 transfected cell lysates (Lane g). Likewise, there is no protein seen at the predicted molecular weight (≈65 kdal) in equine-2 influenza A–infected cell lysates (Lane f). This suggests that the 11B antisera that was raised to an inactivated bivalent vaccine is a poor reagent for NA protein immunoprecipitation. Analysis of pGS20-N8 transfected cell lysates with antisera raised to purified whole equine-2 influenza A virus allowed the detection of the appropriately sized protein (data not shown). Furthermore, when vac-N8 and vac-N7 recombinants were subjected to a biochemical assay for neuraminidase activity, both were positive for sialic acid cleavage activity (date not shown).

After it was verified that the pGS20-EIV vectors were capable of expressing EIV proteins, recombinant vaccinia viruses were generated by homologous recombination in CV-1 cells infected with wild-type vaccinia virus. Pure recombinant virus stocks were obtained and amplified. The vac-EIV stocks were confirmed to be expressing equine influenza A proteins in a manner similar to that described from the transient assay (data not shown). The four recombinant vaccinia viruses are referred to as vac-H7, vac-N7, vac-H3, and vac-N8.

Serological responses. Vac-EIV recombinant viruses were used singly or in combination to immunize horses. Although each horse (except J.T.) was seronegative for both equine-1 and -2 influenza A virus at the beginning of the experiment, their history of exposure to equine influenza A viruses is unknown. The horses were immunized in two groups of four, receiving the following combinations of immunogens: Lola, vac-VSV, a recombinant vaccinia virus expressing the vesicular stomatitis virus glycoprotein G; Fanny, vac H3, vac H7, vac N7, vac N8; Leo and Tiger, vac H3, vac H7; Howard, vac N7, vac N8; Q.D., vac H3; and J.T., vac H7. Each horse was immunized by scarification, receiving a total dose of 4×10^8 PFU of recombinant virus. Calm Storm received a commercially available bivalent inactivated vaccine administered intrasmuscularly. All horses received a second immunization four or five weeks after primary immunization. Horses were bled weekly.

The presence of neutralizing antibody against one or both equine influenza A serotypes was measured in a serum neutralization (SN) assay performed in 96-well microtiter plates. All horses receiving a vac-EIV recombinant mounted some degree of SN titer against the homologous wild-type influenza virus (Table 1), but there was no response to influenza virus in the horse receiving the vac-VSV recombinant. The monovalent SN titers of Q.D., and J.T. indicated serotype-specific responses, as expected. The presence of multiple immunogens did not appear to interfere with response to a

Table 2. Hemagglutination inhibition titers in immunized horses

Weeks after first immunization	Immunogen (horse)							
	VSV (Lola)		H3, H7, N7, N8 (Fanny)		H3, H7 (Leo)		N7, N8 (Howard)	
	Equine-1	Equine-2	Equine-1	Equine-2	Equine-1	Equine-2	Equine-1	Equine-2
0	<8	<8	<8	<8	<8	<8	<8	<8
1	<8	<8	64	16	256	32	<8	<8
3	<8	<8	64	32	128	256	<8	<8
4	<8	<8	64	32	64	64	<8	<8
(Second immunization)								
5	<8	<8	64	256	128	128	<8	<8
6	<8	<8	32	256	128	64	<8	<8
14	<8	<8	16	64	32	64	<8	<8
22	<8	<8	8	32	64	32	<8	<8
	H3 (Q.D.)		H7 (J.T.)		H3, H7 (Tiger)		Equicine[b] (Calm Storm)	
	Equine-1	Equine-2	Equine-1	Equine-2	Equine-1	Equine-2	Equine-1	Equine-2
0	<8	<8	<8	16	<8	<8	<8	<8
1	<8	8	8	16	16	16	64	256
3	<8	32	32	16	128	64	512	128
4	<8	32	32	16	64	128	512	128
5	ND[a]	ND	ND	ND	ND	ND	ND	ND
(Second immunization)								
6	<8	32	128	16	64	128	256	128
14	<8	ND	128	16	64	32	256	32

Notes: Tests performed with Tween 80/ether-treated virus. Equine-1 test virus = A/equine/Prague/56. Equine-2 test virus = A/equine/Kentucky/81.
[a] ND = test not done.

Table 3. Single radial hemolysis test titers in immunized horses

Weeks after first immunization	Immunogen (horse)							
	VSV (Lola)		H3, H7, N7, N8 (Fanny)		H3, H7 (Leo)		N7, N8 (Howard)	
	Equine-1	Equine-2	Equine-1	Equine-2	Equine-1	Equine-2	Equine-1	Equine-2
0	0	0	0	0	0	0	0	TL[a]
1	0	0	79	50	154	133	95	TL
3	0	0	79	133	154	113	177	TL
4	0	0	95	154	133	113	177	TL
(Second immunization)								
5	0	0	113	201	154	113	177	TL
6	0	0	113	177	133	95	177	TL
14	0	0	79	113	79	50	95	TL
22	0	0	79	79	79	59	95	TL
	H3 (Q.D.)		H7 (J.T.)		H3, H7 (Tiger)		Equicine[b] (Calm Storm)	
	Equine-1	Equine-2	Equine-1	Equine-2	Equine-1	Equine-2	Equine-1	Equine-2
0	0	0	0	50	0	0	0	0
1	0	79	0	39	95	64	113	79
3	0	133	113	50	154	154	177	154
4	0	133	95	50	123	113	177	113
5	ND[b]	ND	ND	ND	ND	ND	ND	ND
(Second immunization)								
6	0	133	177	57	113	133	133	113
14	0	ND	113	39	113	79	113	79

Notes: SRH titers expressed in mm^2 areas of hemolysis surrounding wells containing test serum. Equine-1 test virus = A/equine/Prague/56. Equine-2 test virus = A/equine/Kentucky/81.
[a] TL = test too light to read.
[b] ND = test not done.

single component. The horse that received recombinants bearing only the NA (Howard) did mount a measurable SN response, although not as impressive as responses in some of the animals receiving HA recombinants. The ability to boost the SN titer with a second vaccinia immunization varied widely: some animals responded (J.T. and Tiger), some animals did not (Leo and Howard); and some experienced an increase in titer to only one of the serotypes (Fanny). There was no correlation between the vac-EIV titers in these animals and the ability to boost the influenza titers (data not shown). The SN titers in all the vaccinia vaccinees declined fairly rapidly over time, mimicking serological responses in naturally infected horses (Moore & Whalen 1987).

While SN assays directly measure the presence of neutralizing antibody in immune serum, two other serological assays are more often employed to evaluate protective antibody levels and monitor vaccine efficacy: the hemagglutination inhibition assay (HI) (Burki & Sibalin 1973), and the single radial hemolysis test (SRH) (Schild, Pereira & Chakraverty 1975). Sera from the equine vaccinees in this study were analyzed for HI and SRH titers (Tables 2 and 3). As expected, the HI assay measured only HA antibody, while the SRH test measured HA and NA antibody (although not consistently for vac N8). The titers from these assays mirror the general outcome of the SN analysis. For instance, the significant increase in SN titer to equine-2 influenza A exhibited by Fanny after secondary immunization is reflected in both HI and SRH titer. Similarly, J.T.'s response to the equine-1 influenza A antigen during the course of vac H7 immunization was consistent in all three types of analysis. In the case of Howard, however, the SRH titers were quite impressive although the SN titers are fairly low, and, of course, the HI titer was nonexistent. Challenges to animals that have received only NA immunogens will ultimately decide the protective role of NA antibody and will determine the validity of the SRH assay for detecting protective immunity and monitoring vaccine efficacy.

DISCUSSION

Early efforts to understand the role of various influenza virus antigens in inducing protective immunity focused on the surface glycoproteins, the hemagglutinin (HA) and the neuraminidase (NA). In particular, serum antibody to the HA correlates with strain-specific protection against infection by neutralizing virus (Ada & Jones 1986). The role of antibody to the NA, which is also strain-specific, is less clear-cut although passively transferred NA antibody has protected experimental animals (Askonas, McMichael & Webster 1982). In general, antibody to other viral proteins, such as the nucleoprotein (NP) and the matrix protein (M) have no neutralization effect against the virus (Mitchell et al. 1985).

More recently, it has become clear that, in addition to the important B-cell activity, the cytotoxic T lymphocyte (CTL) is important in protection against influenza and recovery from infection. In particular, CTL activity specific for the HA and the NP has been described, with anti-HA being strain-specific and anti-NP exhibiting broad cross-reactivity toward different influenza A subtypes (Ada & Jones 1986).

Among the recombinant vaccinia viruses that allow presentation of isolated influenza virus genes in the context of a "living" infection, a recombinant vaccinia bearing the HA gene of A/Japan/305/57(H2N2) protected hamsters against homologous challenge (Smith et al. 1983). It also stimulated a CTL response in mice (Bennink et al. 1984) that was specific for the H2 subtype (Bennink et al., 1986). Another vaccinia recombinant bearing the NP gene of A/Puerto Rico/8/34(H1N1) stimulated a CTL response in mice that was broadly cross-reactive (Yewdell et al., 1985). These results imply that, whereas the HA protein may constitute an effective immunogen against a particular subtype of A virus, the inclusion of an NP component may lend itself to heterotypic protection.

Most available vaccines for inoculating horses against equine influenza are inactivated preparations containing viruses representative of the two known equine serotypes. These preparations readily generate considerable antibody levels against influenza virus as measured by serum neutralization, hemagglutination inhibition, and single radial hemolysis. However, the duration of immunity following vaccinnation is short-lived, requiring frequent booster vaccinations. The limited duration is quite likely due to the frequent failure of inactivated vaccines to induce a CTL response comparable to that induced by infectious influenza virus and now known to be important in protective immunity against influenza (Ada & Jones 1986).

We have demonstrated that vaccinia recombinants bearing equine influenza surface antigens can induce anti-influenza antibodies with neutralizing capabilities. In the equine host, immunization with vac-EIV recombinants may produce results similar to those in mice, where vaccinia recombinants bearing human HA genes have induced vigorous CTL response. It will first be necessary to assess the level and duration of both humoral and cell-mediated immunity in the horse to develop an effective challenge system to evaluate host protection.

REFERENCES

Ada, G.L., and Jones, F.D. (1986) The immune response to influenza infection. *Curr. Top. Microbiol. Immunol.* **128**, 1-54.

Askonas, B.A.; McMichael, A.J.; and Webster, R.G. (1982) The immune response to influenza virus and the problems of protection against infection. In *Basic and applied influenza research*, pp. 157-188. Ed. P.A.S. Beare. CRC Press, Boca Raton.

Aymard-Henry, M.; Coleman, M.T.; Dowdle, W.R.; Laver, W.G.; Schild, G.C.; and Webster, R.G. (1973) Influenza virus neuraminidase and neuraminidase-inhibition test procedures. *Bull. Wed. Hlth. Org.* **48,** 199-202.

Bennink, J.R.; Yewdell, J.W.; Smith, G.L.; Moller, C.; and Moss, B. (1984). Recombinant vaccinia virus primes and stimulates influenza hemagglutinin specific cytotoxic T cells. Nature, **311,** 578-79.

Bennink, J.R.; Yewdell, J.W.; Smith, G.L.; and Moss, B. (1986). Recognition of cloned influenza virus hemagglutin in gene products by cytotoxic T lymphocytes. J. Virol. **57,** 786-91.

Burki, F., and Sibalin, M. (1973) Standardization of hemagglutination-inhibition test for two equine influenza viruses. Zentralblatt fur Bakteriologie Parasitenkunde Infection skrankbeiten und Hygiene **223,** 163-72.

Cochran, M.A.; Mackett, M.; and Moss, B. (1985) Eukaryotic transient expression system dependent on transcription factors and regulatory DNA sequences of factors and regulatory DNA sequences of vaccinia virus. *Proc. Natl. Acad. Sci. USA* **82,** 19-23.

Coupar, B.E.H.; Andrew, M.E.; Both, G.W., and Boyle, D.B. (1986) Temporal regulation of influenza hemagglutinin expression in vaccinia virus recombinants and effects on the immune response. *Eur. J. Immunol.* **16** 1479-87.

Cranage, M.P.; Kouzarides, T.; Bankier, A.T.; Satchwell, S., Weston, K.; Tomlinson, P.; Barrell, B.; Hart, H.; Bell, S.E.; Minson, A.C.; and Smith G.L. (1986) Identification of the human cytomegalovirus glycoprotein B gene and induction of neutralizing antibodies via its expression in recombinant vaccinia virus. *EMBO J.* **5**, 3057-63.

Dale, B., and Cordell, B. (1986) Methods and compositions useful in preventing equine influenza. U.S. Patent No. 4,631,191.

Dale, B.; Brown, R.; Miller, J.; White, R.T.; Air, G.M.; and Cordell, B. (1986) Nucleotide and deduced amino acid sequence of the influenza neuraminidase genes of two equine serotypes. *Virology* **155**, 460-68.

Mackett, M.; Smith, G.L.; and Moss, B. (1982) Vaccinia virus: A selectable cloning and expression vector. *Proc. Natl. Acad. Sci. USA*, **79,** 7415-19.

———. (1984) General method for production and selection of infecious vaccinia virus recombinants expressing foreign genes. *J. Virol.* **49,** 857-64.

Mackett, M.; Yilma, T.; Rose, J.; and Moss, B. (1985) Vaccinia virus recombinants: Expression of VSV genes and protective immunizations of mice and cattle. *Science* **227,** 433-35.

Mitchell, D.M.; McMichael, A.J.; and Lamb, J.R. (1985) The immunology of influenza. *Br. Med. Bull.* **41,** 80-85.

Moore, B.O., and Whalen, J.W. (1987) An equine influenza virus horse serological study. Fort Dodge Laboratories, Fort Dodge, Iowa.

Olmsted, R.A.; Elango, N.; Prince, G.A.; Murphy, B.R.; Johnson, P.R.; Moss, B.; Chanock, R.M.; and Collins, R.L. (1986) Expression of the F glycoprotein of respiratory syncytial virus by a recombinant vaccinia virus: Comparison of the individual contributions of the F and G glycoproteins to host immunity. *Proc. Natl. Acad. Sci. USA* **83,** 7462-66.

Panicali, D., and Paoletti, E. (1982) Construction of poxviruses as cloning vectors: Insertion of the thymidine kinase gene from herpes simplex virus into the DNA of infectious vaccinia virus. *Proc. Natl. Acad. Sci. USA*, **79,** 4927-31.

Paoletti, E.; Lipinskas, B.R.; Samsonoff, C.; Mercer, S.; and Panicali, D. (1984) Construction of live vaccines using genetically engineered poxviruses: Biological activity of vaccinia virus recombinants expressing the hepatitis B virus surface antigen and the herpes simplex virus glycoprotein D. *Proc. Natl. Acad. Sci. USA* **81,** 193-97.

Schild, G.C.; Periera, M.S.; and Chakraverty, P. (1975) Single-radial hemolysis: A new method for the assay of antibody to influenza hemagglutinin. *Bull. Wld. Hlth. Org.* **52,** 43-50.

Smith, G.L.; Mackett, M.; and Moss, B. (1983) Infectious vaccinia virus recombinants that express hepatitis B virus surface antigen. *Nature* **302,** 490-95.

Smith, G.L.; Murphy, B.R.; and Moss, B. (1983) Construction and characterization of an infectious vaccinia virus recombinant that expresses the influenza hemagglutinin gene and induces immunity to influenza virus infection in hamsters. *Proc. Natl. Acad. Sci. USA* **80,** 7155-59.

Wiktor, T.J.; MacFarlan, R.I.; Reagan, K.J.; Dietzschold, B.; Curtis, P.J.; Wunner, W.H.; Kieny, M.; Lathe, R.; Lecoco, J.; Mackett, M.; Moss, M.; and Koprowski, H. (1984) Protection from rabies by a vaccinia virus recombinant containing the rabies virus glycoprotein gene. *Proc. Natl. Acad. Sci. USA* **81,** 7194-98.

Yewdell, J.W.; Bennink, J.R.; Smith, G.L.; and Moss, B. (1985). Influenza A virus nucleoprotein is a major target antigen for cross-reactive anti-influenza A cytotoxic T lymphocytes. *Proc. Natl. Acad. Sci. USA* **82,** 1785-89.

Live Temperature-Sensitive Equine-1 Influenza A Virus Vaccine: Efficacy in Experimental Ponies

Dorothy F. Holmes, Lucinda M. Lamb, Lynne M. Anguish, Leroy Coggins, Brian R. Murphy, and James H. Gillespie

SUMMARY

A temperature-sensitive (*ts*) reassortant of an equine-1 influenza A virus, when administered by nebulization to experimental ponies, induced subclinical infection as evidenced by the recovery of virus from nasopharyngeal swabs and by a rise in hemagglutination inhibition (HI) antibody. All virus recovered from the nasopharyngeal swabs retained the *ts* phenotype. Ponies challenged by intranasal nebulization with wild-type equine-1 influenza A virus four weeks after *ts* virus administration did not shed challenge virus nor develop a febrile response. For ponies an infectious dose of the *ts* virus was approximately $10^{4.5}$ $TCID_{50}$/0.1 ml of inoculum. Uninoculated ponies did not become infected by their vaccinated stall mates.

INTRODUCTION

As evidenced by epizootiologic studies conducted in groups of horses at horse shows, race meets, and sales and training facilities, the major agent of upper respiratory tract disease is equine influenza A virus (Burrows et al. 1982; Thomson et al. 1977). Because of occasional adverse reactions, some horsemen are reluctant to follow a prescribed vaccination program for their animals, especially those at the peak of training. Even if inoculation takes place, the protection of available vaccines lasts for only a short period.

Although antigenic variation in equine influenza A virus isolates has been reported, it has been limited in nature, making it unlikely that influenza outbreaks in horses can be attributed to antigenic change (Hinshaw et al. 1983). Based on epidemiologic studies, infection of horses with equine influenza A virus confers protection against reinfection with the same subtype. This is supported by the relative resistance of previously exposed older horses in the face of outbreaks among younger animals (Ingram et al. 1978).

In recent years *ts* mutants of human influenza A viruses have been produced, characterized, and evaluated as candidates for live virus influenza vaccines. In replication in vitro, the *ts* reassortant clones are restricted to temperatures of 37-38°C but they multiply efficiently in the cooler environment of the upper respiratory tract in humans and hamsters. There they induce local and systemic immune responses that protect against wild-type influenza A infection (Murphy et al. 1973). Replication is inefficient in the warmer environment of the lower respiratory tract in the horse (38-39°C), and an equine *ts* virus might be expected not to produce the cough and systemic signs of wild-type equine influenza A infection. Rather viral replication might stimulate local and systemic immune response, reducing the need for frequent vaccination.

Two *ts* reassortant equine influenza A viruses have been produced (Brundage-Anguish et al., 1982) by fusing a human influenza A *ts* donor virus with an equine-1 influenza A virus [A/equine/Cornell/16/74(H7N7)], and by isolating a *ts* reassortant virus possessing the equine hemagglutinin (HA) and neuraminidase (NA). The resulting equine reassortant clones, 8B1 and 71A1, had in vitro shutoff temperatures for plaque formation of 38°C and 37°C, respectively. A shutoff temperature is defined as the lowest incubation temperature at which the virus titer is reduced at least 100-fold from the titer at 34°C.

Since the human *ts* donor virus had *ts* mutations on the polymerase 3 (P_3) and nucleoprotein (NP) genes, a *ts* equine reassortant virus would have either or both of these *ts* genes. Complementation analysis indicated that reassortant clone 8B1 had a *ts* lesion on the P_3 gene and clone 71A1 had *ts* lesions on both the P_3 and NP genes. Analysis of the parental origin of the genes in each *ts* equine reassortant virus revealed that clone 8B1 received six of its eight genes, and clone 71A1 three of its eight, from the equine parent virus. The growth of both clones was restricted in the lungs of hamsters but similar to that of the equine wild-type virus in the nasal turbinates. All virus recovered from the hamster lungs or turbinates retained the *ts* phenotype. This paper presents the results of the evaluation of one of the equine *ts* viruses (clone 8B1) for its level of attenuation and immunogenicity in horses.

MATERIALS AND METHODS

Viruses. The *ts* reassortant virus 8B1 was used to vaccinate ponies. It has a 38°C shutoff temperature and grows to at least $10^{6.0}$ $TCID_{50}$/ml titer in the Madin-Darby canine kidney (MDCK) cell line. A/equine/Cornell/16/74(H7N7) was the challenge virus.

Department of Veterinary Microbiology, Immunology and Parasitology, New York State College of Veterinary Medicine, Cornell University, Ithaca, New York 14853.

Tissue culture and infectivity assays. Infectivity and plaque assays were performed in 24-well tissue culture plates (Costar, Cambridge, Mass.). MCDK cell monolayers were used throughout the study. Media was either Eagle's minimal essential medium with Earle's salts for cell growth, or 50% Eagle's No. 2 and 50% medium 199 for infectivity studies. Both contained 0.29 mg/ml of L-glutamine, 2.5µg/ml amphotericin-B, and 66µg/ml of gentamycin. For cell growth, 10% fetal bovine serum (screened for suitability for replication of influenza virus) was included. For virus growth medium, serum was deleted and trypsin (TPCK, Worthington Biochemical, Malvern, Pa.) was added at a final concentration of 2µ/ml. Nasopharyngeal swab samples from infected ponies were collected in a transport medium consisting of 50% Eagle's No. 2 and 50% medium 199 and containing 0.5% gelatin and twice the above concentration of antibiotics. Plaque overlay media was L_{15} medium with L-glutamine, trypsin, and antibiotics at the given concentrations plus 0.75% carboxymethyl cellulose (Hercules Powder Co., Wilmington, Del.). Infectivity and plaque assays were performed by adsorbing tenfold dilutions of virus in 0.1 ml amounts onto washed monolayers of MDCK cells for 30 min at room temperature, after which maintenance medium was added for infectivity studies and overlay medium for plaque assays. Plates were incubated at 34°C or 39°C in a 5% CO_2 atmosphere and read after four days. Plaques were visualized by staining the monolayers with a 1% solution of crystal violet in formaldehyde.

Experimental animals. The mixed-breed ponies of Welsh Mountain type used as subjects were unvaccinated yearlings and two-year-olds from a closed herd at the equine isolation facility at Cornell. None of the animals had preexisting serum antibody titers against equine-1 influenza A virus as measured by a standard hemagglutination inhibition test performed in microtiter plates.

Vaccination and challenge study. During the animal studies, ponies were maintained in individual pens in the equine isolation facilities under conditions (positive air pressure, clothing change between units of caretakers, etc.) designed to prevent spread of infectious disease agents between units. Ponies were introduced into the units at least two weeks before any experimental procedure to permit them to become acclimated. Rectal temperatures were obtained twice daily (midmorning and midafternoon) for each pony whether it was under experiment or not. Because average rectal temperatures showed as much as 1.2°F variation from pony to pony, a baseline rectal temperature for each pony was calculated by averaging the daily readings for a two-week period prior to vaccination or challenge. Deviations from the baseline were used to measure the febrile response to vaccination and challenge.

Ponies were vaccinated by nebulizing a suspension of the equine-1 *ts* virus 8B1, containing at least 10^5 $TCID_{50}$/ml, into the upper respiratory tract by means of a compressor-driven Model 645 nebulizer (De Vilbiss, Somerset, PA) attached to a cone covering the pony's nose and mouth. Nebulization took place over a 3 min period. A few animals were revaccinated one or two times at 28-day intervals.

Blood samples were obtained from each animal prior to vaccination and daily thereafter until the termination of the experiment. Tiegland swabs (HL-206400; Haver Lockhart, Shawnee, Kans.) were used to obtain samples for virus isolation from the posterior nasopharyngeal area on Days 0-7 postvaccination. Swabs were broken off into 5 ml of transport media and transported on ice to the laboratory. They were titrated by making ten-fold dilutions of the transport media sample from 10^0 through 10^{-4} (10^0, being the undiluted sample) prior to inoculation into MDCK monolayers grown in 24-well plates. Virus isolated from any of the nasopharyngeal samples was plaque-assayed at 34°C, a temperature permissive for growth of the *ts* virus, and at 39°C, a growth-restrictive temperature, to determine whether the *ts* phenotype was retained after passage through ponies. Virus recovered from one vaccinated pony was plaque-purified and back-passaged a single time by aerosolizing a series of eight ponies using the same protocol as above.

At Day 28 postvaccination, ponies were challenged by nebulization with A/equine/Cornell/16/74, and postchallenge nasopharyngeal swabs and serum samples were obtained as previously described. A nonvaccinated pony was included as control in most groups of challenged vaccinees.

Deviations from the fever baselines were recorded for each animal in both the vaccinated and the challenge control groups, and an average was obtained for each group.

Serum samples obtained throughout the course of the study (Days 0-28 postvaccination and Days 0-28 postchallenge) were assayed in a standard microhemagglutination inhibition test for HI antibody against equine-1 influenza A virus.

Dose response. Three groups of two ponies each were used to make an approximate determination of the pony-infectious dose of the vaccine virus. In each group, ponies were inoculated by aerosol with 3 ml of three suspensions containing, respectively, $10^{4.5}$ (Ponies 675, 680), $10^{3.5}$ (Ponies 677, 679), and $10^{2.5}$ (Ponies 676, 678) infectious particles per 0.1 ml. The ponies were handled as described with respect to nasopharyngeal swab samples, temperature recording, and monitoring of antibody response. After four weeks these animals were challenged with wild-type virus and the same postchallenge protocol followed.

Contact controls. In contact control studies, Ponies 684 and 685 were nebulized with 8B1 vaccine virus, and each was placed in an isolation unit with a contact control animal (Ponies 683 and 686). All four animals were sampled for virus shedding, observed for clinical signs, and had blood samples drawn for antibody assay. Four weeks after vaccina-

Table 1. Response of ponies to vaccination and challenge with equine-1 influenza A virus

Pony no.	No. of vaccine doses	Day, post-vaccination, of seroconversion	Days, post-inoculation, of vaccine virus isolation	Days, post-challenge, of challenge virus isolation	Day, post-challenge, of seroconversion
Vaccinees					
600	1	14	2, 3, 4, 5, 6	–	0
601	1	29	2, 3	–	0
603	3	7[a]	–	–	0
605	3	14[a]	–	–	0
606	2	27[a]	–	–	14[b]
617	2	13[a]	–	–	0
616	1	21	3	3	14[b]
625	1	15	3	–	0
624	1	21	3	–	7
622	1	15	3, 5	–	0
483F_6	1	12	2	–	0
619	1	19	2, 3, 4	–	0
621	1	19	2, 3, 4	–	0
623	1	–	–	–	26
650	1	–	–	–	5
651	1	–	2, 3, 6	2, 3	5
633	1	14	1, 2, 4	–	0
667	1	–	2	–	5
668	1	14	2, 3	1, 2	0
669	1	–	2, 3	1	6
675	1	–	2, 3	1	6
676	1	–	4	1	8
677	1	–	–	1	7
680	1	–	–	–	6
678	1	–	–	1	2
679	1	–	–	1	12
684	1	–	2	1	8
685	1	–	–	–	5
671	2	7[a]	1, 2, 3, 4, 5	–	0
681	2	8[a]	–	–	0
722	1	–	–	1	7
723	1	14	–	–	0
721	1	28	–	1, 2, 4	5
719	1	18	–	1	0
720	1		–	1, 2	0
709	1	7	–	–	0
724	1	–	4	1, 2	5
693	1	–	2, 5, 6	–	6
695	1	–	2, 3, 4, 5, 6	1, 2	5
708	1	13	–	1	5
Challenge Controls					
611	–	–	–	2, 3, 5	21
618	–	–	–	2, 5	14
620	–	–	–	2, 3, 5	14
451F_6	–	–	–	1, 2, 3, 4, 5, 6	9
632	–	–	–	2, 4, 5, 6	14
670	–	–	–	1, 2	14
683	–	–	–	1, 2, 4, 5	42
686	–	–	–	1, 2, 3, 4, 5, 6	10
692	–	–	–	1, 2, 3, 4, 5, 6	7
674	–	–	–	1, 2, 3, 4, 5, 6	7

[a] Seroconverted after 2nd and 3rd inoculation.

[b] Positive postvaccination titers had dropped to <10 by day of challenge.

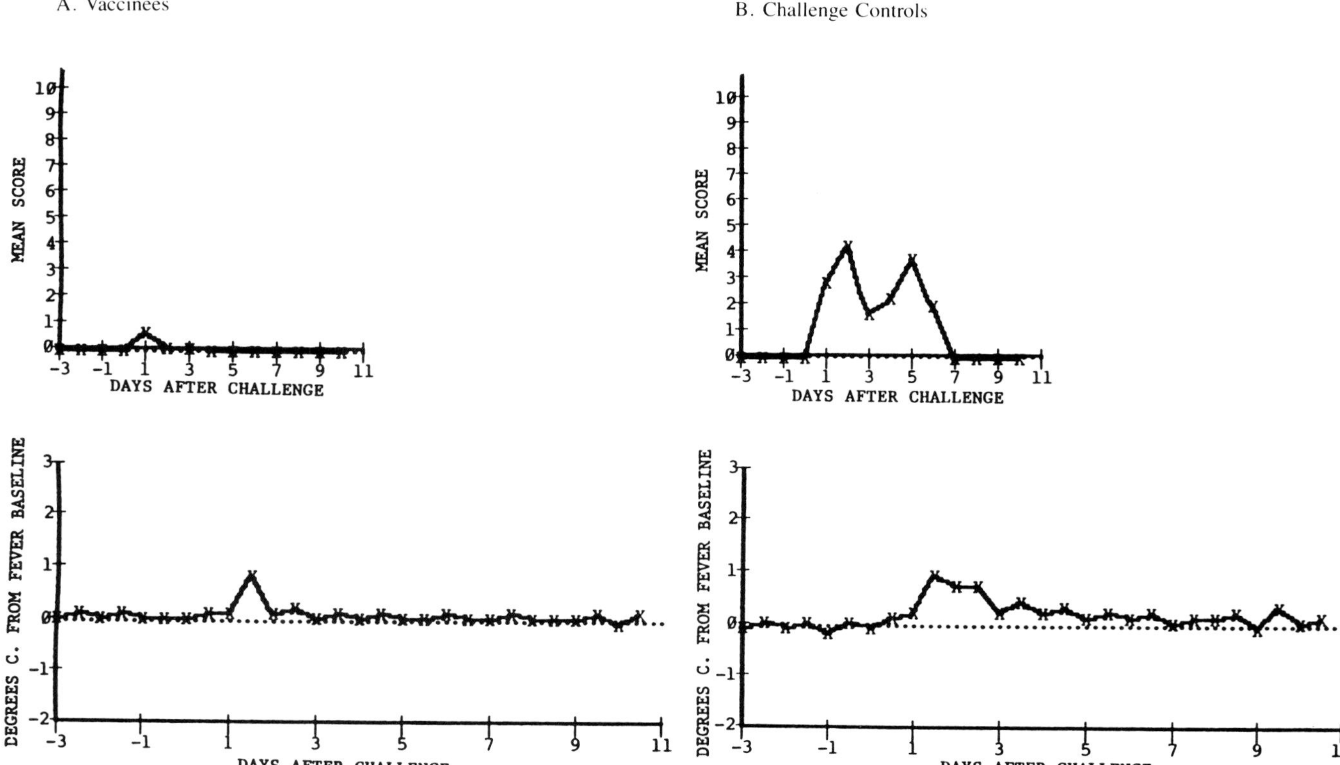

Fig. 1. Febrile response and mean scores of vaccinated and nonvaccinated ponies after virus challenge.

tion, both the vaccinees and the contact controls were challenged with A/equine/Cornell/16/74 and monitored as previously described.

Weanling study. Eight conventionally reared weanling ponies were nebulized for 3 min with a suspension of equine-1 influenza A *ts* virus 8B1. Two animals served as controls. Simultaneously with influenza vaccination, all 10 ponies were vaccinated with tetanus toxoid and equine herpesvirus-1 vaccine, as well as being wormed with an injectable medication and removed from their dams. Nasopharyngeal swabs were obtained from all animals on Days 0, 3, and 7 postinoculation, and blood samples were drawn on Days 0, 7, 12, and 21. On Day 28 postvaccination, three ponies (two vaccinees and one control) were moved into the equine isolation units and challenged by nebulization with A/equine/Cornell/16/74 virus. Serum and nasopharyngeal swab samples were obtained and assayed as in other challenge studies.

RESULTS

Response to vaccination. Forty ponies nebulized with the equine-1 influenza A *ts* virus 8B1 showed no febrile response or coughing. Some animals had mild nasal hyperemia, and occasional serous nasal discharge was noted. All maintained a bright and alert attitude and appetite was unaffected.

Virus was recovered from the nasopharyngeal swabs of 21 of 40 of the experimentally vaccinated ponies (Table 1). Virus was recovered as late as Day 6 postinoculation but most frequently on Days 2 and 3. The maximum titer of recovered virus was 3200 $TCID_{50}$/0.1 ml, but the majority of animals shed at lower levels (5 to 100 $TCID_{50}$/0.1 ml). All virus recovered from the vaccinated ponies maintained the *ts* phenotype as evidenced by its failure to grow at 39°C. Twenty-two of the vaccinated ponies developed measurable serum HI titers against A/equine/Cornell/16/74 within 30 days following vaccination. This number included six animals that were vaccinated two or three times and seroconverted after the last vaccination. The HI titers ranged from 10 to 40-80.

Response to challenge. Following challenge, 23 of the vaccinated ponies shed no challenge virus. Ten ponies shed virus only on Day 1. The titer of virus shed ranged from 0.56 $TCID_{50}$/0.1 ml (Ponies 677, 668, 669) to 1780 $TCID_{50}$/0.1 ml (Pony 722). The challenge virus recovered was shed for an average of 1.6 days postchallenge. Some animals had elevations in body temperatures, but in contrast to challenge control animals fevers were transient (Fig. 1).

Nonvaccinated control animals all shed challenge virus for at least two days and in a number of cases up to six days (average 5.2 days) postchallenge. Virus titers ranged from 32.0 (Pony 670) to 5600 $TCID_{50}$/0.1 ml (Pony 674). Scores assigned to the vaccinated and control animals were a measure of the duration and level (titer) of challenge virus shed (Fig. 1).

Five vaccinated ponies with measurable HI titers shed challenge virus for at least two days after challenge, as did 12 vaccinees with no measurable HI titers. Seventeen seropositive and six seronegative vaccinees did not shed challenge virus.

Dose response. None of the six ponies aerosolized with dilutions of the 8B1 *ts* virus developed detectable HI titers. Shedding of challenge virus was greatly reduced from that seen in unvaccinated challenge controls, being confined to the first day after challenge. The six ponies showed an elevation in temperature of 2.9-4.1°F over their highest prechallenge reading. In the two ponies receiving the highest dose of vaccine virus, $10^{4.5}$ $TCID_{50}$/0.1 ml, fevers lasted less than 12 hr postchallenge, whereas the other four animals were febrile for 36 hr. All six ponies seroconverted after challenge with A/equine/Cornell/16/74.

Ponies receiving the $10^{4.5}$ $TCID_{50}$/0.1 ml dose of vaccine seroconverted on Day 6 postchallenge, earlier than any of the challenge control animals.

Contact control studies. There was no evidence that ponies vaccinated by aerosol with 8B1 virus were capable of infecting unvaccinated ponies in close contact. No vaccine virus was shed by the contact controls, nor did they develop measurable HI antibody titers. When they were challenged with A/equine/Cornell/16/74, they reacted like the challenge control animals, shedding virus for up to six days and taking 10 days or more to develop an antibody response to challenge.

Weanling study. The weanling ponies vaccinated under field conditions and subjected to other stresses showed no clinical signs. One animal shed vaccine virus in low titer on Day 3 postinoculation. The isolate was found to retain the *ts* phenotype. None of the vaccinated weanlings or control developed measurable HI antibody. Following challenge there were no clinical signs in the two vaccinees or the control. The control pony, however, shed challenge virus from Days 1 through 7, and one of the vaccinees shed virus on Day 1 postchallenge.

DISCUSSION

A *ts* reassortant virus containing genes from both a human *ts* influenza A virus and an equine-1 influenza A virus (A/equine/Cornell/16/74) was shown to infect ponies when administered by nebulization. The *ts* virus was recovered from nasopharyngeal swabs, and HI antibody developed.

In response to challenge, animals vaccinated with the *ts* virus showed only transient, if any, elevation in body temperature, and they displayed no clinical signs. In the majority of animals, it was not possible to reisolate challenge virus. Challenge virus that was recovered was shed for an average of 1.6 days postchallenge. Nonvaccinated control ponies shed challenge virus for an average of 5.2 days postchallenge. Challenge controls showed a greater average temperature elevation than vaccinees and displayed occasional clinical signs.

The equine *ts* virus did not cause clinical signs in any of the vaccinated ponies, and all virus reisolated from the nasopharyngeal swabs of vaccinated ponies was found to retain the *ts* phenotype, as did virus back-passaged through ponies a single time and reisolated. In man, loss of the *ts* phenotype with reversion to virulence was reported following intranasal vaccination of a seronegative individual with a human A *ts* reassortant vaccine virus (Tolpin et al. 1981). We have speculated that the body temperature of the horse, being higher than that of humans, may exert a selective pressure against reversion.

Contact control studies indicate that vaccinated animals are not likely to serve as a source of infection for nonvaccinated contacts. The pony-infectious dose of *ts* virus was observed to be in the neighborhood of $10^{4.5}$ $TCID_{50}$/0.1 ml, and vaccinated animals shed *ts* virus below that amount.

Vaccination of animals under field conditions appears to be feasible. No adverse effects after vaccination were apparent in a small group of weanling ponies.

It is recognized that the interval between vaccination and challenge was short. Studies are planned to hold vaccinated ponies in a closed group for a four-month period prior to challenge. The requirement for a bivalent vaccine, containing virus of both equine-1 and -2 influenza A, is recognized. A *ts* equine-2 influenza A virus has been generated and tested, and current studies are addressing the safety, efficacy, and duration of protection of a bivalent *ts* equine influenza A vaccine.

ACKNOWLEDGMENTS

This investigation was made possible through support provided by the Harry M. Zweig Memorial Fund for Equine Research. We appreciate the technical assistance of Robert Graf, Dale Strickland, Susan Quick, Marvin Moore, James Cutler, and Nancy Heisler.

REFERENCES

Brundage-Anguish, L.J.; Holmes, D.F.; Hosier, N.T.; Murphy, B.R.; Massicott, J.G.; Appleyard, G.; and Coggins, L. (1982) Live temperature sensitive equine influenza virus vaccine: Generation of the virus and efficacy in hamsters. *Am. J. Vet. Res.* **43**, 869-74.

Burrows, R.; Goodridge, M.D.; Denyer, M.; Hutchings, G.; and Frank, C.J. (1982) Equine influenza infections in Great Britain, 1979. *Vet. Record* **110**, 494-97.

Hinshaw, V.S.; Naeve, C.W.; Webster, R.G.; Skehel, J.J. and Bryans, J. (1983) Analysis of antigenic variation in equine 2 influenza A viruses. *Bull. Wld Hlth Org.* 61, 153-58.

Ingram, D.G.; Sherman, J.; Mitchell, W.R.; Thorsen, J.; Martin, S.W.; and Barnum, D.A. (1978) The epidemiology and control of respiratory diseases at Ontario racetracks. *Proc. 4th Int. Conf. Equine Infect. Dis.*

Murphy, B.R.; Chalhub, E.G.; Nusinoff, S.R.; Kasal, J.; and Chanock, R.M. (1973) Temperature-sensitive mutants of influenza virus. III. Further characterization of the *ts*-1[E] influenza A recombinant (H_3N_2) virus in man. *J. Infect. Dis.* **128,** 479-87.

Thomson, G.R.; Mumford, J.A.; Spooner, P.R.; Burrows, R.; and Powell, D.G. (1977) The outbreak of equine influenza in England: January 1977. *Vet. Record* **100,** 465-68.

Tolpin, M.D.; Massicott, J.G.; Mullinix, M.G.; Kim, H.W.; Parrott, R.H.; Chanock, R.M.; and Murphy, B.R. (1981) Genetic factors associated with loss of the temperature-sensitive phenotype of influenza A/Alaska/77-ts-1A_2 recombinant during growth *in vivo*. *Virology* **112,** 505-17.

A Study of the Serological Response of Horses to Influenza Vaccination: Comparison of Protocols and Types of Vaccines

Eric Plateau, Aimé Jacquet, and Maurice Cheyroux

SUMMARY

During recent years, outbreaks of equine influenza have occurred in training centers in France where the animals were regularly vaccinated according to the official protocols.

Viruses isolated during these outbreaks showed some antigenic differences from the prototype A/equine/Miami/63 (H3N8) strain and they differed among themselves, but the variations were not sufficient to explain why vaccination failed to protect the horses.

Different vaccination protocols were compared using the vaccines currently available in France. It was observed that a maximum of six months between booster injections was compatible with protection. However, interpretation of the serological results varied according to the analytical techniques used.

The authors also studied the immunological response to different vaccines recently introduced in France.

INTRODUCTION

Immunization against equine influenza virus is still unsatisfactory, many years after the first vaccines were proposed. Equine influenza epidemics occur periodically, and clinical, virological, and serological surveys indicate that outbreaks occur at any time of the year.

At the end of 1978 a widespread epidemic occurred in France and the United Kingdom (Burrows et al. 1981; Cruciere & Plateau 1979) and extended to most other European countries (Klingeborn, Rockborn & Dinter 1980; Van Oirschott et al. 1981). In France, sporadic outbreaks were reported in 1980, 1981, 1983, 1984 (Plateau *et al.*, 1984) and they have been observed every year since. Although serological examination of unvaccinated populations has proven that equine-1 influenza A is still present, all the viruses isolated during the major outbreaks were related to equine-2 influenza A. The outbreaks struck not only young horses in training centers but also adult populations (riding horses, show jumpers) previously polyvaccinated according to the protocols recommended by the manufacturers. The lack of protection was judged to result either from antigenic drift or from deficiences in the immunogenicity of the vaccines.

Antigenic drift among equine-2 influenza A viruses has been reported repeatedly (Burrows et al. 1981; Pereira et al. 1982; Burrows & Denyer 1982; Van Oirschott et al. 1981; Plateau, Cruciere & Gayot 1983). The practical importance of this drift was considered minimal by Burrows and colleagues (1982), who examined strains isolated in the United Kingdom, and a similar conclusion was reached following the study of 20 strains isolated in France from 1963 to 1985. When the strains were compared by cross-hemagglutination inhibition (HI) reaction, the degree of similarity to the reference strain A/equine/Miami/63(H3N8) was lower than 50% for only five strains, isolated in 1978, 1979, 1980, 1981, and 1984. Strains corresponding more closely to the reference strain were isolated during the same epidemic from vaccinated animals with clinical signs of disease (Jacquet et al. 1986; Cruciere et al. 1987). The introduction of A/equine/Fontainebleau/1/79(H3N8) strain in vaccines after 1980 did not prevent the recurrence of influenza. Recently a vaccine including the A/equine/Joinville/1/78(H3N8) strain has become available in France, but we do not yet have sufficient data to evaluate its efficacy under field conditions.

These elements suggest that the way to improve protection is to increase the antigenicity and immunogenicity of the vaccines, rather than to change vaccine antigens frequently.

Equine-2 influenza A is known to be less antigenic than equine-1 influenza A, and it does not induce a long-term serological response even after natural infection. If the response to vaccination remains low, improvement in immune response could be expected from closely repeated vaccinations.

The purpose of this study was to compare different vaccination protocols among horses that had never been vaccinated and also among horses that had been vaccinated regularly. The antibody response to five different vaccines was also compared.

MATERIALS AND METHODS

Experiment 1. Among the 54 horses selected from the Royal Guard of Morocco, 40 had never been vaccinated and 14 had last been vaccinated in 1979. After primary vaccination (two injections at a one-month interval), three groups of 11 horses each were revaccinated at two, three, or six months. Another

Plateau: Ministère de l'Agriculture, Direction Générale de l'Alimentation, Services Vétérinaires de la Santé et de la Protection Animale, Laboratoire Central de Recherches Vétérinaires, B.P. 67, 22 rue Pierre Curie, 94703 Maisons-Alfort Cedex, France. Jacquet: Fédération Nationale des Sociétés de Courses, Bureau de Biologie Equine, 11 rue du Cirque, 75382 Paris Cedex 08, France. Cheyroux: Institut Pasteur, 28 rue du Docteur Roux, 75724 Paris Cedex 15, France.

group was not revaccinated and a control group remained unvaccinated at anytime.

Experiment 2. Forty horses six to 13 years old were selected at the French Centre Sportif d'Equitation Militaire (C.S.E.M.). They had been vaccinated twice a year for several years, receiving a total number of vaccinations ranging from five to 13. The last injection had taken place six months previously. During the experiment, 10 horses were revaccinated every two months (Group 1); 10 every three months (Group 2); ten after six months (Group 3); the remaining 10 received a double dose of vaccine every three months (Group 4).

Experiment 3. Six two-year-old ponies from the Laboratoire Central de Recherches Vétérinaires (L.C.R.V.), which had been isolated from other animals since they were one year old, were experimentally infected with A/equine/Fontainebleau/1/79. They were challenged intranasally after 150 days with homologous virus and at Day 210 with the heterologous A/equine/Joinville/1/78 strain. At the same time, this strain was used to challenge three-year-old nonvaccinated horses. Ponies and horses were subject to regular clinical, virological, and serological examination.

Experiment 4. Fifty-eight horses from the C.S.E.M., all having been vaccinated twice a year, were divided into groups to receive one of five commercial vaccines at the regularly scheduled time. Five groups were vaccinated in this manner, and one group served as controls. The horses were serologically checked before revaccination and one month after.

Vaccines. Five different vaccines were used in the various experiments (Table 1).

Viruses. A/equine/Prague/1/56(H7N7) and A/equine/Miami/1/63(H3N8) were obtained from the American Type Culture Collection (Rockville, Md.). A/equine/Fontainebleau/1/79(H3N8) was given by Dr. A. Moraillon (Moraillon 1980). A/equine/Joinville/1/78(H3N8) was isolated at the L.C.R.V. (Plateau et al. 1979).

Serology. HI tests were performed after treatment of the sera by heat, kaolin 25%, and chick red blood cells, as previously described (Plateau 1983). Influenza antigen was used both without treatment and after ether treatment (Fontaine 1971).

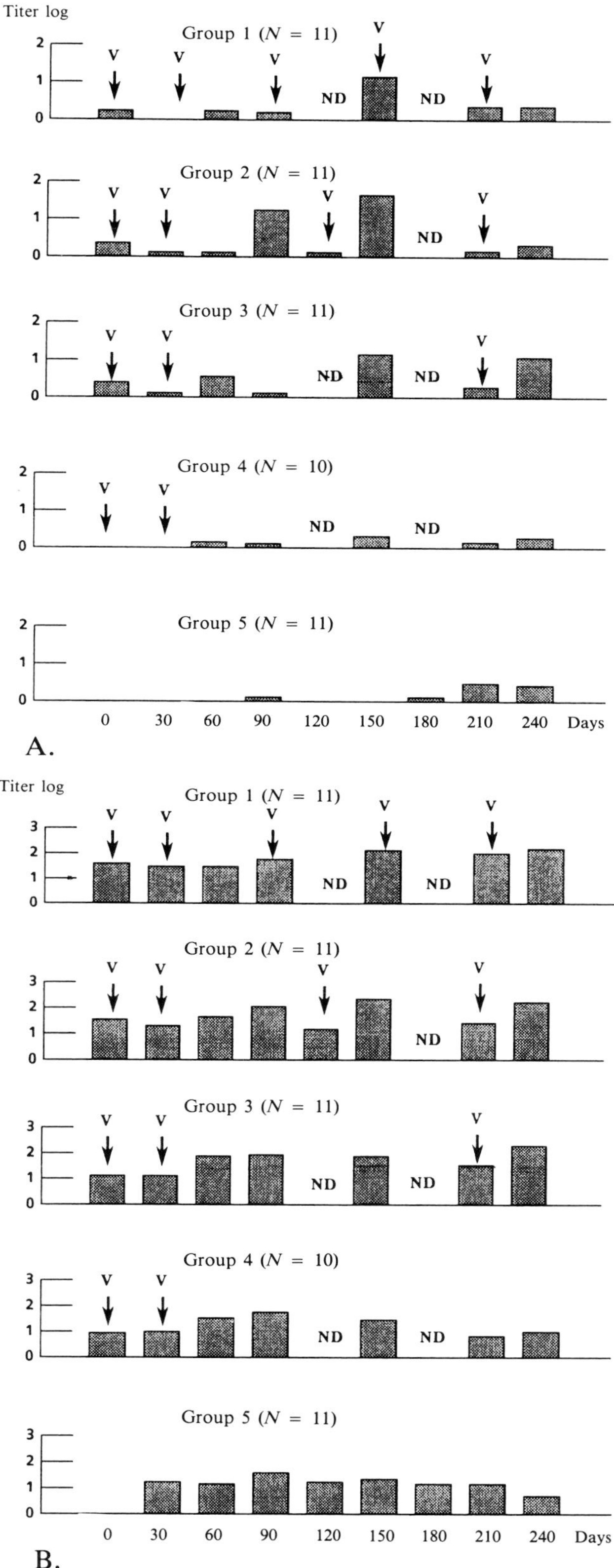

Fig. 1. Mean HI titers against A/equine/Miami/1/63 strain: A. Untreated antigen. B. Ether-treated antigen. V = vaccination; ND = no sample examined.

RESULTS

Only the results concerning the equine-2 influenza A are presented.

Experiment 1. Results of HI tests (mean values) are presented in Figure 1A (untreated antigens) and 1B (treated antigens). Forty animals had a titer lower than 1.6, and three had a titer equal to 1.6 before vaccination (Day 0) when

Table 1. Compositions of vaccines and used

Experiment	Vaccine	Antigenic composition	Adjuvant
1	A	Equine-1 and -2 influenza A	Aluminum hydroxide
2	A	Equine-1 and -2 influenza A	Aluminum hydroxide
4	A	Equine-1 and -2 influenza A	Aluminum hydroxide
	B	Equine-1 and -2 influenza A	Oil
	C	Equine-1 influenza A; Equine-2 influenza A, strains 1 and 2	Aluminum hydroxide
	D	Equine-1 and -2 influenza A	Alumimun phosphate
	E	Equid herpesvirus-1; reovirus 1 and 3; A/equine/Prague/1/56, Miami/1/63, and Fontainebleau/1/79	Aluminum hydroxide

measured with untreated antigen (m = 0.17). With treated antigen, 15 animals were over the limit of 1.9 (m = 1.30). After primary vaccination, the titers measured with untreated antigens remained low even for the groups receiving booster vaccination at two or three months' interval. In contrast, the response measured with treated antigen could be considered satisfactory for Groups 1, 2, and 3.

Experiment 2. Results of HI tests (mean values) are presented in Figure 2*A* (untreated antigens) and 2*B* (treated antigens). Most of the horses had HI titers below 1.6 log before vaccination when measured with untreated antigens A/equine/Miami/1/63 (m = 0.97) and A/equine/Fontainebleau/1/79 (m = 0.69), while the majority had titers close to 1.9 with treated antigens Miami/1/63 (m = 1.9) and Fontainebleau/1/79 (m = 2.07). According to the results with untreated antigens, only protocols 1, 2, and 4 can be considered satisfactory, while the results obtained with ether-treated antigen indicated that a six-month interval (Group 3) could be considered adequate.

An outbreak of equine-2 influenza A occurred in the C.S.E.M. during Experiment 2 around Day 180. A group of young, recently introduced horses and a group of annually vaccinated adults, none included in the experiment, became infected. In contrast, no horses that were part of Experiment 2, even vaccinated six months earlier, were affected.

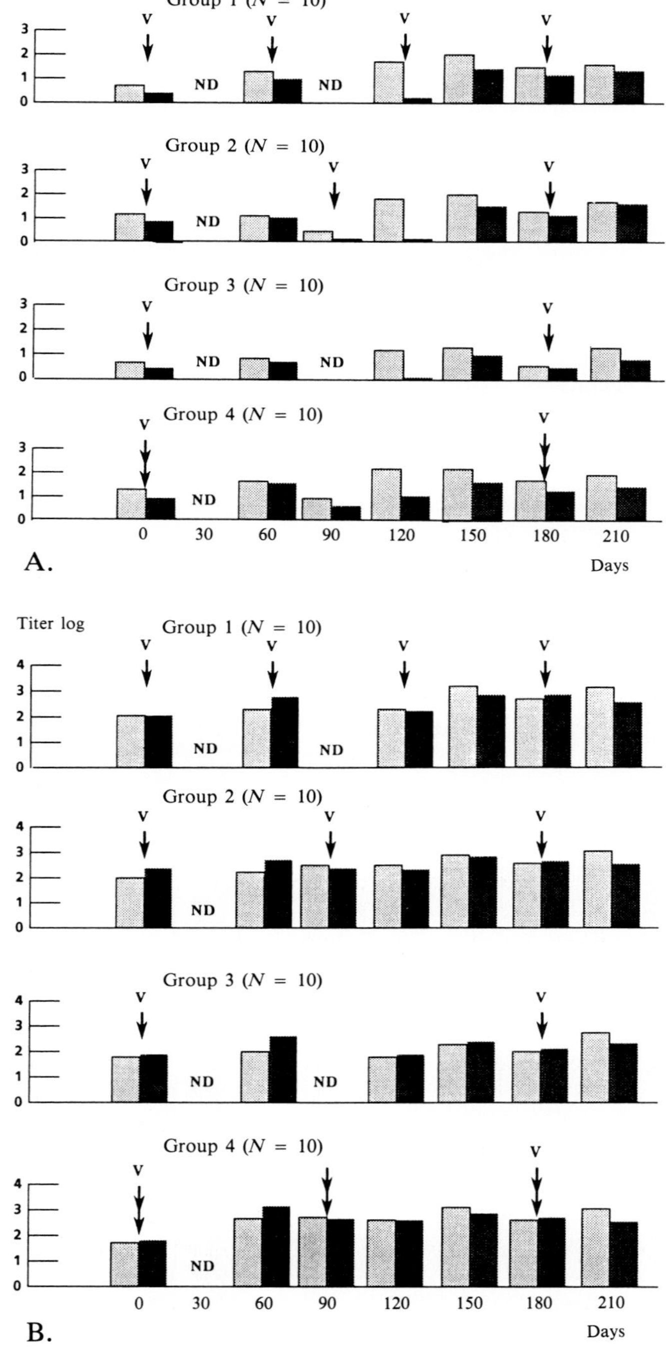

Fig. 2. Mean HI titers against A/equine/Miami/1/63 (*light shading*) and A/equine/Fontainebleau/1/79 (*dark shading*): A. Untreated antigen. B. Ether-treated antigen. V = vaccination; ND = no sample examined.

Experiment 3. Results of HI tests (mean values) are presented in Figure 3. When the six ponies were rechallenged at 150 days with A/equine/Fontainebleau/79, five had a titer of 1.6 log but all developed an anamnestic HI response with no clinical signs. To determine whether antigenic drift would result in clinical disease, three horses were challenged two months later with A/equine/Joinville/1/78 virus. Although their titers were below 1.6 log, they did not exhibit any clinical signs. No anamnestic response was detected, although the pathogenicity of this strain was found to cause clinical disease following the experimental infection of three unprimed control horses (Fig. 3).

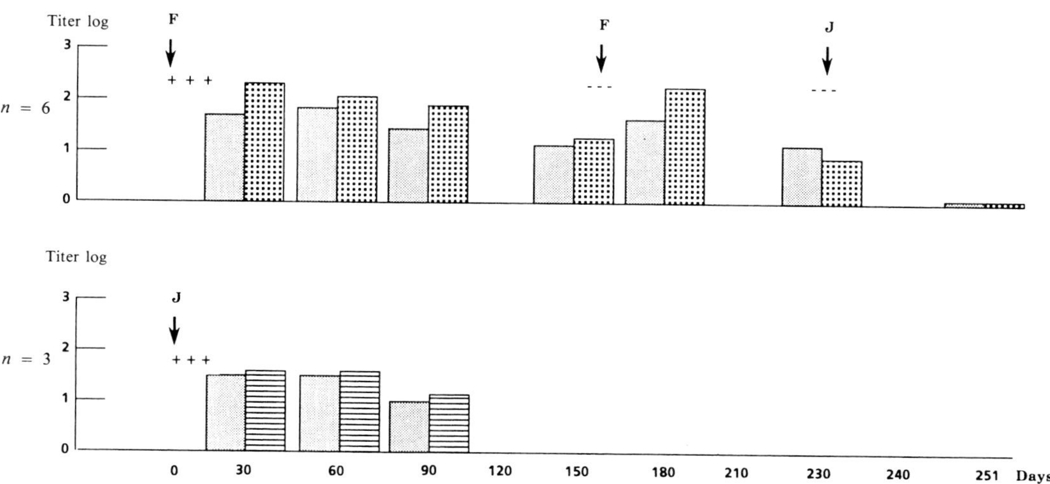

Fig. 3. Serological and clinical response to intranasal infection and challenge by: F, A/equine/Fontainebleau/1/79: J. A/equine/Joinville/1/78. Clinical signs: + + + = present; − − − = absent. HI titers (untreated antigens) against: Miami/1/63, *stippled bars;* Fontainebleau/1/79, *checkered bars;* Joinville/1/78, *ruled bars.*

Experiment 4. Results of the HI test (untreated antigens), before vaccination and 30 days after inoculation with five types of vaccine, are presented in Figure 4. Vaccine A (also used in Experiments 1 and 2) was the least efficient, since only four animals out of nine had a significant increase in titer. Vaccine B was considered the most efficient, as it was followed by a significant increase in HI titer in all the horses.

DISCUSSION

Evaluation of the potency of influenza vaccines is somewhat moot among horses that have demonstrable levels of antibody by way of previous vaccination or natural infection. The response of such horses is anamnestic and subject to individual variations. Under field conditions it is not possible, at least in France and probably in most other countries, to assemble large populations of adult Standardbred and Thoroughbred horses free of previous contact with the virus or the vaccine. Despite vaccination, influenza outbreaks are observed every year in almost every class and breed of horse. Epidemiological observations indicate that the disease is inevitably more acute in nonvaccinated than vaccinated populations. The few groups of horses that regularly escape infection are either kept in isolation or are exposed but vaccinated three or more times a year, according to the risk of mixing with other populations during training, competition, and transportation. The result can be "overvaccination," which is difficult to justify.

During the study it was possible to distinguish between high-risk or susceptible populations, including vaccinated animals or those lacking clinical signs, and low-risk or resistant populations—those either vaccinated frequently or previously exposed to infection.

Animals of Experiment 1 belonged to the high-risk category, and animals of Experiments 2 and 4 were low-risk. Even though the horses in Experiment 1 were not completely seronegative, there is an obvious difference between their titers and the titers of horses in Experiments 2 and 4. One way of evaluating the level of protection is to measure seroconversion after vaccination or challenge. Postvaccination seroconversions are usually measured by the level of circulating HI antibodies. Since the titers with untreated antigens are generally low against equine-2 influenza A, antigens are usually treated with a detergent such as ether, Tween 80, or a combination (Berlin et al. 1963). Using treated antigens, many animals considered free of contact with the virus were revealed as having been inapparently infected, as was the case in Experiment 1. Treated antigens also make it possible to detect weak responses following primary vaccination.

HI titers measured with treated antigens can vary from batch to batch of antigens (Burrows et al. 1981). Nevertheless, the titer generally considered protective is 1.6 log with untreated antigen (Bryans et al. 1966) and 1.9 log with ether-treated antigens (Lucam et al. 1974). Other seriological methods of measuring the antibody response, such as single radial hemolysis (SRH), are considered more sensitive than HI (Mumford et al. 1983; Fontaine et al. 1971). The SRH test is reliable and reproducible but must be carefully standardized between laboratories and, like the HI test, measures only circulating antibody.

The results from Experiment 2 indicated that in the case of untreated antigens HI titers lower than 1.6 log were protective following a six-month interval between booster vaccinations. Vaccination with double doses or vaccination every two or three months was not justified for horses already polyvaccinated, since over a certain limit the response was not dose-dependent. Results from Experiment 3 suggested that for untreated antigen horses with titers were protected, even against challenge with heterologous virus, and that antigenic drift was not a reason for protection failure in primed animals.

It is questionable whether the immunity induced by natural exposure is identical to vaccinal immunity. In particular, local cellular and humoral immunity develops in the respiratory tract after contact with the virus, and neutralization of the

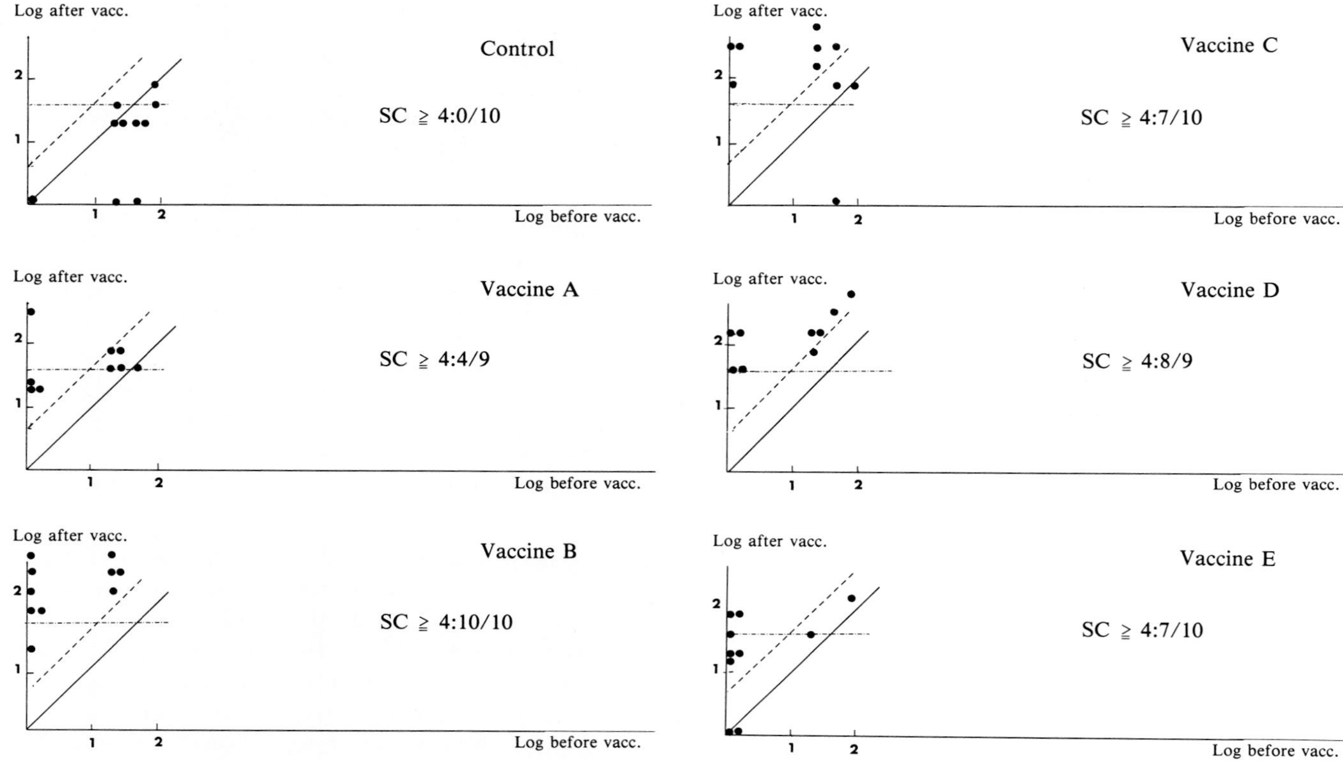

Fig. 4. HI antibodies against untreated A/equine/Miami/1/63 30 days after injection of one dose of vaccine *A, B, C, D,* or *E*. SC>4 = number of animals for which HI titer was multiplied by 4 or more.

virus in situ may explain the absence of a serological response following challenge with A/equine/Joinville/1/78. These mechanisms were investigated by Rouse and Ditchfield (1970a, b), who demonstrated that most horses without nasal neutralizing antibodies were susceptible to challenge even when they were HI-positive. They reported that neutralizing antibodies did not persist beyond 30 days after natural infection, but this does not fully agree with our observations on the duration of natural immunity.

Previous studies (Jacquet et al. 1986) indicated that the high levels of antibody induced by Vaccine B persisted for at least 12 months. Even if field trials cannot resolve the determination of an absolute protection level, they will be useful for veterinarians and their clients and for scientists in charge of licensing vaccines.

ACKNOWLEDGMENTS

We want to thank Dr. H. Marzak, Dr. Moussaoui Souad, Dr. J.M. Krawiecky, and Dr. Sylvie Gerard for their active participation in this study.

REFERENCES

Berlin, B.S.; McQueen, J.L.; Minuse, E.; and Davenport, F.M. (1963) A method for increasing the sensitivity of hemagglutination inhibition test with equine influenza virus. *Virology* **21,** 665-66.

Bryans, J.T.; Doll, E.R.; Wilson, J.C.; and McCollum, W.H. (1966) Immunisation for equine influenza. *J. Am. Vet. Med. Assoc.* **48,** 413-16.

Burrows, R. and Denyer, H. (1982) Antigenic properties of some equine influenza viruses. *Virology* **73,** 15-24.

Burrows, R.; Denyer, H.; Goodridge, D.; and Hamilton, F. (1981) Field and laboratory studies of equine influenza virus isolated in 1979. *Vet. Rec.* **109,** 353-56.

Cruciere, C., and Plateau, E. (1979) L'epizootie de grippe equine 1978-1979. Probleme du diagnostic et de la protection vaccinale. *Bull. Soc. Vét. Pratique, Fr.* **63,** 191-97.

Cruciere, C.; Guillemain, M.C.; Rosetto, A.; and Plateau, E. (1987) Production of monoclonal antibodies against equine influenza: application to a comparative study of various strains of the vaccine. *Ann. Rech. Vet.* Accepted for publication.

Fontaine, M. (1971) La grippe du cheval. *Pratique Vet. Equine* **2,** 9-18.

Jacquet, A.; Plateau, E.; Cheyroux, M.; Brun, A.; Devaux, B.; Krawiecky, J.M.; and Boutte, J. (1986) Etude de l'immunite antigrippale naturelle et post vaccinale chex le cheval. *C.R. 12e Journee d'Etude du C.E.R.E.O.P.A.*, pp. 115-27.

Klingeborn, B.; Rockborn, G.; and Dinter, Z. (1980) Significant antigenic drift within the influenza equi subtype in Sweden. *Vet. Rec.* **106,** 363-64.

Lucam, F.; Fedida, M.; Dannacher, G.; Coudert, M.; and Peillon, M. (1974) La grippe equine, caracteres de la maladie expérimentale et de l'immunité post-vaccinale. *Rev. Med. Vet.* **125,** 1273-93.

Moraillon, A., and Moraillon, R. (1980) Grippe equine 78-79; actualités. *Pratique Vet. Equine* **12,** 85.

Mumford, J.; Wood, J.M.; Scott, A.M.; Folkers, C.; and Schild, G.C. (1983) Studies with inactivated equine influenza vaccine: 2 protection against experimental infection with influenza virus A/equine/Newmarket/79 (H3N8). *J. Hyg. Camb.* **90,** 385-95.

Pereira, H.G.; Takimoto, S.; Piega, N.S.; Riberiro, D.O.; and Valle, L.A. (1982) Antigenic variation of equine (Heq2Neq2) influenza virus. *Bull. Wld. Hlth. Org.* **47**, 465-69.

Plateau, E.; Cruciere, C.; Virat, J.; and Benazet, P. (1979) Grippe equine. Isolement, caractérisation et étude sérologique dans divers foyers au cours de l'epizootie 1978-1979. *Bull. Acad. Vet. Fr.* **52,** 184-94.

Plateau, E.; Cruciére, C.; and Gayot, G. (1983) Dérive antigenique d'une souche de virus influenza equi isolée en France au cours de l'hiver 1978-1979. *Ann. Rech. Vet.* **14**, 71-77.

Plateau, E.; Cruciére, C.; Jacquet, A.; and Cheyroux, M. (1984) Mise au point et recherches an cours nur l'evolution epidemiologique et antigenique de la grippe equine en France. *Bull. Soc. Vet. Pratique, France* **68,** 345-52.

Rouse, B.T., and Ditchfield, W.J.B. (1970a) The response of ponies to myxovirus influenza A Equi 2: III, the protective effect of serum and nasal antibody against experimental challenge. *Res. Vet. Sci.* **11,** 503-7.

———. (1970b) The response of ponies to myxovirus influenza A Equi 2:I. serum and nasal antibody titre following exposure. *Can J. Comp. Med.* **34,** 1-6.

Van Oirschott, J.T.; Masurel, N.; Huffels, A.D.N.H.; and Anker, W.J. (1981) Equine influenza in the Netherlands during the winter of 1978-1979, antigenic drift of the A Equi 2 virus. *Vet. Q.* **3**, 80-83.

Herpes

Equid Herpesvirus-1 Glycoprotein 13 (gp13): Epitope Analysis, Gene Structure, and Expression in *E. coli*

George P. Allen, Michelle R. Yeargan, and Linda D. Coogle

SUMMARY

The virion of equid herpesvirus-1 (EHV-1) contains six high-abundance glycoprotein antigens. One of these EHV-1 glycoproteins, gp13, is presumed on the basis of genetic colinearity, to be the functional and structural homolog of a major glycoprotein (gC-like glycoproteins) shown to be a dominant antigen in the host immune response to several other herpesviruses. In this study, the methods of monoclonal antibody analysis, expression cloning in *E. coli*, and DNA sequencing were applied toward the antigenic and molecular characterization of gp13, the major, gC-like glycoprotein of EHV-1. An immunoaffinity chromatography system was developed for the purification of EHV-1 gp13 as an antigen against which to screen hybridoma supernatants for gp13-specific monoclonal antibodies. Forty-two monoclonal antibodies directed against EHV-1 gp13 were constructed in this manner and used to characterize the epitopes of the viral antigen.

Eighty-five percent of the estimated 16 gp13 epitopes were subtype-specific, 20% elicited neutralizing antibody, and 90% demonstrated intrasubtypic strain variation. Some gp13 epitopes were highly conserved among EHV-1 isolates, while others demonstrated extensive sequence diversity. Laboratory-passaged strains and members of the 1B electropherotype of EHV-1 were antigenically distant from prototype isolates in regard to gp13 epitopes. A recombinant expression library of the EHV-1 BamHI h fragment, which contains the gene for gp13, was constructed in the lambda phage vector λgt11 and screened with all 42 monoclonal antibodies for expression of gp13 sequences. Thirty-six recombinant phage expressing EHV-1 gp13 epitopes were identified and plaque-purified. All 36 phage expressed a fusion protein that reacted with the same subset of 15 monoclonal antibodies, indicating the existence of at least one immunodominant domain of gp13 comprised of continuous epitopes. The partial nucleotide sequence of the 6-kb BamHI-EcoRI restriction fragment containing the coding sequences for gp13 was determined. A region of amino acid sequence homology to herpes simplex virus and pseudorabies virus gC glycoproteins was identified. The data provide basic information on the antigenic structure of a major glycoprotein of EHV-1.

INTRODUCTION

EHV-1 is an alphaherpesvirus of economic importance to the horse breeding industry (Bryans 1980; Bryans & Allen 1986a). Associated with abortion, respiratory tract disease, and encephalomyelopathy, EHV-1 infections are worldwide in distribution and occur in most horses before they reach one year of age (Allen & Bryans 1986). Immunity to the herpesvirus, resulting from either natural infection or vaccination, is both weak and short-lived (Bryans 1969). Horses may become reinfected at frequent intervals throughout their lifetimes despite the implementation of programs of intensive vaccination (Bryans & Allen 1986b). As a consequence, EHV-1 continues to be a cause of significant, perennial loss to the purebred horse industry. The need for improvement in the control of EHV-1 disease and for an increased understanding of the horse's protective immune responses to the virus is evident. Our approach to this research problem has been to identify and characterize the antigens of EHV-1 that stimulate the immune defenses of the horse.

The surface glycoproteins of herpesviruses are the molecules that interact with the immune system of the host and therefore play a pivotal role in either inducing or suppressing the protective immune response (Spear 1985). EHV-1 has been reported to synthesize several major and minor glycoprotein antigens that are localized in the viral envelope as well as the plasma membrane of EHV-1–infected cells (Allen & Bryans 1986; Turtinen & Allen 1982). The coding sequences for the six high-abundance glycoproteins of EHV-1 have recently been mapped on the viral genome (Allen & Yeargan 1987). Three of the major EHV-1 glycoproteins (gp13, 14, and 17/18) are encoded by sequences genetically colinear with those for major glycoproteins of several other herpesviruses (gC-, gB-, and gE-like glycoproteins, respectively). Other major glycoproteins of EHV-1 (gp2, 10, and 21/22a) appear, from the information currently available, to be unique to this herpesvirus of the horse.

EHV-1 gp13, one of the most abundant glycoproteins in the EHV-1 virion (Fig. 1), demonstrates a consistent and marked difference in electrophoretic mobility (i.e., apparent molecular weight) between the two subtypes of EHV-1 (96 versus 110 kdal) and can be used for unambiguous differen-

Department of Veterinary Science, University of Kentucky, Lexington, Kentucky 40546-0099. Published as paper No. 87-4-257 of the Kentucky Agricultural Experiment Station with approval by the Director.

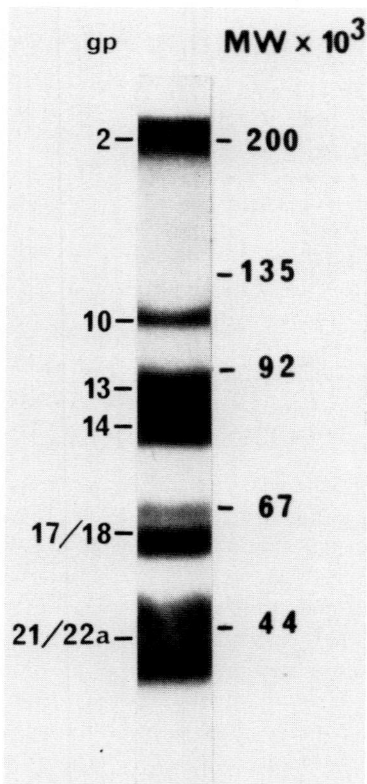

Fig. 1. Autoradiographic images of electrophoretically separated [^{3}H]glucosamine-labeled virion glycoproteins of EHV-1 subtype 1; *left*, designations of six families of high-abundance glycoproteins.

tiation of the two virus subtypes (Allen & Bryans 1986). On the basis of the recently demonstrated genomic location of the gene encoding EHV-1 gp13 at 0.114-0.148 map units (Allen & Yeargan 1987), it seems reasonable to predict that gp13 is the EHV-1 structural homolog of herpes simplex virus glycoprotein gC (Frink et al. 1983).

In eliciting protective immunity, the importance of the molecular homologs of EHV-1 gp13 present in other herpesviruses (i.e., gC-like glycoproteins) has been well documented. The glycoprotein gC of herpes simplex virus, for example, has been shown to be the immunodominant antigen for eliciting cytotoxic T-cell responses in mice (Glorioso et al. 1985; Rosenthal et al. 1987). Likewise, the majority of the virus-neutralizing activity against pseudorabies herpesvirus (PRV) present in convalescent serum of PRV-infected swine was demonstrated to be directed against the PRV counterpart of EHV-1 gp13 (Ben-Porat et al. 1986).

MATERIALS AND METHODS

Virus and cell culture. Both subtype 1 and subtype 2 strains of EHV-1 were propagated in equine dermal cells (KyED) as described previously (Turtinen et al. 1981). Extracellular virus was concentrated from EHV-1–infected cell cultures and purified by isopycnic banding in potassium tartrate gradients.

Hybridoma technology. The methods for producing monoclonal antibodies to the glycoprotein antigens of EHV-1 were those described by Yeargan, Allen, and Bryans (1985). Antibody-producing hybridomas were generated by the fusion of FOX-NY mouse myeloma cells (Taggart & Samloff 1983) with spleen cells from RBF/Dn mice (Jackson Laboratory, Bar Harbor, Maine) that had been immunized with purified EHV-1 virions. Hybrids were selected in growth medium containing adenine, aminopterin, and thymidine. Hybridoma culture supernatants were screened for antibody to specific EHV-1 glycoproteins with a dot-blot immunoassay. Hybrids secreting monoclonal antibodies specific for EHV-1 gp13 were cloned twice by limiting dilution. The clones were then expanded and inoculated into pristane (Aldrich) primed BALB/c mice at a concentration of 2×10^7 cells/mouse for preparation of antibody-containing ascites fluid.

Dot-blot immunoassay. The screening assay for identifying hybridomas secreting antibodies to EHV-1 gp13 was an enzyme-linked immunosorbent assay–based, avidin-biotin amplified dot-blot immunoassay performed with purified gp13 antigen applied as 1-μl dots (25 ng/dot) to the nitrocellulose bottoms of 96-well plates (Millititer HA plates; Millipore Corp., Bedford, Mass.). After blocking of nonspecific sites and incubation of the nitrocellulose-bound antigen with hybridoma supernatants, the plates were washed by filtration and then incubated in succession with biotinylated goat anti-mouse IgG, avidin-biotinylated peroxidase complex (Vectastain ABC reagent; Vector Laboratory, Burlingame, Calif.) and peroxidase substrate (4-chloro-1-napthol/H_2O_2). Control sera consisted of mouse polyclonal antiserum to EHV-1, preimmune mouse serum, FOX-NY myeloma supernatants, known anti-gp13 monoclonal antibody, and monoclonal antibodies directed against other EHV-1 glycoproteins. Control antigens in each assay plate included intact virions; a mixture of EHV-1 glycoproteins Nos. 10, 14, 18, and 22a; and no-antigen wells.

Immunoaffinity chromatography. A monoclonal antibody (14H7) directed against EHV-1 gp13 (Allen and Yeargan 1987) was purified from mouse ascites fluid by Protein A-Sepharose chromatography (MAPS system; Biorad, Richmond, Calif.) and then covalently linked to CNBr-activated Sepharose (Pharmacia, Piscataway, N.J.) to form an antibody-immunoaffinity column specific for gp13 (Dalchau & Fabre, 1982). Detergent extracts of EHV-1 virions were prepared by incubating 15 mg of zonal-purified virus with 1% sodium desoxycholate for 1 hr at 4°C. The mixture was centrifuged at 15,000 g for 30 min, and the detergent-extracted proteins present in the supernatant were slowly passed through the 14H7 antibody affinity column. After extensive washing of the column with 0.1% desoxycholate followed by phosphate-buffered saline (PBS) without detergent, the bound material (gp13) was eluted with 1 M propionic acid and then neutralized with a solution of 2 M Tris-HC1 (pH 9).

Microneutralization assay. EHV-1 neutralizing activity of the monoclonal antibodies present in hybridoma supernatants was assayed by microneutralization in 24-well culture plates. Cell-free virus (100 $TCID_{50}$ units) was incubated for 30 min at 37°C with undiluted antibody in the presence or absence of guinea pig complement. The virus-antibody mixture was then added to monolayer cultures of KyED cells in 24-well plates. The formation of viral cytopathic effect (CPE) in the culture wells was assessed after five days by microscopic examination, and antibodies that completely prevented EHV-1–induced CPE were considered to be neutralizing in nature.

Plaque-reduction assays for neutralizing antibody were performed as described previously (Turtinen et al. 1981).

Enzyme-linked immunosorbent assay (ELISA). Gradient-purified virions of EHV-1 at a concentration of 40 μg/ml viral protein in coating buffer (carbonate buffer, pH 9.0) were allowed to adsorb overnight at 4°C onto polystyrene 96-well microassay plates (Nunc, Roskilde, Denmark). After blocking for 1 hr at room temperature with coating buffer containing 5% (v/v) goat serum, the plates were washed with PBS–0.05% Tween-20. Dilutions of monoclonal antibody were then added to the antigen-coated, blocked wells and incubated for 1 hr at 37°C. After washing, the plates were similarly incubated with peroxidase-conjugated goat anti-mouse IgG and washed again, and the peroxidase substrate, O-phenylenediamine in citrate/H_2O_2 buffer, was added. The reaction was stopped 30 min later with 2 M H_2SO_4, and the A_{495} of each well was measured with an ELISA plate reader (Biotek, Winooski, Vt.).

DNA sequencing. The 7.5-kb BamHI h fragment of EHV-1 DNA was cloned into the plasmid pIBI24 (IBI, Inc., New Haven, Conn.). The recombinant vector was cleaved at the unique EcoRI site within the h fragment to yield a 6-kb BamHI-EcoRI insert, which was subsequently subcloned into M13mp18 and -mp19 for sequencing. The sequencing strategy was based on the procedure developed by Henikoff (1984), in which an ordered set of overlapping deletion subclones of the insert DNA to be sequenced are generated with exonuclease III. Sequencing reactions, with ^{35}S-dATP as the radiolabeled deoxynucleotide, were carried out using the dideoxy chain–termination procedure of Sanger, Nicklen, and Coulson (1977). A 17-nucleotide universal primer (IBI, Inc.) was used for sequencing M13 inserts, and other primers (New England Biolabs, Beverly, Mass.) were used for sequencing EHV-1 DNA cloned into λgt11. Recording and analysis of the DNA sequence data were done with the assistance of the Intelligenetics sequence analysis software programs available through the BIONET network.

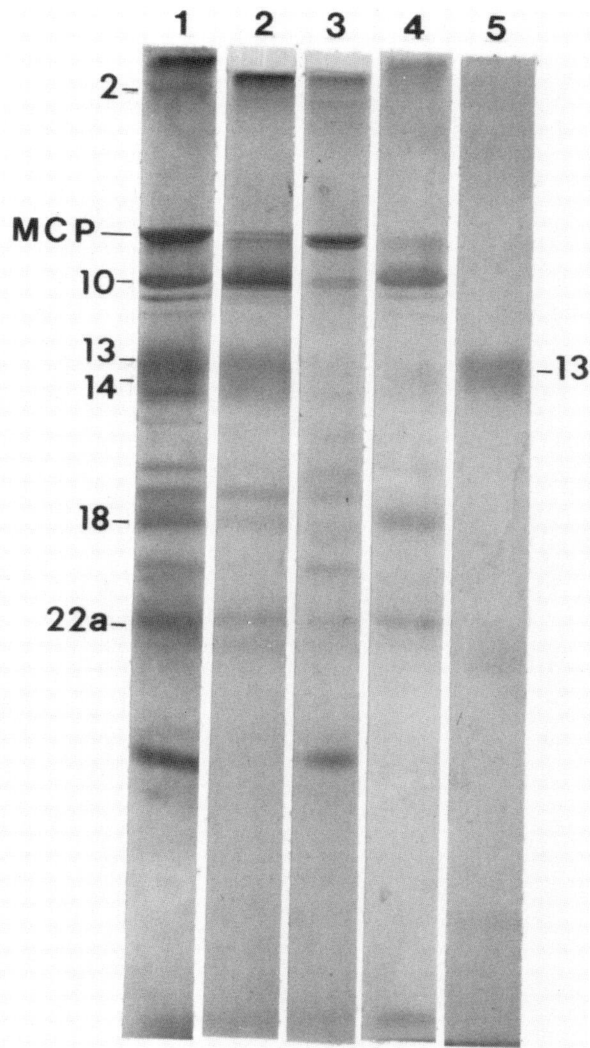

Fig. 2. Sodium dodecyl sulfate–polyacrylamide gel electrophoresis analysis of samples from each step in purification of EHV-1 gp13 by immunoaffinity chromatography. Aliquots of each sample were dissociated and electrophoresed on 7.5% polyacrylamide slab gels, developed with a silver stain (Biorad). The six major envelope glycoproteins and the major capsid protein of EHV-1 are identified at left. *Lane 1*, starting material for purification of gp13 (purified virions); *Lane 2*, material loaded onto monoclonal antibody affinity column (supernatant after incubation of EHV-1 virions with 1% sodium desoxycholate followed by centrifugation); *Lane 3*, pellet after incubation of EHV-1 virions with detergent followed by centrifugation; *Lane 4*, material not bound to affinity column; *Lane 5*, aliquot of pool of affinity column fractions containing material reacting with anti-gp13 monoclonal antibody (fractions 11-14; see *Fig. 3*) after elution of the loaded and washed column with 1 M propionic acid.

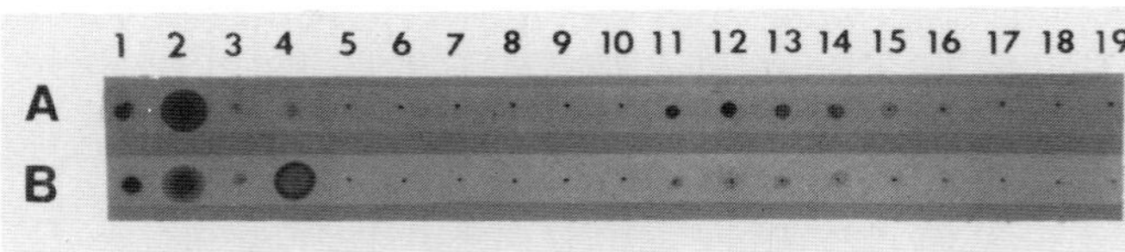

Fig. 3. Dot-blot immunoassay for EHV-1 gp13 in fractions collected from monoclonal antibody-Sepharose affinity column used for purification of gp13. Aliquots of each column fraction were blotted as duplicate, 1-µl dots onto two strips of nitrocellulose. After drying, strips were blocked with 10% goat serum in PBS and then incubated, in succession, with either: *A*, an anti-gp13 monoclonal antibody, or *B*, an anti-gp14 monoclonal, biotinylated goat antimouse IgG, avidin-biotinylated peroxidase complex, and peroxidase substrate. *Dot 1*, starting material for gp13 purification (purified EHV-1 virions); *dot 2*, material applied to immunoaffinity column (supernatant after incubation of EHV-1 virions with desoxycholate followed by centrifugation); *dot 3*, pellet after incubation of EHV-1 virions with desoxycholate followed by centrifugation; *dot 4*, material not bound to column; *dots 5-19*, 0.5-ml fractions collected from column after elution with 1 M propionic acid (pH 2). Fractions 11-14 were pooled, neutralized, dialyzed against PBS, and used as gp13 antigen for screening hybridoma supernatants.

Expression cloning in E. coli. Random DNA fragments 200-400 base pairs in length were generated by sonication of the cloned BamHI h fragment of EHV-1 DNA and then inserted into the lambda vector λgt11 for expression in *E. coli* (Young & Davis, 1983). The expression library was amplified, and recombinant phage expressing gp13 epitopes were identified with monoclonal antibodies and isolated as reported previously (Allen & Yeargan 1987).

RESULTS

Purification by immunoaffinity chromatography. A purification method was developed to isolate EHV-1 gp13 as an antigen against which to screen hybridoma supernatants for specific anti-gp13 monoclonal antibodies. The one-step purification method was based upon antibody-affinity chromatography as a technique for isolation of minor protein components from complex mixtures. EHV-1 glycoproteins extracted from purified virions with sodium desoxycholate were applied to a monoclonal antibody-affinity column specific for gp13. After extensive washing of the column to remove unbound proteins, gp13 was eluted with a low-pH buffer.

Samples of the starting material and of each column fraction were analyzed by electrophoresis on slab gels of 7.5% polyacrylamide–0.1% sodium dodecyl sulphate (SDS), followed by staining with a silver stain (Biorad, Richmond, CA) (Fig. 2). Within the column fractions, gp13 antigenic activity was identified by an avidin-biotin based enzyme immunoassay after spotting 1-µl "dots" of each column fraction into nitrocellulose membranes (Fig. 3).

Table 1. Immunoreactivity of EHV-1 anti-gp13 monoclonal antibodies raised against subtype 1 virions with subtype 2 EHV-1 isolates in an ELISA assay

Category of isolates	Number of reactive monoclonal antibodies/ total number tested	Reactive antibodies, percentage of total
All subtype 2	3/42	7%
Some subtype 2	3/42	7%
No subtype 2	36/42	85%

The results indicated that electrophoretically pure EHV-1 gp13 that retained antigenic activity could be prepared by this one-step immunoaffinity chromatographic procedure. The purified gp13 antigen did not react with monoclonal antibodies directed against any of the other major glycoproteins of EHV-1 (data not shown). The yield from 15 mg of virion protein as the starting material was approximately 100 µg of purified gp13.

Preparation of monoclonal antibodies. Two independent fusions of FOX-NY myeloma cells with splenocytes collected from mice immunized with EHV-1 (either prototype T431 strain or electrophoretic variant 1B strain) were performed. Using an ELISA-based dot-blot immunoassay, the supernatants from 3200 hybridoma colonies growing in wells of 96-well microassay plates were screened for immunoreactivity against affinity-purified gp13.

Sixty hybridomas producing monoclonal antibodies specific for EHV-1 gp13 and stable through two successive cloning steps were isolated and preserved for future studies. High-titered ascites preparations have been prepared in mice for 42 of the anti-gp13 monoclonal antibodies. The monoclonal reagents are currently being used for investigation of the antigenic structure of EHV-1 gp13.

Use of monoclonal antibodies to analyze immunogenic structure. Ascites preparations of the 42 monoclonal antibodies directed against epitopes present on gp13 of subtype 1 strains of EHV-1 were tested in an ELISA assay for reactivity to 12 independent subtype 2 EHV-1 isolates. The results, summarized in Table 1, indicated that the majority of the immunodominant epitopes on EHV-1 gp13 are subtype-specific and are not represented on EHV-1 isolates of the heterologous subtype. Only three of the 42-member monoclonal antibody panel reacted with all 12 subtype 2 isolates, while three others reacted with some but not all. Of the anti-gp13 monoclonal antibodies, prepared by immunization of mice with subtype 1 virions, all those that reacted with subtype 2 EHV-1 isolates demonstrated two- to eightfold lower ELISA titers against the subtype 2 isolates than against subtype 1 strains of the virus.

Culture supernatants from 24 of the hybridoma cell lines

Table 2. Neutralizing activity of anti-gp13 monoclonal antibody 16E4 against strains of EHV-1 in a plaque-reduction neutralization assay

Conditions	50% titer against: Subtype 1 EHV-1 (Army-183)	Subtype 2 EHV-1 (Kentucky T2)
With complement	40,000	6,000
Without complement	<500	<500

secreting anti-gp13 monoclonal antibody were tested for virus-neutralizing activity against EHV-1 in a microneutralization assay. Four of the monoclonals were able to neutralize EHV-1 infectivity, but only in the presence of exogenous complement. The antiviral activity of one of the anti-gp13 neutralizing monoclonals that was reactive against both EHV-1 subtypes (16E4) was investigated further in a plaque-reduction assay (Table 2). An ascites preparation of the monoclonal antibody 16E4 could effect a 50% reduction in the 100-plaque test dose of subtype 1 EHV-1 as a titer of 40,000 but exhibited a 50% plaque-reduction titer of only 6000 against a similar test dose of subtype 2 EHV-1. Other neutralizing anti-gp13 monoclonal antibodies were subtype-specific and were neutralizing against only subtype 1 isolates of EHV-1.

To estimate the minimum number of unique epitopes present on EHV-1 gp13, each member of the panel of 42 antibodies was tested in an ELISA assay for reactivity against a collection of 72 independent subtype 1 field isolates of EHV-1. The 72 viral antigens had been recovered over a period of 25 years in five states from aborted equine fetuses or nasopharyngeal swabs, or from the central nervous system of infected horses. Enveloped virions of each virus isolate were purified and individually adsorbed onto 96-well plates for use as viral antigen in the ELISA.

Any two monoclonal antibodies reacting with different subsets of the 72 EHV-1 isolates were considered to recognize different binding sequences (epitopes) on the gp13 antigen molecule. Using this criterion for differentiating the binding specificities, at least 16 distinct epitopes could be demonstrated. Some isolates of EHV-1 contained all 16 identified gp13 epitopes (i.e., reacted with all 42 monoclonal antibodies) and were apparently closely related antigenically (with respect to gp13 epitopes) to the EHV-1 strains used for preparation of the monoclonal antibody reagents. However, the majority of the 72 isolates differed from the immunizing strains at one or more gp13 epitopes. No specific set of gp13 epitopes could be correlated with disease manifestation. However, it was obvious that strains of EHV-1 that had undergone extensive laboratory passage in non-equine cells (such as hamster-adapted strains and attenuated vaccine strains) were antigenically distinguishable within their gp13 epitopes from prototype strains of EHV-1 (Table 3). Likewise, the majority of the isolates screened that possessed the DNA restriction endonuclease cleavage pattern categorized as electropherotype 1B (Allen et al. 1985) were devoid of several immunodominant gp13 epitopes present on prototype isolates (Table 3).

Examination of the reactivity profiles of the 72 EHV-1 isolates with the panel of monoclonal antibodies representing 16 discrete gp13 epitopes revealed the existence of both conserved and divergent epitopes on the glycoprotein antigen. Some epitopes on gp13 (e.g., those recognized by monoclonal antibodies 16E4, 14H7, 16H9, etc.) were highly conserved among EHV-1 isolates and were present on all 72 strains of the virus that were examined. At the opposite pole of reactivity were gp13 determinants found in no isolates of EHV-1 other than the immunizing virus strain used for preparation of the monoclonal antibodies. The majority of gp13 epitopes, however, fell between these two extremes in their variability, being present on the majority, but not all, of the 72 isolates of EHV-1.

Expression of EHV-1 gp13 epitopes in *E. coli*. Young and Davis (1983) have developed the phage vector λgt11, which expresses foreign, inserted DNA as a protein fused to β-

Table 3. ELISA immunoreactivity of 9 selected isolates of EHV-1 with 9 selected monoclonal antibodies (representative of patterns in testing 72 EHV-1 isolates with 42 monoclonal antibodies)

EHV-1 subtype 1 isolate	Description	Anti-gp13 monoclonal antibody: 14H7	27E5	49G12	52B6	48F4	26A5	36F3	35G6	60D8
T431	1P	+	+	+	+	+	+	+	+	+
T242	Army-183 strain	+	+	+	+	+	+	+	+	+
T252	1P	+	−	+	+	+	+	+	+	+
T186	Extensive passage in non-equine cells	+	−	−	−	−	+	+	+	+
T373	1B	+	−	+	−	+	−	−	−	−
T275	1B	+	−	+	+	+	−	−	−	+
T636	CNS isolate	+	−	+	+	+	−	−	−	−
T509	CNS isolate	+	+	+	+	+	+	+	+	+
T538	1P	+	−	+	−	−	−	+	+	+

Note: Negative titer = at least 32-fold lower than the ELISA titer of the same antibody when tested against the immunizing strain of EHV-1.

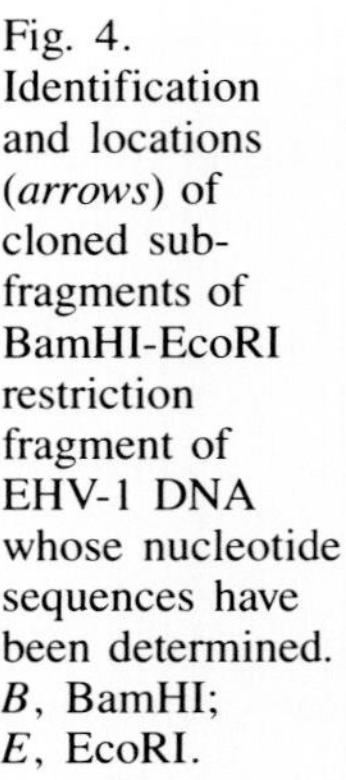

Fig. 4. Identification and locations (*arrows*) of cloned subfragments of BamHI-EcoRI restriction fragment of EHV-1 DNA whose nucleotide sequences have been determined. *B*, BamHI; *E*, EcoRI.

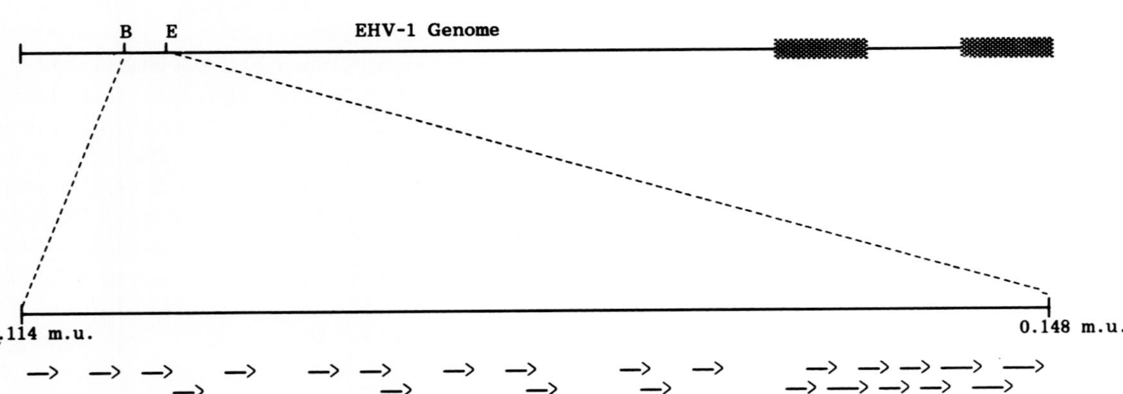

galactosidase. The λgt11 vector system allows efficient expression of the inserted DNA as well as convenient screening of a large number of recombinant phage for expression of the sequences of interest. As an approach to identifying the precise subregions of EHV-1 gp13 that comprise the antigenic domains of the molecule, an expression library of the sequences contained within the BamHI h fragment of EHV-1 DNA was constructed in λgt11. The BamHI h fragment encompasses the EHV-1 DNA sequences that encode gp13 (Allen & Yeargan 1987).

Four pools, each containing 10-12 different anti-gp13 monoclonal antibodies, were used for immunodetecting λgt11 recombinants expressing gp13 antigenic determinants. Thirty-six such λgt11 clones expressing gp13 sequences were plaque-purified and individually screened for immunoreactivity with each of the 42 anti-gp13 monoclonal antibodies. Each of the lambda recombinants containing and expressing inserts of EHV-1 DNA as gp13 epitopes reacted with the same subset of 15 monoclonal antibodies. Among the antibodies recognizing the immunodominant domain expressed in *E. coli* were both neutralizing and nonneutralizing monoclonals and the group of monoclonal antibodies directed against epitopes absent from most 1B electropherotypes of EHV-1. Sequencing of the EHV-1 insert DNA present within the λgt11 clones is underway to localize and determine the amino acid sequence of this immunodominant, epitope-encoding region of the gp13 gene.

Determination of partial nucleotide sequence of restriction endonuclease fragment containing gene for EHV-1 gp13. A project to determine the nucleotide sequence of the 6-kb BamHI-EcoRI fragment of EHV-1 DNA that contains the coding sequences for gp13 was begun. A nested set of overlapping subclones of the fragment was prepared in M13mp18 and -mp19 for sequencing. The locations of the cloned subfragments of the BamHI-EcoRI fragment whose nucleotide sequences have been determined to date are shown in Figure 4. More than 60% of the 6000 nucleotides that comprise the fragment have been sequenced. The coding DNA strand and the correct translational reading frame were identified by sequencing inserts present in λgt11 expressing gp13 determinants.

No homology was detected between the EHV-1 gp13 DNA sequences and those encoding glycoprotein C of herpes simplex virus or pseudorabies virus. However, a search for homology at the amino acid level among the three herpesvirus glycoproteins revealed several regions of limited sequence homology (Fig. 5). The observed homology was in the same range, 15% to 30%, among all three herpesviral glycoproteins (Robbins et al. 1986).

DISCUSSION

As part of long-range research to characterize the antigens of EHV-1 responsible for stimulating or suppressing protective immunity in the horse, we have begun to examine the antigenic properties of the major glycoproteins of EHV-1. The genome of EHV-1 encodes six families of high-abundance glycoproteins. In this report, we have described the results, to date, of our analysis of the epitopes of one of these major EHV-1 glycoproteins, gp13. This viral glycoprotein, which is the homolog of herpes simplex virus gC, is one of the immunodominant species in the equine immune response to experimentally acquired-EHV-1 infection.

A monoclonal antibody immunoaffinity system was optimized to purify gp13 for use an an antigen for screening hybridoma supernatants. The large panel of monoclonal antibodies thus raised against EHV-1 gp13 was then used to characterize the antigenic determinants of the glycoprotein.

As demonstrated by these studies, 85% of the immunogenic regions of gp13 have undergone extensive sequence alteration during the divergent evolution of the two biotypes of EHV-1. This alteration, along with the observation that gp13 homologs of other herpesviruses are nonessential for growth in cell culture, does not suggest a conserved, essential replicative function for this glycoprotein (as is the case with gB-like glycoproteins of herpesviruses), but one that contributes to the adaptation of the particular EHV-1 subtype to its

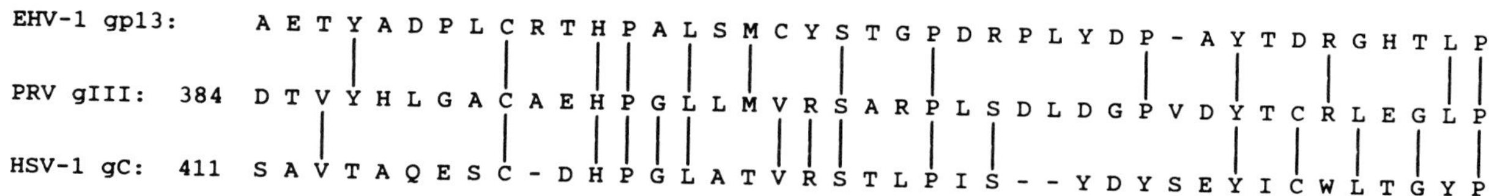

Fig. 5. Illustration of a region of sequence homology among HSV-1 glycoprotein C, PRV glycoprotein III, and gp13 of EHV-1.

unique ecological niche within the horse (Longnecker & Roizman 1987). Likewise, considerable antigenic variation was observed within the majority of gp13 epitopes found among different isolates of the same subtype of EHV-1. It seems feasible that such divergence of select gp13 epitopes has occurred during the adaptation of particular strains of the virus to a more efficient existence within the biochemical and immunologic milieu of the horse.

The antigenic divergence within gp13 determinants of 1B isolates of EHV-1 is particularly intriguing. Isolates with DNA of the 1B electropherotype have, within the past six years, emerged as the dominant cause of herpesvirus abortion in vaccinated mares (Allen et al. 1985). There is need to investigate such antigenic variation for its role, if any, in making 1B isolates better able to circumvent the immune defenses of horses vaccinated with prototype strains of the virus.

It was shown by these investigations that EHV-1 neutralizing antibodies with specificity for gp13 are directed against both highly conserved and highly divergent epitopes. The effect of such antigenic diversity on the successfulness of vaccine control of EHV-1 infections must eventually be addressed.

Expression in *E. coli* of short fragments of the gene encoding gp13 revealed, unexpectedly, the existence of only a single epitope-encoding domain within the gene. Six of the 16 identified epitopes of gp13 were coded from this region of the gene. Whether the anti-gp13 monoclonal antibodies recognizing discontinuous epitopes are directed against amino acid sequences within the same antigenic domain or in other antigenic regions of the gp13 molecule could not be determined by these investigations. However, it is noteworthy that immunodominant, continuous epitopes are a prerequisite for the synthetic peptide approach to vaccine development.

The homology observed between EHV-1 gp13 coding sequences that have been determined thus far and those encoding gC-like glycoproteins of other herpesviruses was limited and restricted to the amino acid level. This finding is consistent with the view that herpesvirus gC-like glycoproteins are evolutionarily dynamic proteins that have undergone extensive sequence divergence both among different herpesvirus types of the alphaherpesvirinae subfamily as well as among different alphaherpesviruses of the same host species (e.g., HSV-1 and -2; EHV-1 subtypes 1 and 2).

It is not yet clear which host immune responses or which viral epitopes will ultimately prove most useful in protection against EHV-1. Current studies in our laboratory are directed at defining and characterizing the importance of specific viral glycoprotein antigens and their respective epitopes in triggering different host immune responses, both stimulatory and suppressive. Further molecular characterization of the determinants of EHV-1 glycoproteins should provide information essential for development of more effective vaccines for herpesviral diseases of the horse.

ACKNOWLEDGMENTS

These studies were supported by research grants from The Grayson Foundation, Inc., and from the United States Department of Agriculture.

REFERENCES

Allen, G.P., and Bryans, J.T. (1986) Molecular epizootiology, pathogenesis, and prophylaxis of equine herpesvirus 1 infections. In *Progress in Veterinary Microbiology and Immunology*, Vol. 2, pp. 78-144. Ed. R. Pandey. S. Karger, Basel.

Allen, G.P., and Yeargan, M.R. (1987) Use of λgt11 and monoclonal antibodies to map the genes for the six major glycoproteins of equine herpesvirus 1. *J. Virol.* **61**, 2454-61.

Allen, G.; Yeargan, M.; Turtinen, L.; Bryans, J.; and McCollum, W. (1983) Molecular epizootiologic studies of equine herpesvirus 1 infections by restriction endonuclease fingerprinting of viral DNA. *Am. J. Vet. Res.* **44**, 263-71.

Allen, G.; Yeargan, M.; Turtinen, L., and Bryans, J. (1985) Emergence of a new field strain of equine abortion virus (equine herpesvirus 1). *Am. J. Vet. Res.* **46**, 138-40.

Ben-Porat, T.; DeMarchi, J.; Lomniczi, B.; and Kaplan, A. (1986) Role of glycoproteins of pseudorabies virus in eliciting neutralizing antibodies. *Virology* **154**, 325-34.

Bryans, J.T. (1969) On immunity to disease caused by equine herpesvirus 1. *J. Am. Vet. Med. Assoc.* **155**, 294-300.

———. (1980) Herpesviral disease affecting reproduction in the horse. *Vet. Clin. N. Am. Large Anim. Pract.* **2**, 303-12.

Bryans, J.T., and Allen, G.P. (1986a) Equine viral rhinopneumonitis. *Rev. Sci. Tech. Off. Intl. Epzoot.* **5**, 837-47.

———. (1986b) Control of abortigenic herpesviral infections. In *Current Therapy in Theriogenology*, Vol. 2, pp. 711-14. Ed. D. Morrow. W.B. Saunders, Philadelphia.

Dalchau, R., and Fabre, J. (1982) The purification of antigens with monoclonal antibody affinity columns. In *Monoclonal Antibodies in Clinical Medicine*, pp. 519-56. Ed. A. McMichale and J. Fabre. Academic Press, New York.

Frink, R.J.; Eisenberg, G.; Cohen, G.; and Wagner, E.K. (1983) Detailed analysis of the portion of the herpes simplex virus type 1 genome encoding glycoprotein C. *J. Virol.* **45**, 634-47.

Glorioso, J.; Kess, U.; Kumel, G.; Kirchner, H.; and Krammer, P. (1985) Identification of herpes simplex virus type 1 (HSV-1) glycoprotein gC as the immunodominant antigen for HSV-1-specific memory cytotoxic T lymphocytes. *J. Immunol.* **135**, 575-82.

Henikoff, S. (1984) Unidirectional digestion with exonuclease III creates targeted breakpoints for DNA sequencing. *Gene* **28**, 351-59.

Longnecker, R., and Roizman, B. (1987) Clustering of genes dispensable for growth in culture in the S component of the HSV-1 genome. *Science* **236**, 573-76.

Robbins, A.K.; Watson, R.J.; Whealy, M.E.; Hays, W.W.; and Enquist, L.W. (1986) Characterization of a pseudorabies virus glycoprotein gene with homology to herpes simplex virus type 1 and type 2 glycoprotein C. *J. Virol.* **58**, 33-347.

Rosenthal, K.L.; Smiley, J.R.; South, S.; and Johnson, D.C. (1987) Cells expressing herpes simplex virus glycoprotein gC but not gB, gD, or gE are recognized by murine virus-specific cytotoxic T lymphocytes. *J. Virol.* **61**, 2438-47.

Sanger, F.; Nicklen, S.; and Coulson, A. (1977) DNA sequencing with chain terminating inhibitors. *Proc. Natl. Acad. Sci. USA* **74**, 5463-67.

Spear, P.G. (1985) Glycoproteins specified by herpes simplex viruses. In *The Herpesviruses*, Vol. 3, pp. 315-56. Ed. B. Roizman. Plenum, New York.

Taggart, R.T., and Samloff, I. (1983) Stable antibody-producing murine hybridomas. *Science* **219**, 1228-30.

Turtinen, L.W., and Allen, G.P. (1982) Identification of the envelope surface glycoproteins of equine herpesvirus type 1. *J. Gen. Virol.* **63**, 481-85.

Turtinen, L.; Allen, G.; Darlington, R.; and Bryans, J. (1981) Molecular and serological comparisons of several strains of equine herpesvirus 1. *Am. J. Vet. Res.* **42**, 2099-2104.

Yeargan, M.R.; Allen, G.P.; and Bryans, J.T. (1985) Rapid subtyping of equine herpesvirus 1 with monoclonal antibodies. *J. Clin. Microbiol.* **21**, 694-97.

Young, R.A., and Davis, R.W. (1983) Efficient isolation of genes by using antibody probes. *Proc. Natl. Acad. Sci. USA* 80, 1194-98.

Identification and Location of a Gene in Equid Herpesvirus-1 Analogous to the Major Glycoprotein gB of Herpes Simplex Virus

G.C. Hudson, James M. Whalley, G.R. Robertson, N.A. Scott, Margaret M. Sabine, and Daria N. Love

SUMMARY

As part of the analysis of the equine herpesvirus-1 (EHV-1) genome structure and function, we have identified and located a major EHV-1 glycoprotein gene equivalent to the herpes simplex virus (HSV) gB. This glycoprotein has been shown for HSV and other herpesviruses to invoke an antiviral immune response and is currently a favored candidate for a genetically engineered or subunit vaccine. In this study, the EHV-1 gB gene has been mapped using restriction enzymes, molecular hybridization, and nucleotide sequencing to a region of the genome around 0.4 map units, extending from the end of a BamHI A restriction fragment into the adjacent BamHI I fragment. Computer homology programs using sequence generated at the 3′ end of the gene have shown that there are regions of nucleotide and amino acid sequence analogous to domains in both HSV-1 gB and varicella zoster virus gp-II (gB). A comparison of hydrophobicity profiles of the predicted polypeptides suggests considerable secondary structural similarities between the different herpesviruses, and implications of these findings for potential development of EHV-1 vaccines are discussed.

INTRODUCTION

EHV-1, also variously known as equine abortion virus, EHV-1 subtype 1, or the abortigenic subtype of EHV-1, is a major cause worldwide of abortion in mares and severe neonatal disease in foals. Serious neurological disorders may also be a consequence of EHV-1 infection. The epidemiology, pathogenesis, and molecular biology of EHV-1 have been the subject of a number of reviews over the last few years (e.g., O'Callaghan, Gentry & Randall 1983; Campbell & Studdert 1983; Sabine et al. 1983; Allen & Bryans 1986). Of the current approaches to development of a new generation of herpesvirus vaccines, one is based on the use of envelope glycoproteins (Spear 1985) as immunogens. In the case of herpes simplex virus (HSV), several individual glycoproteins have been shown to invoke circulating antibody and/or cell-mediated immune (CMI) responses that are capable of protecting mice against lethal challenge with virus (Chan, Lukig & Liew 1985; Berman et al. 1985; Long et al. 1984; Blacklaws, Nash & Darby 1987). Immunopurified HSV-1 envelope glycoprotein gB was shown to be a more effective protective immunogen, through CMI, than similarly prepared gD or gH (Chan et al. 1985). However, cell lines constitutively expressing gD were found to induce both CMI and a neutralizing antibody response and to be a stronger protective antigen than cells expressing gB (Blacklaws et al. 1987).

Based on molecular hybridization and sequence data, genes analogous to HSV-1 gB have been identified in some other herpesviruses (HSV-2, Bzik et al. 1986; VZV, Keller et al. 1986; EBV, Pellet et al. 1985a; HCMV, Mach, Utz & Fleckenstein 1986; Cranage et al. 1986), and antigenic studies and peptide analysis have indicated that EHV-1–infected cells contain polypeptides analogous to and cross-reactive with HSV-1 gB (Snowden et al. 1985; Snowden & Halliburton 1985). This apparent conservation of gB-like sequences, along with the known colinearity (Davison & Wilkie 1983) of the HSV-1 and EHV-1 genomes, forms a basis for identification and location of the EHV-1 gene equivalent to the HSV gB. Consistent with this is the assignment of a major EHV-1 glycoprotein (gp14) gene to a genome location colinear with the HSV gB gene (Allen & Yeargan 1987). In this paper we present evidence for the existence of a "gB" gene in the EHV-1 genome, and define its exact position on the genome, using molecular hybridization and DNA sequencing of part of the EHV-1 gB gene. Some of the features of the gene are discussed with reference to the equivalent gene in other herpesviruses and to its potential for development as a subunit vaccine for EHV-1.

MATERIALS AND METHODS

Viral and plasmid DNA preparation. EHV-1 (isolate HVS 25A) was grown in BHK21 cells and DNA was prepared by a standard method (Whalley, Robertson & Davison 1981). Recombinant plasmids pMAC209 and pMAC221 containing EHV-1 BamHI-I and BamHI-IBG fragments inserted in pBR322 (Robertson & Whalley 1985) were grown in *E. coli* HB101 cells. pGX37, donated by V. Preston and J. Subak-Sharpe (University of Glasgow), contained the BamHI G fragment of HSV-1 inserted in pAT153. Plasmids were amplfied with chloramphenicol and purified by sodium dodecyl sulphate (SDS) lysis and cesium chloride gradient

Hudson, Whalley, Robertson, Scott: School of Biological Sciences, Macquarie University, Sydney, Australia 2109. Sabine, Love: Department of Veterinary Pathology, University of Sydney, Sydney, Australia 2006.

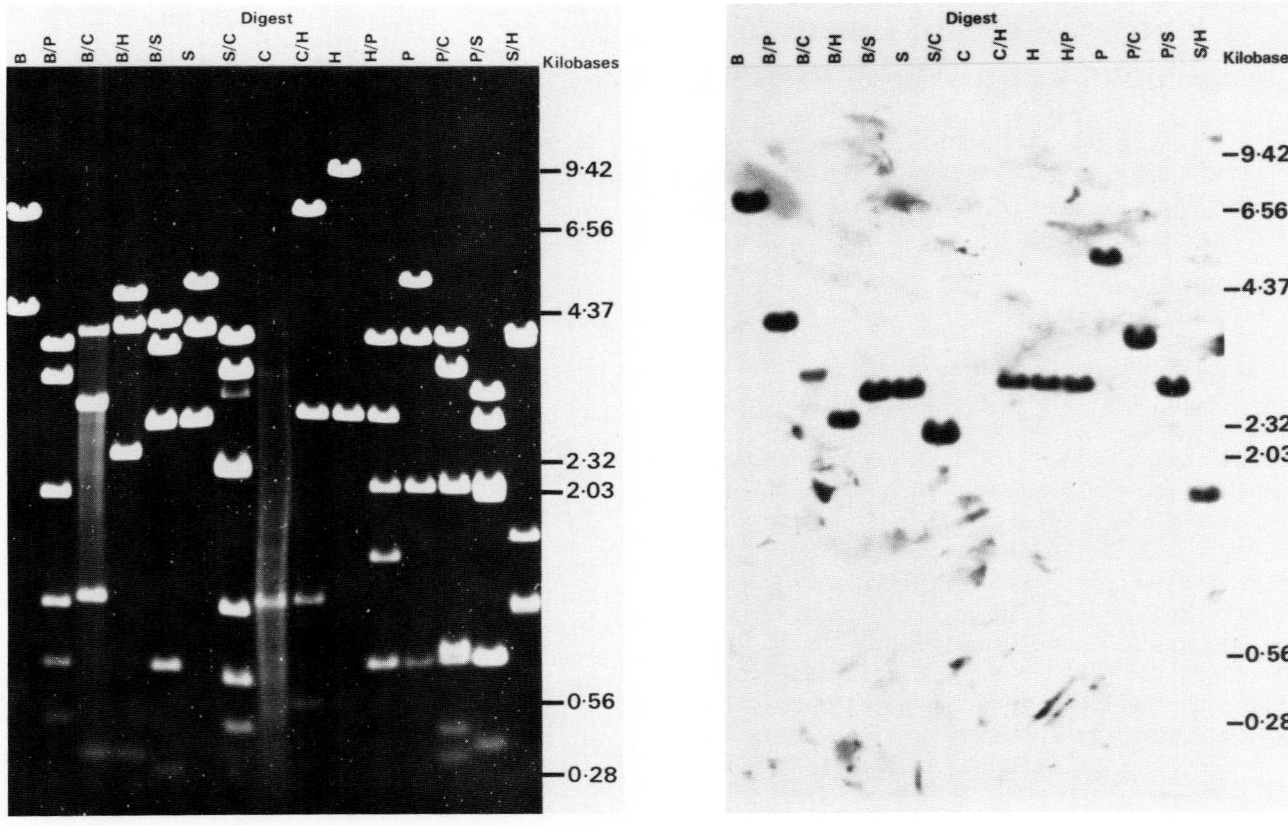

Fig. 1. A(left). 0.75% agarose gel of EHV-1 BamHI I fragment (pMAC209) cleaved with all combinations of single and double digests of restriction endonucleases BamHI (*B*), SalI (*S*), ClaI (*C*), HindIII (*H*), and PstI (*P*). B(right). Autoradiograph of Southern blot of same gel probed with M13/pGX37 subclone containing HSV-1 gB sequences.

ultracentrifugation, essentially as described by Maniatis, Fritsch, and Sambrook (1982). To remove HSV sequences not coding for gB, PGX37 was digested with the restriction enzymes BamHI and SalI and ligated into M13, followed by selection of a subclone containing a 1.74-kb region of HSV-1 gB gene (deduced from Bzik et al. 1986).

For initial EHV-1 DNA sequencing and identification of gB-like regions, a 0.6-kb HindIII/ClaI fragment and a 2.9-kb BamHI/ClaI fragment of pMAC209 were subcloned in defined orientations into M13 vectors.

DNA analysis. Restriction endonucleases BamHI, SalI, ClaI, HindIII and PstI (Boehringer-Mannheim, North Ryde, N.S.W.) were used to digest DNA samples for 4-6 hr in conditions recommended by the manufacturer, and the resulting DNA fragments were characterized by electrophoresis through gels of 0.75% agarose (Type 1, Sigma) in E buffer (40 mM Tris, 30 mM NaH_2PO_4, 1 mM EDTA). Vizualization and photography of DNA bands was by UV light using an orange filter. For hybridization experiments DNA bands were transferred from agarose gels to nitrocellulose sheets (Schleicher & Schuell BA85) according to the method of Southern (1975). Plasmid DNA was labeled with ^{32}P-labeled dATP by nick translation (Rigby et al. 1977) using a kit (Biotechnology Research Enterprises, Adelaide). Recombinant M13 template DNA was also used in hybridization experiments and was labeled using a modified sequencing reaction mix that lacked any dideoxynucleotide. Labeled DNA from both reactions was separated from unincorporated nucleotides by elution through Sephadex G-50 with 10 mM Tris-HC1, pH 8.0, 1 mM EDTA. Labeled denatured DNA probes and DNA immobilized on nitrocellulose were incubated in hybridization solutions containing 6× SSC, 0.5% sodium dodecyl sulphate (SDS), 5× Denhardt's solution and 100 μg/ml denatured salmon sperm DNA at 55°C for 16-20 hr. Washes were 2× SSC, 0.1% SDS at 55°C, after which the nitrocellulose was dried and autoradiographed.

DNA sequencing. DNA from recombinant M13 phages was sequenced by the dideoxynucleotide chain termination method of Sanger and colleagues (1980). For the initial identification of the EHV-1 "gB" gene, sequence was obtained from BamHI, ClaI, or HindIII restriction sites using forced clones. Subsequent sequencing aimed at characterizing the complete EHV-1 gB sequence is based on the method of Dale, McClure & Houchins (1985), with the generation of several series of

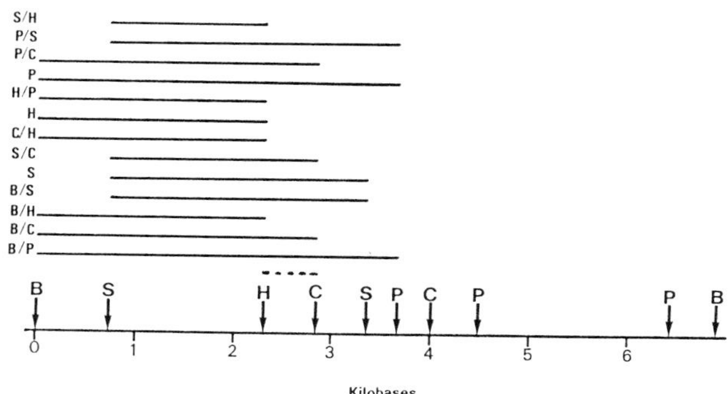

Fig. 2. Physical map of EHV-1 BamHI I fragment for restriction endonucleases BamHI (*B*), SalI (*S*), ClaI (*C*), HindIII (*H*), and PstI (*P*), showing (bars) fragments to which M13/pGX subclone hybridized. *Dotted line*, region sequenced and detailed in *Figure 3*.

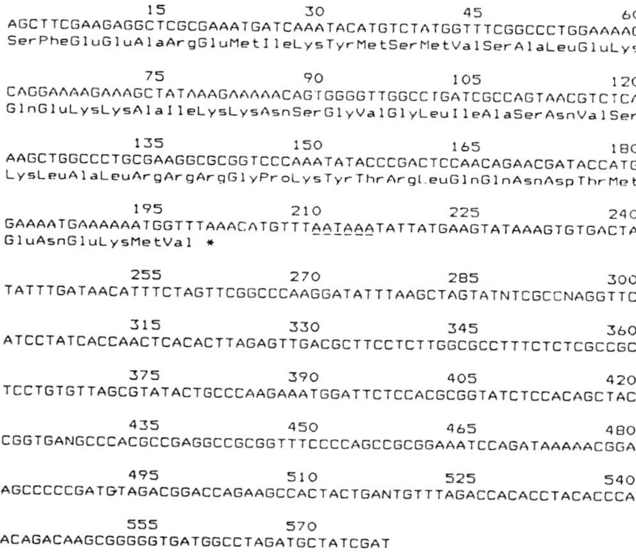
15 30 45 60
AGCTTCGAAGAGGCTCGCGAAATGATCAAATACATGTCTATGGTTTCGGCCCTGGAAAAG
SerPheGluGluAlaArgGluMetIleLysTyrMetSerMetValSerAlaLeuGluLys
75 90 105 120
CAGGAAAAGAAAGCTATAAAGAAAAACAGTGGGGTTGGCCTGATCGCCAGTAACGTCTCA
GlnGluLysLysAlaIleLysLysAsnSerGlyValGlyLeuIleAlaSerAsnValSer
135 150 165 180
AAGCTGGCCCTGCGAAGGCGCGGTCCCAAATATACCCGACTCCAACAGAACGATACCATG
LysLeuAlaLeuArgArgArgGlyProLysTyrThrArgLeuGlnGlnAsnAspThrMet
195 210 225 240
GAAAATGAAAAAATGGTTTAAACATGTTTAATAAATATTATGAAGTATAAAGTGTGACTA
GluAsnGluLysMetVal *
255 270 285 300
TATTTGATAACATTTCTAGTTCGGCCCAAGGATATTTAAGCTAGTATNTCGCCNAGGTTC
315 330 345 360
ATCCTATCACCAACTCACACTTAGAGTTGACGCTTCCTCTTGGCGCCTTTCTCTCGCCGC
375 390 405 420
TCCTGTGTTAGCGTATACTGCCCAAGAAATGGATTCTCCACGCGGTATCTCCACAGCTAC
435 450 465 480
CGGTGANGCCCACGCCGAGGCCGCGGTTTCCCCAGCCGCGGAAATCCAGATAAAAACGGA
495 510 525 540
AGCCCCCGATGTAGACGGACCAGAAGCCACTACTGANTGTTTAGACCACACCTACACCCA
555 570
ACAGACAAGCGGGGGTGATGGCCTAGATGCTATCGAT

Fig. 3. EHV-1 nucleotide sequence between HindIII site and adjacent ClaI site of the BamHI I fragment; sequence starts from HindIII site and is shown in 5′ to 3′ direction. Possible polyadenylation site close to 3′ end of gene is underlined; amino acid sequence predicted from inspection of three possible reading frames.

M13 overlapping clones deleted sequentially from one end of the inserted fragments. The Cornell DNA sequence analysis package (Fristensky et al. 1982) was used for sequence data processing, including identification of nucleotide and amino acid homologies.

RESULTS

The M13 clone possessing the SalI/BamHI fragment of pGX37, containing 1.74 kb of HSV-1 gB sequence (Bzik et al. 1984), was found in initial hybridization experiments (not shown) to anneal to the EHV-1 BamHI I fragment of BamHI-digested total viral DNA. The complete plasmid pGX37 containing these gB sequences and also part of the HSV-1 DNA-binding protein was likewise found to hybridize strongly to the EHV-1 BamHI A fragment and also to the BamHI I fragment. If the orientation of the genes coding for gB and the DNA-binding protein is conserved between EHV-1 and HSV-1, this hybridization data indicated that the gB gene homolog in EHV-1 codes in the 5′ to 3′ direction from the BamHI A fragment into the BamHI I fragment. To locate more precisely the gB homologous regions, the DNA of clone pMAC209 was digested with single and double digests of BamHI, PstI, ClaI, HindIII, and SalI, the resulting fragments were separated by agarose gel electrophoresis (Fig. 1A), and the data used to derive a restriction enzyme map for the EHV-1 BamHI I fragment (Fig. 2). Hybridization of the M13 recombinant SalI/BamHI subclone of pGX137 to a Southern transfer of the gel of Figure 1A revealed homology with single bands for each digest (Fig. 1B). The common region of hybridization was defined as a sequence of approximately 1.5 kb between the left-hand SalI site and the adjacent HindIII site (Fig. 2). This region of homology, and thus the EHV-1 gene analogous to gB, mapped to 0.42 map units, is similar to the location of the gene in HSV-1.

Sequence data were obtained initially for the 573-bp HindIII/ClaI fragment (Fig. 3). Using this sequence, homology was found between the first 200 nucleotides from the HindIII site of the EHV-1 sequence and regions of the last 200 nucleotides (at the C-terminus) of the protein-coding regions of the genes for HSV-1 gB (Bzik et al. 1984) and VZV gp-II (gB) (Keller et al. 1986). These results indicated that this region of EHV-1 represented the C-terminal 200 nucleotides of the coding region of a homologous gene, and that the EHV-1 gene was more similar to the HSV-1 gB gene than to the VZV gp-II gene. The longest open reading frame in this EHV-1 sequence was a stretch of 198 nucleotides from the HindIII site representing 66 amino acids (Fig. 4), corresponding to the region of nucleotide sequence homology with both HSV-1 and VZV. A potential polyadenylation site was found about 10 nucleotides downstream from the stop codon, and was in a position similar to the predicted sites in HSV-1 and VZV. The G+C content of this EHV-1 sequence was 47%, which is substantially lower than the total genomic estimate of 56% (Goodheart & Plummer 1975), and contrasts with an overall G+C content of 66% for HSV-1 gB (Bzik et al. 1984).

Amino acid sequence comparisons (Figs. 4 and 5) confirmed the existence of the gB equivalent protein in EHV-1 but revealed more homology of EHV-1 with VZV than with HSV-1 at this level, in contrast to the result for the nucleotide sequences. The number of conserved amino acids, out of 66, were 26 for EHV-1 and HSV-1, 33 for EHV-1 and VZV, and 28 for VZV and HSV-1, with a highly conserved domain being particularly evident in the first 28 amino acids of the sequence. A few deletions (particularly for VZV) were apparent relative to the other two sequences. A graphical represen-

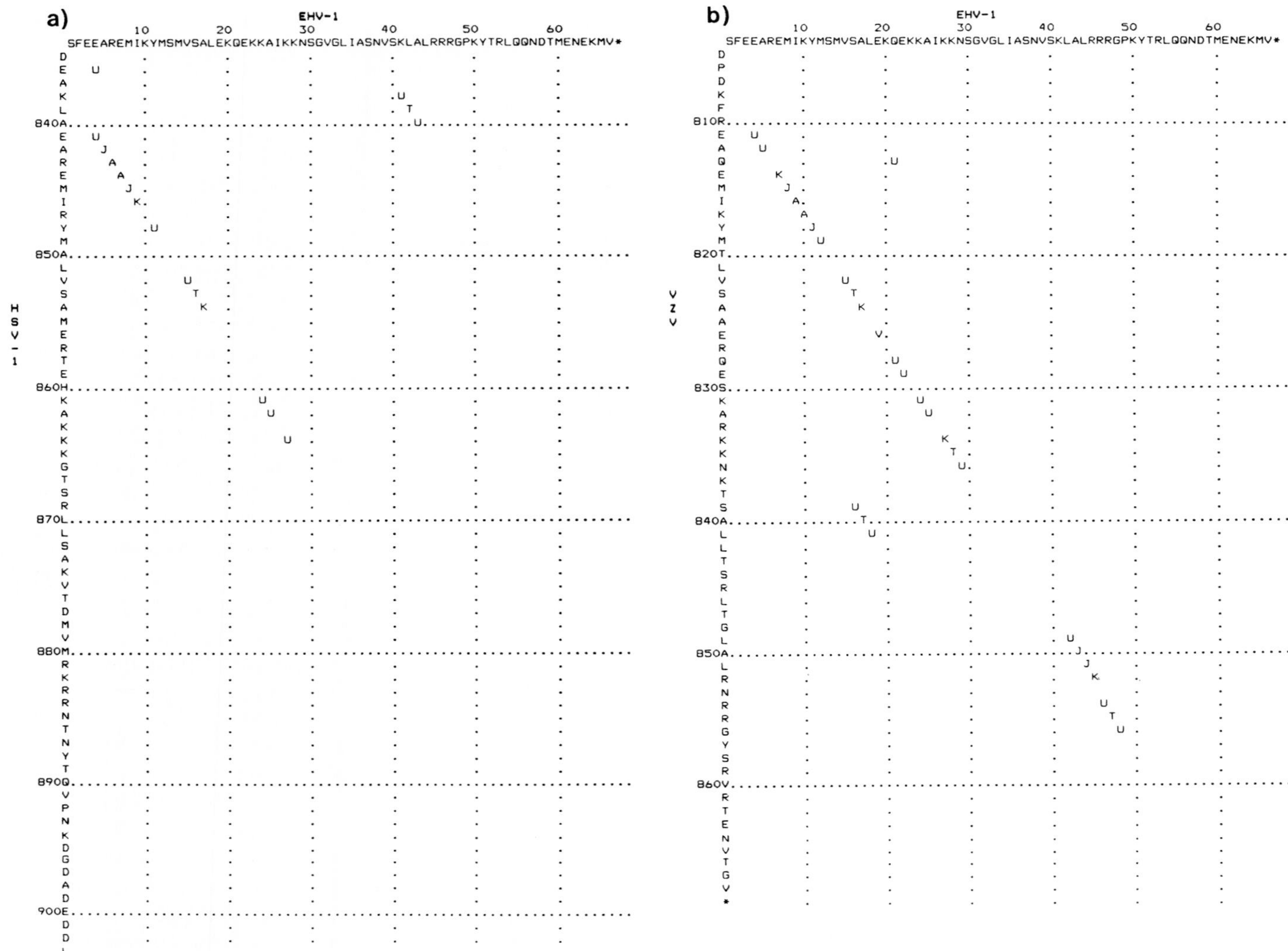

Fig. 4. Amino acid sequence homology between 3′ ends of EHV-1 "gB" gene and those of HSV-1 and VZV. Parameters: homology range, two residues; minimum percent homology printed, 60%; graph compression, 1; scale factor, 0.90. Standard one-letter amino acid symbols along each axis. Homology symbols (Fristensky et al. 1982): *A* = 100% homology, *B* = 98-99% homology, . . ., *U* = 60-61% homology. Colinearity appears as diagonal between sequences. *A*. Horizontal axis: EHV-1 predicted sequence; vertical axis: HSV-1 gB (Bzik et al. 1984) between residue 835 and stop codon. *B*. Horizontal axis: EHV-1 predicted sequence; vertical axis: VZV gp-II (Keller et al. 1986) between residue 805 and stop codon.

tation of the percentage of nonpolar amino acids across the region was used to depict the hydrophobicity profiles of the C-terminus of the three gB polypeptides. Figure 6 shows that the profiles of the analogous domains are very similar; in particular, the initial nonpolar peaks, representing the most highly conserved portion of the sequences, are identical.

The complete EHV-1 gB gene is being sequenced, and homology with HSV-1 and VZV gB genes of sequence 3′ of the BamHI site between A and I fragments has confirmed the location of the gene on the EHV-1 genome. The segment of the gene from this BamHI site to the stop codon contains 2,485 nucleotides and has substantial regions of nucleotide and amino acid homology in addition to those described above. From the alignment of homologous sequences, it is predicted that the translation start signal for the EHV-1 gB gene is approximately 350 nucleotides upstream from the A-I BamHI site in the BamHI A fragment, with all promoter sequences likely to be within 1 kb of this site.

DISCUSSION

In this paper we have provided evidence for the existence of an EHV-1 gene with homology to the gene encoding the glycoprotein gB of HSV-1, and have assigned the EHV-1 gene to 0.41-0.43 map units on the viral genome. Sequence analysis has shown the general similarity of these proteins, with the implication that their antigenic properties are also likely to be comparable. Key immunogenic domains or seg-

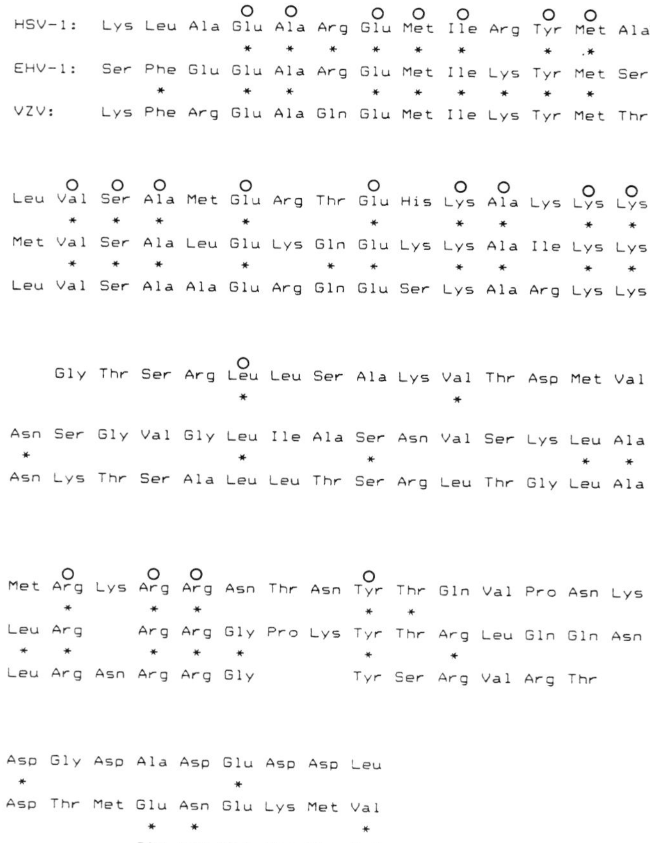

Fig. 5. Comparison of predicted EHV-1 amino acid sequence with analogous domains of HSV-1 gB and VZV gp-II. Sequences aligned to maximize amino acid homologies between sequences. *Identity between EHV-1 and HSV-1 or VZV residues; *open circle*, position of triple homology.

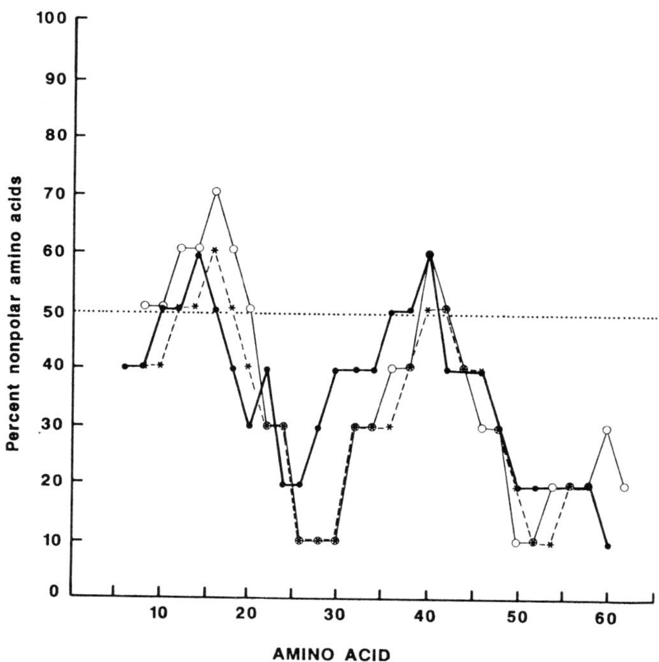

Fig. 6. Percentages of nonpolar amino acid residues across analogous domains at 3′ end of genes of EHV-1 predicted sequence (*solid circle*); HSV-1 gB (*open circle*); and VZV gp-II (*star*). Regions searched: five residues on each side of every second residue (Region = 10, Skip = 2).

ments of the protein identified for HSV or other herpesviruses can therefore be predicted for EHV-1, and vice versa.

In related studies on other EHV-1 genes in this region of the genome, we have also identified the genes coding for EHV-1 thymidine kinase (TK), the major capsid protein, and at least two other genes. Figure 7 shows the relative locations of these genes and the gB gene in the EHV-1 genome. Comparison of this arrangement shows that the gene order in this region is highly conserved between EHV-1 and HSV-1 genomes, but that the levels of sequence homology vary considerably from gene to gene. For example, the gB glycoprotein appears to have large regions of homologous sequence in HSV-1, EHV-1, and VZV, whereas the regions of homology of the TK gene are much less extensive. Presumably the degree and regions of homology reflect the functional significance of certain domains in the polypeptide product. The HSV-1 gB polypeptide is believed to contain 903 amino acids in four major domains: a hydrophobic 29–amino acid signal sequence at the N-terminal, which is cleaved after translocation of the peptide across the endoplasmic reticulum membrane; a hydrophilic cell-surface domain of 695 amino acids; a hydrophobic transmembrane domain of 70 amino acids that probably contains three antiparallel segments traversing the membrane; and a cytoplasmic domain that comprises the remaining 109 C-terminal amino acids (Pellett et al. 1985b). It is this C-terminal domain to which the EHV-1 sequence described here shows homology. It is a highly conserved region of the predicted amino acid sequences of HSV-1 gB, VZV gp-II (Keller et al. 1986), and the EHV-1 gene, and a cell membrane fusing function has been mapped to this region of HSV-1 gB (Deluca et al. 1982).

Envelope proteins of EHV-1 have been analyzed by Turtinen and Allen (1982), and also summarized by O'Callaghan and colleagues (1983). From map locations, it is evident that the gB gene described here is the same as the gp14 gene identified by Allen and Yeargan (1987) using a λgt11 expression system and EHV-1 specific monoclonal antibodies. The glycoprotein g14 (apparent molecular weight of 90,000 kilodaltons) has been shown to be one of four subtype-common antigens, and was also one of the dominant immunogens for EHV-1 in both horses and rabbits (Allen & Bryans 1986).

Knowledge of the complete sequence of the EHV-1 gB

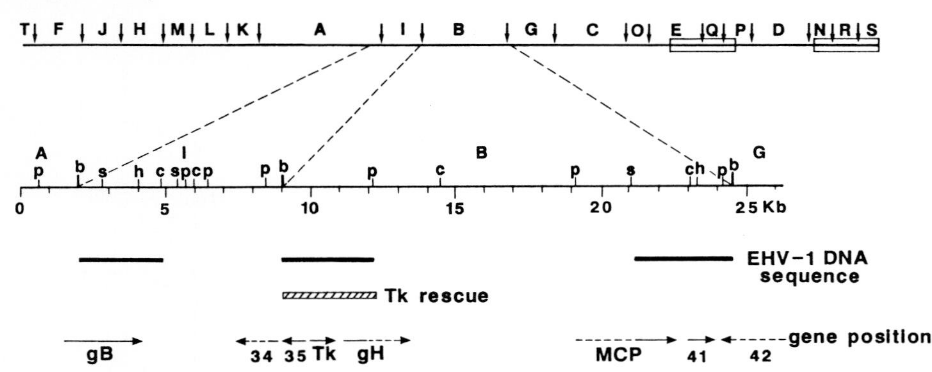

Fig. 7. Gene organization in central region of EHV-1 genome (BamHI map, Whalley et al., 1981). Detailed restriction site map of BamHI I and B fragments: regions that have been sequenced shown as solid bars; TK rescue was by transfection of LMTK⁻ cells. *Solid lines*, known gene sequence; *dotted lines*, predicted gene sequence; *arrows*, direction of transcription.

gene and of its genome location makes possible a range of subsequent experiments to assess the potential of the gB gene product in development of an EHV-1 vaccine. Expression of the cloned gene in bacterial or animal cells, followed by immunization in animals, can provide information on cell-mediated or circulating antibody responses. One useful approach to obtaining satisfactory expression of glycoprotein genes is to use a recombinant poxvirus as a vector (Mackett & Smith 1986). The inserted "foreign" glycoprotein genes may be expressed on the surface of infected cells (along with vaccinia virus products), where they are highly immunogenic. The recombinant virus has the added advantage of in vivo delivery of antigens in the vaccinated animal. Directly relevant to this study on EHV-1 is the report by Cranage and colleagues (1986), who described the expression of the human cytomegalovirus (HCMV) glycoprotein gB in such a recombinant vaccinia virus, which was able to induce neutralizing antibody against HCMV in rabbits. Glycosylation appears to occur as in the original "foreign" virus, hence the recombinant poxvirus system has considerable potential in the development of vaccines, including polyvalent vaccines, in which several genes from the same or different viruses are inserted in tandem (Paoletti et al. 1984).

In the case of EHV, for example, such a polyvalent vaccine could include genes for the two glycoproteins gB and gD, possibly for both abortigenic and respiratory equine herpesviruses. The sequence data also allows the chemical synthesis of oligopeptides that may comprise key antigenic domains of the gB protein. It may be possible to create a multipronged attack on the virus by using mixtures of immunogenic peptides with a range of antigenic determinants.

ACKNOWLEDGMENTS

This research was supported in part by grants from the Australian Research Grants Scheme and the Australian Equine Research Foundation.

REFERENCES

Allen, G.P., and Bryans, J.T. (1986) Molecular epizootology, pathogenesis, and prophylaxis of equine herpesvirus-1 infections. In *Progress in Veterinary Microbiology and Immunology,* Vol. 2, pp. 78-144. Ed. R. Pandey. S. Karger, Basel.

Allen, G.P., and Yeargan, M.R. (1987) Use of λgt11 and monoclonal antibodies to map the genes for the six major glycoproteins of equine herpesvirus 1. *J. Virol.* **61**, 2454-61.

Berman, P.W.; Gregory, T.; Crase, D.; and Lasky, L.A. (1985) Protection from genital herpes simplex virus type 2 infection by vaccination with cloned type 1 glycoprotein D. *Science* **227**, 1490-92.

Blacklaws, B.A.; Nash, A.A.; and Darby, G. (1987) Specificity of the immune response of mice to herpes simplex virus glycoproteins B and D constitutively expressed on L cell lines. *J. Gen. Virol.* **68**, 1103-14.

Bzik, D.J.; Fox, B.A.; Deluca, N.A.; and Person, S. (1984) Nucleotide sequence specifying the glycoprotein gene, gB, of herpes simplex virus type 1. *Virology* **133**, 301-314.

Bzik, D.J.; Debroy, C.; Fox, B.A.; Pederson, N.E.; and Person, S. (1986) The nucleotide sequence of the gB glycoprotein gene of HSV-2 and comparison with the corresponding gene of HSV-1. *Virology* **155**, 322-33.

Campbell, T.M., and Studdert, M.J. (1983) Equine herpesvirus type-1 (EHV-1). *Vet. Bull.* **53**, 135-46.

Chan, W.L.; Lukig, M.L.; and Liew, F.Y. (1985) Helper T cells induced by an immunopurified herpes simplex virus type 1 (HSV-1) 115 kilodalton glycoprotein (gB) protect mice against HSV-1 infection. *J. Exp. Med.* **162**, 1304-18.

Cranage, M.P.; Kouzarides, T.; Bankier, A.T.; Satchwell, S.; Weston, K.; Tomlinson, P.; Barrell, B.; Hart, H.; Bell, S.E.; Minson, A.C.; and Smith, G.L. (1986) Identification of the human cytomegalovirus glycoprotein B gene and induction of neutralizing antibodies via its expression in recombinant vaccinia virus. *EMBO J.* **5**, 3057-63.

Dale, R.M.K.; McClure, B.A.; and Houchins, J.P. (1985) A rapid single-stranded cloning strategy for producing a series of overlapping clones for use in DNA sequencing. *Plasmid* **13**, 31-40.

Davison, A.J., and Scott, J.E. (1986) The complete DNA sequence of varicella-zoster virus. *J. Gen. Virol.* **67**, 1759-1816.

Davison, A.J., and Wilkie, N.M. (1983) Location and orientation of homologous sequences in the genomes of five herpesviruses. *J. Gen. Virol.* **64**, 1927-42.

Deluca, N.; Bzik, D.J.; Bond, V.C.; Person, S.; and Snipes, W. (1982) Nucleotide sequences of herpes simplex virus type 1 (HSV-1) affecting virus entry, cell fusion, and production of glycoprotein gB (VP7). *Virology* **122**, 411-23.

Fristensky, B.; Lis, J.; and Wu, R. (1982) Portable microcomputer software for nucleotide sequence analysis. *Nucl. Acids Res.* **10**, 6451-63.

Goodheart, C.R., and Plummer, G. (1975) The densities of herpesviral DNAs. *Prog. Med. Virol.* **19**, 324-52.

Keller, P.M.; Davison, A.J.; Lowe, R.S.; Bennet, C.D.; and Ellis, R.W. (1986) Identification and structure of the gene encoding gpII, a major glycoprotein of varicella-zoster virus. *Virology* **152**, 181-91.

Long, D.; Madara, T.J.; Ponce de Leon, M.; Cohen, G.H.; Montgomery, P.C.; and Eisenberg, R.J. (1984) Glycoprotein D protects mice against lethal challenge with herpes simplex virus types 1 and 2. *Infect. Immun.* **43**, 761-64.

Mach, M.; Utz, U.; and Fleckenstein, B. (1986) Mapping of the major glycoprotein gene of human cytomegalovirus. *J. Gen. Virol.* **67**, 1461-67.

Mackett, M., and Smith, G.L. (1986) Vaccinia virus expression vectors. *J. Gen. Virol.* **67**, 2067.

Maniatis, T.; Fritsch, E.F.; and Sambrook, J. (1982) In *Molecular Cloning: A Laboratory Manual*, pp. 92-94. Cold Spring Harbor Laboratory, Cold Spring Harbor, N.Y.

O'Callaghan, D.J.; Gentry, G.A.; and Randall, C.C. (1983) The equine herpesviruses. In *The Herpesviruses*, Vol. 2, pp. 215-318. Ed. B. Roizman. Plenum Press, New York.

Paoletti, E.; Lipinskas, B.R.; Samsonoff, C.; Mercer, S.; and Panicali, D. (1984) Construction of live vaccines using genetically engineered poxviruses: biological activity of vaccinia virus recombinants expressing the hepatitis B virus surface antigen and the herpes simplex virus glycoprotein D. *Proc. Natl. Acad. Sci. USA* **81**, 193-97.

Pellett, P.E.; Biggin, M.D.; Barrell, B.; and Roizman, B. (1985a) Epstein-Barr virus genome may encode a protein showing significant amino acid and predicted secondary structure homology with glycoprotein B of herpes simplex virus 1. *J. Virol.* **56**, 807-13.

Pellett, P.E.; Kousoulas, K.G.; Pereira, L.; and Roizman, B. (1985b) Anatomy of the herpes simplex virus 1 strain F glycoprotein B gene: primary sequence and predicted protein structure of the wild type and of monoclonal antibody-resistant mutants. *J. Virol.* **53**, 243-53.

Rigby, P.W.J.; Dieckmann, M.; Rhodes, C.; and Berg, P. (1977) Labelling deoxyribonucleic acid to high specific activity *in vitro* by nicktranslation with DNA polymerase I. *J. Mol. Biol.* **113**, 237-51.

Robertson, G.R., and Whalley, J.M. (1985) Molecular cloning and physical mapping of the equine herpesvirus I genome. In *Veterinary Viral Diseases: Their Significance in South East Asia and the Western Pacific*, pp. 471-72. Ed. A.J. Della Porta. Academic Press, Sydney, Australia.

Sabine, M.; Feilen, C.; Herbert, L.; Jones, R.; Lomas, S.; Love, D.; and Wild, J. (1983) Equine herpesvirus abortion in Australia (1977-1982). *Equine Vet. J.* **15**, 366-70.

Sanger, F.; Coulson, A.R.; Barrell, B.G.; Smith, A.J.H.; and Roe, B.A. (1980). Cloning in single stranded bacteriophage as an aid to rapid DNA sequencing. *J. Mol. Biol.* **143**, 161-78.

Snowden, B.W., and Halliburton, I.W. (1985) Identification of cross-reacting glycoproteins of four herpesviruses by western blotting. *J. Gen. Virol.* **66**, 2039-44.

Snowden, B.W.; Kinchington, P.R.; Powell, K.L.; and Halliburton, I.W. (1985) Antigenic and biochemical analysis of gB of herpes simplex virus type 1 and type 2 and of cross-reacting glycoproteins induced by bovine mammillitis virus and equine herpes virus type 1. *J. Gen. Virol.* **66**, 231-47.

Southern, E. (1975) Detection of specific sequences among DNA fragments separated by gel electrophoresis. *J. Mol. Biol.* **98**, 503-17.

Spear, P.G. (1985) Glycoproteins specified by herpes simplex viruses. In *The Herpesviruses*, Vol. 3, pp. 315-356. Ed. B. Roizman. Plenum Press, New York.

Turtinen, L.W., and Allen, G.P. (1982) Identification of the envelope surface glycoproteins of equine herpesvirus type 1. *J. Gen. Virol.* **63**, 481-85.

Whalley, J.M.; Robertson, G.R.; and Davison, A.J. (1981) Analysis of the genome of equine herpesvirus type I: arrangement of cleavage sites for restriction endonucleases EcoRI, BglII and BamHI. *J. Gen. Virol.* **57**, 307-23.

Skin Explant Targets in the Genetic Restriction of Cytolysis during Equid Herpesvirus-1 Subtype 2 Infection

Neil Edington, Charles Gordon Bridges, Simon Broad, and Lyn Griffiths

SUMMARY

Fragments of skin biopsies cocultivated with autologous monocytes in the presence of arginine, cystine, histidine, methionine, lysine, and cysteine proved reliable in obtaining autologous monolayers that would propagate to at least 15 passages and act as targets for assaying cytotoxic lymphocyte activity against equid herpesvirus-1 (EHV-1) infection. In six ponies, genetically restricted cytolysis was demonstrated at Days 7 and 21 following a second exposure to subtype 2 EHV-1. Killing of subtype 2 antigen–labeled cells was more efficient than killing those labeled with subtype 1 virus.

INTRODUCTION

The immune response to EHV-1 is apparently short-lived or inappropriate, as reinfection can take place as early as two to three months after natural or experimental infection (Allen & Bryans 1986). Investigation of cell-mediated immunity in horses infected with EHV-1 has been predominantly restricted to lymphocyte proliferation assays (Gerber et al. 1977; Dutta, Myrup & Bumgardner 1980), with Wilks and Coggins (1976) recording natural killer cytolysis of EHV-1–infected cell lines. A major problem in investigating cytotoxic T-lymphocyte (CTL) activity is that in an outbred population of animals autologous targets must be developed. While explants of skin biopsies or monocyte cultures have been established readily from cattle and pigs (Findlay & Jenkinson 1960; Nunn & Johnson 1979; Asagaba 1979; Hammer & Halprin 1981; Hebda et al. 1986), similar equine explants have failed to thrive (Wardley, Lawman & Hamilton 1980 and unpublished observations). After considerable manipulation, Moore and Katada (1978) cultured equine monocytes as monolayers but only in the presence of 60% sheep serum and with a supplement of arginine, cystine, and histidine. With the goal of developing a CTL assay to investigate the immune response to EHV-1 (Bridges & Edington 1987), preliminary studies were made in culturing monocytes and/or skin biopsies. The objective was a reproducible technique for establishing targets in the form of autologous cultures that would passage and would be sensitive to infection by both subtypes of EHV-1. The results describe the optimal conditions for such targets and their use in investigating CTL activity against EHV-1 subtype 2.

Department of Microbiology and Parasitology, Royal Veterinary College, Royal College Street, London NW1 OTU, England.

MATERIALS AND METHODS

Skin explants. Disposable 4-mm sterile punches (Stiefel Laboratories, Woodburn Green, England) were used to take skin biopsies from outbred Welsh ponies, sampling the hairless ventral aspect at the base of the tail. An appropriate area was swabbed with alcohol and anaesthetized with a lignocaine spray and a subcutaneous inoculation of 0.5 ml of a 0.5% solution of lignocaine HC1 (Xylocaine). The biopsy was immediately transferred with sterile instruments into 2.5 ml of growth medium in 5-ml containers. The excised skin was cut into approximately 0.5-mm cubes in a sterile petri dish and transferred on the tip of a 10-cm needle into a 25.0 cm^2 plastic disposable flask and allowed to adhere for 10 min at 37°C. Duplicate flasks, each containing approximately 20 explants, were made and to one of the flasks 7×10^6 washed leucocytes were added. The medium (with or without autologous monocytes) was dropped directly onto the explants to avoid dislodging them. In all cases the medium was MEM supplemented with 10% fetal bovine serum, arginine, cystine, and histidine, as described by Moore and Katada (1978), and with 14.5 μg/ml lysine HC1, 3.0 μg/ml methionine, and 5.7 μg/ml cysteine. The three amino acids promoted the growth of squamous epithelial cells from equine epidermal explants (unpublished observation). Twice the normal levels of penicillin, streptomycin, and fungizone were included in the medium, since contamination, particularly by fungus, was a problem in early samples. The medium was changed after 24 hr using gentle agitation to resuspend the majority of the lymphocyte population in those flasks seeded with leucocytes.

Monocytes. Twenty milliliters of venous blood was collected using 10 i.u/ml heparin; the mononuclear leucocyte fraction was obtained using Lympho Hypaque (Nycomed UK Ltd., Birmingham, England) and the cells were washed twice with phosphate-buffered saline (PBS). Cells were seeded at 10^6 ml^{-1} onto one of the two flasks of skin explants, and a third flask was seeded with a similar aliquot of leucocytes alone.

Virus isolation and EHV-1–specific antibody. Virus isolation from nasal swabs and leucocytes was attempted daily, according to Patel, Edington & Mumford (1982), as detailed previously (Bridges & Edington 1986). Complement-fixing (CF) and virus-neutralizing (VN) antibody were measured by the method of Thomson and colleagues (1976).

Leucocytes for CTL. Equine peripheral blood mononuclear cells (MNCs) were isolated from heparinized venous blood as described previously (Bridges & Edington 1986).

Viral antigen for CTL. Virus-infected equine embryonic kidney (EEK) monolayers in 75 cm^2 flasks exhibiting >90% cytopathic effect were collected and rinsed four times in ice-cold Dulbecco's PBS. The final 1.0-ml suspension was inactivated with B-propriolactone (0.1% Sigma) for 16 hr at 80°C and 3 hr at 37°C (Campbell, Studdert & Blackney 1982).

Preparation of interleukin. Equine MNCs (5×10^6 ml^{-1}) were stimulated for 48 hr at 37°C in 20 mM hepes buffered RPMI 1640 containing 1% autologous plasma and 2 µg/ml Concanavalin A (Sigma, St. Louis, Mo.). Excess Con A was removed by PBS-swollen Sephadex G50 as described by Bridges and Edington (1987). The resultant filtered supernatant was able to augment antigen-driven responses at least 17-fold.

Statistics. Animals were analyzed on an individual basis and as a cohort, for changes in responses with time or between antigens (Bridges & Edington 1987).

In vitro stimulation of effector cells. Mononuclear cells at a final concentration of 1-2 $\times$ 10^7 ml^{-1} were cultured with EHV-1 subtype 2 antigen (1 µg/ml) for 65 hr in 3-ml volumes of medium containing 10% interleukin and 2% autologous plasma. At the end of this incubation the viable cell yield was 60% to 105% of the original number (Bridges & Edington 1986).

Labeling of target cells. Autologous equine skin fibroblasts seeded at 5×10^4 cells per well of a flat-bottomed microtiter plate, in a volume of 150µl, were incubated with antigen (final concentration 10µg/ml^{-1}) and Cr-51 (1-2µCi/well) (CJSI; Amersham International, Aylesbury, England) for 20 hr at 37°C in serum-free RPMI 1640. The medium was removed and the cell monolayers rinsed four times in PBS immediately before the cytotoxicity assay.

Cytotoxicity assay. Washed cells harvested from antigen-stimulated cultures were tested for cytolytic activity in a conventional Cr-51 release assay (Bridges & Edington 1987). Assays were conducted against autologous fibroblasts coated with subtype 1, subtype 2, or mock antigen, as well as subtype 2 antigen-coated allogeneic cells.

Animals, viruses, and experimental infections. Six healthy Welsh Mountain pony foals, kept in isolation, were given $10^{6.8}$ tissue culture infective doses of sixth-passage EHV-1 subtype 2 by intranasal swab and nebulizer. These animals received an identical exposure to the same isolate 165 days later, when their complement-fixing antibody levels had declined to resting values. The foals were examined on both occasions for the parameters described above. Concurrent field infection was excluded by serological monitoring for a minimum of three weeks preceding the first infection and at appropriate intervals prior to the second exposure. Cytotoxicity and lymphoproliferation were examined at Days 3, 7, and 18 after the primary exposure, and at Days 3, 7, and 21 after the second infection.

Table 1. Outgrowths of monocytes and skin explants from six ponies

Pony no.	Monoctyes[a] (7 $\times$ 10^6 cells)	Skin[b]	Skin + autologous monocytes[b]
1	3	10/12	17/17
2	0	5/16	11/20
3	8	4/22	14/27
4	1	11/21	23/23
5	2	0/16	13/14
6	0	8/19	19/20

[a] Number of foci growing at 28 days in vitro.
[b] Number of outgrowths/number of explants made.

RESULTS

Skin explants. Macrophage-like cells were seen to move out from skin explants after three to seven days in vitro. There was a similar clustering of macrophages around explants in the flasks containing both explants and leucocytes, but the source of the cells could not be distinguished (Fig. 1). The first outgrowths of fibroblast and/or epithelial cells occurred at seven to 10 days (Fig. 1) and individual biopsies continued to produce cells up to 21 days after explantation (Fig. 2). Because of the numbers of epidermal explants giving rise to exfoliation (Table 1), it was generally advisable to make the first passage of the cells by 14-28 days, as early outgrowths were tending to overgrow. Where confluent monolayers were obtained, they usually made a 1:3 or 1:4 increase each week for up to 15 passages, seeding at 2×10^6 cells per 25 cm^2. They were sensitive to both subtypes of EHV-1, to EHV-2, and to equine adenovirus, with the yield of virus being equivalent to that in EEK.

In every case, it was the fibroblast-like component of mixed outgrowths that trypsinized most easily and divided most rapidly. Squamous epithelial cells required up to 20 minutes' exposure to ATV to disrupt desmosomes, and they did not passage successfully. Each system yielded some cultures that persisted for at least 12-15 passages and supported replication of equine viruses (Table 1).

Cocultivation with autologous monocytes produced outgrowths from all six ponies and cells grew from 80% of explants, whereas cell growth was limited to 37% if mono-

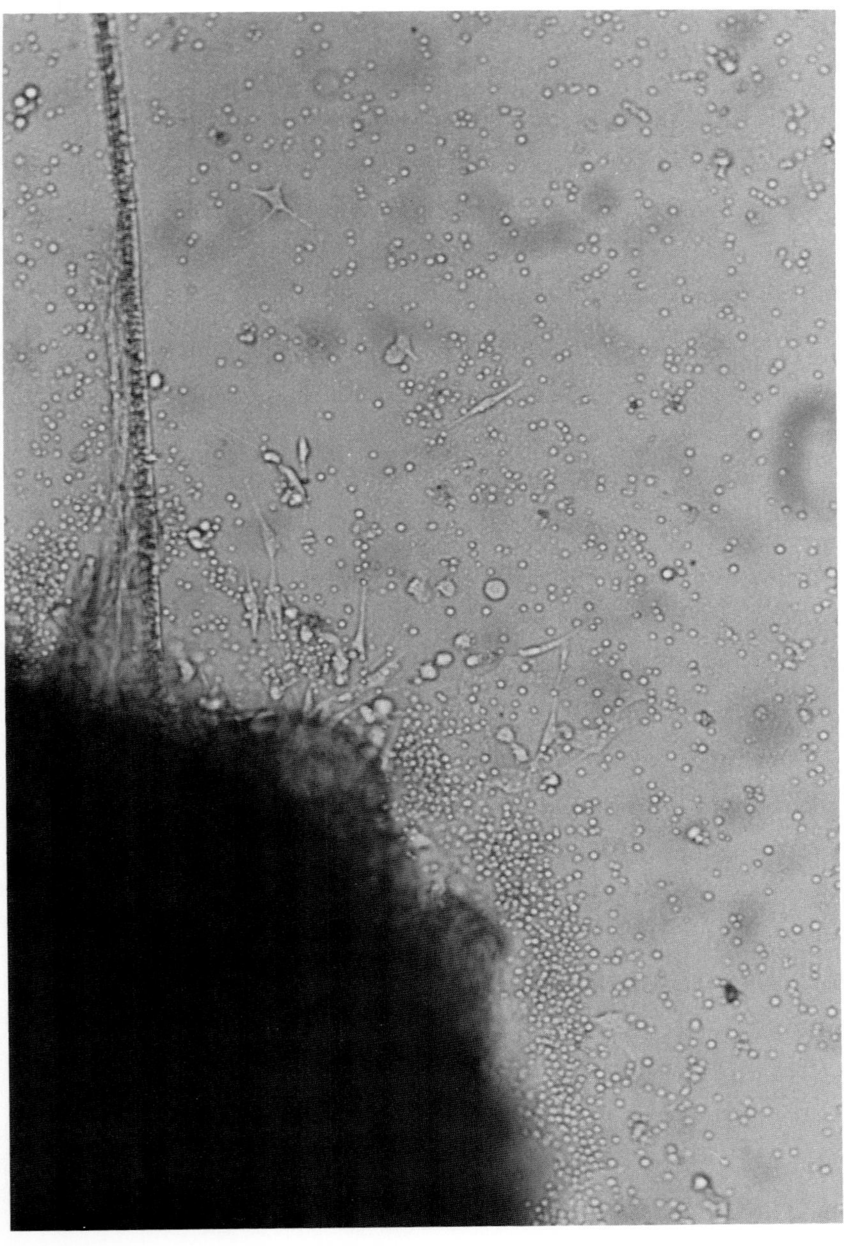

Fig. 1. Explant of equine skin biopsy after 8 days' culture with autologous monocytes. Macrophages have moved out of tissue to form dense accumulation 3-4 cells deep; elongated fibroblasts are just beginning to grow out of explant (mag 400×).

cytes were omitted (Table 1). The cocultivation also established more rapidly, with the mean incubation to first trypsinization being 16 ± 2.2 days compared with 25 ± 3.1 days in skin-only explants. Among the monocytes cultured alone, distinct foci of ellipsoid confluent cells developed in monocytes from only three of the six animals and then only in low numbers. Monocytes did not appear to divide in the presence of autologous skin explants. Thus while cocultivation increased outgrowth from the dermis ($P > .001$), it appeared to inhibit the nondermal monocytes from changing into confluent monolayers.

Virus isolation. The pattern of virus isolation from nasal swabs is shown in Figure 3. The mean length of virus excretion was 8.5 days for the first infection but was limited to 2.2 days for the second exposure ($P < 0.001$). Virus was not recovered from the peripheral blood leucocytes on any occasion.

Cytotoxicity. There was no evidence of EHV-1–specific cytotoxicity at Days 3 and 7 postexposure during the primary subtype 2 infection (data not shown). Unfortunately, technical difficulties prevented assessment of the samples at Day 18 postinfection. On the other hand, virus-specific cytolysis was observed at Days 7 and 21 after the second exposure (Fig. 4). Cytolysis appeared to be genetically restricted, as killing of subtype 2–labeled allogeneic targets was significantly less (Day 7, $0.02 > P > 0.01$; Day 21, $0.05 > P > 0.02$). The

Fig. 2. After 20 days in vitro, fibroblastic outgrowths are extensive, as cells divide in situ; rounded cells are migrating fibroblasts (mag 400 ×). Cultures will passage readily, whereas epithelial outgrowths fail to passage.

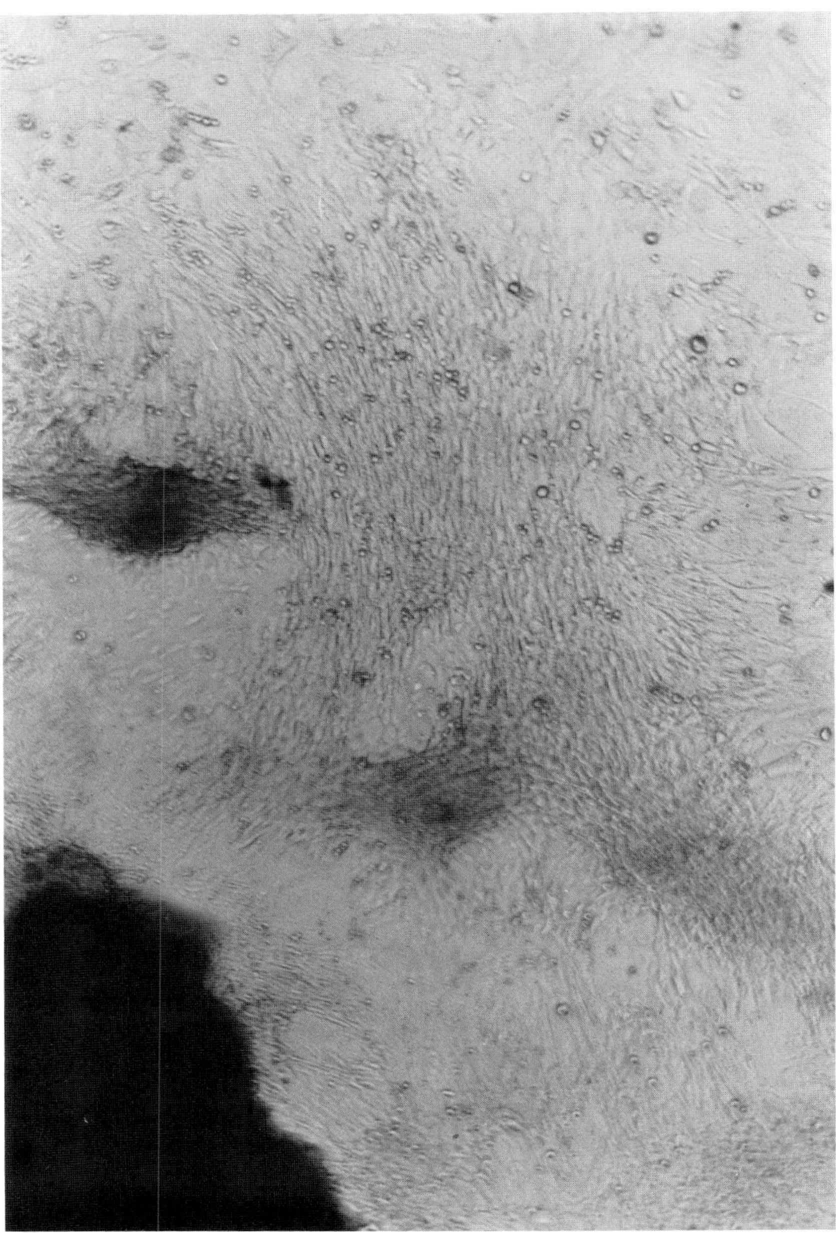

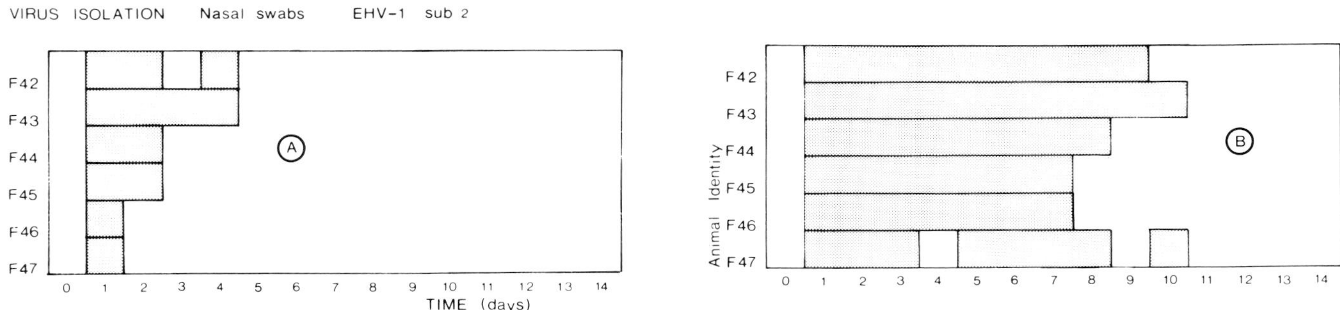

Fig. 3. Virus isolation (nasal swabs) from horses after experimental infections with EHV-1 subtype 2: *A*. second exposure; *B*. first exposure.

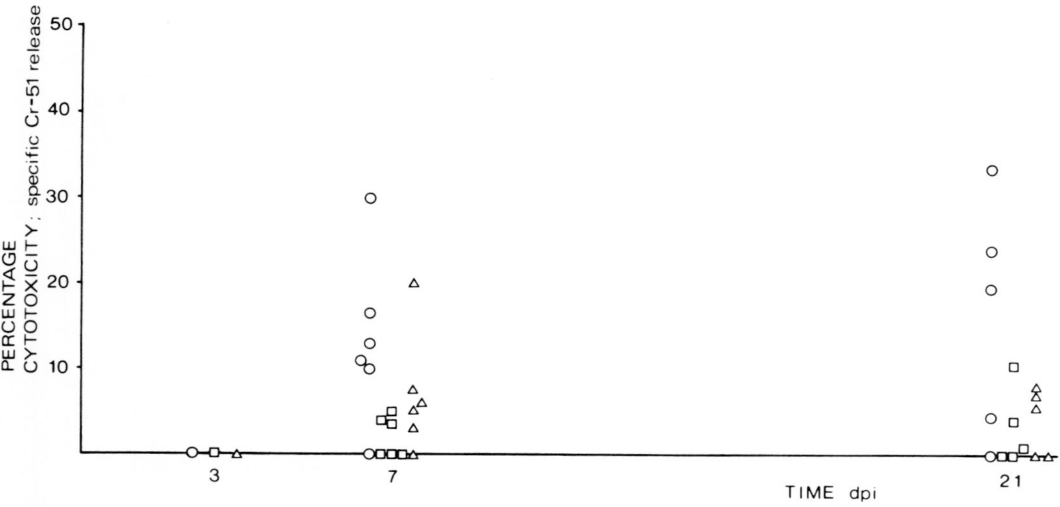

Fig. 4. Equine cell-mediated cytotoxicity during second EHV-1 subtype 2 infection: *circles*, EHV-1 subtype 2 coated autologous targets; *squares*, EHV-1 subtype 2 coated allogeneic targets; *triangles*, EHV-1 subtype 1 coated autologous targets. $N = 5$ at Day 21 postinfection. Effector: target ratio = 30:1.

cytotoxic response to subtype 1 virus on autologous target cells was also measurable in several animals at Days 7 and 21 postinfection, but did not attain the efficiency of subtype 2–directed cytolysis (Day 7, $0.01 > P > 0.001$; Day 21, $0.05 > P > 0.02$).

Circulating antibody levels. Changes in VN and CF antibody are recorded in Table 2. The primary infection produced significant increases in the levels of neutralizing subtype 2 antibody, whereas subtype 1 VN antibody levels remained static. Complement-fixing antibody to either subtype was initially inapparent, but by Day 14 measurable amounts were found against both subtypes. By Day 21, CF antibody was significantly higher against subtype 2. The second infection produced an increase in VN antibody to subtype 1 virus, as well as to the challenge subtype. As in the first exposure, CF antibody was present against both subtypes but reached higher levels against EHV-1 subtype 2.

DISCUSSION

Previous researchers have indicated that humoral responses and lymphocyte transformation following primary exposure to EHV-1 are subtype-specific (Fitzpatrick & Studdert 1984; Allen & Bryans 1986). However, these parameters do not readily relate to protection. If effective control programs are to be developed for EHV-1, it is imperative that the CTL and T-helper functions are delineated in the horse as they have been for herpes simplex virus (HSV) infection both in mice (Sethi et al. 1983; Nash & Gell 1983) and, more recently, in man (Yasukawa & Zarling 1984; Williamson et al. 1986). The development of reliable autologous targets is fundamental to such investigations. In the present experiments, cocultivation of host monocytes with skin explants significantly enhanced ($P > .001$) outgrowth of cells so that confluent cultures could be rapidly and reliably established. No attempt was made to investigate whether the synergistic effect could be reproduced by interleukins (Schmidt et al. 1982) or by platelet factors (Hebda et al. 1986), nor whether the presence of autologous, as opposed to homologous, cells was essential to evoke the synergism. As our interest was to investigate CTL activity, autologous cells were necessary in every case.

The established monolayers were successfully used to demonstrate the genetic restriction of CTL activity in six ponies in two sequential infections with subtype 2 EHV-1. While the cells were sensitive to both subtypes of EHV-1, the attachment of inactivated virus produced lower background in the CTL assays and was therefore used in these assays. Propagation of the cells to at least 15 passages meant that they were available for consecutive investigations. Similar monolayers have been prepared successfully from a further 12 ponies. In two of them equid herpesvirus-2 was recovered at the fifth passage, indicating that it is advisable to monitor the cells using indirect immunofluorescence as described by Mumford and Thomson (1978).

The experiments using these cells as targets led us to conclude that a genetically restricted CTL component does occur in EHV-1 infections but can only be detected in expanded populations of cells, as in humans with HSV infection (Yasukawa & Zarling 1984). As with the antibody response and lymphocyte proliferation assays, the CTL assay to EHV-1 showed subtype specificity in unprimed animals, with a definite indication that this was broadening by the second exposure to same subtype. The CTL activity after secondary exposure followed a peak of virus-mediated lymphoproliferation at Day 3 postinfection, with rapid curtailment (Bridges & Edington 1988). After primary exposure the lymphoproliferation was only observed at Day 18, suggesting that activation is a later event.

Further work is needed to identify the components of the virus that elicit the CTL response and to define the onset, duration, and specificity of CTL activity in animals exposed to a controlled sequence of infections. A more comprehensive understanding of the regulation of EHV-1 infection, and of

Table 2. Mean antibody levels against EHV-1 during primary and secondary infections with EHV-1 subtype 2

	subtype 1 antibody				subtype 2 antibody			
	CF		VN		CF		VN	
	(1)	(2)	(1)	(2)	(1)	(2)	(1)	(2)
Preinfection	0	0.90	<0.90	0.95	0	1.1	0.95	0.95
Day postinfection								
7	0	1.40	<0.90	1.05	0	2.0	1.05	1.05
14	0.9	1.60	<0.90	1.40	1.4	2.1	1.6	1.60
21	1.0	1.50	0.90	1.40	1.7	1.9	2.2	1.70

Note: Results expressed as log transformation reciprocal of titer. CF = complement fixing; VN = virus neutralization.

the interrelationship between the two subtypes, will be the basis for more rational control programs.

ACKNOWLEDGMENTS

Thanks are due to Neil Ledger for technical assistance and to the staff of the gnotobiotic unit for the care of the ponies. Generous financial support from the Horserace Betting Levy Board is gratefully acknowledged.

REFERENCES

Allen, G.P., and Bryans, J.T. (1986) Molecular epizootiology, pathogenesis and prophylaxis of equine herpesvirus-1 infections. In *Progress in Veterinary Microbiology and Immunology*, Vol. 2, pp. 78-144. Ed. R. Pandey. S. Karger, Basel.

Asagaba, M.O. (1979) Establishment of a bovine macrophage cell line. MSc. thesis, James Cook University, Queensland.

Bridges, C.G., and Edington, N. (1986) Innate immunity during equine herpesvirus-1 (EHV-1) infection. *Clin. Exp. Immunol.* **65**, 172-81.

———. (1987) Genetic restriction of cytolysis following infection with equid herpesvirus-1, subtype 2. *Clin. Exp. Immunol.* **70**, 276-82.

Campbell, T.M.; Studdert, M.J.; and Blackney, M.H. (1982) Immunogenicity of equine herpesvirus type 1 (EHV-1) and equine rhinovirus type 1 (ERhV-1) following inactivation by beta-propriolactone (BPL) and ultraviolet (UV) light. *Vet. Micro.* **7**, 535-44.

Dutta, S.K.; Myrup, A.; and Bumgardner, M.K. (1980) Lymphocyte responses to virus and mitogen in ponies during experimental infection with equine herpesvirus-1. *Am. J. Vet. Res.* **41**, 2066-2068.

Findlay, J.D., and Jenkinson, D.M. (1960) The morphology of bovine sweat glands and the effect of heat on the sweat glands of the Ayrshire calf. *J. Agric. Sci.* **55**, 247-49.

Fitzpatrick, D.R., and Studdert, M.J. (1984) Immunologic relationships between equine herpesvirus type 1 (equine abortion virus) and type 4 (equine rhinopneumonitis virus). *Am. J. Vet. Res.* **45**, 1947-52.

Gerber, J.D.; Marron, A.E.; Bass, E.P.; and Beckenhauer, W.H. (1977) Effect of age and pregnancy on the antibody and cell-mediated immune responses of horses to equine herpesvirus-1. *Can. J. Comp. Med.* **41**, 471-78.

Hammer, H., and Halprin, K. (1981) Epidermal cell growth. In *The Epidermis in Disease*, pp. 243-65. Eds. R. Marks and E. Christophers. MTB Press, Lancaster.

Hebda, P.A.; Alstadt, S.P.; Hileman, W.T.; and Eaglestein, W.H. (1986) Support and stimulation of epidermal outgrowth from porcine skin explants by platelet factors. *Br. J. Dermatol.* **115**, 529-41.

Moore, R.W., and Katada, M. (1978) The nutritional needs of a continuous passage horse leucocyte culture. *Vet. Micro.* **3**, 71-76.

Mumford, J.A., and Thomson, G.R. (1978) Serological methods for identification of slowly growing herpesviruses isolated from the respiratory tract of horses. *Proc. 4th Int. Conf. Equine Infect. Dis.*, pp. 49-55.

Nash, A.A., and Gell, P.G.H. (1983) Membrane phenotype of murine effector and suppressor T cells involved in delayed hypersensitivity and protective immunity to herpes simplex virus. *Cell Immunol.* **75**, 348-53.

Nunn, M., and Johnson, R.H. (1979) A simple technique for establishing cell lines from porcine blood. *Aust. Vet. J.* **55**, 446.

Patel, J.R.; Edington, N.; and Mumford, J.A. (1982) Variation in cellular tropism between isolates of Equine herpesvirus-1 in foals. *Arch. Virol.* **74**, 41-51.

Schmidt, J.A.; Mizel, S.B.; Cohen, D.; and Green, I. (1982) Interleukin 1, a potential regulator of fibroblast proliferation. *J. Immunol.* **128**, 2177-82.

Sethi, K.K.; Omata, Y.; and Schneweis, K.C. (1983) Protection of mice from fatal herpes simplex virus type 1 by adoptive transfer of cloned virus-specific and H-2 restricted cytotoxic T lymphocytes. *J. Gen. Virol.* **64**, 443-47.

Thomson, G.R.; Mumford, J.A.; Campbell, J.; and Griffiths, L. (1976) Serological detection of Equine herpesvirus-1 infections of the respiratory tract. *Equine Vet. J.* **8**, 58-65.

Wardley, R.C.; Lawman, M.J.; and Hamilton, F. (1980) The establishment of continuous macrophage cell lines from peripheral blood leucocytes. *Immunology* **39**, 67-73.

Wilks, C.R., and Coggins, L. (1976) In vitro cytotoxicity of serum and peripheral blood leukocytes for Equine herpesvirus type 1-infected target cells. *Am. J. Vet. Res.* **38**, 117-21.

Williamson, S.A.; Parish, N.; Chambers, J.D.; and Knight, R.A. (1986) Human immune responses to herpes simplex virus, varicella-zoster and cytomegalovirus in vitro. *Immunology* **57**, 437-42.

Yasukawa, M., and Zarling, J.M. (1984) Human cytotoxic T cell clones directed against herpes simplex virus-infected cells. I. Lysis restricted by HLA class II MB and Dr antigens. *J. Immunol.* **133**, 422-27.

The Derivation of Restriction Endonuclease Maps of the Equid Herpesvirus-1 Subtype 2 Genome

Ann Cullinane and Andrew Davison

SUMMARY

Electron microscopy of EHV-1 subtype 2 DNA that had been denatured and self-annealed indicated that a sequence of one genome terminus is repeated in inverse orientation at one internal site. The inverted repeats were shown to be separated by a unique sequence of approximately 13 kilobase-pairs (kbp). The presence of the repeated sequence within the EHV-1 subtype 2 genome was confirmed by hybridization studies using DNA probes isolated from virion DNA. A library of plasmid clones containing BamHI fragments representing approximately 75% of the genome was prepared, and the clones were used to derive BamHI and EcoRI restriction endonuclease maps for EHV-1 subtype 2 DNA. The results show that the EHV-1 subtype 2 genome consists of two segments, L (109 kbp) and S (35 kbp). The S component consists of a unique sequence (U_S; 9.6-16 kbp) flanked by inverted repeats (TR_S and IR_S; 9.5-12.7 kbp). Published data indicate that the EHV-1 subtype 1 genome has a similar structure.

INTRODUCTION

Equid herpesvirus-1 (EHV-1), a member of the alphaherpesvirinae, is a major cause of abortion and respiratory disease in horses worldwide. It is also associated with a neurological syndrome, neonatal foal disease, and more rarely with coital exanthema (O'Callaghan, Allen & Randall 1979; O'Callaghan, Gentry & Randall 1983; Campbell & Studdert 1983; Allen & Bryans, 1986). Two antigenically and genetically distinct subtypes of EHV-1 can be unequivocally differentiated by restriction endonuclease analysis of their DNAs (Sabine, Robertson & Whalley 1981; Studdert, Simpson & Roizman 1981). Restriction endonuclease analysis has been used in epizootiological studies of EHV-1 in Kentucky (Allen et al. 1983) and Australia (Studdert 1983). Although subtype 2—unlike subtype 1—does not appear to be associated with abortion storms or with the neurological syndrome, these studies indicate that it is a major cause of epizootics of respiratory disease in young horses and that it has the potential to cause abortion. It has been suggested that EHV-1 subtype 2 be renamed EHV-4 (Studdert et al. 1981).

MRC Virology Unit, Institute of Virology, University of Glasgow, Church Street, Glasgow G11 5JR, U.K. Present address, Cullinane: Irish Equine Centre, Johnstown Naas, Co. Kildare, Ireland.

Restriction endonuclease maps of EHV-1 subtype 1 DNA have been published (Whalley, Robertson & Davison 1981; Henry et al. 1981). The genome comprises two covalently linked segments designated L (Long) and S (Short). The S segment consists of a unique region (U_S) bracketed by inverted repeat sequences (TR_S, IR_S). This arrangement allows the S segment to invert relative to the L segment, which is a unique sequence in a fixed orientation. A combination of electron microscopy, restriction endonuclease analysis, and molecular hybridization was used to determine whether the two subtypes of EHV-1 share a common genome structure and to construct the first restriction endonuclease maps of EHV-1 subtype 2.

MATERIALS AND METHODS

Cells and virus. EHV-1 subtype 2 isolate 1942, kindly supplied by J.A. Mumford (Animal Health Trust, Newmarket), was propagated in an SV40-transformed cell line derived from sheep lung fibroblasts, a generous gift of Dr. J. Macnab (Institute of Virology). The cells were grown in Glasgow's modified BHK medium, supplemented with 10% fetal calf serum.

Virus DNA preparation and restriction endonuclease analysis. Cell-released virus was purified by rate zonal centrifugation through a Percoll gradient (Sigma), and the DNA was extracted according to the method of Wilkie (1973) for herpes simplex virus. Restriction endonuclease digestion of DNA was performed under the conditions recommended (Boehringer, Lewes, England). DNA fragments resulting from restriction endonuclease cleavage were fractionated by electrophoresis through gels with agarose concentrations of 0.5-1.0% stained with 0.5 μg/ml ethidium bromide. When specific DNA fragments were required as probes for hybridization studies, individual bands were sliced from a 0.7% low-melting-point agarose gel and the DNA was purified as described by Weislander (1979).

Electron microscopy of DNA. Intramolecular annealing studies were performed by the method of Ruyechan, Dauenhauer, and O'Callaghan (1982). Both single-stranded and double-stranded circular Phi X174 DNAs were added as size markers. Samples were prepared for electron microscopy, the grids examined, and the lengths of DNA molecules measured as described by Rixon, Taylor, and Desselberger (1984).

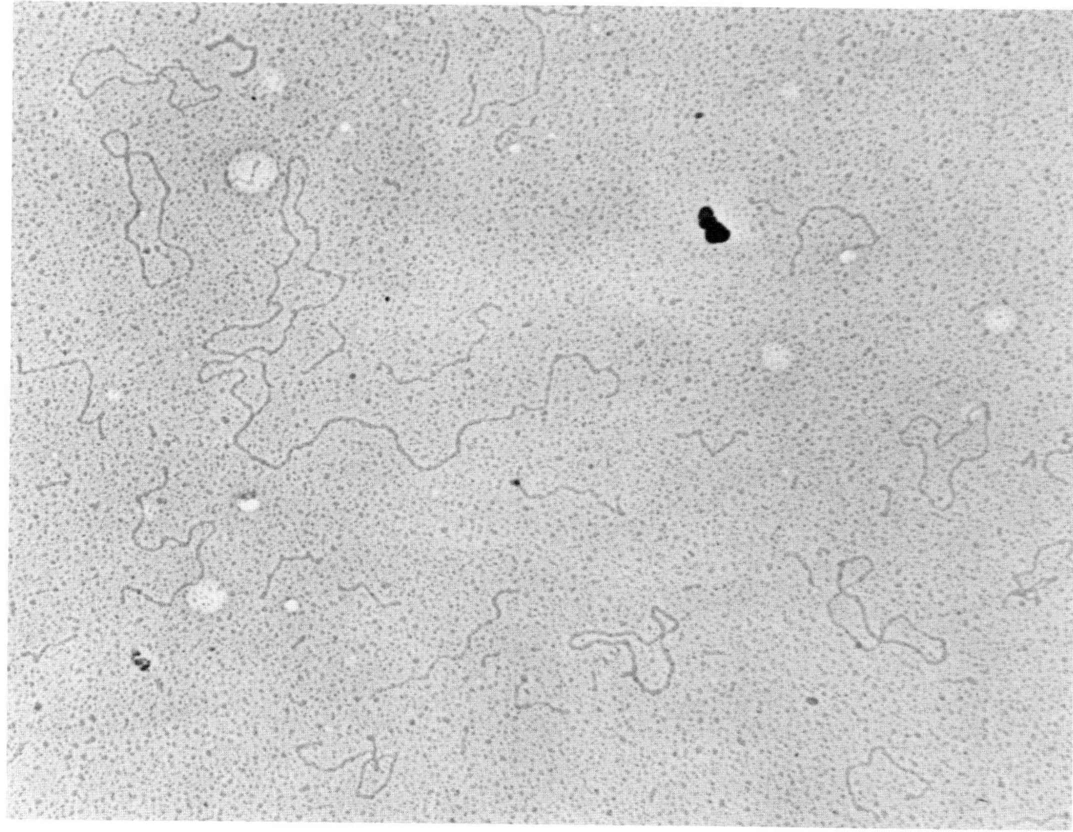

Fig. 1. Electron micrograph of annealed single-stranded EHV-1 subtype 2 DNA molecule: a single-stranded loop (U_S) with a double-stranded stem (TR_S/IR_S) contiguous with a single-stranded tail. *Arrows*, single-stranded Phi X174 DNA molecules.

Cloning. The DNA cloning methods were those described by Maniatis, Fritsch, and Sambrook (1982). Viral DNA was digested to completion with BamHI and shotgun-cloned into pUC9 (Vieira & Messing 1982). Calcium-shocked *Escherichia coli* DHI (Hanahan 1983) were transformed with recombinant DNA as described by Cohen and colleagues (1972). The recombinant plasmids were harvested from mini-cultures (Holmes & Quigley 1981) and analyzed by restriction enzyme digestion and electrophoresis of the resultant fragments.

Molecular hybridization analysis. The transfer of DNA fragments from agarose gels to nitrocellulose membranes (Schleicher & Schuell, Keene, N.H.) was accomplished by the technique of Southern (1975). Filters were prehybridized at 42°C for at least 2 hr in a hybridization solution consisting of 3× standard saline citrate, 5× Denhardt's solution 0.02% (w/v) Ficoll 400, 0.02% (w/v) polyvinylpyrrolidone, 0.02% (w/v) bovine serum albumin and 100 μg/ml denatured salmon sperm DNA in 50% (v/v) formamide. The filters were then treated overnight at 42°C in fresh hybridization solution with ^{32}P-labeled denatured viral DNA fragments. Radioactive labeling of probes was by nick translation (Rigby et al. 1977). After hybridization, the filters were washed in 3× SSC, 0.2% sodium dodecyl sulphate, 10 mM sodium phosphate (pH 7.5) at 50°C for at least 3 hr. The buffer was changed every hour. The filters were air-dried and exposed to Kodak X-Omat film at −70°C.

RESULTS

Electron microscopy of EHV-1 DNA. To identify inverted repeat sequences in the genome of EHV-1 subtype 2, DNA was denatured and the single strands allowed to self-anneal. Electron microscopy then revealed structures consisting of single-stranded loops joined to a double-stranded region contiguous with a single strand (Fig. 1). The structures were interpreted as the result of annealing of a terminal sequence to an internal inverted complementary sequence. The single-stranded loop connecting these sequences and the long single-stranded tail thus represent unique sequences. The lengths of 27 single-stranded loops were measured. On the basis of the ratio of these lengths to those of single-stranded Phi X174, the size of the short unique sequence was calculated as approximately 13.3 kbp.

Molecular weights of restriction digest fragments of EHV-1 subtype 2 DNA. EHV-1 subtype 2 DNA was digested with restriction endonucleases BamHI and EcoRI, and the molecular weights of the fragments were determined by comparison with a HindIII digest of phage lambda DNA (Maniatis, Jeffrey & Van de Sande 1975). Fragments of both

Table 1. Sizes (kbp) of EHV-1 subtype 2 DNA fragments

BamHI			EcoRI		
Fragments	Estimated size	Estimated molarity	Fragments	Estimated size	Estimated molarity
a	18.5	1	ab	27.5	2
bcd	14.1	3	c	18.5	1
e	12.7	1	d	14.1	1
f	11.0	1	e	12.0	1
g	9.5	1	f	9.5	1
h	8.4	1	g	7.3	1
i	6.4	1	h	6.3	1
jkl	4.6	3	ij	6.0	2
mno	4.5	3	k	3.4	1
o	4.2	1	l	2.9	1
p	3.6	1	m	2.2	1

Table 2. Results of hybridizing nick-translated BamHI and EcoRI fragments from EHV-1 subtype 2 virion DNA, to fragments of EHV-1 subtype 2 DNA

BamHI probe	Hybridizing BamHI fragment	Hybridizing EcoRI fragment	EcoRI probe	Hybridizing EcoRI fragments	Hybridizing BamHI fragments
a	a	c,h	ab	ab,f	bcd,e,f,i,jkl,mnn,o,p
bcd	bcd,jkl	ab,d,e,f,g,ij,l,m,n,q	c	c	a,h
e	e	ab	d	d	bcd,g
f	f	ab	e	e	bcd,jkl,mnn
g	g	d,h	f	f,ab	bcd,jkl,mnn,p
h	h	c,k,p	g	g,i,j	bcd,bjkl
i	i	ab	h	h	a,g
jkl	jkl,bcd,p	ab,e,f,g,ij,o,p	ij	ij,g	bcd,jkl
mnn	mnn	ab,e,f	k	k	h
o	o	ab	l	l	bcd
p	jkl,p	ab,f	m	m	bcd

Table 3. Hybridization data for BamHI clones

BamHI cloned probes	Hybridizing BamHI bands	Hybridizing EcoRI bands
a	a	c, h
b	bcd	d, ij, l
c	bcd	ab, e
4	bcd, jkl, p	ab, d, f, ij, l
f	f	ab
g	g	d, h
h	h	p, k, c
i	i	ab
j	jkl	e, o, p
l	bcd, jkl	ab, f, g, ij
m	mnn	e
n	mnn	ab, f
n+o	mnn, o	ab, f
q	—	e

Table 4. Sizes (kbp) of fragments generated by digesting cloned EHV-1 subtype 2 DNA fragments with BamHI and EcoRI

Clones	Products of BamHI digestion	Products of BamHI + EcoRI digestion	Products of EcoRI digestion
a	18.5, 2.7	13.7, 4.8, 2.7	13.7, 7.5
b	14.1, 2.7	6.3, 5.0, 2.8, 2.7	6.3, 7.8, 2.7
c	14.1, 2.7	10.0, 3.1, 2.7, 1.0	12.6, 3.2, 1.0
f	11.0, 2.7	11.0, 2.7	13.7
g	9.5, 2.7	8.0, 2.7, 1.5	1.5, 10.7
h	8.4, 2.7	4.7, 3.3, 2.7	7.4, 3.3
i	6.4, 2.7	6.4, 2.7	9.1
j	4.6, 2.7	3.4, 2.7, 1.0	7.3
l	4.6, 2.7	3.0, 2.7, 1.6	4.3, 3.0
m	4.5, 2.7	4.5, 2.7	7.2
n	4.5, 2.7	4.5, 2.7	7.2
o	4.2, 2.7	4.2, 2.7	6.9
q	1.0, 2.7	1.0, 2.7	3.7

Note: pUC9 = 2.7 kbp.

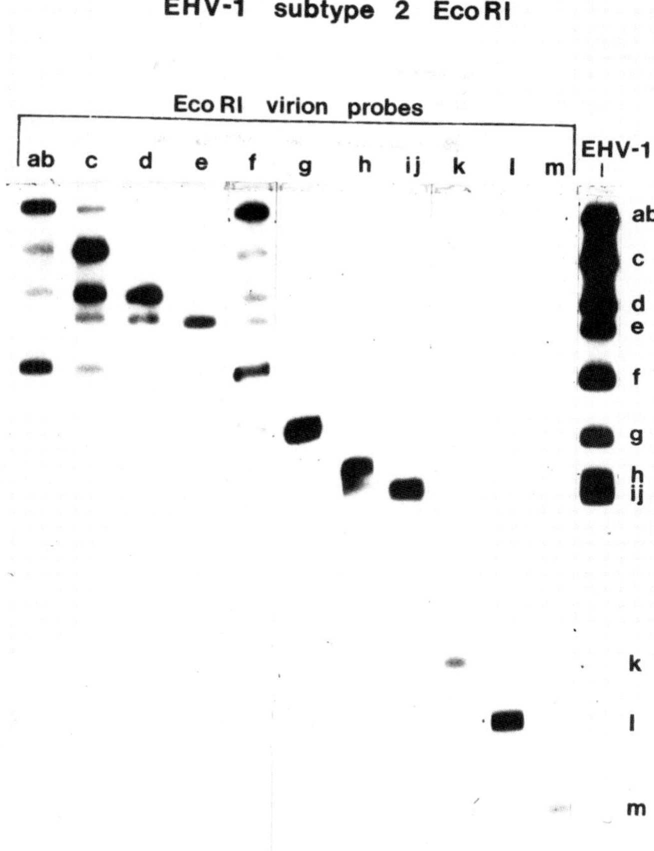

Fig. 2. Autoradiograph of results of hybridizing ^{32}P-labeled EcoRI fragments of EHV-1 subtype 2 DNA to an EcoRI digest of the same DNA.

digests were assigned letters alphabetically in descending order of molecular weight (Table 1). The relative molarity of the bands of EHV-1 subtype 2 DNA visualized in agarose gels was estimated from densitometric traces (Table 1) and taken into account when estimating the size of the genome as 144 kbp.

Hybridization using virion DNA probes. ^{32}P-labeled BamHI and EcoRI fragments of EHV-1 subtype 2 DNA were hybridized to restriction enzyme digests of the same DNA (Table 2). The presence of a repeated sequence within the genome was confirmed by such studies. For example, in hybridizing ^{32}P-labeled EcoRI fragments of EHV-1 subtype 2 DNA to an EcoRI digest of the same DNA, each DNA probe as expected, hybridized to the equivalent fragment in the EcoRI digest. However, probe ab hybridized also to f and vice versa. The results are consistent with the presence of fragments in the repeated regions of the genome.

Probes isolated from virion DNA in the derivation of restriction endonuclease linkage maps were contaminated by comigrating fragments in the restriction enzyme digests. Fragment contamination, an unavoidable feature of these experiments, complicated the interpretation of results. To overcome these problems, BamHI fragments representing approximately 75% of the genome were cloned into plasmid vector pUC9. The clones were used in two ways to derive BamHI and EcoRI restriction endonuclease maps of EHV-1 subtype 2 DNA. First, they were used in hybridization studies (Table 3) to determine the order of restriction fragments in the genome. Second, the products of simultaneous digestion by two restriction endonucleases (Table 4) were analyzed to determine the location of BamHI and EcoRI cleavage sites in the genome.

Derivation of restriction endonuclease map for S region of EHV-1 subtype 2 genome. The hybridization of BamHI virion DNA fragments to a BamHI digest of EHV-1 subtype 2 DNA (Table 2) showed that, in addition to hybridizing to themselves, BamHI bcd hybridized to jkl, BamHI jkl hybridized to bcd and to p, and BamHI p hybridized to jkl. These data indicate the presence of portions of the fragments in these bands in repeated DNA sequences. The use of cloned DNA as hybridization probes helped to identify the individual fragments mapping in the repeats. Cloned BamHI l

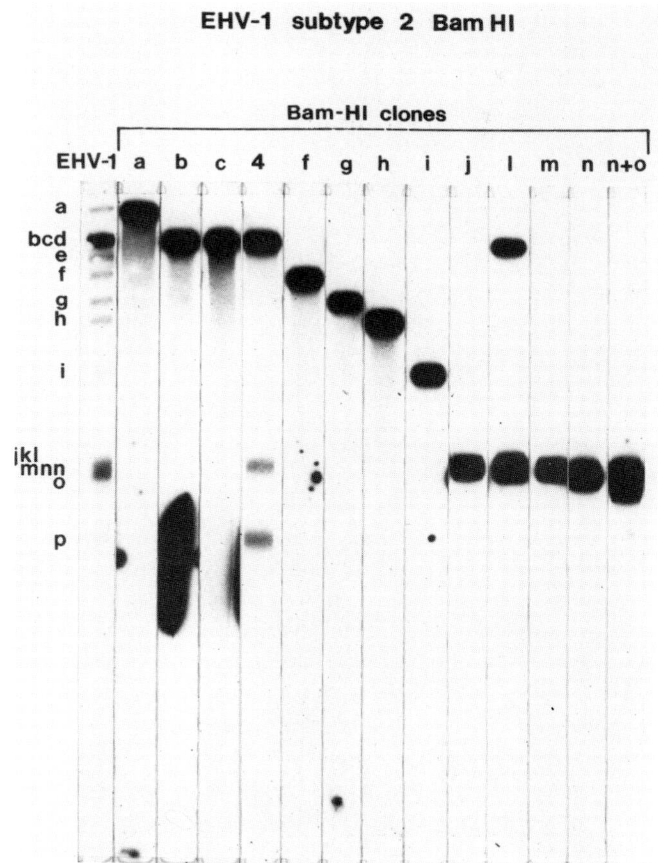

Fig. 3. Autoradiograph of results of hybridizing ^{32}P-labeled BamHI cloned fragments of EHV-1 subtype 2 DNA to a BamHI digest of the same DNA; clone 4 of undetermined structure. (Faint band common to all tracks may be a contaminant, perhaps pUC9, in the dye.)

hybridized to BamHI jkl and bcd, but neither cloned BamHI b nor cloned BamHI c hybridized to BamHI jkl (Fig. 3). The implication is that BamHI l hybridizes only to BamHI d, which was not cloned. BamHI p from virion DNA hybridized to BamHI jkl (Table 2) and, since neither cloned BamHI l nor cloned BamHI j hybridized to p, BamHI k, which was not cloned, must hybridize to p (Fig. 3).

The hybridization of EcoRI virion DNA probes to an EcoRI digest of EHV-1 subtype 2 DNA (Fig. 2) indicated the presence of portions of EcoRI f and one or both of EcoRI ab in the repeated regions. Similarly, the results in Figure 2 suggest that EcoRI g and either or both of ij hybridized to each other. However, the weak hybridization between EcoRI g and ij indicates that hybridizing fragments share only a short sequence. The interpretation is that, first of all, EcoRI b and f, which show a high degree of homology, originate from the S terminus and L-S joint. EcoRI f, being the smaller of the fragments, represents the S terminal fragment, and EcoRI b contains the L-S joint. Beyond that, EcoRI g and j contain the Tr_S/U_S and IR_S/U_S junctions. The proposed arrangement of EcoRI fragments in S, illustrated in Figure 4A, does not exclude the presence of additional EcoRI fragments between b and g, g and j, and j and f. Hybridization of cloned BamHI l to EcoRI ab, f, g, and ij (Fig. 5) shows that this fragment spans the junction between EcoRI b and g or j and f. The stronger hybridization to EcoRI ij than to g indicates that BamHI l shares more sequence with the former, and therefore that BamHI l spans the junction between EcoRI j and f (Fig. 4B). Restriction endonuclease analysis showed that BamHI l is cleaved by EcoRI to give fragments of 3 kbp and 1.6 kbp (Table 4). The stronger hybridization of BamHI l to EcoRI ij than to EcoRI f (Fig. 5) suggests that the EcoRI site is nearer the right end of BamHI l. The BamHI site that divides l and n is located approximately 8 kbp from the S terminus, and an equivalent BamHI site is located in IR_S. The genome location of BamHI d, which hybridized to BamHI l (Table 4), is shown in Figure 4B.

EcoRI f hybridized to BamHI bands bcd, jkl, mnn, and p (Fig. 2). Cloned BamHI n hybridized to EcoRI ab and f, and BamHI mnn, verifying the location of this fragment completely within TR_S/IR_S (Figs. 3 and 5). BamHI n was not cleaved by EcoRI (Table 4), and is unlikely to be the S terminal fragment because it was cloned. EcoRI f also hybridized to BamHI p, which hybridized to itself and to BamHI k (Table 2). Neither BamHI p nor BamHI k was cloned, but on the basis of size it is proposed that p is at the S terminus and k at the L-S joint. The data are consistent with the location of BamHI n between l and p (Fig. 4C). The sum of the sizes of BamHI p, n, and the portion of l within EcoRI f corresponds to the size of EcoRI f, implying that all large BamHI fragments in TR_S/IR_S have been accounted for. However, the sum of the sizes of BamHI d and l is 18.7 kbp, whereas the sum of the sizes of EcoRI j and g, plus twice the size of the portion of BamHI l to the right of the EcoRI site, is only 16.5 kbp. The difference between these sizes implies

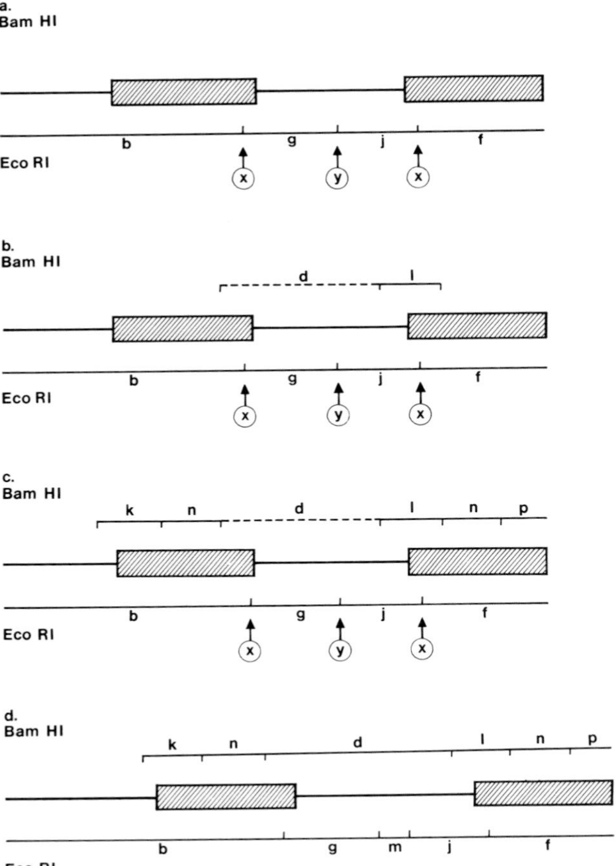

Fig. 4. Derivation of BamHI and EcoRI linkage maps for *S* segment of EHV-1 subtype 2 genome: *hatched rectangles*, inverted repeats; *broken lines*, fragments, not drawn to scale; *x* and *y*, possible additional EcoRI fragments.

that there is a 2.2-kbp fragment between EcoRI g and j. BamHI bcd from virion DNA hybridized to EcoRI ab, d, e, f, g, ij, l, m, and n (Table 2). Cloned BamHI b hybridized to EcoRI d, ij, and l, while clone BamHI c hybridized to EcoRI ab and e (Fig. 5). Thus EcoRI m and n are candidates for the small fragment between EcoRI g and j. EcoRI n is anomalous in being present in reduced molarity on control filters and is possibly related to another fragment such as EcoRI m. EcoRI m, having a size of 2.2 kbp, is the best candidate for the small fragment between EcoRI g and j. The complete BamHI and EcoRI restriction endonuclease maps for the S segment of the genome of EHV-1 subtype 2 are shown in Figure 4D.

Derivation of restriction endonuclease map for L segment of EHV-1 subtype 2 genome. EcoRI b contains the L-S joint and a portion of this fragment makes up the major part of IR_S (Fig. 4D). The hybridization data concerning EcoRI ab were analyzed in an attempt to determine the relationship of EcoRI b to other fragments in U_L and to ascertain which BamHI fragments hybridized to EcoRI a but not to b. Probe EcoRI ab

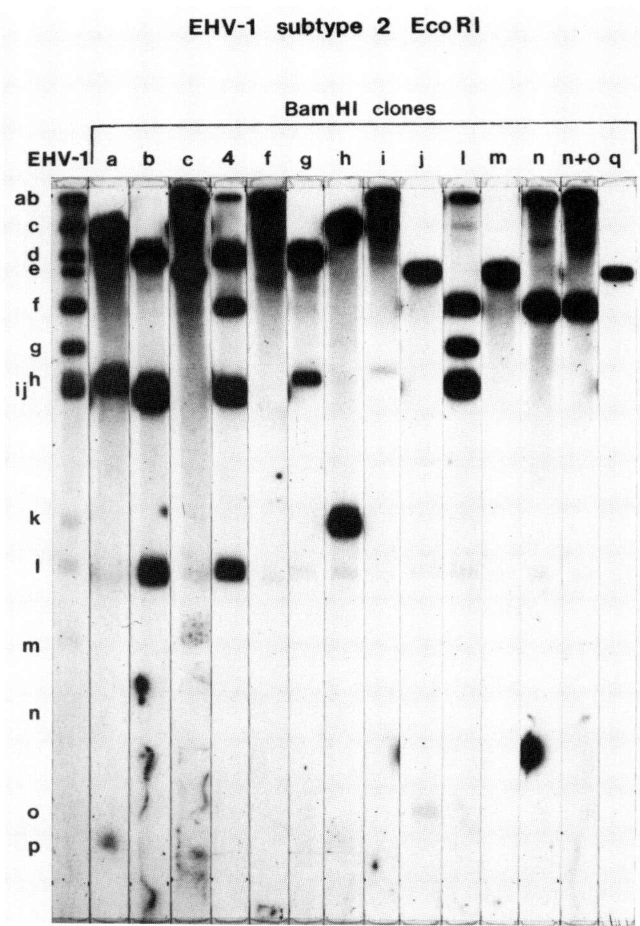

Fig. 5. Autoradiograph of results of hybridizing ^{32}P-labeled BamHI cloned fragments of EHV-1 subtype 2 DNA to EcoRI digest of same DNA (see *Table 3*); clone 4 of undetermined structure. (Faint band migrating below EcoRI l in all tracks may represent contaminating pUC9 in the dye.)

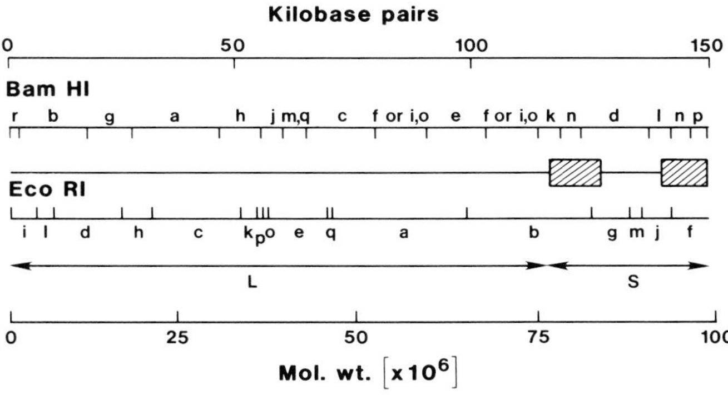

Fig. 6. BamHI and EcoRI maps of EHV-1 subtype 2 DNA; *hatched rectangles*, inverted repeat sequences. The relative order of BamHI f, i, and o, and BamHI m and q were not determined.

hybridized to BamHI bcd, e, f, i, jkl, mnn, o, and p (Table 2). BamHI d, k, l, n, and p hybridized to a portion of EcoRI b in IR_S. Cloned BamHI fragments b, j, and m did not hybridize to EcoRI ab (Fig. 5). Thus, BamHI c, e, f, i, and o overlap EcoRI a or the portion of b in U_L. The hybridization patterns of these BamHI fragments were studied to elucidate the location of EcoRI a. Cloned BamHI c hybridized to EcoRI ab and e (Fig. 5) and produced fragments of 10 kbp, 1.0 kbp, and 3.1 kbp on digestion with EcoRI and BamHI (Table 4). These data imply that the left end of EcoRI b or one end of EcoRI a is contiguous with a small EcoRI fragment of approximately 1.0 kbp contiguous with EcoRI e. Cloned BamHI f and i hybridized only to band ab of an EcoRI digest (Fig. 5). Similarly, virion probe BamHI o hybridized only to EcoRI ab (Table 2). None of these three BamHI fragments possesses an EcoRI site (Table 4), implying that they are wholly contained within EcoRI a and b. Thus, adjacent locations of EcoRI a and b are indicated, since the only fragment unaccounted for is BamHI e, which is proposed as the fragment containing the EcoRI site between a and b. The sum of the sizes of BamHI n, k, o, i, e, f, and the 1.6 kbp of d within EcoRI b, plus the 10-kbp EcoRI product of BamHI c, correlates well with the sizes of EcoRI a and b.

BamHI e was not cloned and subjected to restriction endonuclease analysis to locate the proposed EcoRI site in BamHI e. It was thus not possible to map unequivocally the relative positions of BamHI f, i, and o. The size of BamHI i plus f eliminates the possibility that these two fragments are adjacent to each other on either side of BamHI e.

Cloned BamHI c hybridized to EcoRI ab and e (Fig. 5) and yielded products of 10, 1.0 and 3.1 kbp on digestion with EcoRI (Table 4). The 1.0-kbp fragment contained within BamHI c and located between EcoRI e and a were identified as EcoRI q on the basis of hybridization of BamHI bcd to an EcoRI digest of EHV-1 subtype 2 DNA (Table 2). Probe EcoRI e hybridized to BamHI bcd, jkl, and mnn. Cloned BamHI q and m hybridized only to EcoRI e, and cloned BamHI j hybridized to EcoRI e and to two smaller fragments, EcoRI o and p. Therefore, BamHI fragments m and q, which were not cleaved by EcoRI, are located between BamHI j and c. It was not possible to determine the order of BamHI m and q from these data.

Cloned BamHI j and h hybridized to EcoRI p, but only BamHI j hybridized to EcoRI o, implying that EcoRI o is contained completely within BamHI j and maps adjacent to EcoRI e. Digestion of cloned BamHI j with BamHI and EcoRI resulted in fragments of 3.4 kbp and 1 kbp, which represent a portion of EcoRI e and the whole of EcoRI o, respectively. EcoRI p contains the BamHI site between j and h, but the small portion of this fragment within BamHI j was not detected by restriction endonuclease digestion.

Cloned BamHI h hybridized to EcoRI p, k, and c. EcoRI k hybridized only to BamHI h, and one of the fragments resulting from digestion of cloned BamHI h with BamHI and EcoRI is equivalent in size to EcoRI k (Table 4). This indicates that EcoRI k is contained wholly within BamHI h, and is thus located between EcoRI p and c (Fig. 6). Hybridization of EcoRI c to a BamHI digest of EHV-1 subtype 2 DNA (Table 2) showed that BamHI a and h are adjacent. Cloned BamHI a hybridized to EcoRI c and h (Fig. 5), thus locating EcoRI h next to EcoRI c, and EcoRI h hybridized to BamHI g and a (Table 2), indicating that BamHI g is next to BamHI a (Fig. 6). These fragment locations were confirmed by double digestion of cloned BamHI a and g (Table 4).

EcoRI d hybridized to BamHI bcd and g (Table 2). As BamHI c and d were mapped previously, BamHI b must be adjacent to BamHI g (Fig. 7). Cloned BamHI b hybridized to EcoRI d, ij, and l (Fig. 5) and on digestion with BamHI and EcoRI yielded products of 6.3, 5, and 2.8 kbp (Table 4). The 6.3-kbp product plus the 8-kbp product of cloned BamHI g is equivalent in size to EcoRI d. The 2.8-kbp product represents the whole of l, and the remaining 5 kbp is equivalent to the portion of EcoRI i that overlaps BamHI b. BamHI b was cloned and is therefore unlikely to be the fragment at the L terminus. The restriction endonuclease digestion results suggest that the 1 kbp of EcoRI i that does not map in BamHI b is present in a small BamHI fragment at the L terminus. The complete BamHI and EcoRI restriction endonuclease maps of the EHV-1 subtype 2 genome are shown in Figure 6.

DISCUSSION

The analysis of EHV-1 subtype 2 DNA is consistent with a model for the genome structure similar to that for EHV-1 subtype 1. However, the two subtypes are quite different in the arrangement of restriction sites.

The EHV-1 subtype 2 genome (144 kbp) consists of two segments: L (109 kbp) and S (35 kbp). The S segment comprises a unique sequence (U_S) flanked by inverted repeat sequences (TR_S/IR_S). From estimates of fragment size, $TR/_S$ and $IR/_S$ are larger than 9.5 kbp (EcoRI f) and less than 12.7 kbp (BamHI $l + n + p$). The electron microscopy data indicate a size of 13.3 kbp for U_S, suggesting that TR_S and IR_S are 10.8 kbp in size, a value which falls within this range.

The hybridization data do not indicate the presence of an inverted repeat flanking U_L of EHV-1 subtype 2. However, a very small repeat, such as that present in the VZV genome (Davison 1984) cannot be ruled out at present. Similarly, no indication of a terminal redundancy akin to the HSV-1 a sequence was found.

Since both EcoRI and BamHI cleave within the inverted repeat sequences of the subtype 2 genome, it is not known whether U_S inverts relative to a fixed orientation of L, as occurs in subtype 1.

ACKNOWLEDGMENTS

We are grateful to Dr. F. Rixon for expert assistance with the electron microscopy, and Ms. C. O'Brien and Ms. S. Toyias for efficient typing of the manuscript. During her time at the Institute of Virology, Glasgow, Ann Cullinane was supported by a Horserace Betting Levy Board Veterinary Research Training Scholarship.

REFERENCES

Allen, G.P., and Bryans, J.T. (1986) Molecular epizootiology, pathogenesis and prophylaxis of equine herpesvirus-1 infections. In *Progress in Veterinary Microbiology and Immunology*, Vol. 2, pp. 78-144. Ed. R. Pandey. Karger, Basel.

Allen, G.P.; Yeargan, M.R.; Turtinen, L.W.; Bryans, J.T.; and McCollum, W.H. (1983) Molecular epizootiologic studies of equine herpesvirus-1 infections by restriction endonuclease finger printing of viral DNA. *Am. J. Vet. Res.* **44**, 263-71.

Campbell, K.M., and Studdert, M.J. (1983) Equine herpesvirus type 1 (EHV-1). *Vet. Bull.* **53**, 135-45.

Cohen, S.N.; Chang, A.C.Y.; and Hsu, L. (1972) Nonchromosomal antibiotic resistance in bacteria: genetic transformation of *Escherichia coli* by R-factor DNA. *Proc. Natl. Acad. Sci. USA* **69**, 2110-14.

Davison, A.J. (1984) Structure of the genome termini of varicella-zoster virus. *J. Gen. Virol.* **65**, 1969-77.

Hanahan, D. (1983) Studies on transformation of *Escherichia coli* with plasmids. *J. Mol. Biol.* **166**, 557-80.

Henry, B.E.; Robinson, R.A.; Dauenhauer, S.A.; Atherton, S.S.; Hayward, G.S.; and O'Callaghan, D.J. (1981) Structure of the genome of equine herpesvirus type 1. *Virology* **115**, 97-114.

Holmes, D.S., and Quigley, M. (1981) A rapid boiling method for the preparation of bacterial plasmids. *Analyt. Biochem.* **114**, 193-97.

Maniatis, T.; Jeffrey, A.; and Van de Sande, H. (1975) Chain length determination of small double and single-stranded DNA molecules by polyacrylamide gel electrophoresis. *Biochemistry* **14**, 3787-94.

Maniatis, T.; Fritsch, E.F.; and Sambrook, J. (1982) *Molecular cloning: A laboratory manual*. Cold Spring Harbor Laboratory, Cold Spring Harbor, N.Y.

O'Callaghan, D.J.; Allen, G.P.; and Randall, C.C. (1978) Structure and replication of the equine herpesviruses. In *Proc. 4th Int. Conf. Equine Infect. Dis.*, pp. 1-32.

O'Callaghan, D.J.; Gentry, G.A.; and Randall, C.C. (1983) The equine herpesviruses. In *The Herpesviruses*, Vol. 2, pp. 215-318. Ed. B. Roizman. Plenum Press, New York.

Rigby, P.W.J.; Dieckmann, M.; Rhodes, C.; and Berg, P. (1987) Labeling deoxyribonucleotide acid to high specific activity *in vitro* by nick-translation with DNA polymerase I. *J. Mol. Biol.* **113**, 237-51.

Rixon, F.J.; Taylor, P.; and Desselberger, U. (1984) Rotavirus RNA segments sized by electron microscopy. *J. Gen. Virol.* **65**, 233-39.

Ruyechan, W.T.; Dauenhauer, S.A.; and O'Callaghan, D.J. (1982) Electron microscopic study of equine herpesvirus type 1 DNA. *J. Virol.* **42**, 297-99.

Sabine, M.; Robertson, G.R.; and Whalley, J.M. (1981) Differentiation of subtypes of equine herpesvirus 1 by restriction endonuclease analysis. *Aust. Vet. J.* **57**, 148-49.

Southern, E.M. (1975) Detection of specific sequences among DNA fragments separated by gel electrophoresis. *J. Mol. Biol.* **90**, 503-33.

Studdert, M.J. (1983) Restriction endonuclease DNA fingerprinting of respiratory, fetal and perinatal foal isolates of equine herpesvirus type 1, *Arch. Virol.* **77**, 249-58.

Studdert, M.J.; Simpson, T.; and Roizman, B. (1981) Differentiation of respiratory and abortogenic isolates of equine herpesvirus 1 by restriction endonucleases. *Science* **214**, 562-64.

Vieria, J., and Messing, J. (1982) The pUC plasmids, and M13mp7-derived system for insertion mutagenesis and sequencing with synthetic universal primers. *Gene* **19**, 259-68.

Weislander, L. (1979) A simple method to recover intact high molecular weight RNA and DNA after electrophoretic separation in low gelling temperature agarose gels. *Analyt. Biochem.* **98**, 305-9.

Whalley, J.M.; Robertson, G.R.; and Davison, A.J. (1981) Analysis of the genome of equine herpesvirus type 1: arrangement of cleavage sites for restriction of endonucleases Eco RI, Bgl II and Bam HI. *J. Gen. Virol.* **57**, 307-23.

Wilkie, N.M. (1973) The synthesis and substructure of herpesvirus DNA: the distribution of alkali-labile single-strand interruptions in HSV-1 DNA. *J. Gen. Virol.* **49**, 1-21.

Molecular Characterization of the Gene Products of the Short Region of the Equid Herpesvirus-1 Genome

Alice T. Robertson, Raymond P. Baumann, John Staczek, and Dennis J. O'Callaghan

SUMMARY

To further our understanding of the molecular biology of equid herpesvirus-1 (EHV-1), we have undertaken a series of experiments aimed at mapping individual gene products to specific locations on the viral genome. In this study, we have concentrated on identifying viral proteins that map specifically within the Short (S) region of the viral genome, by means of in vitro translation of viral-specific messages that had been hybrid-selected using cloned EHV-1 DNA fragments. Poly(A)+ mRNA for hybrid selection was isolated from infected cells at either early or late stages of the infection cycle using the guanidinium isothiocyanate/CsC1 centrifugation procedure. Following selection, viral-specific mRNA species were either identified by Northern blot analysis or translated in vitro in the presence of ^{35}S-methionine. Labeled translation products were separated by polyacrylamide gel electrophoresis and visualized by fluorography. As many as 10 different viral-specific polypeptides were mapped to DNA fragments within the Short region of the EHV-1 genome. Of these, one nonstructural protein of particular interest was the 31.5-kilodalton (kdal) "very early" protein, which is encoded by a 1.2-kb mRNA transcript originating from the internal termini of the Short region inverted repeat sequences.

INTRODUCTION

EHV-1 was first described more than 50 years ago as the etiologic agent of a contagious disease of horses, which resulted in "abortion storms" in seemingly healthy pregnant mares (Dimock & Edwards, 1936). It has since been documented as a cause of respiratory infections and neurological disorders in the Equidae family (Allen & Bryans 1986). Using permissive, primary hamster embryo cell culture systems to explore additional biological outcomes of infection, previous investigations from this laboratory have demonstrated the ability of EHV-1 to mediate the coestablishment of persistent infection and oncogenic transformation (Dauenhauer et al. 1982; O'Callaghan et al. 1983; Robinson et al. 1980a, b). To circumvent the lytic cycle and achieve these altered outcomes of infection, the virus preparations used were UV-irradiated or were propagated to enrich for the presence of defective interfering particles (DIPs). In addition, viral-mediated oncogenic transformation of nonpermissive mouse embryo cells was accomplished using standard viral preparations (Allen et al. 1978). In an effort to understand the molecular events that mediate the various biological outcomes, we have initiated studies aimed at defining the underlying molecular mechanisms that regulate the EHV-1 cytolytic infection cycle.

EHV-1 has a 94-megadalton, double-standard DNA genome that is subdivided into a Long (L) and a Short (S) region (Fig. 1). The L region is composed exclusively of unique sequences, whereas in the S region, the unique sequences (U_S) are bracketed by inverted repeat sequences (IR_S) (Baumann et al. 1986b; Henry et al. 1981; O'Callaghan et al. 1983; Whalley et al. 1981). Earlier investigations of EHV-1 gene expression demonstrated that the production of viral gene products is coordinated in a temporal fashion such that the immediate early (IE) mRNA and proteins are produced first during an infection cycle, as they are required for production of subsequent gene products (Caughman et al. 1985; Gray et al. 1987a). Beta, or early, genes are transcribed following synthesis of functional IE polypeptides. Last, transcription and translation of the gamma, or late, genes occur concomitantly with, or immediately following, the onset of viral DNA replication.

Initial investigations of the molecular anatomy of the EHV-1 genome have shown that the S region is of particular interest, for two reasons. First, two copies of the key regulatory gene, the IE gene, are located within the IR_S, at map units 0.78-0.83 and 0.95-1.0 (Gray et al. 1987a, b; Robertson et al. 1987). Second, specific areas of the S region are conserved within the DIP genome (Baumann et al. 1984; 1986a, b; 1987), and thus may be involved in the mediation of persistent infection and/or oncogenic transformation. Our investigations have therefore centered on molecular analyses of the S region. In this report, we describe initial results using in vitro translation of hybrid-selected viral messages, which have enabled us to define and orient gene products mapping within both the U_S and IR_S segments.

MATERIALS AND METHODS

Virus propagation, infection, and in vivo labeling of viral proteins. Stock virus preparations of the Kentucky A strain of EHV-1, propagated in mouse LM cell cultures (O'Callaghan et al. 1968; Perdue et al. 1974; Gray et al. 1987a), were

---

Department of Microbiology and Immunology, Louisiana State University Medical Center, Shreveport, Louisiana 71130-3932.

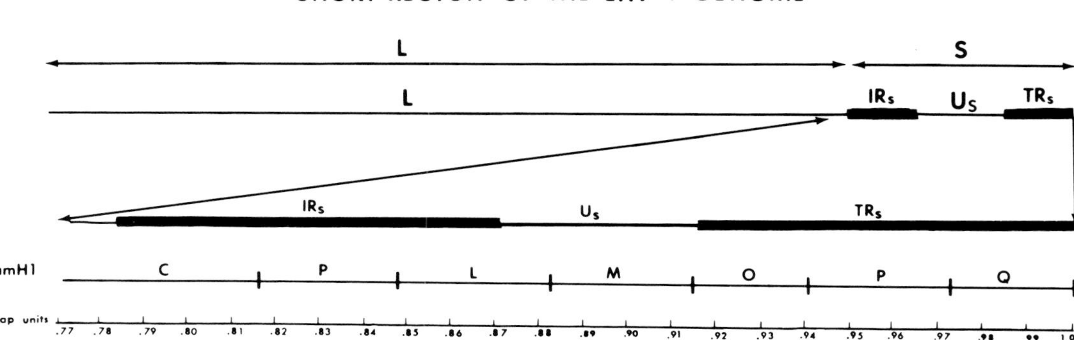

Fig. 1. Long (*L*) and Short (*S*) regions of EHV-1 genome; diagram of *S* region shows placement of inverted (IR_S) and unique (U_S) sequences. (BamHI restriction enzyme map described by Henry and colleagues, 1981, and Baumann and colleagues, 1986b.)

used for these studies. EHV-1, at a multiplicity of infection of 10-15 plaque-forming units (PFU)/cell, was allowed to adsorb onto confluent rabbit kidney cell monolayers in the presence (to isolate early RNA or proteins) or absence (to isolate late RNA or proteins) of 150 µg/ml of phosphonacetic acid (PAA; Sigma Chemical Corp., St. Louis, Mo.). After 1-1/2 hr, the inoculum was replaced with fresh medium (with or without PAA), and the infection was allowed to proceed for 8 hr. For mock infections, the inoculum consisted of Eagle's minimal essential medium (MEM). To label viral proteins in vivo, infected rabbit kidney cell monolayers were incubated in the presence of MEM containing 0.10 the normal concentration of methionine and 5% dialyzed fetal bovine serum. Two hours prior to harvest, ^{35}S-methionine (1180 Ci/mmole; New England Nuclear, Boston, Mass.) was added to a final concentration of 25 µCi/ml. At 8 hr postinfection, the cells were washed twice with ice-cold phosphate-buffered saline (PBS), overlaid with 1.0 ml of extraction buffer (50 mM Tris-HC1, pH 7.5, 100 mM NaC1, 5 mM EDTA, 0.5% Nonidet-P40 (v/v), 1% aprotinin (v/v), and 30 µg/ml phenylmethylsulphonyl fluoride) and stored at −70°C. Just prior to use, the monolayers were thawed, scraped into 5-ml tubes, and sonicated briefly to ensure cell lysis.

Isolation and Northern analysis of viral mRNA. Total cell RNA was isolated using guanidinium isothiocyanate as described by Chirgwin and colleagues, (1979) and Maniatis and colleagues (1982). Briefly, at 8 hr postinfection, 850 cm^2 roller bottles of EHV-1–infected or mock-infected rabbit kidney cells were rinsed twice with PBS, and any excess PBS was removed by aspiration. After the cells were lysed by the addition of 10 ml of guanidinium lysis buffer (5 M guanidinium isothiocyanate, 50 mM Tris-HC1, pH 7.5, 0.5% N-lauroyl sarcosine, 5 mM EDTA, 0.7 M ß-mercaptoethanol), the lysate was scraped into 50-ml centrifuge tubes and passed through an 18-gauge needle to shear high molecular weight DNA. To pellet RNA, the lysate from two roller bottles was layered over a 15-ml CsC1 cushion (5.7 M CsC1, 0.1 M K $^+$EDTA) in an SW28 centrifuge tube and centrifuged at 25,000 rpm for 28-32 hr in an SW28 rotor (Beckman Instruments, Palo Alto, Calif.). After the supernatant was removed by aspiration, the RNA pellet was immediately overlaid with 0.2 ml of lysis buffer and then resuspended in 4 ml of sterile RNase-free ddH_2O. After ethanol precipitation, the RNA was extracted twice with an equal volume of phenol/chloroform (1:1), reprecipitated, and finally resuspended in 1 mM EDTA. Poly(A)+ mRNA was selected using oligodeoxythymidylate-cellulose (oligo dT) chromatography according to the directions of the manufacturer (Bethesda Research Laboratories, Gaithersburg, Md.) and as described elsewhere (Roberton et al. 1988). Following two ethanol precipitations, mRNA was washed with 70% ethanol, dried in vacuo, and resuspended in ddH_2O containing RNasin (Promega Biotech, Madison, Wis.).

Northern analysis of EHV-1–specific mRNA was performed using 1.2% formaldehyde agarose gels according to the method described by Maniatis and colleagues (1982), as modified by Gray and colleagues (1987a, b). After transfer to Gene Screen Plus membranes (New England Nuclear), viral-specific mRNA species were identified by hybridization with ^{32}P-labeled cloned viral DNA fragments (Baumann et al. 1986b; Gray et al. 1987b). RNA bands were visualized by autoradiography. For each gel, RNA standards used as size markers included 16S, 18S, 23S, and 28S ribosomal RNA species.

Hybrid selection of EHV-1–specific mRNA. Cloned viral DNA fragments bound to diazotized paper were used to select viral-specific messages. BamHI DNA fragments were chosen for these studies since they were small and relatively equal in size (4.8 to 5.8 kilobase pairs), and since one fragment, BamHI M, contained almost all of the U_S segment (Fig. 1). Approximately 15 µg of purified protein-free viral DNA was bound to activated 7-mm aminophenylthieoether (APT) filter disks (Schleicher and Schuell, Keene, N.H.) according to methods described by the manufacturer and by Maniatis and colleagues (1982). Hybrid selection was performed using a combination of procedures (Ricciardi et al. 1979; Robertson et al. 1988; Stinski et al. 1983). For each selection, two disks were incubated in 100 µl of hybridization buffer [50% formamide, 0.4 M NaC1, 0.01 M Pipes, pH 6.4, 2 mM EDTA, 0.2% sodium dodecyl sulphate (SDS)] containing 22.5 µg of calf liver tRNA (Boehringer Mannheim Biochemicals, Indianapolis, Ind.) and poly(A)+ mRNA. The mRNA was isolated from either mock-infected or EHV-1–infected cells under early (+PAA) or late (−PAA) conditions. Routinely, mRNA representing approximately 1.5×10^8 infected cells was used per selection. After incubation for 4 hr at 54°C, the filter disks were washed successively in 20 mM Tris-HC1, pH 7.5, 2% SDS, 2 mM EDTA, two times at room temperature, and then in 0.1X SSC (1X SSC = 0.15 M NaC1, 0.015 M NaCitrate), 0.2% SDS, four times for 15 min each at 65°C. After a brief wash in 0.1 X SSC to remove the SDS, mRNA was eluted by two sequential incubations in 200 µl of 98% formamide, 20 mM Pipes, pH 6.4, at 70°C for 5 min each. The eluates were pooled, diluted with 100 µl of sterile ddH$_2$O, and then ethanol-precipitated in the presence of 15 µg of tRNA and 0.3 M NaAcetate. The precipitates were washed twice with 70% ethanol, dried in vacuo, and resuspended in 10 µl of 1 mM dithiothreitol containing 1 U/µl RNasin. For Northern blot analysis, RNA was either used at this point or was reselected using oligo dT as described above.

In vitro translation and polyacrylamide gel electrophoresis (PAGE). A rabbit reticulocyte lysate system supplemented with 0.3 mM MgAcetate and 80 mM K-Acetate was used to translate in vitro hybrid-selected mRNA according to the protocol recommended by the supplier (New England Nuclear). For each assay, 1.5µl of RNA was used in a 12.5Ml total reaction volume, and ^{35}S-methionine was included to label the protein products. After 90 min at 30°C, the reactions were terminated by the addition of one volume of 2X Laemmli sample buffer (50 mM Tris-HC1, pH 6.5, 2% SDS, 10% β-mercaptoethanol, 1% bromophenol blue; Laemmli 1970), heated to 100°C for 5 min. and analyzed directly by PAGE. Electrophoresis was performed according to the method of Laemmli (1970) except that 6-12% gradient gels were used to facilitate detection of a wide size range of protein products. Following electrophoresis, the gels were fixed in 40% methanol/10% acetic acid, impregnated with Enlightning (New England Nuclear), dried, and exposed to Kodak X-Omat XAR-5 radiographic film. ^{14}C-labeled molecular weight markers (Bethesda Research Laboratories), used to calculate the molecular weight of viral proteins, included myosin (200 kdal), phosphorylase b (97.4 kdal), bovine serum albumin (68 kdal), ovalbumin (43 kdal), and α-chymotrypsinogen (25.7 kdal).

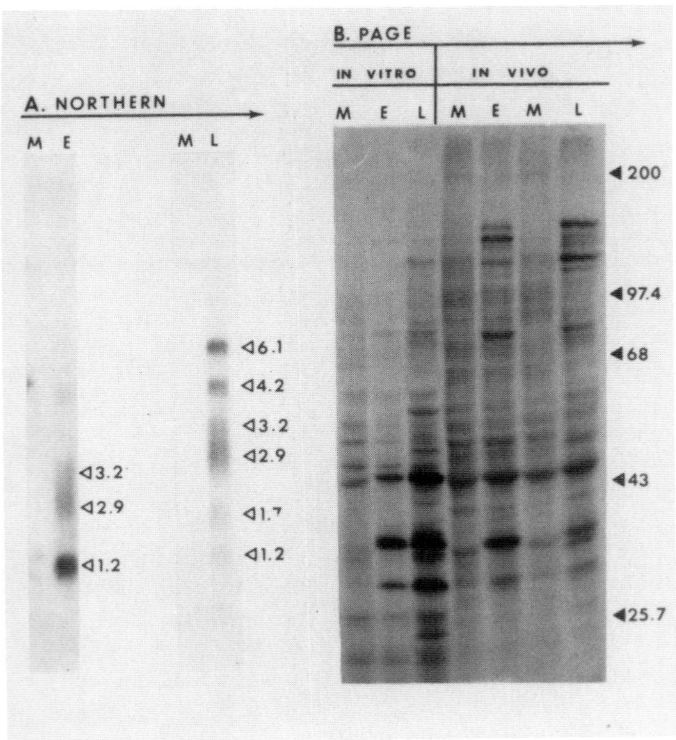

Fig. 2. Early and late transcripts of *S* region. *A*. Northern analyses of early and late mRNAs (see *Materials and Methods*): blots probed with equimolar combination of ^{32} P-labeled BamHI L, M, O, and P fragments. Sizes in kb; *M* = mock, *E* = early, *L* = late. *B*. PAGE analysis of total mock-infected or EHV-1–infected cell proteins: polypeptides, labeled with ^{35}S-methionine either during production in the in vitro translation reaction (in vitro) or during the normal cytolytic infection cycle (in vivo), were electrophoresed on 6-12.5% polyacrylamide gels (see *Materials and Methods*). Molecular weights (kdal) of size markers are at right.

RESULTS

Gene products of the U$_S$ region. Initial characterization of the gene products of the EHV-1 genome demonstrated that viral gene expression was regulated in an alpha, beta, gamma fashion (Caughman et al. 1985). Furthermore, Northern analysis of total infected cell RNA had identified numerous early and late transcripts that mapped to various regions of the viral genome (Gray et al. 1987a, b). Recently, we have shown that the EHV-1 immediate early (IE) gene (map units 0.78 to 0.83 and 0.95 to 1.0) is located within each of the IR$_S$ segments and is transcribed to yield a 6.0-kb mRNA that encodes the family of EHV-1 IE polypeptides (Caughman et al. 1985; Gray et al. 1987a, b; Robertson et al. 1987, 1988). In this investigation, we identify the major early and late gene products mapping within the S region. These products include seven poly(A)+ mRNA species (identified in Fig. 2A) and as many as 10 different viral-specific polypeptides.

To define poly(A)+ mRNA species mapping within the IR$_S$ and U$_S$ segments of the S region, nick-translated cloned BamHI P, O, L, and M (Fig. 1) fragments were used to probe Northern blots of infected cell poly(A)+ mRNA. As can be seen in Figure 2A, three early mRNA species (3.2, 2.9, and 1.2 kb) and three late mRNA species (6.1, 4.2, and 1.7 kb) were detected. Of the late mRNAs, both the 6.1- and 1.7-kb mRNAs could be detected in greatly reduced quantities in RNA preparations isolated under early conditions. Hence, these mRNAs may represent beta/gamma, or λ_1, genes (Roizman & Batterson 1985) rather than true late, or λ_2, gene

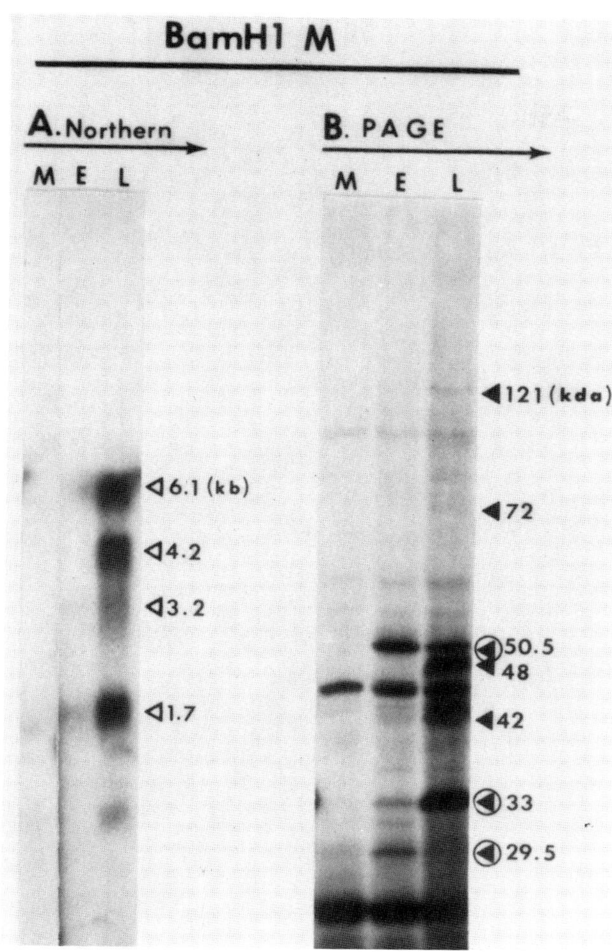

Fig. 3. EHV-1 gene products encoded within BamHI M fragment (map units 0.87-0.91). *A*. Northern blot analysis of BamHI M hybrid-selected mRNA species. *B*. PAGE analysis of BamHI M specific polypeptides. *M* = mock, *E* = early, *L* = late; *circled arrows*, early proteins.

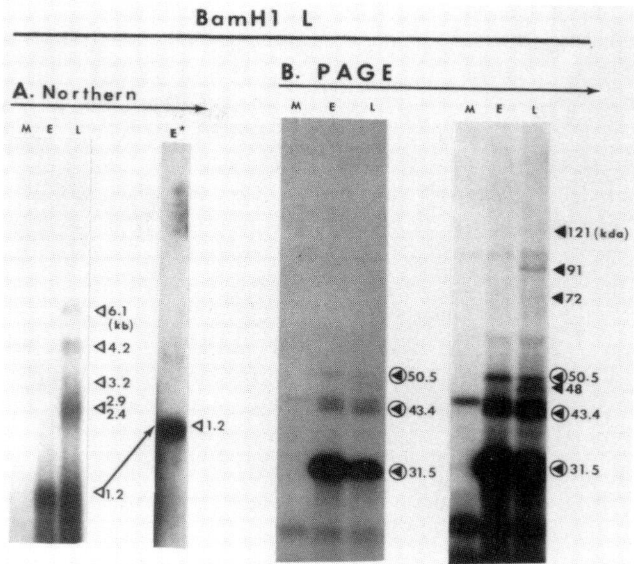

Fig. 4. Gene products mapping within BamHI L fragment (map units, 0.91-0.84). *A*. BamHI L selected mRNA analyzed directly on Northern blots (Lanes M, E, and L) or after reselection over oligo dT (Lane E*); probe was ^{32}P-labeled BamHI L DNA. *B*. BamHI L hybrid-selected mRNA translated in vitro and products analyzed by PAGE; gel at left, exposed for 4 hr; at right, exposed overnight. *M* = mock, *E* = early, *L* = Late; *circled arrows*, early proteins.

products. Finally, when pooled poly(A)+ reselected mRNA preparations were analyzed, an additional 2.4-kb mRNA species was detected at both early and late times during infection. Although this 2.4-kb mRNA species appears early, it is often indistinguishable from the 2.9-kb species during late stages of the infection cycle. (The bands are thus labeled 2.9/2.4 mRNA species in the figures throughout this paper).

In Figure 2B, proteins derived from in vitro translation of total poly(A)+ mRNA are compared with polypeptides labeled in EHV-1–infected RK cells. As expected, there was a good correlation between the polypeptides synthesized by in vitro translation and those made in vivo. However, while some of the proteins were more highly labeled in vivo (e.g., the 148-kdal protein), others were produced in higher concentrations in vitro. Of major interest, the 31.5-kdal polypeptide was produced in large quantities in the in vitro translation reactions. This polypeptide is also made in large quantities in EHV-1–infected cells and is synthesized very early in the infection cycle. Although it is not synthesized under conditions that select for the production of IE polypeptides, it is the first protein produced in significant concentrations in uninhibited infected cells. The 31.5-kdal nonstructural protein is thus referred to as the "very early" polypeptide.

Identification of gene products mapping within U_S. To analyze the mRNA and protein species mapping within the unique Short region, poly(A)+ RNA from mock-infected or EHV-1–infected cells was hybrid-selected with the BamHI M fragment. Northern blots of the hybrid-selected mRNA were then probed with ^{32}P-labeled BamHI M DNA, and the resulting bands were visualized by autoradiography. As shown in Fig. 3A, one early mRNA species (3.2) and three late viral mRNAs (6.1, 4.2, and 1.7 kb) mapped to this genomic segment. As discussed above, two of the late mRNAs (6.1 and 1.7 kb) could be detected in minor amounts in mRNA preparations isolated under early conditions (Fig. 3A, Lane E). Therefore, it may be more appropriate to classify these species as beta/gamma (λ_1) rather than true gamma, or late (λ_2), gene products. The smallest mRNA species (<1 kb) present on this blot may represent a degradation product, as it was not reproduced from blot to blot.

PAGE analysis of the in vitro translation products of these BamHI M hybrid-selected mRNAs (Fig. 3B) identified three viral-specific early proteins (50.5, 33, and 29.5 kdal) and four late proteins (121, 72, 48, and 42 kdal). The appearance of in vitro translation products for which no RNA was detectable by Northern analysis is not unexpected under these conditions since in vitro reaction is more sensitive than Northern analysis (unpublished observation). In addition, several other proteins smaller than 42 kdal can be seen. These proteins are always produced in reduced quantities and are not detected as consistently as the major products. Finally, of the proteins depicted in Figure 3B, four (50.5, 42, 33, and 29.5 kdal) appear to be encoded exclusively by U_S region sequences. The others apparently overlap with IR_S sequences as will be shown below.

Identification of RNA and proteins encoded within IR_S. To define the gene products mapping within the IR_S, the BamHI clones O, L, and P were used. While the BamHI O and L fragments contain both unique and repeat sequences, the BamHI P fragment lies exclusively within the IR_S (Fig. 1; Baumann et al., 1986b and 1987). The gene products encoded within the BamHI L fragment are shown in Figure 4. As identified by Northern analysis, the early mRNA species include a 3.2- and a 1.2-kb transcript. An additional 2.4-kb mRNA is detectable on longer exposures. Late specific mRNAs derived from the BamHI L segment are 6.1, 4.2, and 2.9 kb in size. On the Northern blot in Fig. 4A, the smear at the bottom of the gel results from hybridization to DNA, minor amounts of which elute from the filter during hybrid selection. Therefore, to ensure that no mRNAs smaller than 1.2 kb mapped within the BamHI L fragment, hybrid-selected early RNA was reselected over oligo dT and analyzed using Northern blots (Fig. 4A, Lane E*). Although there was a loss of RNA after the second oligo dT column, no additional viral-specific RNAs were detected.

PAGE analyses of the protein products obtained by in vitro translation of BamHI L hybrid-selected mRNA are shown in Fig. 4B. On the shorter exposure, three early proteins (50.5, 43.4, and 31.5 kdal) were detected, while on the longer exposure (Fig. 4B) the four late proteins of 121, 91, 72, and 48 kdal were more easily visualized. Of the early proteins, the 50.5-kdal species also mapped within the BamHI M fragment. Since the mRNA for this protein was not hybrid-selected by the BamHI O, this protein must map exclusively within the unique sequences of the BamHI L and M fragments. It is interesting to note that the appearance of this protein closely corresponds with the appearance of the 3.2-kb mRNA, suggesting that the 3.2-kb mRNA may code for the 50.5 kdal protein. In addition, there are several late proteins (121, 72, and 48 kdal) that map within S region unique and repeat sequences. Finally, there are three proteins that map within the IR_S but not within the BamHI M. These include the early 43.4- and 31.5-kdal species and the late 91-kdal protein.

The major early protein, mapping within the BamHI L and BamHI O fragments (Fig. 5B), is the 31.5-kdal "very early" polypeptide described earlier. The synthesis of this protein correlates with the presence of the 1.2-kb mRNA in both the

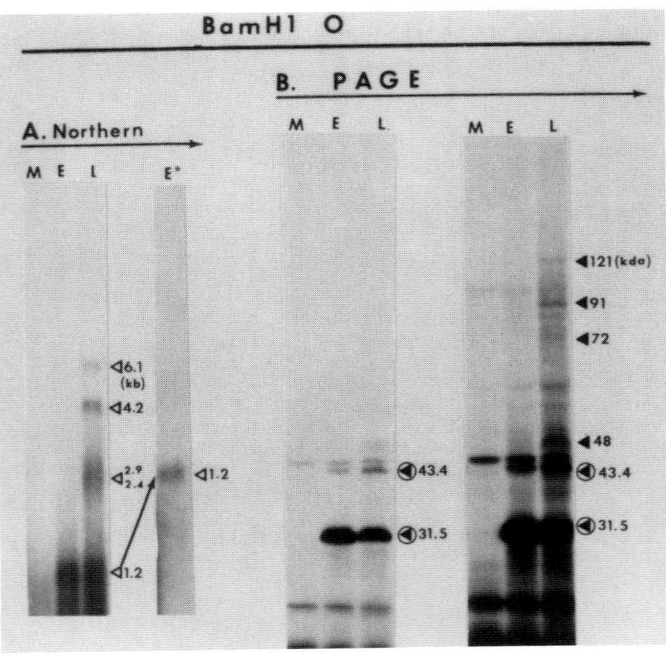

Fig. 5. Gene products mapping within BamHI O fragment (map units 0.84-0.87). *A*. Northern blots of BamHI O hybrid-selected mRNA assayed directly (*Lanes M*, *E*, and *L*) or after reselection over oligo dT cellulose (*Lane E**); probe was ^{32}P-labeled BamHI O DNA. *B*. PAGE of BamHI O specific polypeptides; BamHI O hybrid-selected mRNA translated in vitro, and products analyzed by PAGE. Gel at left, exposed for 4 hr; at right, exposed overnight. *M* = mock, *E* = early, *L* = late; *circled arrows*, early proteins.

in vitro translation reactions and the in vivo infection in cell culture systems (Caughman et al. 1985; Gray et al. 1987a, b). The DNA sequences encoding this nonstructural "very early" polypeptide lie within the internal termini of the IR_S segments, and thus this gene, like the IE gene, is present in two copies within the EHV-1 genome.

The BamHI O and BamHI L fragments share considerable amounts of IR_S sequences and, as a result, coselect many of the same mRNA species that are translated into proteins of the same size (compare Figure 4 and Figure 5). In fact, no gene products that map within the BamHI O but not within the BamHI L can be identified by these methods. Of particular interest is the 2.4-kb early mRNA species, which is selected in minor amounts by both DNA fragments, and which correlates in appearance with the 43.4-kdal protein.

In contrast, results obtained with the BamHI P are less straightforward. Previous studies (Gray et al. 1987b) analyzing early and late infected cell RNA that mapped within the BamHI P fragment defined one RNA species that always appeared as a large smear on Northern blots, the center of which was approximately 3.0 kb in size. In these studies using hybrid-selected poly(A)+ mRNA, this band also is visualized early, but appears smaller (approximately 2.5 kb in size) and much less diffuse (Fig. 6A). In addition, when late RNA from several hybrid selections is pooled and re-

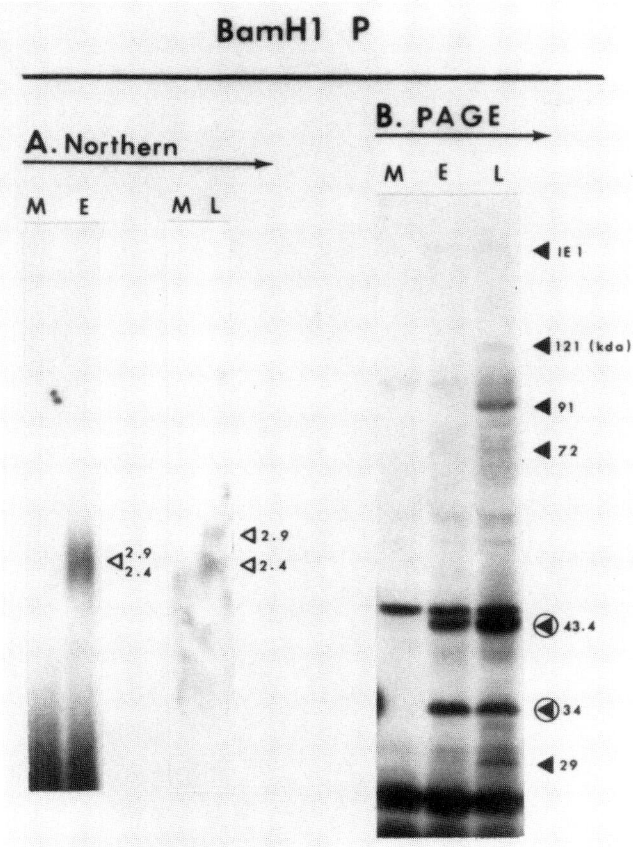

Fig. 6. Analysis of gene products mapping within the BamHI P fragment (map units, 0.81-0.84 and 0.94-0.97). *A*. Northern analysis of mRNAs hybrid-selected from mock-infected or EHV-1 infected cells: early (*E*) mRNA analyzed on Northern blots after hybrid selection; late (*L*) mRNA reselected over oligo dT cellulose prior to electrophoresis; nick-translated BamHI P–cloned DNA used as probe. *B*. PAGE of in vitro translation products of BamHi P–specific RNA.M = mock, *E* = early, *L* = late; *circled arrows*, early proteins.

selected over oligo dT, two mRNA species of approximately 2.9 and 2.4 kb are detected. Translation of the early hybrid-selected mRNA yielded the 43.4-kdal protein which also mapped within the BamHI O and BamHI L region, as well as an additional 34-kdal protein that had not been detected earlier. This result was unexpected in that the mRNAs mapping within the BamHI P were routinely less homogeneous than the corresponding mRNAs that mapped to the BamHI O and BamH1 L fragments (Fig. 6A; Gray et al. 1987b). However, the result of the in vitro translation indicated that the early 2.4-kb message mapping within the BamHI O and BamHI L fragments also mapped within the BamHI P fragment along with a heterogeneous population of mRNAs that may or may not be translatable. Whatever the case, the in vitro translation products of BamHI P hybrid-selected early mRNA do not reflect the heterogeneity of the mRNA species detected by Northern analysis (Fig. 6; Gray et al. 1987b). Finally, in vitro translation of BamHI P late mRNA consistently resulted in the production of the 121-, 91-, 72-, and 29-kdal proteins, but only the 2.9- and 2.4-kb mRNAs could be detected by blot analysis.

The immediate early proteins of the EHV-1 genome also map within the BamHI P fragment (Gray et al. 1987a, b). Of the four IE proteins (IE1, IE2, IE3, and IE4) produced both in vivo and in vitro, the major product is the 195- to 200-kdal IE1 species (Caughman et al. 1985; Robertson et al. 1987). During early and late times of the infection cycle, these IE proteins are expressed in very low quantities, and thus only the major IE1 protein is visible under these conditions (Fig. 6B). This was not unexpected since detection of IE RNA at early and late times was difficult and required large quantities of RNA and lengthy exposure times.

DISCUSSION

Our initial studies mapped various EHV-1 mRNAs and in vivo translation products to specific fragments within the IR_S and U_S segments of the S region (Table 1). Overall, seven poly(A)+ mRNA species and 10 distinct proteins have been assigned a map location on the viral genome. While additional work is in progress to extend these findings, there are possible correlations between several of the EHV-1 polypeptides and certain individual transcripts. These correlates include the 3.2-kb early mRNA and the 50.5-kdal early protein; the 2.4-kb early mRNA and the 43.4-kdal protein; the 1.2-kb mRNA and the 31.5-kdal very early protein; and the 2.9-kb late RNA and the 91-kdal protein. Furthermore, the appearance of the 6.1- and 4.2-kb mRNAs correlate with the detection of both the 121- and 72-kdal proteins, except in the case of the BamHI P fragment. Under the conditions of hybridization used, the Northern blots are less sensitive than the hybrid-selection procedures since hybrid selection can detect homologies as small as 50 bp (Ricciardi et al. 1979). As a result, it is possible that the 6.1- and 4.2-kb messages overlap only a very small portion of the BamHI P, presumably 150 bp or less. If so, since both messages also extend into the BamHI M sequences, then both transcripts, particularly the 4.2-kb species, may be spliced. Consequently, the only message without an assigned translation product would be the 1.7-kb mRNA mapping within the BamHI M. However, there are several smaller proteins (42, 33, and 29.5 kdal) that are unique to the BamHI M, and any of these could be the product of the 1.7-kb mRNA. Of these, the 33-kda protein would be the most likely candidate, since levels of this protein correspond with the levels of detectable mRNA.

There are several other proteins for which no mRNA could be directly correlated, including the 48-kdal protein and the 34- and 29-kdal proteins mapping within the BamHI P. The 48-kdal protein was found to vary in electrophoretic mobility and was not selected consistently by BamHI M sequences. This puzzling finding is under further investigation.

The 34-kdal protein mapping within the BamHI P fragment may be a premature termination product related to the

Table 1. Major in vitro translation products of Short region of EHV-1 viral genome

Location (map units)	Hybrid-selected poly(A)+ mRNA	Early and late viral-specific protein products
BamHI P (0.81-0.84 and 0.94-0.97)	2.9/2.4[a]	121,* 91,* 72,* 43.4, 34, 29*
BamHI O (0.84-0.87)	6.1,* 4.2,* 2.9/2.4,[a] 1.2	121,* 91,* 72,* 48,* 43.4, 31.5
BamHI M (0.87-0.91)	6.1,* 4.2,* 3.2, 1.7	121,* 72,* 50.5, 48,* 42,* 33, 29.5
BamHI L (0.91-0.94)	6.1,* 4.2,* 3.2, 2.9/2.4,[a] 1.2	121,*, 91,* 72,* 50.5, 48,* 31,5

[a] Exact nature of transcripts remains unclear.
* Late gene products.

43.4-kdal species. If so, then it would not be seen as a product of the BamHI O and BamHI L specific mRNAs since the overproduction of the 31.5-kdal protein would make it difficult to detect. However, numerous possible mechanisms would account for the presence of the 34-kdal protein and the other smaller proteins that map within the BamHI M and P fragments. They could arise from RNAs not visible on the Northern blots, or from unique, individual mRNA species that comigrate on formaldehyde gels with those RNAs identified above. Furthermore, it is possible that a single mRNA species could generate more than one primary translation product; in fact, numerous examples are found in both viral and cellular systems. The mechanisms by which additional in vitro products may be generated include use of alternate initiation and/or termination signals (Haarr et al. 1985; Hughes et al. 1986; Kozak 1986; Nagashima et al. 1986; Strubin et al. 1986); posttranslational proteolytic processing (De Varennes et al. 1986; Tian & Shih 1986); and, finally, premature termination (Hughes et al. 1986). While the first several mechanisms are known to occur in vivo, premature termination may be unique to the in vitro system.

Prior to this study, the only other protein mapped to sequences within the Short region of the EHV-1 genome was the glycoprotein gp17/18, identified by Allen and Yeargan (1987) using the Army-183 strain of EHV-1. As defined by restriction enzyme analysis, this virus strain is only slightly different from the Kentucky A strain used in these studies. Therefore, assuming colinearity between the genomes, it is possible that one of the proteins defined in this report is the unglycosylated precursor form of the S region glycoprotein. Two proteins, in particular, meet the criteria of size and map location: the 50.5- and 42-kdal proteins that map within the BamHI M fragment.

In combination with ongoing studies on the IE proteins and gene products that map within the BamH1 Q fragment (Robertson et al. 1988) these investigations represent the initial identification and mapping of gene products of the EHV-1 S region. Experiments now in progress are aimed at fine-mapping the EHV-1 S region, identifying additional gene products that may map within this region, and assigning translation products to specific viral mRNA species using size-fractionated mRNA and hybrid-arrest translation.

ACKNOWLEDGMENTS

These studies were supported by research grants AI22001, AI21996, and F32-CA07700 from the National Institutes of Health; research grant 86-CRCR-1-2257 from the United States Department of Agriculture; a research grant from The Grayson Foundation, Inc.; and a research grant from the LSU System Biotechnology Institute.

REFERENCES

Allen, G.P., and Bryans, J.T. (1986) Molecular epizootiology, pathogenesis, and prophylaxsis of equine herpesvirus 1 infections. In *Progress in Veterinary Microbiology and Immunology*, Vol. 2, pp. 78-144. Ed. R. Pandey. S. Karger, Basel.

Allen, G.P., and Yeargan, M.R. (1987) Use of λgt11 and monoclonal antibodies to map the genes for the six major glycoproteins of equine herpesvirus 1. *J. Virol.* **61,** 2454-61.

Allen, G.P.; O'Callaghan, D.J.; and Randall, C.C. (1978) Oncogenic transformation of non-permissive murine cells by viable equine herpesvirus type 1 (EHV-1) and EHV-1 DNA. In *Oncogenesis and Herpesviruses III,* Part 1, pp. 509-516. Eds. G. de The and F. Rapp. International Agency for Research on Cancer, Lyons, France.

Baumann, R.P.; Dauenhauer, S.A.; Caughman, G.B.; Staczek, J.; and O'Callaghan, D.J. (1985) Structure and genetic complexity of the genomes of herpesvirus defective-interfering particles associated with oncogenic transformation and persistent infection. *J. Virol.* **50**, 13-21.

Baumann, R.P.; Staczek, J.; and O'Callaghan, D.J. (1986a) Cloning and fine mapping the DNA of herpesvirus type one defective interfering particles. *Virology* **153,** 188-200.

Baumann, R.P.; Sullivan, D.C.; Staczek, J.; and O'Callaghan, D.J. (1986b) Genetic relatedness and colinearity of the genomes of equine herpesvirus types one and three. *J. Virol.* **57,** 816-25.

Baumann, R.P.; Staczek, J.; and O'Callaghan, D.J. (1987) Equine herpesvirus type 1 defective-interfering (DI) particle DNA structure: The central region of the inverted repeat is deleted from DI DNA. *Virology* **159**, 137-46.

Caughman G.B.; Staczek, J.; and O'Callaghan D.J. (1985) Equine herpesvirus type 1 infected cell polypeptides: Evidence for immediate early/early/late regulation of viral gene expression. *Virology* **145,** 49-61.

Chirgwin, J.M.; Przybyla, A.E.; MacDonald, R.J.; and Rutter, W.J. (1979) Isolation of biologically active ribonucleic acid from sources enriched in ribonuclease. *Biochemistry* **18,** 5294-99.

Dauenhauer, S.A.; Robinson, R.A.; and O'Callaghan, D.J. (1982) Chronic production of defective-interfering particles by hamster embryo cultures of herpesvirus persistently infected and oncogenically transformed cells. *J. Gen. Virol.* **60**, 1-14.

De Varennes, A.; Lomonossoff, G.P.; Shanks, M.; and Maule, A.J. (1986) The stability of cowpea mosaic virus VPg in reticulocyte lysates. *J. Gen. Virol.* **67,** 2347-54.

Dimock, W.W., and Edwards, P.R. (1936) The differential diagnosis of equine abortion with special reference to a hitherto undescribed form of epizootic abortion of mares. *Cornell Vet.* **26,** 231-39.

Gray, W.L.; Baumann, R.P.; Robertson, A.T.; Caughman, G.B.; O'Callaghan, D.J.; and Staczek, J. (1987a) Regulation of equine herpesvirus type 1 gene expression: Characterization of immediate early, early, and late transcription. *Virology* **158**, 79-87.

Gray, W.L.; Baumann, R.P.; Robertson, A.T.; O'Callaghan, D.J.; and Staczek, J. (1987b) Characterization and mapping of equine herpesvirus type 1 immediate early, early, and late transcripts. *Virus Res.* **8,** 233-44.

Haarr, L.; Marsden, H.S.; Preston, C.M.; Smiley, J.R.; Summers, W.C.; and Summers, W.P. (1985) Utilization of internal AUG codons for initiation of protein synthesis directed by mRNAs from normal and mutant genes encoding herpes simplex virus-specified thymidine kinase. *J. Virol.* **56,** 512-19.

Henry, B.E.; Robinson, R.A.; Dauenhauer, S.A.; Atherton, S.S.; Hayward, G.S.; and O'Callaghan, D.J. (1981) Structure of the genome of equine herpesvirus type 1. *Virology* **115**, 97-114.

Hughes, G.; Davies, J.W.; and Wood, K.R. (1986) In vitro translation of the bipartite genomic RNA of pea early browning virus. *J. Gen. Virol.* **67,** 2125-33.

Kozak, M. (1986) Bifunctional messenger RNAs in eukaryotes. *Cell* **47,** 481-83.

Laemmli, U.K. (1970) Cleavage of structural proteins during the assembly of the head of bacteriophage T4. *Nature* **227,** 680-85.

Maniatis, T.; Fritsch, E.R.; and Sambrook, J. (1982) *Molecular Cloning: A Laboratory Manual.* Cold Spring Harbor Laboratory, Cold Spring Harbor, N.Y.

Nagashima, K.; Yoshida, M.; and Seiki, M. (1986) A single species of pX mRNA of human T-cell leukemia virus type 1 encodes trans-activator $p40^x$ and two other phosphoproteins. *J. Virol.* **60,** 394-99.

O'Callaghan, D.J.; Cheevers, W.P.; Gentry, G.A.; and Randall, C.C. (1968) Kinetics of cellular and viral DNA synthesis in equine abortion (herpes) virus-infection of L-M cells. *Virology* **36,** 104-114.

O'Callaghan, D.J.; Gentry, G.A.; and Randall, C.C. (1983) The equine herpesviruses. In *The Herpesviruses.* Vol. 2, pp. 215-305. Eds. H. Fraenkel-Conrat and R.R. Wagner. Plenum, New York.

Perdue, M.L.; Kemp, M.C.; Randall, C.C.; and O'Callaghan, D.J. (1974) Studies of the molecular anatomy of the L-M cell strain of equine herpesvirus type 1: Proteins of the nucleocapsid and intact virion. *Virology* **59**, 210-16.

Ricciardi, R.P.; Miller, J.S.; and Roberts, B.E. (1979) Purification and mapping of specific mRNAs by hybridization-selection and cell-free translation. *Proc. Natl. Acad. Sci. USA* **76**, 4927-31.

Robertson, A.T.; Colacino, J.M.; Baumann, R.P.; Gray, W.L.; and O'Callaghan, D.J. (1987) Mapping EHV-1 specific polypeptides to the unique long region of the viral genome (abstract). *Proc. 12th Int. Herpesvirus Workshop,* p. 318.

Robertson, A.T.; Caughman, G.B.; Gray, W.L.; Baumann, R.P.; Staczek, J.; and O'Callaghan, D.J. (1988) Analysis of the in vitro translation products of the immediate-early RNA of equine herpesvirus type 1. *Virology.* In press.

Robinson, R.A.; Henry, B.E.; Dugg, R.G.; and O'Callaghan, D.J. (1980a) Oncogenic transformation by equine herpesviruses (EHV-1) I. Properties of hamster embryo cells transformed by UV-irradiated EHV-1. *Virology* **101,** 335-62.

Robinson, R.A.; Vance, R.B.; and O'Callaghan, D.J. (1980b) Oncogenic transformation by equine herpesviruses. II. Coestablishment of persistent infection and oncogenic transformation of hamster embryo cells by equine herpesvirus type 1 preparations enriched for defective interfering particles. *J. Virol.* **36,** 204-219.

Roizman, B., and Batterson, W. (1985) Herpesviruses and their replication. In *Virology,* pp. 497-526. Eds. B.N. Fields, D.M. Knipe, R.M. Chanock, J.L. Melnick, B. Roizman, and R.E. Shope. Raven Press, New York.

Stinski, M.F.; Thomson, D.R.; Steinberg, R.M.; and Goldstein, L.C. (1983) Organization and expression of the immediate early genes of human cytomegalovirus. *J. Virol.* **46**, 1-14.

Strubin, M.; Long, E.O.; and Mach, B. (1986) Two forms of the Ia antigen-associated invariant chain result from alternative initiations at two in-phase AUGs. *Cell* **47**, 619-25.

Tian, Y.C.; and Shih, D.S. (1986) Cleavage of a viral polyprotein by a cellular proteolytic activity. *J. Virol.* **57**, 547-51.

Whalley, J.M.; Robertson, G.R.; and Davison, A.J. (1981) Analysis of the genome of equine herpesvirus type 1: Arrangement of cleavage sites for restriction endonuclease EcoRI, BglII, and BamHI. *J. Gen. Virol.* **57,** 307-323.

Molecular Pathogenesis of Equine Coital Exanthema: Identification of a New Equine Herpesvirus Isolated from Lesions Reminiscent of Coital Exanthema in a Donkey

Robert J. Jacob, D. Cohen, D. Bouchey, T. Davis, and J. Borchelt

SUMMARY

DNA purified from an equid herpesvirus (EHV) isolated (Burrows 1973) from lesions reminiscent of equine coital exanthema in a donkey (*E. asinus*) appears to differ in some characteristics from the DNAs of the other equid herpesviruses (EHV-1, -2, and -3). The DNA is 92 md ± 12, G+C content of 69-70%, and does not contain any XbaI restriction endonuclease (RE) digestion sites. The fragment patterns seen when this DNA is digested with other REs indicates that it is different from the DNA of the EHV-3 virus, the causative agent of equine coital exanthema in the horse (*E. cabalus*), and unique also when compared with the patterns reported for digestion products of the DNAs of EHV-1, and -2. Southern blot hybridization of the products from RE digestions indicates that there is only minor sequence homology between this DNA and the DNA of EHV-3 large-plaque (LP) and small-plaque (sp) strains. Neutralizing antisera, produced in rabbits sensitized to purified virus, underscored the unique features of this isolate within the EHV group. It is suggested that this isolate be temporarily referred to as donkey herpesvirus-1 or be considered a candidate for EHV-5.

INTRODUCTION

Three herpesviruses are known to infect equines (Bryans 1969; Mathews 1981; O'Callaghan, Allen & Randall 1978; O'Callaghan, Gentry & Randall 1984a; O'Callaghan et al. 1984b; Plummer, Goodheart & Studdert 1973; Sabine, Robertson & Whalley, 1981). The members of this triad differ in their pathogenicity for their host. EHV-1 is known to cause upper respiratory infections, abortions in pregnant mares, and encephalomyopathy. Research indicates that EHV-1 may be two viruses that are now referred to as subtypes (Burrows & Goodridge 1973; Sabine et al. 1981; Shimizu et al. 1959; Studdert et al. 1981; Turtinen et al. 1982). EHV-2 is considered a cytomegalovirus in both its growth and culture characteristics. Equid herpesvirus 3 (EHV-3) is known to be the causative agent of equine coital exanthema (ECE), a sexually transmitted disease usually limited to the external genitalia of both stallions and mares. However, evidence has been presented that a noncoital transmission may occur (Crandell & Davis 1985; Krogsrud & Onstad 1971).

Several years ago, a virus with the physiochemical properties of a herpesvirus and the cultural characteristics of EHV-3 was isolated by Burrows (1973) from the nares of a donkey foal and the teats of its dam. The clinical presentation was reminiscent of ECE as seen in the horse. Antibodies raised against EHV-1 and EHV-2 would not cross-react with this new isolate, and it differed when compared serologically with all other EHV-3 strains. This virus was found to be antigenically distinct from other horse viruses, as well from EHV-1 and -2. Because of its clinical presentation, it was suggested that this isolate was an EHV-3 isolate. In this report we confirm that this isolate is serologically distinct from the other EHVs; the DNA isolated from purified virions of this isolate has a higher G+C content, and the RE digestion pattern is different from that of the other EHVs (Allen & Turtinen 1982; O'Callaghan et al. 1984b). Southern blot hybridizations indicate only minor sequence homology between the DNA of this isolate and the DNA of EHV-3 strains LP and sp; the most striking characteristic is that the DNA is not digested with the RE XbaI. This report suggests that the isolate be considered a new and, as yet, uncharacterized member of the EHVs, to be temporarily referred to as donkey herpesvirus-1 or be considered, by the Herpesvirus Study Group, International Committee on Nomenclature of Vires, as a candidate for EHV-5.

MATERIALS AND METHODS

Cells and virus growth. Monolayer cultures of a diploid strain of equine embryo dermal fibroblasts (KYED) cells were used in these studies. The cells were grown in Eagle's minimal essential medium supplemented with 10% fetal bovine serum and 50 µg/ml of kanamycin. The EHV-3 large plaque (1118 LP) and small plaque (1118 sp) were cloned by plaque purification (G.P. Allen, personal communication, 1980). The virus, dky, was isolated from "ECE-like" lesions on a donkey mare and foal in England (Burrows 1973). This virus has been plaque-purified in our laboratory; all strains and cells were procured from G.P. Allen (University of Kentucky). Conditions for purification of these strains in KYED cells and preparation of stocks by low multiplicity (5×10^{-4}

Department of Microbiology and Immunology, Albert B. Chandler Medical Center, University of Kentucky, Lexington, Kentucky 40536-0084.

plaque-forming units (PFU)/cell) infections have been described elsewhere (Allen & Randall 1979).

Purification of virus, preparation of antisera, and neutralization assays. Infectious virus was purified from the cytoplasm of infected KYED cells by the method of Allen and Randall (1979). Briefly, cytoplasmic fractions were layered on top of a 28-40% (w/v) potassium tartrate gradient. The gradients were centrifuged in an SW27 rotor (Beckman, Palo Alto, Calif.) at 15°C, 26,000 rpm, for 1 hr. The appropriate viral band was removed, diluted with twice the volume of distilled water, and pelleted in an SW41 rotor (Beckman) at 15°C, 25,000 rpm, for 2 hr. The viral pellet was washed, eluted in phosphate buffered saline (PBS; 137 mM NaC1, 8 mM Na_2HPO_4, 27 mM KC1, pH 7.4), and stored at −90°C. All stocks were titered as previously described (Jacob 1986).

Purified virions (1-3 × 10^7 PFU/ml) suspended in PBS were emulsified at a 1:1 ratio with Freund's complete adjuvant. Three young adult New Zealand white rabbits were injected subcutaneously with 1 ml of the mixture at the nape of the neck and 0.5 ml of the mixture over both hips. Booster injections were administered every two weeks by the same protocol. A total of three injections were performed. Two weeks after the last injection, rabbits were exsanguinated and the serum was collected from clotted blood. The serum was separated by low-speed centrifugation and heat-inactivated at 56°C for 1 hr. The serum was then filtered through a 0.2-μm nitrocellulose filter. The serum samples were serially diluted with PBS and mixed with a known concentration of plaque-forming units. These mixtures were incubated at 37°C for 1 hr, then assayed on KYED cells as previously described (Jacob 1986).

Labeling and purification of viral DNA. Viral DNA was labeled in vivo as described (Jacob, 1984) using either ^{3}H-Thymidine (New England Nuclear, Boston, Massachusetts) at 5μCi/ml or ^{32}P-labeled orthophosphate (New England Nuclear) at 10-20 μCi/ml. KYED cells infected at 5 PFU/cell were harvested at 24-36 hr postinfection and centrifuged at 7,000 rpm, 20°C for 15 min in a J2-21 centrifuge (Beckman) to separate cell-free virions from cell-associated viral particles. Cell-free virions were pelleted from supernatant by centrifugation at 27,000 rpm and 20°C, for 2 hr in an SW27 rotor. Virion DNA was purified by phenol extraction and ethanol precipitation. Purification of viral DNA from the infected cell pellets has been described previously (Jacob 1984). Briefly, infected cell pellets were resuspended in TE buffer (0.01M Tris-HC1, 0.001M EDTA, pH 7.4), 2% sodium dodecyl sulphate (SDS), 1% sarcosyl, and 1 mg/ml pronase and incubated at 39°C for 3-6 hr. Infected cell DNA was purified in a CsC1 gradient, followed by 18 hr of dialysis against TE buffer and ethanol precipitation.

Centrifugation of viral DNA. Isodense (1.726 gm/cc) CsC1 solution containing viral DNA was centrifuged in Quickseal tubes in an VTI-50 rotor (Beckman), at 40,000 rpm, 20°C, for 18-24 hr. The labeled DNA was recovered by dripping the gradient in 0.75ml fractions from the bottom of the tube. Radioactivity was monitored by acid precipitable counts per fraction, as previously described (Jacob 1984).

RE digestions and agarose gel electrophoresis. The restriction enzymes used were BamHI (GGATCC), Bgl II (AGATCT), EcoRI (GAATTC), HindIII (AAGCTT), PstI (CTGCAG), and XbaI (TCTAGA). Reaction mixtures were incubated at 37°C for 6 hr and stopped by adding 10 μl of 0.2M EDTA and 10 μl of 60% sucrose–0.25% bromophenol blue tracking dye per 100 μl of reaction mixture (Jacob 1984). The products of RE digestions were electrophoresed in 0.5% agarose slab gels, submersed in Loewing's buffer (0.3M NaH_2PO_4, 0.5 M Tris-HC1, 0.01M EDTA, pH 7.2), prepared on a 30-cm × 13-cm horizontal unit, for 18-24 hr at 25°C, 28 volts. RE digestion products of lambda DNA were included as markers in all gels. The resulting gels were stained in ethidium bromide and photographed under UV illumination using Kodak Tri X Pan film. Autoradiography using Wolf cassettes, Cronex 4 (DuPont) medical X-ray film, and Cronex Lightning Plus screens was performed on gels containing ^{32}P-labeled DNA as described previously (Jacob 1984).

Transfers and blot hybridizations. Agarose slab gels were transferred onto nitrocellulose filter paper (Schleicher and Schuell, Keene, N.H.) according to the method of Southern (1975). Transfers were prehybridized in 6X standard saline citrate (SSC), 5X Denhardt's solution, 0.5% SDS, 0.01M EDTA, and 100 μg/ml salmon sperm DNA at 68°C for 24 hr. Hybridization conditions were similar, but 5% dextran sulfate and 0.5 μg probe (EHV-3 LP DNA, Sp. Act. 2 × 10^8 cpm/μgM) were also added. The probe was nick-translated (BRL, Inc. Bethesda, Md.) using ^{32}P-labeled dCTP in the alpha position (3,000 Ci/mM specific activity). After hybridization, the transfer was washed twice with 2X SSC plus 0.5% SDS at 25°C for 20 min, then three times with 0.1X SSC, 0.1% SDS at 68°C for 45 min, dried, and mounted for autoradiography.

RESULTS

Serum neutralization assays. The following experiments were based on a report (Burrows 1973) indicating that the newly isolated dky virus was unique when compared with other equine viruses in serum neutralization tests. Figure 1A shows that serial dilutions of antiserum prepared against purified dky virus were most effective when tested with dky virus and gave a 50% titer reduction at a dilution of 1:600. This antiserum was much less effective against members of the EHV group, giving a 50% reduction in titer at 1:25 for EHV-1 and -3 and at less than 1:100 dilution for EHV-2. Neutralization of EHV strains was not much greater than against unrelated viruses, polio virus or herpes simplex

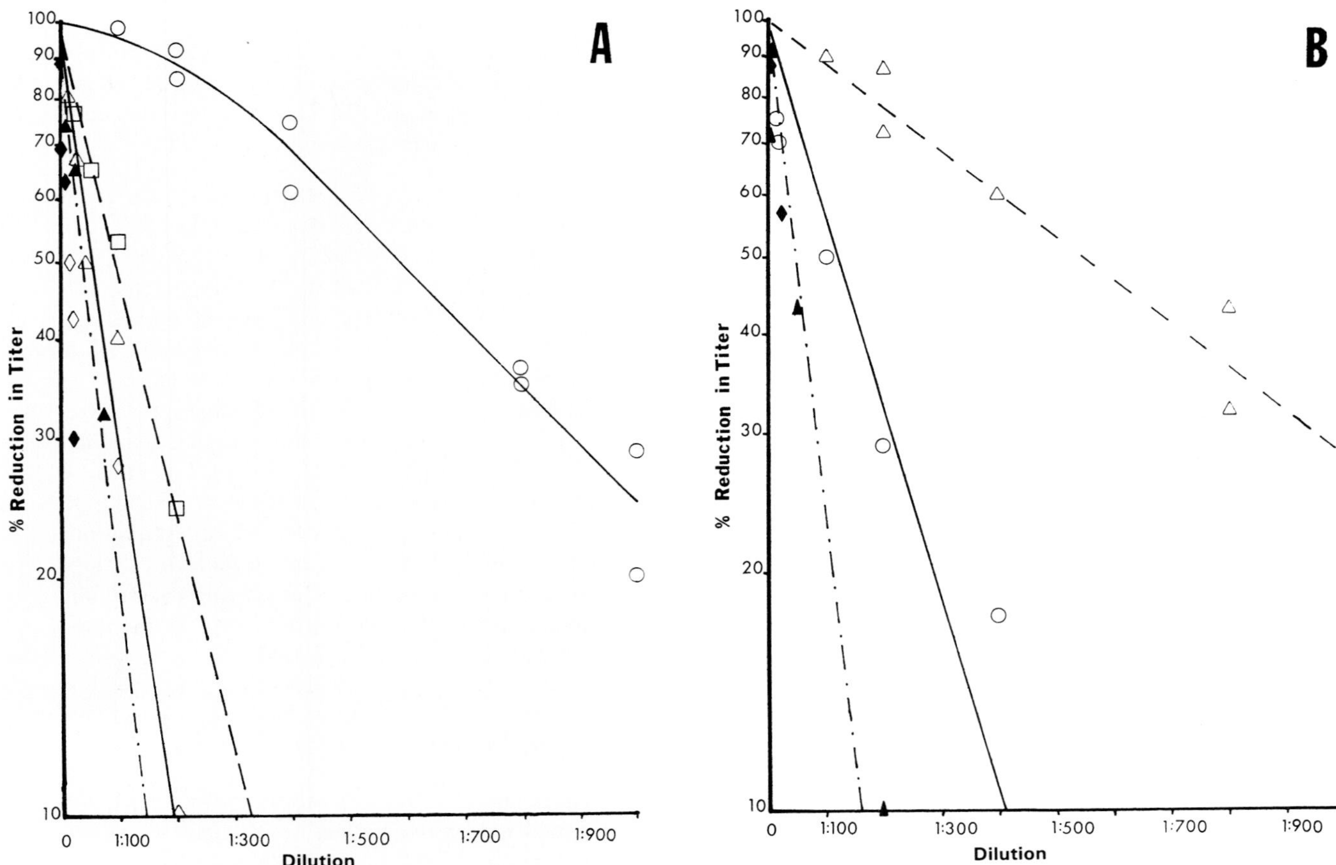

Fig. 1. Neutralization of viral infectivity by rabbit antiserum produced against purified virions and measured by reduction in plaque-forming units on cultured KYED cells. Reduction in titer is percentage of control titer measured in presence of preimmune rabbit serum. A. Results of neutralization assays using antiserum to purified dky virus; virus neutralized: (○) dky, (◇) EHV-1, (□) EHV-2, (△) EHV-3, (◆) Polio, and (▲) HSV-1. B. Results of neutralization assays using antiserum to purified EHV-3 (1118 LP); Virus neutralized: (○) dky, (△) EHV-3, and (▲) preimmune rabbit serum.

virus-I (HSV-1), indicating that the antiserum was specific for dky virus. Figure 1B shows the results of serially diluted antiserum prepared against EHV-3 (1118 LP) and then used to neutralize infectivity of dky virus. The antiserum that gave a 50% reduction of infectious titer was in excess of 1:500 dilution for the immunizing virus, EHV-3. In contrast, a titer of 1:100 was seen against the dky virus, indicating minimal cross-reactivity between EHV-3 and dky viruses. This antiserum did not do much better in neutralizing the infectivity of dky than in neutralizing polio virus, and both neutralization curves were in the range seen for the effect of preimmune rabbit serum against the infectivity of EHV-3 (1118 LP). Inasmuch as antiserum against dky virus was not effective against other viruses tested, and inasmuch as antiserum against EHV-3 (1118 LP) was not effective against dky virus infectivity, the dky virus isolated from coital exanthema-like lesions on a donkey appears to be unrelated to EHV-3, the agent of ECE in the horse.

Sedimentation equilibrium analysis of viral DNA. The following experiments were designed to characterize the DNA extracted from the dky virus and to compare its characteristics with those reported for EHV-3 DNA. Figure 2 shows the radioactivity profiles of viral DNA in CsC1 equilibrium gradients used to compare the density of dky DNA with that of known marker DNAs (Allen & Randall 1979; Atherton et al. 1982; Jacob, Price & Allen 1981; Jacob et al. 1985; Sullivan et al. 1984). Figure 2A shows that dky DNA bands one fraction heavier in density than does the DNA of the 1118 (LP) strain of EHV-3. Figure 2B indicates that dky DNA cobands with DNA isolated from herpes simplex-2 (HSV-2) DNA (Kieff, Bachenheimer and Roizman 1971). Figure 2C indicates that in these equilibrium CsC1 gradients, the DNAs of HSV-2 (1.729 gm/cc) and EHV-3 (1.726 gm/cc) band one fraction apart.

Restriction endonuclease analysis. At this point it became of interest to know whether the dky DNA, when digested with different RE, would give a fragment profile, after agarose gel electrophoresis, similar to those previously reported for the LP or sp strains of EHV-3 DNA (Allen et al. 1979; Atherton et al. 1982; Jacob et al. 1981, 1985; Kamada

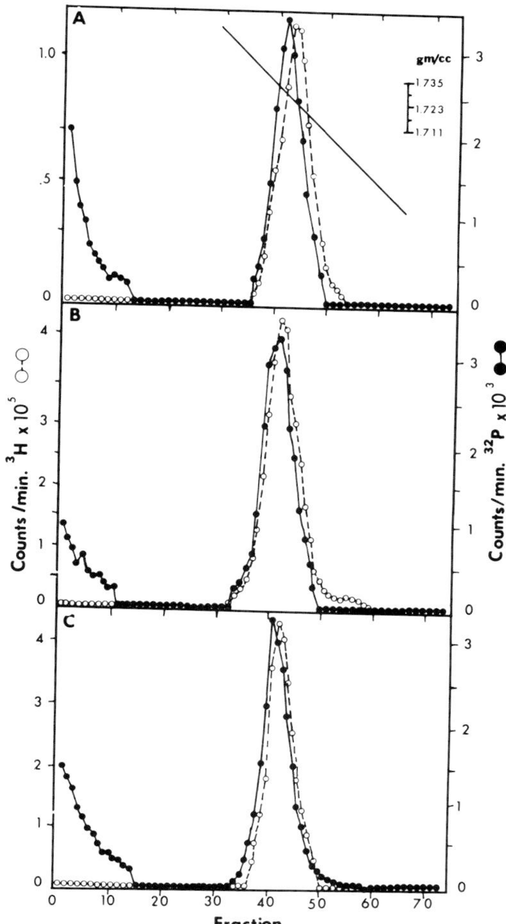

Fig. 2. Radioactivity profiles of labeled DNA extracted from dky virions and centrifuged to equilibrium in CsCl density gradient. A. dky [^{32}P]-DNA (●); EHV-3 (LP) ^{3}H-DNA (○). B. dky [^{32}P]-DNA (●) cosedimented with HSV-2 ^{3}H-DNA (○). C. HSV-2 [^{32}P]-DNA (●) cosedimented with EHV-3(LP) ^{3}H-DNA (○). Bottom of gradient is at left; density distribution of CsCl inset in A.

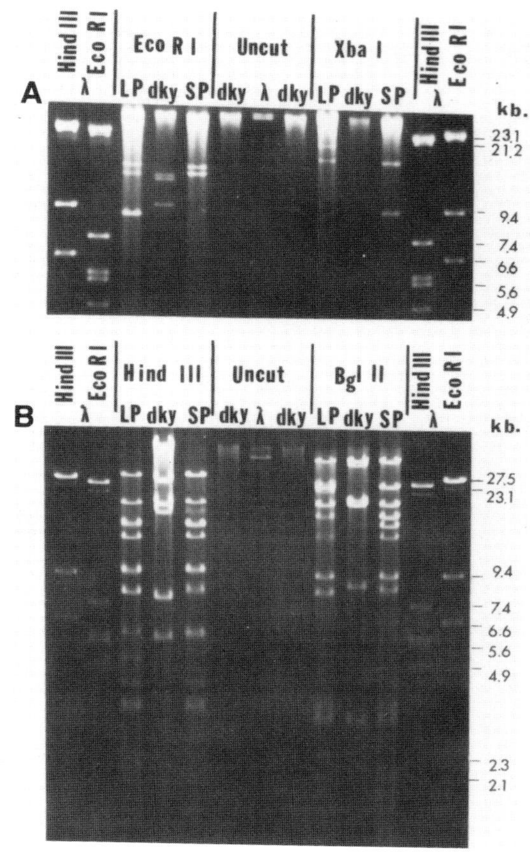

Fig. 3. Ethidium bromide–strained 0.5% agarose gels showing results of electrophoresis of products of EHV DNA digested with restriction endonucleases: *A*. EcoRI and XbaI; *B*. HindIII and BglII. Outside two lanes are products of HindIII and EcoRI digestions of phage λ DNA, respectively, and were used as markers to determine fragment sizes (33) recorded in kilobase pairs (kb). Center lanes are uncut DNA from dky and λ virions, taken to be 146 ± 4 and 48 ± 2 kb, respectively.

& Studdert 1983; Sullivan et al. 1984). Figure 3 shows the fragment profiles for LP, sp, and dky DNA, digested with four different REs and electrophoresed on agarose gel with DNA markers. Figure 3A demonstrates the fragment profile for dky DNA digested with EcoRI and XbaI REs. The overall patterns for EcoRI are not strikingly different from LP and sp DNA. The XbaI does not appear to cut the dky DNA. It has been previously reported (Jacob et al. 1985) that EHV-3 (LP) DNA contains a unique XbaI site in the unique S component of the DNA. Figure 3B shows the profile for the products of HindIII and BglII digests. The patterns for the dky DNA products are markedly different from those for either of the EHV-3 strains. The profile of the HindIII digest of dky DNA products are markedly different from those for either of the EHV-3 strains. The profile of the HindIII digest of dky DNA contained at least eight fragment bands, while the LP and sp profiles contained at least 18 fragment bands. The difference is just as striking for the profiles for BglII digests: BglII digest of dky DNA contained seven fragment bands, while sp and LP DNA digests contained 16 and 17 bands, respectively.

Southern blot hybridization analysis. Figure 4A demonstrates agarose gel analysis of the BamHI and PstI RE digestions. Even though these REs cut dky DNA at a greater frequency than the REs in the previous assay, their fragment profiles reveal few bands that comigrate with bands in the LP and sp digestion products. At this point, it became of interest to know whether the difference between the fragment profiles is a reflection of minor sequence differences, and whether localized sequence homology exists between these DNAs. Figure 4B shows results of Southern blot hybridizations (Southern 1975) of EHV-3 (1118) LP DNA, radioactively labeled and hybridized to the products in Figure 4A that were

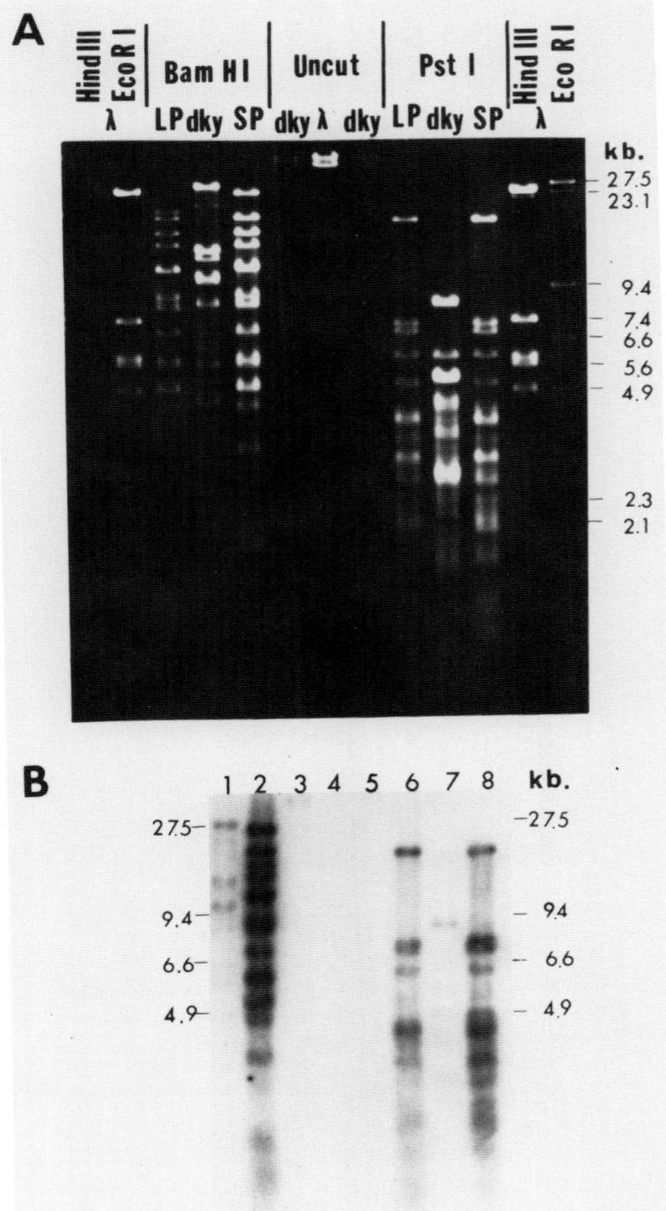

Fig. 4. Products of EHV DNA digested with restriction endonucleases BamHI and PsTI, electrophoresed on 0.5% agarose slab gel: *A*. Ethidium bromide stain of gel; *B*. Autoradiographic image of gel transferred to nitrocellulose paper and hybridized with ^{32}P-labeled EHV-3 (LP) DNA (specific activity 2 × 10^8 cpm/µgM), according to the procedure of Southern (1985). Lanes in B correspond to lanes directly above in *A;* DNA from dky isolate is located in Lanes 1, 3, 5, and 7. (For molecular weight markers, see legend to *Figure 3*.)

transferred to nitrocellulose. As expected, the products from digestions of LP and sp DNA hybridized to give fragment patterns identical with those in Figure 4A. However, the lane that contained the products of the dky DNA digestions did not show significant hybridizations with the EHV-3 DNA probe. The level of hybridization between the EHV-3 DNA probe and dky DNA is reminiscent of that previously seen for EHV-1 and EHV-3 DNA, when hybridized under similar conditions (Allen, O'Callaghan & Randall 1977; Allen and Turtinen 1982; Staczek, Atherton & O'Callaghan 1983).

DISCUSSION

The results in this report indicate that: (1) antiserum generated against the dky virus shows little, if any, specificity for the other equine herpesviruses; (2) antiserum specific for EHV-3 (1118 LP) shows little cross-reactivity with dky virus; and (3) DNA isolated from dky virus is substantially different in G + C content, restriction endonuclease digestion patterns, and sequence content from the DNAs isolated from other EHV-3 viruses. The G + C content is expected to be 69-70% as compared with 66% previously reported for EHV-DNA (Allen and Randall 1979; Atherton et al. 1982; Jacob et al. 1981, 1985; Kamada and Studdert 1983; Sullivan et al. 1984). Parenthetically, the DNA from this virus cobands in sucrose gradients with other EHV-3 DNAs (data not shown), indicating its size at 92 Md ± 12 (Allen and Randall 1979; Atherton et al. 1982; Jacob et al 1981, 1985; Kamada and Studdert 1983; Sullivan et al. 1984). Analysis of the RE digestion profiles indicates that few sites are identical, and that fragment size polymorphism and RE site heterogeneity seen in other herpesviruses (Buchman et al. 1978) are not explanations for the differences in the electrophoretic profiles. The difference in RE fragment patterns is most likely due to extensive sequence differences between the DNAs. Hybridization analysis reveals a minimal amount of homology between these DNAs. Any homology that does exist would be considered to be distributed along the DNA molecule and not localized in any specific regions. Reassociation kinetic analysis (Allen et al. 1977; Allen and Turtinen 1982; O'Callaghan et al. 1984b), a more accurate method of determining the extent of the sequence homology, has recently been initiated in our laboratory.

These findings indicate a significant difference between the DNA of dky virus and DNA isolated from a prototype strain of EHV-3. A comparison of these findings with those describing the characteristics of EHV-1 and 2 (O'Callaghan et al. 1984b) underscores the uniqueness of the DNA. It is unlikely that this virus is an intertypic recombinant (Halliburton 1980) of other EHVs. For these reasons, we suggest that this isolate is a new, as yet uncharacterized, equid herpesvirus.

It has been suggested that the use of subtypes for EHV-1 is no longer valid nomenclature and that subtype 2 should be renamed EHV-4 (Studdert et al. 1981). Our findings indicate that the DNA of the dky isolate is significantly different from the DNAs of other EHVs. It is therefore suggested that it either be referred to as donkey herpesvirus-1 or be considered a candidate for EHV-5. Further comparative studies between the new isolate and EHV-3 appear warranted, since the two contain divergent DNAs and cause similar diseases in divergent species of Equus. Both of these viruses appear to have acquired a natural attenuation, in that they are temperature-sensitive at the body temperature of their hosts (Bouchey, Evermann & Jacob, 1987; Jacob 1986). This may be responsible in part, for such a mild and benign clinical presentation following infection (Bryans 1969; Mathews 1981; O'Callaghan et al. 1978; O'Callaghan et al. 1984a,b). It would be important to examine those differences in gene regulation seen during infection and to compare, at the molecular level, the basis of their temperature restrictions. It is hoped that examining the molecular events leading to the pathogenesis of equine coital exanthema may improve our understanding of naturally acquired attenuation in EHVs.

REFERENCES

Allen, G.P., and Randall, C.C., (1979) Proteins of equine herpesvirus type 3-polypeptides of the purified virion. *Virol.* **92**, 252-57.

Allen, G.P., and Turtinen, L.W. (1982) Assessment of the base sequence homology between the two subtypes of equine herpesvirus 1. *J. Virol.* **44**, 249-55.

Allen, G.P.; O'Callaghan, D.; and Randall, C. (1977) Genetic relatedness of equine herpesvirus types 1 and 3. *J. Virol.* **24**, 761-67.

Atherton, S.; Sullivan, D.G.; Dauenhauer, S.A.; Ruyechan, W.T.; and O'Callaghan, D.J. (1982) Properties of the genome of equine herpesvirus type 3. *Virol.* **120,** 13-32.

Bouchey, D.; Evermann, J.; and Jacob, R.J. (1987) Molecular pathogenesis of Equine Coital Exanthema (ECE): Temperature sensitive (TS) and restriction endonuclease (RE) fragment profiles of several field isolates. *Arch. Virol.* **92,** 293-99.

Bryans, J.T. (1969) The herpesvirus in disease of the horse. *Proc. 14th Ann. Conv. Am. Assoc. Equine Practnr.*, pp. 119-25.

Bryans, J.T., and Allen, G.P. (1973) In vitro and in vivo studies of equine coital exanthema. *Proc. 3d Int. Conf. Equine Dis.*, pp. 322-36.

Buchman, T.G.; Roizman, B.; Adams, G.; and Stover, B.H. (1978) Restriction endonuclease fingerprinting of herpes simplex virus DNA; A novel epidemiological tool applied to nosocomial outbreaks. *J. Infect. Dis.* **132,** 488-98.

Burki, F.; Lorin, D.; and Sibalin, M. (1974) Experimental genitale and nasale infektion von pferden mit den viros des equine coital exanthems. *Zbl. Veterin. Armed.* **21,** 362-75.

Burrows, R. (1973) Discussion on equine coital exanthema infections. *Proc. 3d Int. Conf. Equine Infect. Dis.*, pp. 337-42.

Burrows, R., and Goodridge, D. (1973) In vivo and in vitro studies of equine rhinopneumonitis virus strains. *Proc. 3d Int. Conf. Equine Infect. Dis.* pp. 306-21.

Crandell, R., and Davis, E.R. (1985) Isolation of equine coital exanthema virus (equine herpesvirus 3) from the nostril of a foal. *J. Am. Vet. Med. Assoc.* **187,** 503-4.

Halliburton, I.W. (1980) Intertypic recombinants of herpes simplex viruses. *J. Gen. Virol.* **48,** 1-23.

Jacob, R.J. (1984) DNA labeled during phosphonoacetate inhibitions and following its reversal in herpesvirus infected cells. *Arch. Virol.* **79,** 221-40.

———. (1986) Molecular pathogenesis of equine coital exanthema (ECE): temperature-sensitive function(s) in cells infected with equine herpesviruses. *Vet. Microbiol.* **11,** 11-27.

Jacob, R.J., and Roizman, B. (1977) Anatomy of herpes simplex virus DNA VIII. Properties of the replicating DNA. *J. Virol.* **23,** 394-411.

Jacob, R.J.; Morse, L.S.; and Roizman, B. (1979) Anatomy of herpes simplex DNA XII. Accumulation of head-to-tail concatemers in nuclei of infected cells and their role in the generation of the four isomeric arrangements of viral DNA. *J. Virol.* **29,** 448-57.

Jacob, R.J.; Price, R.; and Allen, G.P. (1981) Restriction endonuclease digestions of equine herpesvirus III DNA: Evidence for isomeric forms of virion DNA. 6th *Proc. Int. Workshop Herpesviruses*, pp. 16-17.

———. (1985) Molecular pathogenesis of equine coital exanthema: Restriction endonuclease digestions of EHV-3 DNA and indications of a unique Xba-1 cleavage site. *Intervirology* **23,** 172-80.

Kamada, M.; and Studdert, M.J. (1983) Analysis of small and large plaque variants of equine herpesvirus type 3 by restriction endonucleases. *Arch. Virol.* **77,** 259-64.

Kieff, E.D.; Bachenheimer, S.L.; and Roizman, B., (1971) Size, composition and structure of the DNA of herpes simplex virus subtypes 1 and 2. *J. Virol.* **8,** 125-32.

Krogsrud, J., and Onstad, O. (1971) Equine coital exanthema—Isolation of a virus and transmission experiments. *Acta. Vet. Scand.* **12,** 1-14.

Mathews, R.E.F. (1981) Classification and nomenclature of viruses; summary of results of International Meeting on Taxonomy of viruses in Strasburg. *Intervirology* **16,** 53-60.

O'Callaghan, D.; Allen, G.P.; and Randall, C.C. (1978) Structure and replication of the herpesviruses. *Proc. 4th Int. Conf. Equine Infect. Dis.*, pp. 1-31.

O'Callaghan, D.; Gentry, G.A.; and Randall, C.C. (1984a) The equine herpesviruses. In *The Herpesvirus,* Vol. 2, pp. 215-318. Ed. B. Roizman. Plenum Press, New York.

O'Callaghan, D.J.; Sullivan, D.C.; Baumann, R.P.; Caughman, G.B.; Flowers, C.C.; Robertson, A.T.; and Staczek, J. (1984b) Genomes of the equine herpesvirus, molecular structure, regions of homology and DNA sequences associated with transformation. In *Herpesvirus,* pp. 507-22. Ed. F. Rapp. Alan R. Liss Inc., New York.

Plummer, G.; Goodheart, C.R.; and Studdert, M.J. (1973) Equine herpesvirus, antigenic relationships and DNA densities. *Infect. Immun.* **8,** 621-27.

Sabine, M.; Robertson, G.R.; and Whalley, J.M. (1981) Differentiation of subtypes of equine herpesvirus 1 by restriction endonuclease analysis. *Aust. Vet. J.* **57,** 148-49.

Shimizu, T.; Ishizaki, R.; Ishii, S.; Kawakami, Y.; Kagi, T.; Sugimuia, K.; and Matumoto, M. (1959) Isolation of equine abortion virus from natural cases of equine abortion in horse kidney cell culture. *Jpn. J. Exp. Med.* **29,** 643-49.

Southern, E. (1975) Detection of specific sequences among DNA fragments separated by gel electrophoresis. *J. Mol. Biol.* **93,** 503-15.

Staczek, J.; Atherton, S.S.; and O'Callaghan, D.J. (1983) Genetic relatedness of the genomes of equine herpesvirus types 1, 2, and 3. *J. Virol.* **45,** 855-58.

Studdert, M. (1974) Comparative aspects of equine herpesviruses. *Cornell Vet.* **64,** 94-122.

Studdert, M.; Simpson, T.; and Roizman, B. (1981) Differentiation of respiratory and abortigenic isolates of equine herpesvirus 1 by restriction endonucleases. *Science* **214,** 562-64.

Sullivan, D.; Atherton, S.S.; Staczek, J.; and O'Callaghan, D.J. (1984) Structure of the genome of equine herpesvirus type 3. *Virology* **132,** 352-67.

Thomas, M.; and Davis, R.W. (1975) Studies on the cleavage of bacteriophage lambda DNA with EcoRI restriction endonuclease. *J. Mol. Biol.* **91,** 315-25.

Turtinen, L.; Allen, G.P.; Darlington, R.W.; and Bryans, J.T. (1982) Serologic and molecular comparisons of several equine herpesvirus type 1 strains. *Am. J. Vet. Res.* **42,** 2099-2104.

Infections of the Reproductive System

Persistent Infection of the Reproductive Tract in Stallions Experimentally Infected with Equine Arteritis Virus

Suzanne M. Neu, Peter J. Timoney, and William H. McCollum

SUMMARY

Sixteen stallions were infected intranasally with equine arteritis virus (EAV) and monitored for evidence of persistent infection. All stallions developed clinical signs of equine viral arteritis. Virus was recovered repeatedly from the nasopharynx, urethra, semen, urine, and buffy coat of the blood during the acute phase of the infection. Thirteen stallions were shedding virus at the time they were killed, six to 148 days after inoculation. All five horses killed between 92 and 148 days after inoculation were shedding virus in the semen just prior to being killed. Of the eight experimentally infected stallions studied for eight weeks or more, a total of five (62%) developed the long-term carrier state. On the basis of attempts to isolate virus from tissues, EAV had been eliminated from most sites during the first 40 days after inoculation. Tissues from the genitourinary tract remained virus-positive in stallions that were shedding virus in the semen at the time of death. The areas where virus was detected most frequently were the ampulla of the vas deferens (73.3%), the vas deferens (68.8%), and the bulbourethral glands (62.5%).

INTRODUCTION

Equine viral arteritis (EVA) was first recognized as a specific disease of the horse after the etiologic agent was isolated from the lung of an aborted fetus during an outbreak of abortion in Bucyrus, Ohio, in 1953 (Doll et al. 1957a; Doll, Knappenberger & Bryans, 1957b). The chief mode of transmission during that outbreak was direct contact via nasal droplet or spray (McCollum et al. 1961). An investigation of an epizootic of EVA on Thoroughbred breeding farms in Kentucky in 1984 found that a high percentage (36%) of affected stallions continued to shed equine arteritis virus in the semen (Timoney 1985). The result was venereal transmission of the virus to susceptible mares to which they were bred. Various investigations of equine arteritis virus following natural infection have documented not only the occurrence of persistent seminal shedding but also the absence of persistent shedding from other sources such as the nasopharynx, urine, and buffy coat (Timoney et al. 1987). There is evidence of two carrier states: a short-term state during convalescence and a long-term chronic condition (Timoney & McCollum 1985; Timoney et al. 1986b; Timoney et al. 1987).

The purpose of the present study was to establish persistent EAV infection in stallions, to investigate the route(s) and temporal pattern of virus shedding during the convalescent and postconvalescent periods, and to determine the anatomic site(s) of viral persistence.

Department of Veterinary Science, University of Kentucky, Lexington, Kentucky 40506. Published as paper No. 87-4-220 by permission of the Dean and Director, College of Agriculture and Kentucky Agricultural Experiment Station.

MATERIALS AND METHODS

Horses. The 17 sexually mature stallions in the experiment ranged in age from three to ten years or more. Stallions 1 through 15 were obtained from a local commercial vendor, fourteen of them being crossbred and one (No. 12) a Thoroughbred. Two additional crossbred horses were obtained from the resident horse population of the University of Kentucky Agricultural Experiment Station. Neutralizing antibodies to EAV were not detected in serum collected from the stallions on several occasions prior to inoculation.

Virus. The source of the virus inoculum was a citrated blood sample pooled from three Thoroughbred stallions naturally infected during the 1984 outbreak of EVA in Kentucky. The pooled blood was inoculated intravenously into a susceptible mare that was killed six days later. A homogenized tissue suspension made from the mesenteric lymph node of this mare was used to inoculate a second susceptible mare, also killed on the sixth day after inoculation. The spleen from the second mare was harvested and portions were homogenized in Eagle's minimal essential medium containing 2% fetal calf serum to form a 10% tissue suspension. The supernate of this suspension was stored at $-80°$ and used as the inoculum in this study.

Experimental design. The study was conducted in two experiments. The first experiment studied eight stallions (Nos. 1-8) from the day of intranasal inoculation with EAV to Day 49 afterward, during the period from November 1985 to January 1986. One stallion was killed on each of Days 6, 10, 14, 20, 27, 34, 41, and 49. In the second experiment, eight stallions (Nos. 10-17) were studied from the day after inoculation to Day 148, beginning in June 1986 and continuing through November 1986. One stallion was killed on each of Days 57, 64, 78, 92, 105, 120, 134, and 148. Stallion 9 served as a control for both experimental groups. It was vaccinated intramuscularly with a commercial modified-live virus vaccine (Arvac; Fort Dodge Labs, Fort Dodge, Iowa) at 14 days and at three days before the first experiment began.

Animal inoculation. The experimental animals were inoculated via the nasopharynx with 5 ml of a splenic suspension containing 10^4 plaque-forming units (PFU) of EAV per milliliter. The control stallion was inoculated in an identical manner with 5 ml of sterile saline.

Collection of specimens. Rectal temperatures and clinical signs were monitored twice daily, at approximately 7:00 A.M. and 3:00 P.M. during the period of acute illness. Blood, semen, urine, nasal swabs, rectal swabs, and urethral swabs were collected prior to inoculation two to four times per week throughout both experiments. The following tissues and bodily fluids were collected from each animal at necropsy for virus isolation: peritoneal fluid, pleural fluid, pericardial fluid, urine, lymph nodes (mesenteric, colonic, splenic, deep inguinal, superficial inguinal, retropharyngeal, and tracheobronchial), pharyngeal tonsil, spleen, lung, liver, kidneys, adrenal glands, ureters, urinary bladder, urethra (proximal, middle, and distal), testes, epididymes, vasa deferentia, ampullae of the vasa deferentia, seminal vesicles, vesicular fluid, prostate gland, and bulbourethral glands.

Blood and nasal, rectal, and urethral swabs were collected by methods previously described (McCollum, Prickett & Bryans, 1971). Midstream urine samples were collected in sterile containers following intravenous administration of 150 mg furosemide (Butler Company, Columbus, Ohio) on days alternating with semen collection. Semen was collected using a modified Colorado artificial vagina (Lane Manufacturing Co., Denver, Colo.) with sterile disposable plastic liners and collection bottles and a teaser mare. Samples were refrigerated on ice for transport to the laboratory, where they were either processed immediately for virus isolation or frozen at −80°C and processed later. Urine samples from Experiment 2 were frozen at −20°C prior to processing. At necropsy, stallions were immobilized with succinyl choline followed immediately by an overdose of pentobarbitol sodium or gunshot to the head. The major vessels were transected at the thoracic inlet for exsanguination. Tissues and body fluids were collected aseptically as quickly after death as possible and placed immediately on ice.

Virus isolation. Nasal swabs, buffy coat preparations, tissues, and bodily fluids were processed for virus isolation as previously described (McCollum et al 1971). Urethral and rectal swabs were processed in the same manner as nasal swabs. Urine was concentrated against an 8% solution of polyethylene glycol (PEG) of molecular weight 15,000 to 20,000 daltons (J.T. Baker Chemical Company, Phillipsburg, N.J.). Two to four dialysis sacks (Sigma, St. Louis, Mo.) per sample were filled with 30 ml of urine each, placed in 800 ml of PEG and refrigerated at 4°C. Sixteen to 24 hours of dialysis were required to obtain a sufficiently concentrated urine sample. Urine was harvested aseptically from the dialysis sacks and inoculated undiluted onto cell cultures. Samples of gel-free semen were subjected to sonication and centrifugation as described by Timoney and colleagues (1987).

Isolation of EAV was attempted using monolayer cell cultures of the RK-13 cell line of rabbit kidney (ATCC CCL37), passage levels 185-210, in 12-well culture plates (Costar, Cambridge, Mass.). Cultures with no evidence of cytopathic effect (CPE) after seven days' incubation at 37°C were frozen at −20°C, thawed, and passaged a second time. Cultures were considered negative for EAV if CPE was not observed after seven days' incubation on the second passage. Identity of any isolated virus was confirmed by a plaque-reduction assay in monolayer cultures of RK-13 cells in the presence of an excess of guinea pig complement (Pel-Freez Biologicals, Rogers, Alaska), using equine antiserum prepared against the strain of EAV associated with the 1984 Kentucky epizootic.

Viral assay. Serial decimal dilutions were made of sonicated seminal plasma and tissue suspensions for determination of virus concentration in semen and selected tissues. Titration assays were performed in quadruplicate, utilizing monolayer cultures of RK-13 cells in 12-well plates, with 0.1 ml of inoculum per well. Plaques were counted microscopically after five days' incubation at 37°C.

Serum neutralization test. Serum-neutralizing antibodies to EAV were detected in a microneutralization test using RK-13 cells in the presence of guinea pig complement (Senne, Pearson & Carbrey 1985).

RESULTS

Clinical signs. All 16 stallions developed clinical signs of EVA from one to six days following inoculation of the virus. Clinical signs were variable in range and severity; they included fever; edema of the limbs, scrotum, prepuce, and periorbital tissues; conjunctivitis; papular skin eruptions on the neck; reluctance to move; and decreased libido. Fever of three to nine days' duration was present in all horses, with maximal temperatures of 39.7°C to 40.9°C (mean, 40.3°C). Clinical signs subsided in most cases after 10 to 14 days. Limb edema persisted in Stallion 2 until termination on Day 27.

Virus isolation (Tables 1-3). *Nasal swabs.* Virus was first isolated from the nasopharynx on Day 1 following inoculation. Nasal shedding of virus continued until Day 19 in Experiment 1 (one horse) and up to Day 21 in Experiment 2 (three horses). The average duration of nasal shedding, ex-

Table 1. Days of first isolation and last isolation of virus from clinical specimens from stallions inoculated intranasally with a 1984 Kentucky strain of equine arteritis virus (Experiment 1)

		Source of specimen					
Horse no.	Day killed	Naso-pharynx	Urethra	Rectum	Buffy coat	Urine	Semen
1	6	Day 3/Day 5	Day 5/Day 5	—	Day 3/Day 5	Day 6/Day 6	Day 5/Day 5
5	10	Day 1/Day 9	Day 7/Day 9	—	Day 3/Day 9	Day 8/Day 10	-/-
3	14	Day 1/Day 11	Day 5/Day 11	—	Day 3/Day 13	Day 6/Day 14	Day 5/Day 13
4	20	Day 1/Day 9	Day 5/Day 9	—	Day 2/Day 17	Day 4/Day 18	Day 5/Day 19
2	27	Day 3/Day 19	Day 5/Day 17	—	Day 3/Day 24	Day 6/Day 18	Day 5/Day 26
6	34	Day 1/Day 17	Day 5/Day 9	Day 7/Day 7	Day 3/Day 31	Day 6/Day 16	Day 5/Day 33
7	41	Day 3/Day 11	Day 9/Day 11	—	Day 3/Day 28	Day 8/Day 8	Day 9/Day 39
8	49	Day 1/Day 11	Day 9/Day 11	—	Day 5/Day 45	Day 6/Day 10	Day 7/Day 48

Note: Virus isolation attempted in monolayer cultures of RK-13 cells.

Table 2. Days of first isolation and last isolation of virus from clinical specimens from stallions inoculated intranasally with a 1984 Kentucky strain of equine arteritis virus (Experiment 2)

		Source of specimen					
Horse no.	Day killed	Naso-pharynx	Urethra	Rectum	Buffy coat	Urine	Semen
14	57	Day 2/Day 19	Day 12/Day 12	—	Day 7/Day 40	-/-	Day 12/Day 28
10	64	Day 5/Day 14	Day 7/Day 14	—	Day 5/Day 21	Day 8/Day 8	Day 7/Day 21
13	78	Day 2/Day 12	Day 5/Day 14	—	Day 2/Day 26	Day 8/Day 8	Day 7/Day 19
12	92	Day 2/Day 21	Day 5/Day 12	Day 7/Day 7	Day 2/Day 26	Day 6/Day 15	Day 7/Day 89
17	105	Day 5/Day 21	Day 5/Day 14	—	Day 2/Day 33	Day 6/Day 22	Day 9/Day 100
15	120	Day 2/Day 21	Day 5/Day 7	—	Day 5/Day 40	Day 8/Day 20	Day 7/Day 117
11	134	Day 5/Day 16	Day 7/Day 7	—	Day 7/Day 58	Day 6/Day 8	Day 7/Day 131
16	148	Day 5/Day 21	Day 5/Day 7	Day 9/Day 9	Day 2/Day 111	Day 6/Day 20	Day 7/Day 135

Note: Virus isolation attempted in monolayer cultures of RK-13 cells.

Table 3. Virus isolations from genitourinary tract tissues of stallions inoculated intranasally with a 1984 Kentucky strain of equine arteritis virus

	Horse No. (and day killed)															
	1	5	3	4	2	6	7	8	14	10	13	12	17	15	11	16
	(6)	(10)	(14)	(20)	(27)	(34)	(41)	(49)	(57)	(64)	(78)	(92)	(105)	(120)	(134)	(148)
Tissue																
Testis	3.8	5.9	3.8	+	–	–	–	–	–	–	–	–	–	–	–	–
Epididymis	4.5	1.7	3.1	5.2	+	–	–	–	–	–	+	2.4	+	–	–	1.7
Vas deferens	5.1	2.6	4.0	4.4	1.4	+	+	4.0	–	–	–	4.6	–	2.0	–	+
Ampulla	ND[a]	6.0	–	4.5	+	2.5	2.8	4.7	–	–	–	4.3	3.5	4.7	4.5	4.9
Seminal vesicle	3.3	3.3	–	2.5	+	–	–	2.8	–	–	–	2.1	–	3.6	–	2.8
Bulbourethral gl.	6.0	6.0	3.3	+	+	–	+	–	–	–	–	–	1.4	1.4	+	1.4
Prostate	3.0	–	–	2.2	–	–	–	2.5	–	–	–	+	2.2	3.2	–	2.4
Kidney	+	2.6	4.3	2.7	3.6	+	–	–	+	–	–	–	–	–	–	–
Ureter	+	–	–	–	–	–	–	–	–	–	–	–	–	–	–	–
Urinary bladder	+	+	–	–	–	–	–	–	–	–	–	–	–	2.0	–	2.5
Prox. urethra	+	4.6	–	3.3	–	–	2.1	–	–	–	–	+	2.2	2.9	2.5	2.8
Mid. urethra	+	–	–	+	+	–	–	–	–	–	–	–	–	+	–	–
Dist. urethra	+	+	–	–	–	–	–	–	–	–	–	–	–	+	–	+

Note: Virus isolations attempted in monolayer cultures of RK-13 cells; virus titers expressed as $\log_{10}$ PFU/gm of tissue; + = virus isolated, concentration not determined.

[a] ND = not done.

cluding the two stallions killed during this period, was 12.9 days.

Buffy coat. Virus was isolated from buffy coat preparations beginning on Day 2 in both experiments. EAV was recovered from 64 of 73 samples (88%) collected from Day 3 to Day 48 in Experiment 1. Stallions 1-6 had virus in the buffy coat at the time they were killed, six to thirty-four days after inoculation. Stallion 7 was positive by virus isolation until Day 28 and was killed Day 41; Stallion 8 was positive by virus isolation on Day 45 and was killed on Day 49. In Experiment 2, EAV was isolated from the buffy coat until Day 21 in one horse (No. 10), Day 26 in two horses (Nos. 12 and 13), Day 33 in one horse (No. 17), and Day 40 in two horses (Nos. 14 and 15). Virus isolation from the buffy coat continued sporadically in the remaining two horses until Day 58 (No. 11) and Day 111 (No. 16). The median duration of virus persistence in buffy coat cells was 25.5 days.

Urine. Virus was detected in urine beginning four to eight days after inoculation. Four horses in Experiment 1 (Nos. 1, 3, 5, and 4) had virus in the last urine sample obtained before they were killed. The remaining horses ceased shedding virus in the urine between Days 8 and 18. The horses in Experiment 2 began shedding virus in the urine on Days 6-8. A single isolation was obtained from each of two horses (Nos. 10 and 13) on Day 8. The remaining stallions ceased shedding virus in the urine on Day 20 or 22. Virus was not isolated from the urine of Stallion 14.

Semen. EAV was isolated from 70 of 76 semen samples (92%) collected from Days 5 to 48 in Experiment 1. Virus isolation attempts were unsuccessful on samples obtained prior to Day 5. Seven stallions shed virus in the semen continuously until the time they were killed. Semen could not be obtained from one horse (No. 5). Stallions in Experiment 2 began shedding virus in the semen on Day 7. Three stallions ceased shedding virus during Experiment 2, on Day 19 (No. 13), Day 21 (No. 10), and Day 28 (No. 14) respectively. Of 170 semen samples collected from the remaining five stallions from Day 7 to Day 135, 167 (98%) contained EAV on virus isolation. These five stallions shed virus in the semen continuously from Day 7 until they were killed.

Urethral swabs. Virus was isolated from the urethra of stallions in both experiments beginning on Day 5. In Experiment 1, stallions ceased shedding virus from the urethra between Days 9 and 17; in Experiment 2, between Days 7 and 14.

Rectal swabs. Three isolations were made from rectal swabs, two on Day 7 (Nos. 6 and 12) and one on Day 9 (No. 16).

Tissues and body fluids. Virus was isolated from tissues of all of the experimental animals after death (Tables 3 and 4). All tissues and body fluids assayed from Stallion 1, killed on Day 6, contained EAV. Most tissues and fluids, including all lymphoid tissues examined, still contained virus on Day 10 (No. 5). Results of virus isolation attempts from tissues of Stallions 3, 4, 2, 6 and 7, killed on Days 14, 20, 27, 34 and 41, indicated a gradual elimination of virus from most sites in the body. However, a variety of tissues taken from the genitourinary tract remained virus-positive in the stallions that were shedding virus in the semen at the time of death. The colonic lymph node was the only site outside the reproductive tract that contained EAV by virus isolation in Stallion 8, killed on Day 49. Stallions 12, 17, 15, 11, and 16, killed on Days 92, 105, 120, 134, and 148, respectively, contained detectable amounts of virus in the reproductive tract and lower urinary tract only. EAV was most frequently isolated from the ampulla of the vas deferens (positive in 73.3% of the stallions), from the vas deferens itself (68.8%), and from the bulbourethral glands (62.5%). In the five stallions that shed virus in the semen for 89 days or longer, virus was found to be present in the ampulla of the vas deferens and the proximal urethra of all. EAV was isolated from the prostate and bulbourethral glands of four (80%); the vas deferens, epididymis, and seminal vesicle of three (60%); the urinary bladder and distal urethra of two (40%); and the middle urethra of one (20%). No other tissues contained virus in this group of animals. Virus was not isolated from the testes of any horse killed later than Day 20.

In Experiment 2, EAV was isolated from certain tissues collected at necropsy of three horses (10, 13, and 14) that had ceased shedding detectable quantities of virus via the nasopharynx, rectum, urethra, urine, buffy coat, and semen. After Stallion 14 was killed on Day 57, EAV was isolated from the kidney, 17 days after the last antemortem virus

Table 4. Virus isolations from seminal plasma from stallions inoculated intranasally with a 1984 Kentucky strain of equine arteritis virus

Horse No.	No. of days after inoculation							
	5-9	12-19	26-33	39-46	56	86-89	114	135
1	2.1	*	*	*	*	*	*	*
3	+	3.3	*	*	*	*	*	*
4	3.7	4.7	*	*	*	*	*	*
2	4.0	2.9	3.0	*	*	*	*	*
6	2.2	2.9	+	*	*	*	*	*
7	4.2	2.9	2.9	+	*	*	*	*
8	5.9	3.3	4.3	3.3	*	*	*	*
10	5.1	+	+	+	+	*	*	*
13	3.7	+	+	+	4.2	*	*	*
12	+	+	1.7	+	3.5	3.7	*	*
17	+	3.7	+	4.0	2.7	2.9	*	*
15	3.7	+	4.6	4.4	4.6	5.1	4.4	*
11	5.7	+	+	4.9	4.2	4.6	5.2	*
16	+	5.7	3.7	5.9	4.5	5.2	4.8	3.9

Note: Virus titers expressed as $\log_{10}$ PFU/ml of sonicated seminal plasma; + = virus isolated, concentration not determined.

* Indicated animal had been euthanized.

isolation (buffy coat, Day 40). Stallion 10, killed on Day 64, contained virus in a deep inguinal lymph node, 43 days after the last virus isolation was made from semen (Day 21). Pericardial fluid and epididymis from Stallion 13 contained virus on Day 78, 52 days after the last virus isolation (buffy coat, Day 26). These results were confirmed by reisolation of EAV from the original specimens obtained at necropsy and stored at $-80°C$.

Viral assay. The concentration of virus in the semen varied among horses; however, each horse maintained a relatively constant amount of virus per milliliter of sonicated seminal plasma throughout the period of seminal shedding. The viral content of the semen ranged from $10^{1.7}$ plaque–forming units (PFU) per milliliter to $10^{5.9}$ PFU/ml of sonicated seminal plasma (Table 4). Concentration of EAV in genitourinary tissues was also variable and tended to be greater in those animals killed during the acute phase of the infection (Nos. 1 and 5). The highest concentration of virus per gram of tissue in the remaining horses was found in the ampulla of the vas deferens, which in most cases contained between $10^{2.5}$ and $10^{4.9}$ PFU/gm of tissue (Table 3).

Identity of virus. Viral isolates from all animals were neutralized by equine antiserum prepared against the same strain of EAV as used in this study.

DISCUSSION

The long-term carrier state with EAV was successfully established in five of the eight (62.5%) experimentally infected stallions studied for eight weeks or more. These stallions exhibited persistent virus shedding in the semen after clinical recovery. Virus shedding from other sites was not detectable after 30-45 days, with the exception of sporadic isolations from the buffy coat of two horses. The sites of virus persistence in the carrier stallions were found to be the excretory ducts and accessory glands of the reproductive tract. The ampulla of the vas deferens was the most common site from which virus was isolated, and it contained the highest concentration of virus among the tissues and fluids collected from the carriers. Results of virus isolations indicated a gradual elimination of virus from most body sites within 28-34 days after infection, with localization of the virus in the genitourinary tract of those horses that became chronic carriers. The most frequent sites of virus isolation in these horses were the ampulla of the vas deferens, proximal urethra, prostate, bulbourethral glands, vas deferens, epididymis, and seminal vesicles. According to titration studies, the ampulla of the vas deferens had the highest concentration of virus ($10^{2.5}$ to $10^{6.0}$ PFU/gm). Isolation of virus from the proximal urethra may have resulted from contamination of this site by secretions from the accessory glands entering the proximal urethra in the region of the seminal colliculus. The urinary bladders of two persistently infected horses contained virus, possibly the result of retrograde passage of the virus from the proximal urethra. Postmorten urine samples from these two stallions did not, however, contain EAV. Virus was isolated from genitourinary tissues up to 148 days after virus inoculation, when this study was terminated. The longest duration of viral persistence within tissues was previously reported as 19 days in the kidney, lung, and bronchial lymph node (McCollum et al 1971), and 36 days in the lung (Fukunaga et al. 1981). The results of the present study do not support earlier speculation that EAV may persist for long periods of time in the kidney (McCollum et al. 1971). With one exception (No. 14), virus was not isolated from the kidney of any horse killed after Day 34.

The isolation of EAV from tissues of the three nonshedding stallions was somewhat unexpected, considering the length of time (17-52 days) since the previous antemortem isolation of virus from blood, semen, urine, nasopharanyx, rectum, and urethra. The sources of the viral isolates were the kidney (Day 57), a deep inguinal lymph node (Day 64), and epididymis and pericardial fluid (Day 78). The isolations from these horses were confirmed by reisolation of EAV from the original specimens collected at necropsy. The presence of virus in the pericardial fluid of Stallion 13 is not easily explained. Virus was not detected in other bodily fluids or in the thoracic lymph nodes of this horse. With the exception of epididymis, virus was not isolated from these sites in any of the long-term carriers. It is possible that, while virus is localized in the reproductive tract of the majority of persistently infected horses, others may develop viral persistence in sites that are less easily detected clinically. Had it been known that these animals still harbored the virus, immunosuppressive agents could have been administered in attempts to induce resumption of virus shedding. Animals have not been reported to resume shedding EAV after a period of quiescence (Timoney and McCollum, unpublished data). It is more likely, therefore, that these animals were in the process of eliminating the virus from their tissues. The duration of virus persistence in these tissues is surprising nonetheless, and determination of its significance warrants further investigation.

Virus first appeared in the semen of most of the stallions two to seven days after intranasal inoculation of EAV. In all but three stallions, virus was recovered from nearly every semen sample obtained until the horses were killed. Five stallions in Experiment 1 (Nos. 4, 2, 6, 7, and 8) shed virus in the semen for one to five weeks after clinical recovery and could thus be considered at least short-term convalescent carriers according to Timoney and colleagues (1986a). The additional five stallions in Experiment 2 that shed virus for 89 days or longer were considered to be long-term chronic carriers. Three stallions ceased shedding virus in the semen during the second experiment. The duration of seminal shedding in these animals averaged 17.3 days (range, 15-20 days) and was roughly equivalent to the duration of shedding via the nasopharynx and urine; these animals were considered noncarriers. The concentration of virus in the semen of noncarriers was similar to that for carriers. There was no apparent decline in the amount of virus shed in the semen of carrier stallions over the course of the experiment. Timoney and colleagues (1987) reported similar results, with virus concentrations ranging from 3.7×10^2 to 4.4×10^6 PFU/ml in two naturally infected carrier stallions sampled intensively for three months. It is the constant high concentration of EAV in the semen of carrier stallions that ensures perpetuation of the virus in an equine population. It also facilitates detection of the carrier state (Timoney et al., 1986a). There has been only one report of a long-term carrier stallion that subsequently ceased shedding virus in the semen (Timoney et al. 1987). Virus was isolated from the buffy coat of all the stallions in this study, persisting for periods from three to 110 days (median, 25.5 days). Isolations of EAV from the buffy coat after Day 45 of the experiment were sporadic and occurred in only two horses (Nos. 11 and 16). In two short-term studies, virus was recovered from the buffy coat for 10 to 19 days after inoculation (McCollum & Timoney 1985; McCollum et al. 1971). In a third study virus was recovered sporadically from two horses for 30 to 36 days, respectively, before the experiment was terminated (Fukunaga et al. 1981). These results, together with the findings of the present study, indicate that individual animals may harbor the virus in cells of the buffy coat for extended periods of time following clinical recovery. It is possible that the sporadic isolation of virus from the buffy coat fraction of the blood was due to clearance of the virus from persistently infected sites in the body by lymphocytes or other blood leukocytes. Another possible explanation is that occasional horses develop persistent low-grade infection of blood leukocytes in which the number of circulating infected cells exceeds the threshold of detection only on a sporadic basis. Cultures of equine macrophage cells have been shown to support the replication of EAV in vitro (McCollum 1978). More work needs to be done in this area to determine the cell type involved and to provide more detailed information as to the nature of the infection of these cells.

The pattern of virus shedding from the nasopharynx, rectum, and urine was similar to that in previous reports (McCollum et al. 1971; Fukunaga et al. 1981; McCollum & Timoney 1985). Virus isolations from urethral swabs occurred only during the acute phase of illness, ruling out the distal urethra as a possible site of virus persistence and as the source of virus in semen and urine.

The findings of this study are an important step in understanding the pathogenesis and epidemiologic significance of the carrier state of EAV in the stallion. Further study of the disease will be needed to determine the mechanism of virus persistence, the reason for its preferential localization in the male reproductive tract, and the factors influencing development of the carrier state in stallions.

REFERENCES

Doll, E.R.; Bryans, J.T.; McCollum, W.H.; and Crowe, M.E.W. (1957a) Isolation of a filterable agent causing arteritis of horses and abortion of mares. Its differentiation from the equine abortion (influenza) virus. *Cornell Vet.* **47,** 3-41.

Doll, E.R.; Knappenberger, R.E.; and Bryans, J.T. (1957b) An outbreak of abortion caused by equine arteritis virus. *Cornell Vet.* **47,** 69-75.

Fukunaga, Y.; Imagawa, H.; Tabuchi, E.; and Akiyama, Y. (1981) Clinical and virological findings on experimental equine arteritis in horses. *Bull. Equine Res. Inst.* **18,** 110-18.

McCollum, W.H. (1978) Studies of the replication of equine arteritis virus in macrophage cultures. (Abstr.) *Proc. 59th Conf. Res. Workers Anim. Dis.*, p. 23.

McCollum, W.H., and Timoney, P.J. (1985) The pathogenic qualities of the 1984 strain of equine arteritis virus. *Proc. Grayson Found. Intl. Conf. Thoroughbred Breeders Orgs. on Equine Viral Arteritis*, pp. 34-47.

McCollum, W.H.; Doll, E.R.; Wilson, J.C.; and Johnson, C.B. (1961) Propagation of equine arteritis virus in monolayer cultures of equine kidney. *Am. J. Vet. Res.* **89,** 731-35.

McCollum, W.H.; Prickett, M.E.; and Bryans, J.T. (1971) Temporal distribution of equine arteritis virus in respiratory mucosa, tissues and body fluids of horses infected by inhalation. *Res. Vet. Sci.* **2,** 459-64.

Senne, D.A.; Pearson, J.E.; and Carbrey, E.A. (1985) Equine viral arteritis: A standard procedure for the virus neutralization test and comparison of results of a proficiency test performed at five laboratories. *Proc. U.S. Anim. Hlth. Assoc.* pp. 29-34.

Timoney, P. J. (1985) Clinical, virological and epidemiological features of the 1984 outbreak of equine viral arteritis in the thoroughbred population in Kentucky, USA. *Proc. Grayson Found. Intl. Conf. Thoroughbred Breeders Orgs. on Equine Viral Arteritis*, pp. 24-33.

Timoney, P. J., and McCollum, W.H. (1985) The epidemiology of equine viral arteritis. *Proc. 31st Ann. Conv. Am. Assoc. Equine Practnr.*, pp. 545-51.

Timoney, P. J.; McCollum, W. H.; and Roberts, A. W. (1986a) Detection of the carrier state in stallions persistently infected with equine arteritis virus. *Proc. 32d Ann. Conv. Am. Assoc. Equine Practnr.*, pp. 57-65.

Timoney, P. J.; McCollum W. H.; Roberts, A. W.; and Murphy, T. W. (1986b) Demonstration of the carrier state in naturally acquired equine arteritis virus infection in the stallion. *Res. Vet. Sci.* **41,** 279-80.

Timoney, P. J.; McCollum, W. H.; Murphy, T. W.; Roberts, A. W.; Willard, J. G.; and Carswell, G. D. (1987) The carrier state in equine arteritis virus infection in the stallion with specific emphasis on the venereal mode of virus transmission. *J. Reprod. Fert. Suppl.* **35,** pp. 95-102.

Contagious Equine Metritis: The Pathogenicity for Mares of Small and Large Colonial Variants of *Taylorella equigenitalis* Isolated from a Laboratory Strain

Takumi Kanemaru, Masanobu Kamada, Tohru Anzai, and Takeshi Kumanomido

SUMMARY

An experiment was carried out to clarify the pathogenicity for mares of small and large colonial variants of *Taylorella equigenitalis* that had undergone eight passages in vitro since isolation from a laboratory strain. Two groups of three mares were inoculated intrauterinely with 10^6 colony-forming units of either the large or small colonial variant. Both variants were visible on Eugon chocolate agar within three days after cultivation. All mares exposed to the large colonial variant exhibited typical signs of contagious equine metritis, and large colonies were recovered from both cervical and clitoral swabs taken during the experimental period. Mares exposed to the small colonial variant exhibited no clinical signs of disease during the experimental period; small colonies were isolated from clitoral, but not cervical, swabs. Serological and pathological findings indicated that the pathogenicity of the small colonial variant for mares was much weaker than that of the large colonial variant. The results of the experiment indicate that the colonial variations of *T. equigenitalis* are associated with changes in virulence of the organism.

INTRODUCTION

Contagious equine metritis (CEM), a veneral disease of horses (Crowhurst 1977), is caused by a microaerophilic, Gram-negative, nonfermentative coccobacillus or bacillus classified as *Taylorella equigenitalis* (Sugimoto et al. 1983; International Committee on Systemic Bacteriology 1984). Several colonial variants of *T. equigenitalis* have been described (Sahu & Weber 1982; Sahu, Wool & Breeze 1982; Hitchcock et al. 1985). Alterations in the colonial morphology of bacteria are often indicative of changes in antigenicity and virulence (Cooper, Keller & Walters 1957; Walstad Guyman & Sparling 1977; Swanson 1978; Kellogg et al 1968). There have been few reports on such changes in *T. equigenitalis*.

This paper deals with clinical, hematological, bacteriological, serological, and pathological changes that occurred during an experiment with mares to determine whether colonial variations of *T. equigenitalis* were associated with changes in virulence.

Epizootic Research Station, Equine Research Institute, Japan Racing Association, 1400-4, Shiba, Kokubunji-machi, Shimotsuga-gun, Tochigi 329-04, Japan.

MATERIALS AND METHODS

Isolation history of bacteria and inocula. The To-89 strain (Kamada et al. 1981) of *T. equigenitalis* was isolated from a mare with metritis during the 1980 breeding season in Japan. After the third subculture on Eugon chocolate agar (ECA) in an atmosphere containing 10% CO_2, numerous colonial phenotypes varying in opacity and size were observed. Small (To-89S) and large (To-89L) colonial variants were subcultured eight times to ensure a single colony type. Small colonial variants, tranparent in opacity, were initially isolated at a low frequency and grew more slowly on ECA than other colonial variants, reaching a diameter of 0.7 mm or less at seven days of incubation. During subculture, reversion from small to large colonies occurred on ECA at a low frequency after six days of cultivation (Fig. 1). Large, opaque colonial variants 3 to 5 mm in diameter were isolated at a high frequency at seven days of incubation. When cultivated on EGA, both variants were visible within three days. In biochemical and serological tests, both had almost the same characteristics as the To-89 strain (Kamada et al. 1987). After the eighth subculture, the To-89S and To-89L strains were prepared as experimental inocula by means of cultivation on ECA at 37°C for four days in an atmosphere containing 10% CO_2, suspension in phosphate-buffered saline (PBS; pH 7.0), and dilution to 10^6 colony-forming units per 10 ml.

Experimental inoculation. Six Thoroughbred or pony mares, three to 16 years of age, were experimentally inoculated (Table 1). Their ovulation time was synchronized with progesterone, prostaglandin $F_2\ \alpha$, and human chorionic gonadotropin in the manner described by Holtan, Douglas, and Ginther (1977). At the time of estrus, each mare was inoculated with 10 ml of the large or small colonial variants, introduced directly into the uterus with the aid of a catheter. Group 1 (Mares 1, 2, and 3) received To-89L and Group 2 (Mares 4, 5, and 6) received To-89S. After inoculation, each mare was stabled individually in a loose box.

Clinical and hematological examinations. Rectal temperatures were recorded in the morning and afternoon and

Table 1. Severity of clinical signs in genital tract of experimental mares after inoculation with small and large colonial variants of *Taylorella equigenitalis*

Group	Mare no.	Breed	Age (years)	Colonial phenotype inoculated	Day[a] of necropsy	Clinical signs[c]	Days after inoculation						
							1	2	3	5	7	14	28
1	1	TH[b]	4	Large	7	Exudate	−	+	++	++	++		
						Inflammation	−	+++	+++	++	++		
	2	TH	5	Large	14	Exudate	−	−	++	++	++	+++	
						Inflammation	−	++	++	++	++	++	
	3	TH	3	Large	28	Exudate	−	−	++	++	++	+	−
						Inflammation	−	+	++	++	++	++	+
	4	TH	4	Small	7	Exudate	−	−	−	−	−		
						Inflammation	−	−	−	−	−		
2	5	TH	4	Small	14	Exudate	−	−	−	−	−	−	
						Inflammation	−	−	−	−	−	−	
	6	Pony	16	Small	28	Exudate	−	−	−	−	−	−	−
						Inflammation	−	−	−	−	−	−	−

[a] Days after inoculation.
[b] Thoroughbred
[c] Degree of severity: +++ severe; ++ moderate; + mild; − absent.

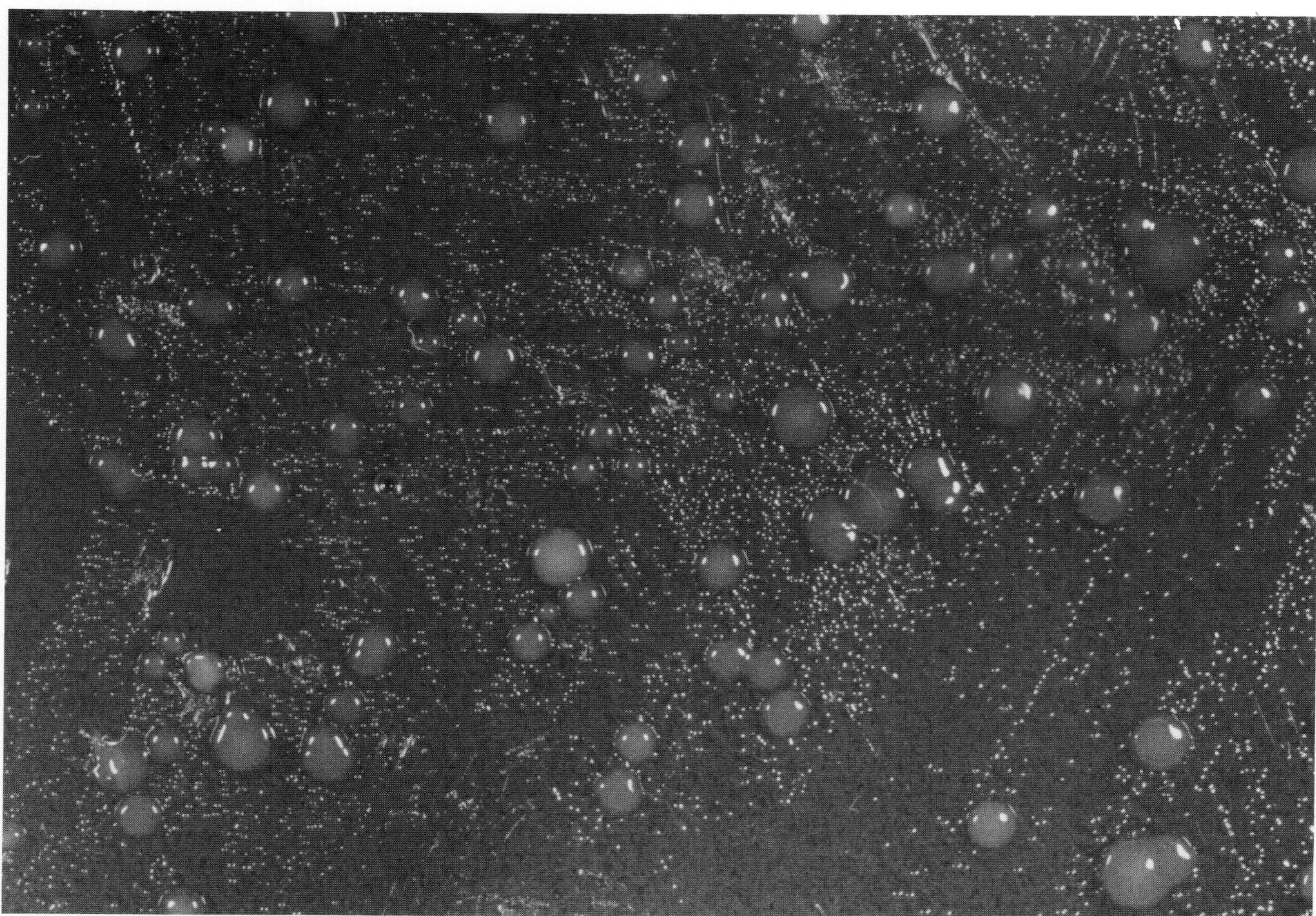

Fig. 1. Reversion from small to large colonial colonial variants of To-89S strain of *T. equigenitalis* on Eugon chocolate agar after eight days of cultivation (low magnification).

clinical signs observed as described previously (Wada et al. 1983). A blood sample was collected from the jugular vein of each mare before inoculation. After inoculation, a blood sample was collected daily for seven consecutive days and then at three- or four-day intervals up to the time of necropsy. Hematological examination included erythrocyte count and total and differential leukocyte counts.

Bacteriological examination. Clitoral and cervical swabs were collected daily for seven days after experimental inoculation and then at two- and three-day intervals. The swabs were immersed immediately in 5 ml of PBS, shaken gently, and then centrifuged at 2,000 rpm for 10 minutes. The resulting sediment was streaked on ECA, blood agar, and MacConkey agar, and incubated under aerobic and microaerophilic conditions. Tissues were also collected from each part of the uterus, cervix, vagina, clitoris, fallopian tube, and ovary at the time of necropsy, and suspended in PBS for bacteriological examination.

Serological examination. Serum samples were obtained at intervals as described for hematological examination. Before the complement fixation (CF) and indirect hemagglutination (IHA) tests were performed, the samples were inactivated at 56°C for 30 min. A four-day culture of the To-89L was used for both tests because of its good growth on ECA and the close antigenic relationship between it and the To-89S strain in the cross-CF and cross-IHA tests (Kamada et al. 1987). Antigen was prepared and tests performed in the manner described by Kamada and colleagues (1983) and Sahu and colleagues (1983). The CF titer was expressed as the reciprocal of the highest serum dilution that had reduced hemolysis to 50% or less. The IHA titer was expressed as the reciprocal of the highest serum dilution that agglutinated sheep erythrocytes to 50% or more.

Pathological examination. The three mares of each group were euthanized at 7-, 14- and 28-day intervals after inoculation. After intravenous injection with 0.2 mg of suxamethonium chloride solution per kilogram of body weight, each mare was exsanguinated by severing the carotid arteries. An examination for gross changes paid special attention to the following genital organs: ovary, oviducts, uterine horns, uterine body, cervix, vagina, vaginal vestibule, clitoris, urinary bladder, and urethra. Tissue samples for histopathological examination were collected from the entire body, including the genital organs, fixed in 10% neutral buffered formalin, and embedded in paraffin. Sections 4 μm thick were prepared and stained with hematoxylin and eosin.

RESULTS

Clinical and hematological findings. During the experimental period, no mares of Group 2 showed clinical or hematological changes. All the mares of Group 1 manifested

Table 2. Bacterial counts of small and large colonial variants of *T. equigenitalis* from genital swabs taken from six experimental mares

Mare		Days after inoculation					
no.	Source	1-2	3	5	7	14	28
1	Cervix	+ + +	+ + +	+ + +	+ + +		
	Clitoris	+ + +	+	−	−		
2	Cervix	+ + +	+ + +	+ + +	+ + +	+ + +	
	Clitoris	+ + +	+	−	−	+ + +	
3	Cervix	+ + +	+ + +	+ + +	+ + +	+ + +	+
	Clitoris	+ + +	+	−	+ + +	+ + +	+ + +
4	Cervix	−	−	−	−		
	Clitoris	+ + +	+	−	−		
5	Cervix	−	−	−	−	−	
	Clitoris	+ + +	+	−	−	+ + +	
6	Cervix	−	−	−	−	−	−
	Clitoris	+ + +	+	−	−	+ + +	−

Bacterial counts (cells/swab): + + + = 100, + + = 11-100, + = 1-10, − = 0; for Nos. 4, 5, and 6, small colonial variants were isolated.

clinical changes characterized by exudation, congestion, and edema of the mucous membrane in the vagina and the external orifice of the cervix (Table 1). Within three days after inoculation, they developed varying amounts of vaginal discharge, congestion, and edema of the external orifice of the cervix and the anterior part of the vagina. The amount of vaginal discharge varied and was usually most abundant three to seven days after inoculation. Each mare of Group 1 exhibited inflammatory changes of the external orifice of the cervix and the anterior part of the vagina persisting up to the time of necropsy.

Bacteriological findings. *T. equigenitalis* was isolated from cervical swabs from all the mares of Group 1, but not from any mare in Group 2 (Table 2). Within two days after inoculation, *T. equigenitalis* was isolated from clitoral swabs taken from all mares in both groups. The large colonial variant was isolated only from the mares in Group 1, while only the small colonial variant was found in the mares of Group 2. No difference between the two groups was observed in number or isolation frequency of *T. equigenitalis*.

The large colonial variant was isolated from the uterus, cervix, vagina, and clitoris, but not the fallopian tube or ovaries, of the mares in Group 1 (Table 3). The small colonial variant was isolated only from the vagina and clitoris of Mare 5 in Group 2, necropsied 14 days after inoculation. No reversion from small to large colonial variants was observed in vivo during the experimental period.

Serological findings. CF and IHA antibody levels increased in every mare of both groups seven days after inoculation (Table 4). Titers tended to be higher in the mares of Group 1 than in those of Group 2. The maximum CF and IHA antibody titers were 1:64 and 1:2048, respectively, in mare No. 3

Table 3. Bacterial counts of small and large colonial variants in genital tract of six experimental mares at necropsy

Mare no.	Fallopian tube and ovary	Uterus	Cervix	Vagina	Clitoris
1	–	+++	+++	+	++
2	–	+++	+++	+++	+++
3	–	+	–	+	+++
4	–	–	–	–	–
5	–	–	–	+	+++
6	–	–	–	–	–

Bacterial counts (cells/g): +++ = >100, ++ = 11-100, + = 1-10, – = 0; for No. 5, small colonial variants were isolated.

of Group 1, and 1:16 and 1:256, respectively, in mare No. 6 of Group 2.

Gross findings. Gross lesions were observed only in the genital tract. The results of macroscopic examination of the genital tract reflected the bacteriological findings (Table 5). Mild edema and congestion were observed in the uterus and cervix of mare No. 4 of Group 2, whereas considerable edema, congestion, and petechial hemorrhage were observed in the genital tract of two mares in Group 1. A white, translucent, odorless viscid exudate was also seen in the genital tract of all the Group 1 mares. The amount of intrauterine exudate was largest in mare No. 1, followed by Nos. 2 and 3. In Mares 1 and 2, the uterine horns showed a relatively severe swelling of the endometrial folds, the membrane of which was pale or yellowish-brown. Cut surfaces of the uterus showed obvious thickening on account of edema. The changes seen in the uterus extended to the cervix and vagina in Mares 1 and 2, but not in No. 3. In all six mares, necropsied 7, 14, or 28 days after inoculation, the ovaries and fallopian tubes were normal.

Histopathological findings. The results of histopathological examination corresponded with those of macroscopic examination (Table 6). Histopathological changes in the genital tract were those of subacute endometritis in every mare of Group 1, and of mild endometritis in each of Group 2, except for No. 6, in which there were no histopathological changes.

The epithelial cells of the uteri of mares in Group 1 showed

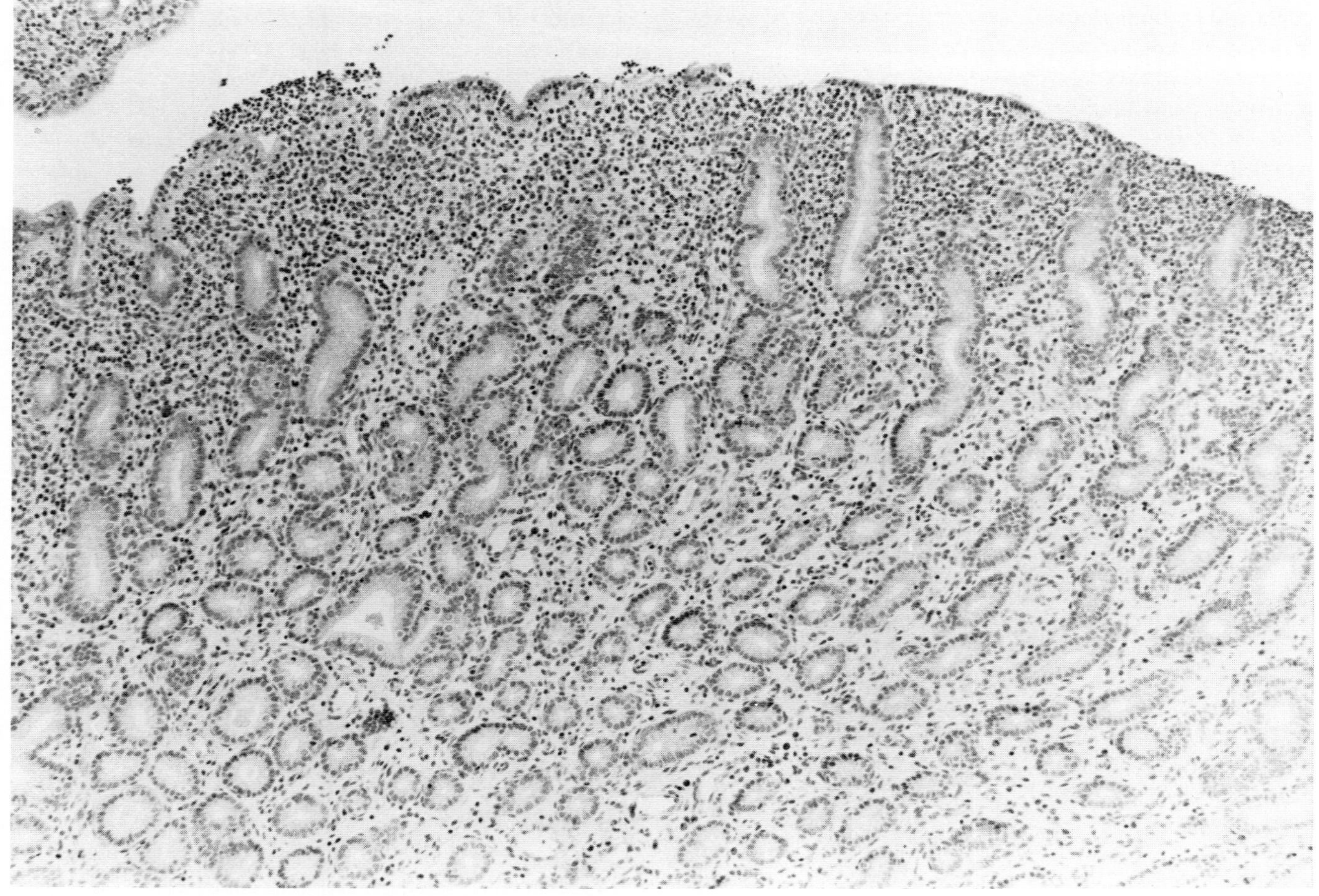

Fig. 2. Uterine body of mare killed seven days after inoculation with the To-89L strain of *T. equigenitalis:* severe diffuse subacute endometritis with degeneration of epithelial cells, epithelial denudation, and hypercellularity of the lamina propria (H&E, mag 136 ×).

Table 4. Development of complement fixing and indirect hemagglutinating antibodies against To-89L strain of *T. equigenitalis* in six experimental mares

Mare no.	Antibody	Days after inoculation 0	5	7	14	21	28
1	CF	<4	<4	4			
	IHA	<16	<16	32			
2	CF	<4	4	4	16		
	IHA	<16	<16	32	1,024		
3	CF	<4	4	4	64	32	32
	IHA	<16	<16	128	2,048	2,048	1,024
4	CF	<4	<4	4			
	IHA	<16	32	64			
5	CF	<4	4	16	8		
	IHA	<16	32	32	64		
6	CF	<4	4	16	8	4	8
	IHA	<16	32	64	128	256	128

CF titer is expressed as reciprocal of highest serum dilution that reduced hemolysis to 50% or less; IHA titer is expressed as reciprocal of highest serum dilution that agglutinated sheep erythrocytes to 50% or over.

degenerative and proliferative changes and were sometimes detached in the lumen. There were numerous polymorphs among epithelial cells, apparently emigrating into the lumen, where an abundant purulent exudate was present. The exudate contained predominantly polymorphs, macrophages, epithelial cells, and a detached portion of the endometrial surface epithelium. The lamina propria contained infiltration of macrophages, lymphocytes, plasma cells, and polymorphs (Fig. 2). Marked edema was seen, with an enlargement of lymphatic vessels and congestion. Two of the mares in Group 2 showed mild degeneration in the epithelial cells of the uterus and infiltration of macrophages, lymphocytes, and plasma cells in the subepithelial and periglandular areas of the lamina propria (Fig. 3).

Table 5. Severity of gross lesions in uterus, cervix, and vagina of six experimental mares

Organ	Mare no.	Amount of exudate in lumen	Inflammation of mucous membrane: Edema	Congestion	Hemorrhage
Uterus	1	+ + +	+ +	+ +	+
	2	+ +	+	+ +	+
	3	+ +	–	–	–
	4	–	±	±	–
	5	–	–	–	–
	6	–	–	–	–
Cervix	1	+ + +	+ +	+ +	+
	2	+ +	+	+	+
	3	+	–	–	–
	4	–	+	±	–
	5	–	–	–	–
	6	–	–	–	–
Vagina	1	+ +	+	+	+
	2	+ +	+	+	+
	3	+	–	+	–
	4	–	–	–	–
	5	–	–	–	–
	6	–	–	–	–

Degree of severity: + + + severe; + + moderate; + mild; ± very mild; – absent.

The cervical and vaginal lumen showed the same changes as the uterine lumen (Table 6). The lamina propria of the cervix was affected with infiltration of lymphocytes, macrophages, plasma cells, polymorphs, and sometimes eosinophils in Mares 1 and 2 (Fig. 4). There was a mild infiltration of lymphocytes, plasma cells, and a very few polymorphs in the mares of Group 2.

Inflammatory cells composed of many lymphocytes, macrophages, and a few neutrophils were noted in the lamina propria of the vagina in all the mares except No. 6. The inflammatory changes were intense in the mares of Group 1 and very mild in Nos. 4 and 5 of Group 2. Lymphocyte stasis of lymphatic vessels was present in the lamina propria of the vagina of mare No. 1 (Fig. 5). Edematous and congestive alterations in the lamina propria of the cervix and vagina were moderate in the mares of Group 1 and very mild in Group 2 except for No. 6. Hemorrhagic foci were present in the uterus, cervix, and vagina in only Nos. 1 and 2. No other parts of the genital tract exhibited any noticeable lesion.

DISCUSSION

Among the studies on colonial variations of *T. equigenitalis* in vitro (Sahu & Weber 1982; Sahu et al. 1982; Hitchcock et al. 1985), there are few reports on changes in its antigenicity or its virulence. The results of clinical, bacteriological, serological, and pathological examinations in this study indicated that the small colonial variant was much weaker in pathogenicity for mares than the large colonial variant. Changes in colonial morphology were closely associated with changes in virulence of *T. equigenitalis*.

Variations of bacteria that in the form of a colony appear either opaque or transparent can be induced by the presence

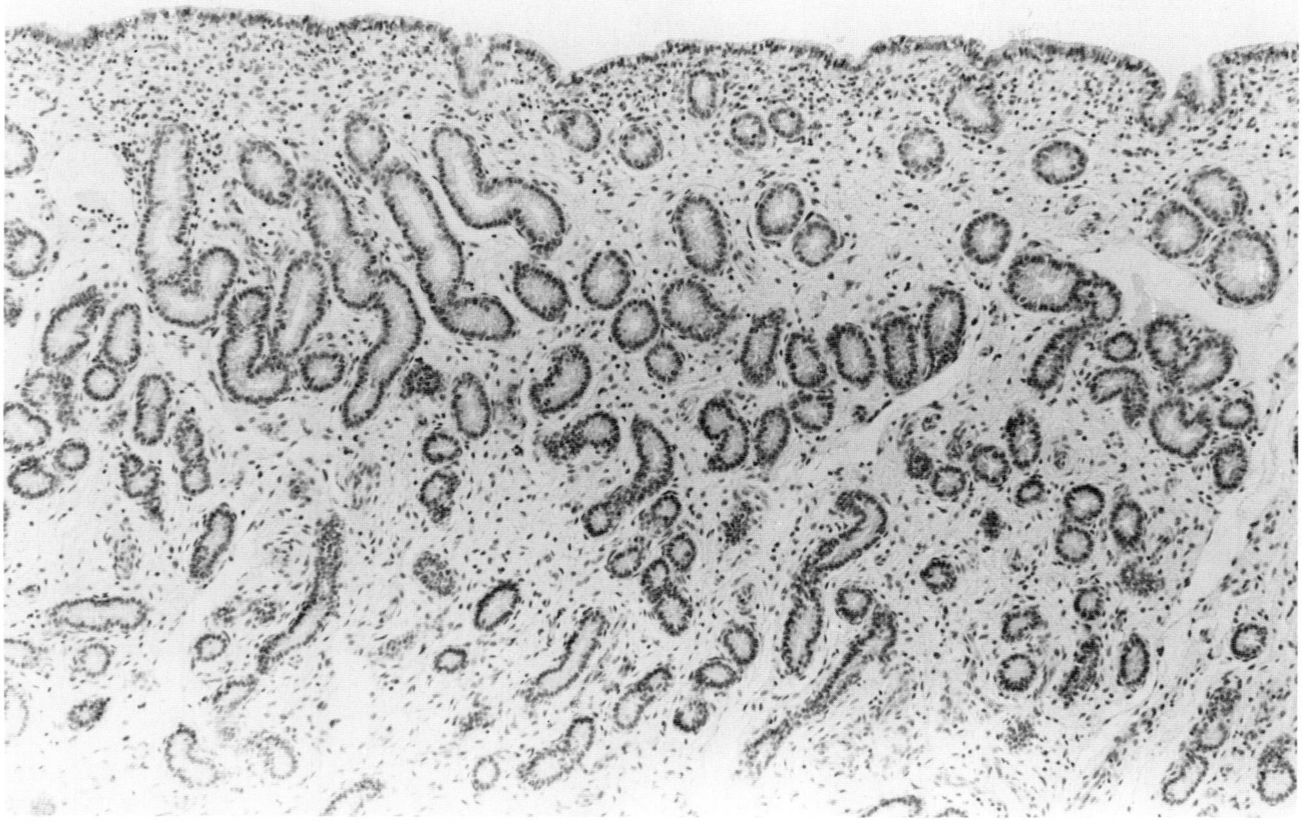

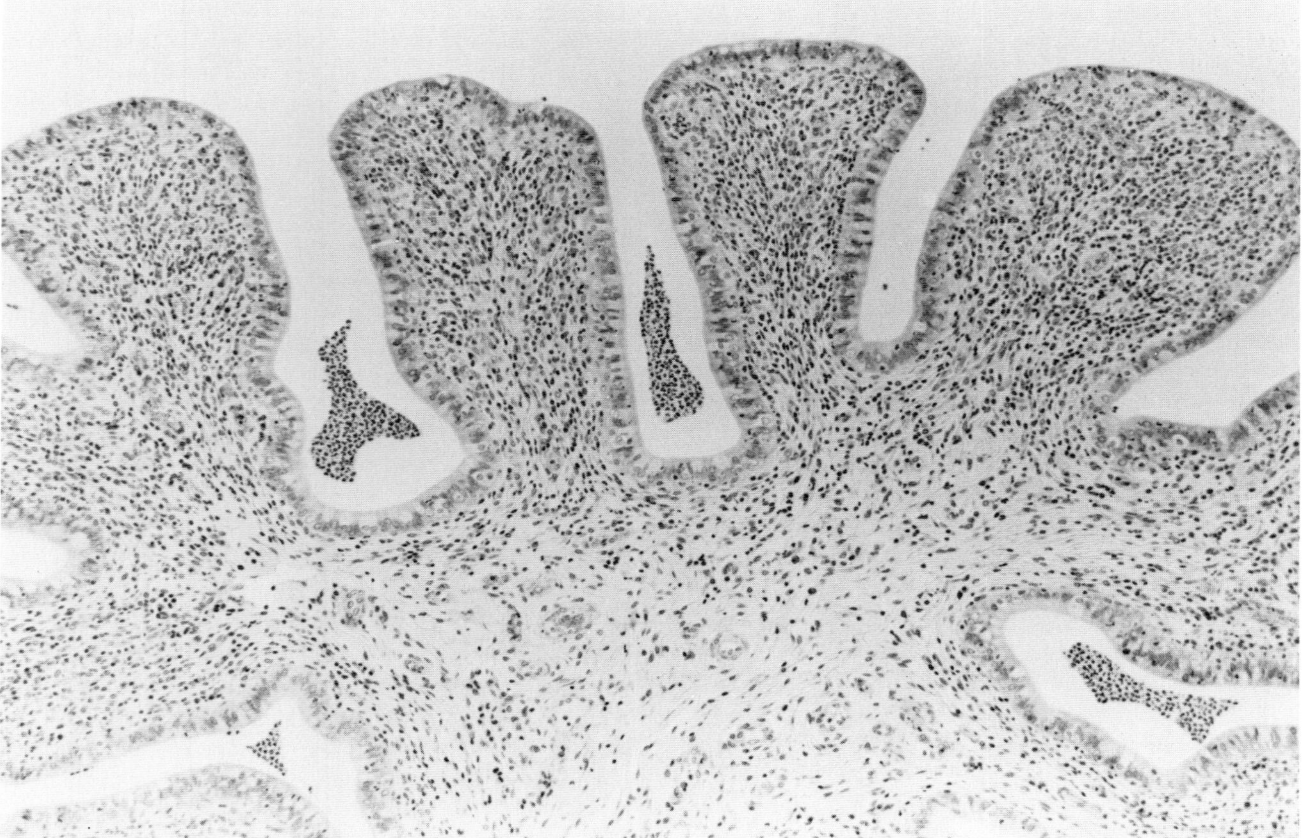

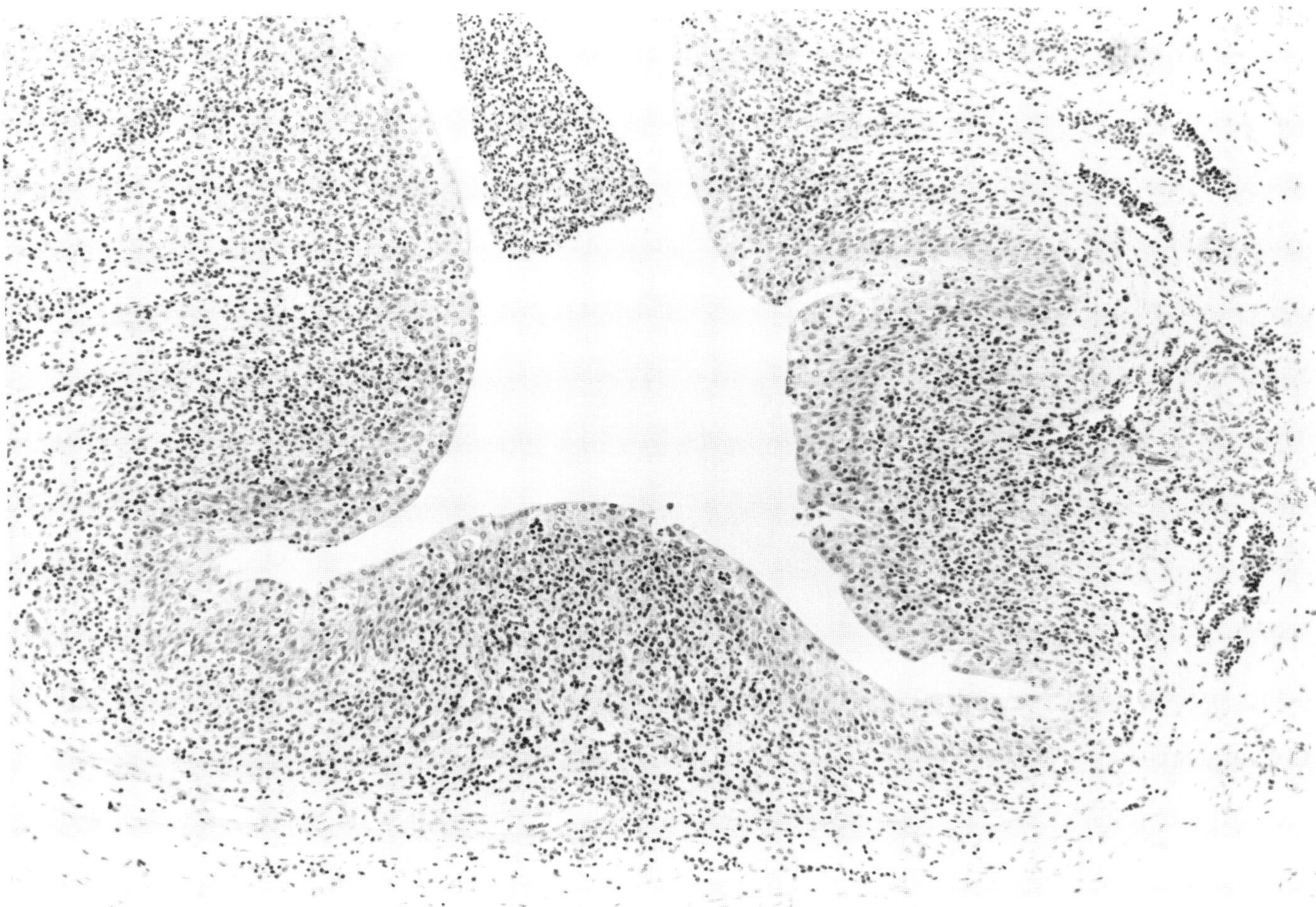

Opposite page, top. Fig. 3. Uterine body of mare killed seven days after inoculation with To-89S strain: very mild subacute endometritis with degeneration of epithelial cells, and mild edema and infiltration of inflammatory cells in the lamina propria (H&E, mag 136 ×). *Bottom.* Fig. 4. Severe subacute cervicitis in mare killed 14 days after inoculation with To-89L strain (H&E, mag 136 ×).

Above. Fig. 5. Severe vaginitis in mare killed seven days after inoculation with To-89L strain: degeneration of squamous epithelium and infiltration of inflammatory cells with lymphocyte stasis in lymphatic vessels (H&E, mag 136 ×).

or absence of a capsule, outer membrane protein, and other surface appendages (Kellogg et al. 1968; Walstad et al. 1977; Swanson 1978; Lambden et al. 1979; Hitchcock et al. 1985). Analysis of colonial variants of *Neisseria gonorrhoeae,* a venereal pathogen in man, revealed that surface constituents, such as pili (Salit, Blake & Gotschlich 1980; Swanson & Barrera 1983) and outer membrane protein (Swanson 1978 and 1982), were correlated with variation in colonial phenotype and virulence. On the other hand, morphological observations of *T. equigenitalis* showed the presence of a fibrillar layer on the outer membrane of various variants, or the presence of intracellular strands in a bleb-forming outer membrane like pili of *N. gonorrheae* (Hitchcock et al. 1985). In this study, no evidence of bacterial shedding from the uterus was observed in three mares intrauterinely inoculated with small colonial variants of *T. equigenitalis*. These variants might be eliminated rapidly from the uterus and cervix, remaining only in the clitoris for an extended time, in contrast to large colonial variants. Small colonial variants are probably closely associated with changes in such adhesive properties of bacteria as pili and outer-membrane proteins.

The small colonial variants used in the present experiment were transparent on ECA and clear typing medium when observed by stereomicroscope. Large colonial variants developed spontaneously in vitro at a low frequency during subculture. During the experimental period, no large colonial variants were isolated from genital swabs taken from any mare inoculated with the small colonial variants. It is possible that small colonial variants give rise to large colonial variants in vivo, as occurs under in vitro conditions.

Observation of the colonial morphology of *T. equigenitalis* grown in ECA revealed small colonial variants in 15 of 33 primary isolations from mares with CEM (unpublished data). To date, pure isolates of small colonial variants have been obtained directly from three cases in the field. When isolates showing transparent phenotypes were subcultured on

Table 6. Histopathological findings in uterus, cervix, and vagina of six experimental mares

Organ	Mare no.	Degeneration of epithelium	Lamina propria			
			Inflammatory cells	Edema	Congestion	Hemorrhage
Uterus	1	++	+++	++	++	+
	2	++	+++	++	++	+
	3	+	++	++	−	−
	4	+	±	+	±	−
	5	±	±	+	±	−
	6	−	−	−	−	−
Cervix	1	++	+++	++	+	+
	2	+	++	+	+	+
	3	+	++	+	+	−
	4	−	±	+	±	−
	5	−	±	±	±	−
	6	−	−	−	−	−
Vagina	1	++	++	++	+	+
	2	++	+++	++	+	+
	3	+	++	++	+	−
	4	±	±	±	±	−
	5	−	±	+	±	−
	6	−	−	−	−	−

Degree of severity: +++ severe; ++ moderate; + mild; ± very mild; − absent.

ECA, large colonial variants grew within eight days. These results indicate that colonial variations of *T. equigenitalis* exhibiting changes in virulence occur in vitro and in vivo and that they have been found among mares in the field. Since CEM was first diagnosed in Japan during the 1980 breeding season, it has been difficult to detect carrier mares because an increasing number of naturally infected mares either present only mild clinical signs of the disease or lack signs entirely. Changes in virulence of colonial variations might have been responsible for the gradual decrease in number of naturally infected horses showing typical clinical signs of CEM in the field.

Success in the control or eradication of CEM in Japan and other countries depends upon the development of a diagnostic method to detect the carrier mare. Usually, the disease is finally diagnosed by isolation of the etiological agent from the genital tract of mares and stallions. In morphology, the small colonial variants have no distinguishing characteristics except that they are transparent and small. It is very difficult to differentiate them from other bacteria showing almost the same colonial appearance at the time of primary isolation. In addition, the presence of slow-growing strains of *T. equigenitalis,* as described in previous reports (Ward et al. 1984; Kamada et al. 1986), makes bacterial differentiation rather difficult. Serological tests, including CF, IHA, and enzyme-linked immunosorbent assay, may be useful for diagnosis of the disease, especially since CF and IHA antibodies were detected in all the mares inoculated, including those with the small colonial variants.

REFERENCES

Cooper, M.L: Keller, H.M.; and Watlers, E.W. (1957) Microscopic characteristics of colonies of *Shigella flexneria* 2a and 2b and their antigenic composition, mouse virulence and immunogenicity. *J. Immunol.* **78,** 160-71.

Crowhurst, R.C. (1977) Genital infection in mares. *Vet. Rec.* **100,** 476.

Hitchcock, P.J.; Brown, T.M.; Corwin, D.; Hayes, S.F.; Olszewski, A.; and Todd, W. (1985) Morphology of three strains of contagious equine metritis organism. *Infect. Immun.* **48,** 94-108.

Holtan, D.W.; Douglas, R.H.; and Ginther, O.J. (1977) Estrus, ovulation and conception following synchronization with progesterone, prostaglandin F_2 and human chorionic gonadotropin in pony mares. *J. Anim. Sci.* **44,** 431-37.

International Committee on Systematic Bacteriology (1984) Validation of the publication of new names and new combinations previously effectively published outside the IJSB. *Int. J. Syst. Bacteriol.* **34,** 503-4.

Kamada, M.; Akiyama, Y.; Oda, T.; and Fukazawa, Y. (1981) Contagious equine metritis: Isolation of Haemophilus equigenitalis from horses with endometritis in Japan. *Jpn. J. Vet. Sci.* **43,** 565-68.

Kamada, M.; Ola, T.; Fukuzawa, Y.; Ohishi, H.; Wada, R.; Fukunaga, Y.; and Kumanomido, T. (1983) Contagious equine metritis: A survey on complement fixing antibody against *Haemophilus equigenitalis* in light horses in Japan. *Bull. Equine Res. Inst.* **20,** 119-25.

Kamada, M.; Kumanomido, T.; Anzai, T.; Kanemaru, T.; Senba, H.; and Ohishi, H. (1986) Isolation and drug sensitivity of streptomycin sensitive *Taylorella equigenitalis* from mares with metritis and infertility in Japan. *Bull. Equine Res. Inst.* **23,** 55-61.

Kamada, M.; Anzai, T.; Kanemaru, T.; Wada, R.; and Kumanomido, T. (1987) Contagious equine metritis: Characterization of small and large colonial variants of Taylorella equigenitalis isolated from a laboratory strain. *Bull. Equine Res. Inst.* **24,** 23-32.

Kellogg, E.S.; Cohen, I.R.; Norins, L.C.; Schroeter, A.L.; and Reising, G. (1968) *Neisseria gonorrheae*. II. Colonial variation and pathogenicity during 35 months *in vitro*. *J. Bacteriol.* **96,** 596-605.

Lambden, P.R.; Heckels, J.E.; James, L.T.; and Watt, P.J. (1979) Variation in surface protein composition associated with virulence properties in opacity types of *Neisseria gonorrhoeae*. *J. Gen. Microbiol.* **114,** 305-12.

Sahu, S.P., and Weber, S. (1982) Contagious equine metritis: Effect of intrauterine inoculation of tiny colony forms in pony mares. *Vet. Rec.* **110,** 250-51.

Sahu, S.P.; Wool, S.; and Breese, S.S. (1982) Observation on the morphology of contagious equine metritis bacterial colonies isolated from infected pony mares. *Am. J. Vet. Res.* **43,** 786-800.

Sahu, S.P.; Rommel, F.A.; Fales, W.H.; Hamdy, F.M.; Swerczek, T.W.; Youngquist, R.S.; and Bryans, J.T. (1983) Evaluation of various serotests to detect antibodies in ponies and horses infected with contagious equine metritis bacteria. *Am. J. Vet. Res.* **44,** 1405-9.

Salit, I.E.; Blake, M.; and Gotschlich, E.C. (1980) Intra-strain heterogeneity of gonococcal pili is related to opacity colony variance. *J. Exp. Med.* **151,** 716-25.

Sugimoto, C.; Isayama, Y.; Sakazaki, R.; and Kuramochi, S. (1983) Transfer of *Haemophilus equigenitalis* Taylor et al. 1978 to the genus *Taylorella* gen. nov. as *Taylorella equigenitalis* com. nov. *Current Microbiol.* **9,** 155-62.

Swanson, J. (1978) Studies on gonococcus infection. XIV. Cell wall protein differences among color/opacity colony variants of *Neisseria gonorrhoeae*. *Infect. Immun.* **21,** 292-302.

———. (1982) Colony opacity and protein II compositions of gonococci. *Infect. Immun.* **37,** 359-68.

Swanson, J., and Barrera, O. (1983) Gonococcal pilus subunit size heterogeneity correlates with transitions in colony piliation phenotype, not with changes in colony opacity. *J. Exp. Med.* **134,** 886-906.

Wada, R.; Kamada, M.; Fukunaga, Y.; and Kumanomido, T. (1983) Studies on contagious equine metritis. IV. Pathology in horses experimentally infected with *Haemophilus equigenitalis*. *Bull. Equine Res. Inst.* **20,** 133-43.

Walstad, D.L.; Guyman, L.F.; and Sparling, P.F. (1977) Altered outer membrane protein in different colonial types of *Neisseria gonorrheae*. *J. Bacteriol.* **129,** 1623-27.

Ward, J.; Hourigan, M.; McGuirk, J.; and Gogarty, A. (1984) Incubation times for primary isolation of the contagious equine metritis organism. *Vet. Rec.* **114,** 298.

Isolation and Characterization of the Outer Membrane of *Taylorella equigenitalis*

Chihiro Sugimoto, Masashi Eguchi, Makoto Haritani, Yasuro Isayama, and Mamoru Kashiwazaki

SUMMARY

The outer membrane of *Taylorella equigenitalis*, the causative organism of contagious equine metritis, was purified by Triton X-100 treatment followed by lysozyme and nucleases treatments. The outer membrane consisted of several major proteins that had molecular weights of 50, 48, 41, 33, 27, and 15 kilodalton (kdal), respectively. Lipopolysaccharide (LPS) and non-LPS antigens of the outer membrane were identified by crossed immunoelectrophoresis using rabbit and horse antisera. By immunoblotting of the outer membrane proteins, antibodies to the 41-kdal protein were demonstrated in sera of mares experimentally infected with *T. equigenitalis*.

INTRODUCTION

The outer membrane (OM) of Gram-negative bacteria constitutes a physical and functional barrier, and a major function of the outer-membrane proteins (OMPs) is uptake of hydrophilic solutes (Brass 1986). OMPs are reported to play a role in bacterial virulence as well; for example, the plasmid-encoded OMP of *Escherichia coli* increases serum resistance (Moll, Manning & Timms 1980), and the expression of iron-repressive OMPs affects bacterial growth in vivo where the amount of iron ion accessible by the bacteria is restricted (Crosa 1984). As hosts infected with Gram-negative bacteria produce antibodies against certain OMPs (Black et al. 1986), OMPs are thought to be possible candidates for vaccine development (Bolin & Jensen 1987; Udhayakumar & Muthakkaruppan 1987). Electrophoresis profiles of OMPs are also useful as epidemiologic and virulence markers (Loeb & Smith 1980).

The outer-membrane proteins of *T. equigenitalis*, the causative organism of contagious equine metritis (CEM) (Taylor et al. 1978) have not previously been studied. The aim of this study was to purify the OM of this organism and analyze it biochemically and immunologically.

MATERIALS AND METHODS

Purification of OM and lipopolysaccharide. The streptomycin-resistant EQ-51 strain of *T. equigenitalis*, isolated in Japan by Sugimoto and colleagues (1980), was cultured on Eugon agar containing 10% heated horse blood in 10% CO_2 for 72 hr. This strain was used throughout these experiments unless otherwise stated. The outer membrane was purified according to the method of Lam and colleagues (1980). Bacterial cells were treated with Tris-hydrochloride buffer (pH 7.0) containing 8 mM $MgSO_4$, 1% (v/v) Triton X-100, and 20% (v/v) sucrose at 4°C overnight. The detergent-insoluble materials were collected by centrifugation at $40,000 \times g$ for 10 min and treated with this solution at room temperature for 1 hr, then with 8 mM $MgSO_4$. The pellet was treated with lysozyme (0.3 mg/ml) for 3 hr at room temperature, then with dioxyribonuclease I (100 μg/ml) and ribonuclease I (100 μg/ml) at 4°C overnight to obtain pure OM. The purified OM was washed twice in distilled water and either utilized immediately for electron microscope examination or frozen at −80°C for other studies. Lipopolysaccharides were extracted from whole cells by phenol as described by Sutherland (1978).

Biochemical assays. Protein concentrations were measured using Folin phenol reagent. Succinate dehydrogenase as a marker of cytoplasmic (inner) membranes was assayed by the method described by Green and Narahara (1980). Sodium dodecyl sulfate-polyacrylamide gel electrophoresis (SDS-PAGE) was done using 11% separating and 3% stacking acrylamide gels (Neville & Glossmann, 1974).

Transmission electron microscopy. The outer membrane was fixed, embedded, and thin-sectioned as described by Lam and colleagues (1980).

Crossed immunoelectrophoresis. Antigens of OM were extracted by 2% SDS solution in phosphate-buffered saline (PBS), and electrophoresed in 1% (w/v) agarose gel in veronal buffer (pH 8.6, ionic strength 0.05) (Ouchterlony & Nilsson 1987) containing 1% (v/v) Triton X-100. After the first electrophoresis, the gel strip containing the antigens was transferred into the second-dimensional gel containing rabbit or horse *T. equigenitalis* antiserum, and electrophoresed at right angles to the first dimension. The gel was washed with PBS and stained with amido black 10 B. The rabbit antiserum was raised by four i.v. inoculations of whole bacterial cells at intervals of one week, and collected one week after final

National Institute of Animal Health, Yatabe Tsukuba, Ibaraki 30S, Japan.

Table 1. Succinate dehydrogenase activity of various membrane fractions

Sample	SDH activity (*N* mol./min. µ g protein
Total membrane[a]	8.3
Triton X-100	0.5
Triton X-100 + lysozyme + nucleases	0.0

[a] Total membrane fraction was obtained from bacterial cells by sonic disruption and ultracentrifugation at 100,000 g for 60 min.

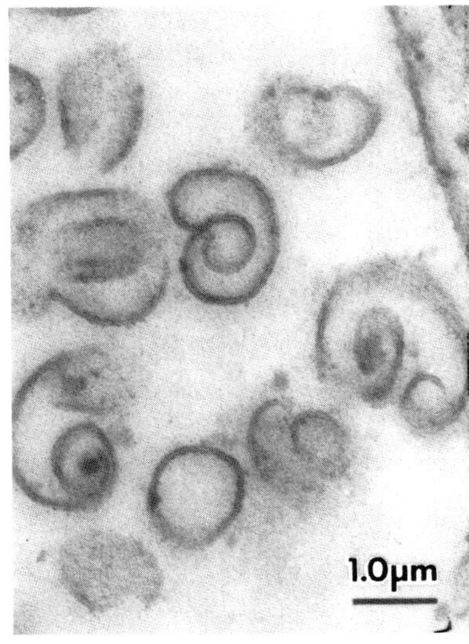

Fig. 1. An electron micrograph of the purified outer membrane of EQ-51 strain of *I. equigenitalis*.

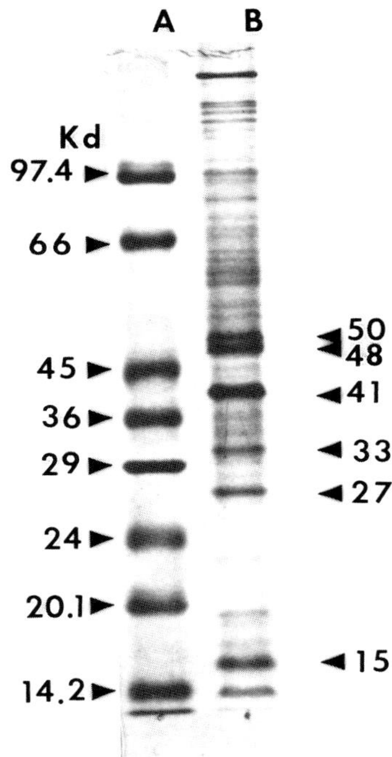

Fig. 2. The outer-membrane protein, profile of EQ-51 is SDS-PAGE. Molecular weights of standard proteins (*Lane A*) and major OMPs (*Lane B*) are indicated.

inoculation. Horse antiserum was collected from a mare experimentally infected with *T. equigenitalis* after three weeks of bacterial inoculation.

Immunoblotting. Proteins separated by SDS-PAGE were electrophoretically transferred to a nitrocellulose sheet (pore size 0.45 µm; Schleicher & Schuell, Keene, N.H.) in 25-mM Tris-192 glycine buffer (pH 9.3) containing 20% methanol at 80 mA for 150 min (Graves et al. 1986; Towbin, Staehelin & Gordon 1979). The sheet was cut into strips, which were incubated in PBS containing 1% Tween 20 for 2hr at 37°C to block nonspecific protein binding. The strips were then incubated in horse serum diluted 1:50 in PBS containing 0.05% Tween 20 (PBS-Tween). Three paired horse sera used for immunoblotting were collected from mares before infection and again about three weeks after bacterial inoculation. After four 10-min washings with PBS-Tween, the strips were incubated for 2 hr at room temperature in peroxidase-conjugated goat antihorse IgG serum (Cooper Biochemical Inc.) diluted 1:1000 in PBS-Tween. Following five 10-min washings, bands were made visible by reacting with 0.025% (w/v) diaminobenzidine and 0.06% (v/v) hydrogen peroxide in 50 mM Tris-hydrochloride buffer (pH 7.5) for 10 min. The reactions were stopped by washing the strips with water. Total OMP bands and molecular weight standard protein bands transferred to the sheet were stained with Aurodye (Janssen Life Science Products, Belgium).

RESULTS

Purification of the OM. Succinate dehydrogenase activity was detected in the membrane fraction after two Triton X-100 treatments (Table 1), and contamination of the inner membrane (IM) in this fraction was also confirmed by electron microscopy (data not shown). The subsequent lysozyme and nuclease treatments of this detergent-insoluble membrane fraction successfully removed succinate dehydrogenase activity. Cytoplasma, capsular materials, and IM were not detected, and the OM retained its single membrane structure, in the form of small broken fragments (Fig. 1).

The OM consisted of a limited number of major proteins of the molecular weights 50, 48, 41, 33, 27, and 15 kdal (Fig. 2), as well as several minor proteins. There was no quantitative or qualitative difference among OMP profiles of three *T. equigenitalis* isolates: EQ-51, Kentucky 188, and NCTC 11184, which were isolated in Japan, the United States, and England, respectively.

Crossed immuno-electrophoresis. Seven peaks were distinguishable when SDS-extract of the OM was reacted with rabbit antiserum in crossed immunoelectrophoresis. Absorption of this serum with LPS eliminated one major peak and one minor peak. Three peaks were observed after the SDS-extract reacted with horse serum, two of which corresponded to the two LPS peaks with rabbit serum. The absorption of horse serum with LPS left one major peak. Phenol-extracted LPS from whole cells formed the same peaks with rabbit and horse sera as those formed when the SDS-extract reacted with sera (data not shown). Preimmune rabbit serum and preinfection horse serum did not react with the SDS-extract of the OM in crossed immunoelectrophoresis.

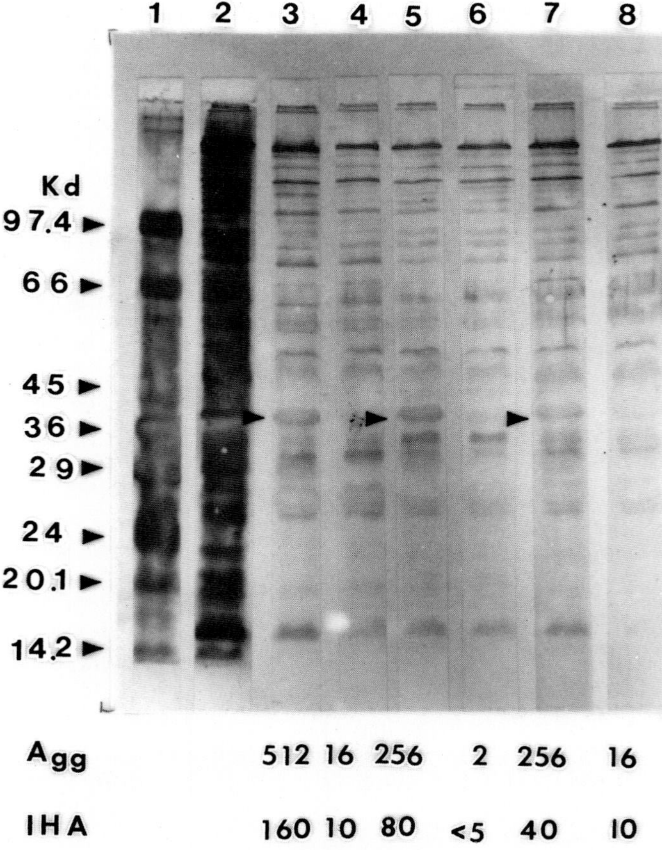

Fig. 3. Immunoblotting of outer-membrane proteins of EQ-51. Molecular weight marker proteins (*Lane 1*) and total OMPs (*Lane 2*) were stained with Aurodye. Three pairs of pre- and post-infection horse sera (*Lanes 3 and 4, 5 and 6, 7 and 8*) were tested. IHA and Agg titers are indicated below lanes; positive reactions with 41-kdal OMP are indicated by arrowhead.

Immunoblotting. Three pairs of sera from Thoroughbred mares experimentally infected by intrauterine inoculation of *T. equigenitalis* were collected before inoculation and three weeks afterward, for testing by immunoblotting. Although nonspecific binding of peroxidase-conjugated secondary antiserum to OMPs was not observed, all three paired sera reacted with a number of OMPs of molecular weights ranging from >200 to 29 kdal, regardless of bacterial inoculation (Fig. 3). The preinfection sera showed positive reactions at lower serum dilutions in the agglutination test (Agg) and indirect hemagglutination test (IHA). On the other hand, antibodies to one of the major OMPs, 41-kdal protein, were detected only in postinfection sera, where they were found in all cases.

DISCUSSION

One of the methods to purify the OM of Gram-negative bacteria is sucrose density gradient centrifugation after treating cells with EDTA/lysozyme and then lysing the spheroplasts by osmotic shock of sonic disruption. This method and its modifications have been applied to purify OM from a wide variety of Gram-negative bacteria (Owen et al. 1982). However, our attempt to isolate OM from *T. equigenitalis* by these methods was unsuccessful because of poor transformation to spheroplasts and poor separations of OM and IM in sucrose gradient.

Another technique to obtain OM is selective solubilization of IM by solutions of Triton X-100/Mg^{2+} or sodium lauryl sarcosinate (Owen et al 1982). The outer membrane of *T. equigenitalis* free of IM and cytoplasmic materials was obtained from materials insoluble in Triton X-100/Mg^{2+} only when the insoluble materials were subsequently treated with lysozyme and nucleases. This purification method has the distinct advantages of simplicity and high yield of ultrastructurally intact OM.

Mares naturally or experimentally infected with *T. equigenitalis* are reported to raise serum antibodies to this organism, measured by Agg, IHA, a complement fixation test, and enzyme-linked immunosorbent assay (ELISA) (Sahu et al. 1983). These serological tests are used as aids in CEM diagnosis. However, the precise nature of bacterial antigens involved in these immune reactions has not been clarified. When antigens obtained from whole cells by sonication were analyzed by immunoelectrophoresis (Corbel & Brewer 1982), the rabbit immune serum recognized 11 antigens of protein nature, one lipopolysaccharide-protein complex antigen, and one polysaccharide antigen. The latter two antigens, which seemed to be exposed on the cell surface, were also recognized by sera of CEM-infected mares. It is likely that these two antigens correspond to some of the antigens detected by us. Our results in crossed immunoelectrophoresis indicate that a major OM antigen recognized by CEM-infected mares is LPS and that a non-LPS component is also immunogenic. The results obtained by immunoblotting revealed that the 41-kdal OMP is an antigen specifically recognized by CEM-infected mares.

In ELISA and passive hemagglutination tests of horse sera, false positive results are occasionally observed (Sahu et al. 1983), and sera from humans and bovines show occasionally positive agglutination reaction to *T. equigenitalis*, even though this organism has never been isolated from the latter two species (Brewer 1983). These reactions are presumed to be due to cross-reactive antibodies to unknown bacterial or nonbacterial antigens. Various Gram-negative species such as *Haemophilus influenzae* and *Acinetobactor calcoacetics* are known to serologically cross-react with *T. equigenitalis* (Taylor et al. 1978), but antigenic components causing these cross-reactions are not specified. Purification of the 41-kdal OMP and further immunological studies on this protein may help to develop more effective, specific, sensitive serological tests for CEM.

At present, the only way of effectively diagnosing CEM is isolation of the causative organism. This organism, however, grows relatively slowly and is often masked by fast-growing bacteria, particularly in the culture from more contaminated sites such as the clitoral sinuses of mares. For effective diagnosis, sensitive and specific methods are needed for early detection of *T. equigenitalis* antigen without cultivation.

It was not expected that positive reactions to various OMPs in immunoblotting would be demonstrated even in sera from mares bacteriologically negative for CEM. These reactions may be partially due to nonspecific binding of equine immunoglobulins to the surface of this organism (Widders et al. 1985). Characterization of the nonspecific immunoglobulin receptor(s) of this organism will lay the groundwork for more specific serological tests for CEM.

REFERENCES

Black, J.R.; Dyer, D.W.; Thompson, M.K.; and Sparling, P.F. (1986) Human immune response to iron repressive outer membrane proteins of *Neisseria meningitidis*. *Infect. Immun.* **54,** 710-13.

Bolin, C.A., and Jensen, A.E. (1987). Passive immunization with antibodies against iron-regulated outer membrane proteins protects turkeys from *Escherichia coli* septicemia. *Infect. Immun.* **55,** 1239-42.

Brass, J.M. (1986) The cell envelope of Gram-negative bacteria: New aspects of its function in transport and chemotoxis. *Curr. Top. Microbiol. Immunol.* **129,** 1-92.

Brewer, R.A. (1983) Contagious equine metritis. *Vet. Bull., Weybridge* **53,** 881-91.

Corbel, M.J., and Brewer, R.A. (1982) Characterization of the major antigens of *Haemophilus equigenitalis* (contagious equine metritis organism). *J. Hyg., Camb.* **89,** 529-38.

Crosa, J.H. (1984) The relationship of plasmid-mediated iron transport and bacterial virulence. *Ann. Rev. Microbiol.* **38,** 69-89.

Graves, D.C.; McNabb, S.J.N.; Worley, M.A.; Downs, T.D.; and Ivey, M.H. (1986) Analysis of rat *Pneumocystis carinii* antigens recognized by human and rat antibodies by using western immunoblotting. *Infect. Immun.* **54,** 96-103.

Green, J.D., and Narahara, H. T. (1980) Assay of succinate dehydrogenase activity by the tetrazolium method: Evaluation of an improved technique in skeletal muscle fractions. *J. Histochem. Cytochem.* **28,** 408-12.

Lam, J.S.; Grannoff, D.M.; Gilsdorf, J.R.; and Costerton, J.W. (1980) Immunogenicity of outer membrane derivatives of *Haemophilus influenzae* type b. *Curr. Microbiol.* **3**, 359-64.

Loeb, M.R., and Smith, D.H. (1980) Outer membrane protein composition in disease isolates of *Haemophilus influenzae:* Pathogenic and epidemiological implications. *Infect. Immun.* **30,** 709-17.

Moll, A.; Manning, P.A.; and Timms, K.N. (1980) Plasmid determined resistance to serum bacteriocidal activity: A major outer membrane protein, the *tra* T gene product, is responsible for plasmid specified serum resistance in *Escherichia coli*. *Infect. Immun.* **28,** 359-67.

Neville, D.M., Jr., and Glossman, H. (1974) Molecular weight determination of membrane protein and glycoprotein subunits by discontinuous gel electrophoresis in dodecyl sulfate. In *Methods in Enzymology,* Vol. 32, pp. 92-102. Eds. S.K. Fleisher and L. Packer. Academic Press, New York.

Ouchterlony, Ö, and Nilsson, L.A. (1978) Immunodiffusion and immunoelectrophoresis. In *Handbook of Experimental Immunology*, 3d ed., pp. 19.1-19.44, Ed. D.M. Weir, Blackwell Scientific, Oxford.

Leptospirosis in Horses

William A. Ellis and John J. O'Brien

SUMMARY

In this study carried out in Northern Ireland, the prevalence of *Leptospira* infection in aborted equine fetuses (24 out of 50 positive) and fatal jaundice cases (seven out of nine positive) was assessed by culture and immunofluorescence.

The strains that were isolated belong to six serogroups of *Leptospira interrogans:* the Australis, Ballum, Canicola, Icterohaemorrhagiae, Pomona, and Sejroe serogroups.

INTRODUCTION

Knowledge of the epidemiology and clinical importance of equine leptospirosis has been severely curtailed by the difficulties of demonstrating infection either by culturing these very fastidious organisms or by demonstrating their presence in equine tissues by immunochemical methods. As a result, undue reliance is placed on the use of serology as a means of diagnosis.

Serological surveys have indicated that exposure of horses to infection by parasitic leptospires is widespread throughout the world. The predominant serogroup has varied with the country surveyed and the leptospiral antigens used in the survey. In Ireland, antibodies to the serogroups Australis (serovar *bratislava*), Icterohaemorrhagiae, Pyrogens, Sejroe (serovar *hardjo*), Ballum, Canicola, and Autumnalis have been detected in horse sera (Ellis et al. 1983a; Egan & Yearsley 1986). Strains belonging to four of these groups (Australis, Icterhaemorrhagiae, Sejroe, and Autumnalis) plus strains of the Pomona group have been recovered from horses there (Ellis et al. 1983a,b).

The reported clinical features of acute leptospirosis in horses include pyrexia, depression, anorexia, and jaundice, while chronic infection is characterized by abortion, premature foaling, and periodic ophthalmia (Morter et al. 1969; Williams et al. 1971). However, despite the widespread serological evidence of horses being exposed to *Leptospira* infection, the paucity of published reports would indicate that clinical cases of leptospirosis are rarely seen in horses. This is certainly the case in the British Isles, where reports on the role of leptospiral infections in the etiology of clinical disease have been limited to: the observation of a high prevalence of leptospiral antibodies in horses with liver disfunction and jaundice (Twigg, Hughes & McDiarmid 1971; Hathaway et al. 1981); limited serological evidence of an association with uveitis (Hathaway et al. 1981; Matthews, Waitkins & Palmer 1987); and the occasional isolation of leptospires from aborted fetuses (Ellis, Bryson & McFerran 1976; Ellis et al. 1983b).

The purpose of the present study was to assess the prevalence of leptospiral infection in aborted equine fetuses and in horses with gross evidence of jaundice at autopsy.

MATERIALS AND METHODS

Animals. Two groups of animals were examined in this study: fifty aborted or stillborn fetuses from Thoroughbred or hunter-type mares submitted to this laboratory between January 1979 and April 1987; six dead neonates and three adult horses that showed gross evidence of jaundice on postmortem examination.

Both groups were examined by culture, serology, and immunofluorescence for evidence of leptospiral infection, by culture for other bacteria and viruses, and by histological methods.

Serological investigation. Blood samples were collected from both groups where possible. Serum was obtained and stored at −20°C until tested. The sera were tested for leptospiral antibodies by the microscopic agglutination test (Wolff, 1954) using live antigens grown in liquid medium (Johnson & Harris 1967). Antigens representing the following *Leptospira* serogroups were used (where the serovar used was not the one that gives its name to the serogroup, its name is indicated in parentheses): Australis (*bratislava*), Autumnalis, Ballum, Bataviae, Canicola, Celledoni (*whitcombi*), Cynopteri, Grippetyphosa, Sejroe (*harjo*), Icterohaemorrhagia (*copenhageni*), Javanica, Panama, Pomona, Pyrogenes, Shermani, and Tarassovi. The test was interpreted as described by Ellis and colleagues (1978).

Leptospire isolation technique. Fetal eye, kidney, and occasionally lung from 32 fetuses were cultured as described by Ellis and colleagues (1983b). Liver, lung, and kidney from the nine jaundiced horses and foals were cultured as described by Ellis and others (1986). All cultures were incubated, examined, and manipulated as described by Ellis and others (1983b).

Antisera to the leptospires isolated were prepared in rabbits and the organisms identified to serogroup level by cross-agglutination reactions as recommended by Dikken and

Veterinary Research Laboratories, Stoney Road, Stormont, Belfast BT4 3SD, Northern Ireland.

Table 1. Isolation of leptospires from aborted fetuses

Serogroup	Number of isolates	Serovar
Icterohaemorrhagiae	2	Not determined
Australis	6	*bratislava* (5); *muenchen* (1)
Pomona	2	*pomona*
Canicola	3	*canicola*
Sejroe	1	*hardjo*
Mixed Australis-Canicola culture	1	*bratislava; canicola*

Kmety (1978). The isolates were identified to serovar level where possible by restriction endonuclease analysis.

Immunofluorescence studies. Tissue homogenate smears and cryostat sections of liver, lung, and kidney, as well as cryostat sections of fetal brain and adrenal, were examined for the presence of leptospiral antigen by a double staining immunofluorescence (FA) technique using a pooled serovar *hardjo-copenhageni-bratislava* antiserum as described by Ellis and colleagues (1983b). A positive diagnosis was made only where fluorescing organisms with typical leptospiral morphology were observed in tissues.

Other microbiological examinations. Isolation of other bacteria and viruses was attempted from brain, liver, lung, kidney, stomach contents (fetuses only), and thoracic fluid as described previously (Neill et al. 1978; Ellis et al. 1983b).

Histopathological examination. Liver, kidney, lung, and brain, and in the case of fetuses thymus and placenta, were collected for histopathological examination. They were fixed in 10% buffered formalin and embedded in paraffin, sectioned, and stained with hematoxylin and eosin.

RESULTS

Fetuses. Leptospiral infection was demonstrated in 24 aborted fetuses by FA (21/48) and/or culture (15/32). The maturity of infected fetuses ranged from six months' gestation to term. The leptospires isolated belonged to five different serogroups, with the Australis serogroup being most prevalent (Table 1).

Leptospiral antibodies were not detected in any of the fetal sera.

Bacteria of possible significance, other than leptospires, were not demonstrated in any of the leptospire-infected fetuses, and the histopathological findings in the fetuses were similar to those reported previously (Ellis et al. 1983b). In one leptospire-infected fetus, the presence of intranuclear inclusion bodies was detected in the hepatocytes, suggestive of equine rhinopneumonitis infection, and equid herpes virus-1 was isolated from that fetus. Histopathological evidence of fungal placentitis was present in the fetal membranes of another leptospire-infected fetus.

Table 2. Isolation of leptospires from jaundiced horses

Horse no.	Age	Culture-positive organs	Serogroup (serovar) of isolate
1	1 day	Lung, kidney	Australis (*bratislava*)
2	1 day	Lung, kidney	Pomona (*pomona*)
3	1 day	None[a]	
4	2 days	Lung, kidney	Icterohaemorrhagiae (not typed to serovar level)
5	5 days	Liver, lung, kidney	Ballum (*arboreae*)
6	10 days	Lung, kidney	Ballum (arboreae)
7	Yearling	Lung, kidney	Ballum (*arboreae*)
8	Adult	Liver, lung	Pomona (*pomona*)
9	Adult	None[a]	

[a] Also negative on immunofluorescent staining.

Jaundiced horses. Leptospiral infection was found by both FA and culture in seven of the nine horses examined, and leptospires were the only possible causal agent demonstrated. Strains belonging to four different serogroups were isolated (Table 2).

DISCUSSIONS

Specific infections have been considered to play a relatively minor role in abortion in the mare. However, the demonstration of leptospires in 24 out of the 50 fetuses examined suggests that leptospiral infection may be an important factor in equine abortions that has been largely ignored because of the absence of adequate techniques for demonstrating letospires in fetuses. The hypothesis that leptospires may cause abortion in mares requires experimental verification but it may be noted that the abortifacient nature of leptospires has been recognized in cattle and pigs for many years (Roberts 1971), and strains belonging to all the serogroups isolated from equine fetuses in this study have been shown to be abortifacient in other domestic species.

The technical difficulties in growing leptospires from fetal material appear to have been off-putting for many investigators. Apart from the Northern Ireland, parasitic leptospires have been isolated from equine fetuses only in Brazil, where de Freitas et al. (1960) isolated an untyped strain by guinea pig inoculation, while Giorgi et al. (1981) isolated *icterohaemorrhagiae* from a fetus.

The results also indicate that in utero infection may result not only in abortion and stillbirth but also in the birth of live foals that succumb shortly after birth. Leptospires were isolated from five out of six neonatal icteric foals no more than 10 days old, and since the incubation period for clinical leptospirosis is usually five to fourteen days (Michna 1970), the foals were probably infected in utero. While this would appear to be the first report of such isolations, it has been suspected for many years that Pomona infection could cause such a syndrome in horses. During an outbreak of Pomona infection on a breeding farm in New York State, Roberts, York, and Robinson (1952) observed a premature foal that died 48 hours after birth with marked icterus. A similar observation was made by Crane (1956) in California. In Australia, Hogg (1974) isolated Pomona from the urine of an 11-week-old foal on a studfarm with a neonatal mortality problem.

Pomona is the *Leptospira* serogroup most commonly incriminated in jaundice and abortion in horses, and high serological prevalences have been reported in horse sera from many parts of the world. Pomona infection in Ireland remains an enigma. There have now been seven isolations of serovar *pomona* from horses (present study and Ellis unpublished data), yet *pomona* antibodies have not been detected in serological surveys conducted on horse sera from Northern Ireland (Ellis et al. 1983a) and from the Republic of Ireland (Egan & Yearsley 1986). No antibodies to it have been detected in extensive surveys of cattle, pig, and sheep sera, nor has a wild animal host been identified. The only other isolation of *pomona* in Ireland came from a sheep, and circumstantial evidence indicated that the source of the infection was contact with a ram imported from France. With the frequent international movement of Thoroughbred and sport horses, it could be speculated that the horse *pomona* infections arose through similar direct or indirect contact with animals infected outside Ireland.

The isolation of Icterohaemorrhagiae strains could have been anticipated since serological prevalences of 10% and 21% have been reported in Irish horses by Ellis and colleagues (1983a) and Egan and Yearsley (1986), respectively. The maintenance host for such strains (the brown rat) is commonly found on horse premises. Icterohaemorrhagiae strains have previously been isolated from aborted equine fetuses by Ellis and others (1976) in Northern Ireland and by Giorgi and colleagues (1981) in Brazil, while a similar strain was recovered from a jaundiced horse in France (Rossi & Kolochine-Erber 1955).

The isolation of *arboreae* (Ballum serogroup) from cases of jaundice in this study appears to be the first such report, although the potential for strains of this group to cause jaundice in horses has been recognized for almost 30 years; in Czechoslovakia, Sova (1958) reported liver damage in a horse that subsequently developed antibodies to *ballum*. Ballum antibodies have been detected in 10% to 16% of horse sera tested in Ireland (Ellis et al. 1983a; Egan & Yearsley 1986).

The recovery of *bratislava* (Australis serogroup) from a jaundiced horse is the first such report. Together with the isolation of *bratislava* strains from aborted fetuses, this indicates a potentially serious problem for the horse industry. In recent years there has been increasing serological evidence of widespread infection in horse populations from different parts of the world, including England (Hathaway et al. 1981), the United States (Hanson 1982), Sweden (Sandstedt & Engvall 1985), and Argentina (Bordoy 1985). The epidemiology of *bratislava* is as yet poorly understood, but strains of this serovar appear to be present in pigs, dogs, and a number of wild animal hosts as well as in horses.

The isolation of serovar *canicola* strains from horses in the present study is apparently the first reported. Infection is presumed to have occurred as a result of contact with dogs, which are the maintenance host for *canicola*. Serological prevalences of 2% and 11%, respectively, have been recorded in horses in Ireland (Ellis et al. 1983a; Egan & Yearsley 1986).

The isolation of *hardjo* from a fetus was not surprising because broodmares in Northern Ireland are usually kept on farms that maintain other livestock, in particular cattle, and the mares frequently graze alongside cattle or succeed them in a pasture. Broodmares will therefore continue to be at risk from incidental infection by the cattle-maintained serovar (*hardjo*). Ellis and colleagues (1983a) found that such incidental infections are common, as almost one-third of broodmares tested had antibodies to *hardjo*.

The finding that as many as six serogroups are involved in clinical disease in horses in Ireland complicates the control of leptospirosis, which is typically pursued by limiting the contact with maintenance hosts and by vaccination. The combined host range for the strains isolated in this study is so wide that it would mean preventing contact with all other animals—an impractical measure. Available vaccines do not include all the necessary serovars, severely limiting their use. Currently, only a serovar *hardjo* (for cattle) and a combined *icterohaemorrhagiae-canicola* vaccine (for dogs) are licensed for use in the British Isles. Not even the American five-way vaccines contain *bratislava* or a Ballum group strain. Future work must pursue a suitable multivalent vaccine for use in horses.

REFERENCES

Bordoy, A.M.R. de (1985) Leptospirosis in horses in three provinces of north-eastern Argentina. *Vet. Arg.* **2,** 978-81.

Crane, C.S. (1956) A report on Leptospirosis in a herd of Shetland ponies, *J. Am. Vet. Med. Assoc.* **129,** 260-62.

Dikken, H. and Kmety, E. (1978) In *Methods in Microbiology,* Vol. 11, p. 259. Academic Press, London.

Egan, J., and Yearsley, D. (1986) A serological survey of leptospiral infection in horses in the Republic of Ireland. *Vet. Rec.* **119,** 306.

Ellis, W.A.; Bryson, D.G.; and McFerran, J.B. (1976) Abortion associated with mixed Leptospira/equid herpes virus 1 infection. *Vet. Rec.* **98,** 218-29.

Ellis, W.A.; Logan, E.F.; O'Brien, J.J.; Neill, S.D.; Ferguson, H.W.; and Hanna, J. (1978) Antibodies to *Leptospira* in the sera of aborted bovine fetuses. *Vet. Rec.* **103**, 237-39.

Ellis, W.A.; O'Brien, J.J.; Neill, S.D.; Ferguson, H.W.; and Hanna, J. (1982) Bovine leptospirosis: microbiological and serological findings in aborted fetuses. *Vet. Rec.* **110,** 147-50.

Ellis, W.A.; O'Brien, J.J.; Cassells, J.A.; and Montgomery, J.

(1983a) Leptospiral infection in horses in Northern Ireland: serological and microbiological findings. *Equine Vet. J.* **15,** 317-20.

Ellis, W.A.; Bryson, D.G.; O'Brien, J.J.; and Neill; S.D. (1983b) Leptospiral infection in aborted equine fetuses. *Equine Vet. J.* **15,** 321-24.

Ellis, W.A.; McParland, P.J.; Bryson, D.G.; and Cassells, J.A. (1986) Prevalence of *Leptospira* infection in aborted pigs in Northern Ireland. *Vet. Rec.* **118,** 63-65.

Freitas, D.C. de; Salles-Gomes, C.E. de; Lacerda, J.P.G. de; and Perevra Lima, F. (1960) Leptospirosis in horses in Brazil. *Arg. Inst. Biol. S. Paulo.* **27,** 93-96.

Giorgi, W.; Teruya, J.M.; Macruz, R.; Genovez, M.E.; Silva, A.S.; and Borgo, F. (1981) Serological survey for equine leptospirosis and the isolation of Leptospira icterohaemorrhagiae from an aborted fetus. *Biologico* **47,** 47-53.

Hanson, L.E. (1982) Leptospirosis in domestic animals: the public health perspective. *J. Am. Vet. Med. Assoc.* **181,** 1505-9.

Hathaway, S.C.; Little, T.W.A.; Finch, S.M.; and Stevens, A.E. (1981) Leptospiral infection in horses in England: a serological study. *Vet. Rec.* **108,** 396-98.

Hogg, G.G. (1974) The isolation of *Leptospira pomona* from a sick foal. *Aust. Vet. J.* **50,** 326.

Johnston, R.C., and Harris, V.G. (1967) Differentiation of pathogenic and saprophytic leptospires. 1. Growth at low temperature. *J. Bact.* **94,** 27-31.

Matthews, A.G.; Waitkins, S.A.; and Palmer, M.F. (1987) Serological study of leptospiral infectious and endogenous uveitis among horses and ponies in the United Kingdom. *Equine Vet. J.* **19,** 125-28.

Mitchna, S.W. (1970) Leptospirosis. *Vet. Rec.* **86,** 484-96.

Morter, R.L.; Williams, R.D.; Bolte, H.; and Freeman, M.J. (1969) Equine Leptospirosis. *J. Am. Vet. Med. Assoc.* **155,** 436-42.

Neill, S.D.; Ellis, W.A.; O'Brien, J.J.; and Cassells, J.A. (1978) Isolation of *Neisseria ovis* from an aborted bovine fetus *J. Comp. Path.* **88,** 473-76.

Roberts, S.J. (1971) *Veterinary Obstetrics and Genital Disease.* Roberts, Ithaca, N.Y.

Roberts, S.J.; York, C.J.; and Robinson, J.W. (1952) An outbreak of leptospirosis in horses on a small farm. *J. Am. Vet. Med. Assoc.* **121,** 237-42.

Rossi, P., and Kolochine-Erber (1955) The relationship of leptospira to encephalitis in horses. *Bull. Acad. Vét. Fr.* **28,** 257-63.

Sandstedt, K., and Engvall, A. (1985) Serum antibodies to *Leptospira bratislava* in Swedish pigs and horses. *Nord. Vet. Med.* **37,** 312-13.

Sova, Z. (1958) Acute hepatitis in horses caused by Leptospira ballum. *Vet. Cas.* **7,** 447-53.

Twigg, G.I.; Hughes, D.M.; McDiarmid, A. (1971) Occurrence of leptospirosis in thoroughbred horses. *Equine Vet. J.* **3,** 52-55.

Williams, R.D.; Morter, R.L.; Freeman, M.J.; Lavignette, A.M. (1971) Experimental chronic uveitis: Opthalmic signs following equine leptospirosis. *Invest. Ophthalmol.* **10,** 948-54.

Wolff, J.W. (1954) *The Laboratory Diagnosis of Leptospirosis,* p. 39, Thomas, Springfield, Ill.

Infective Placentitis in the Mare

Katherine E. Whitwell

SUMMARY

This paper reviews 200 cases of infective placentitis examined during the period 1969-87 at the pathology unit of the Animal Health Trust, Newmarket, England. Placentitis was diagnosed in the placentas of fetuses from 75 days' gestation to term. Thirty-two foals were born alive. There were approximately equal numbers of bacterial and fungal infections. Chlamydial and mycoplasma cultures from limited numbers of cases were negative. In 88% of cases, placentitis was recognized macroscopically by discoloration and thickening of the chorion. In 12%, mainly the most recent and most acute infections, diagnosis depended on histological assessment. In three mares with placentitis attributable to *Taylorella equigenitalis,* the changes were subacute and low-grade, and the foals were normal.

Fetal lesions varied according to the duration of the infection; granulomas were present in some fungal infections. Fetal sera showed an increase in IgG and a decrease in albumin levels. Premonitory signs of impending abortion, usually premature lactation and vaginal discharge, were seen in many mares. Studbook records indicated an increase in pregnancy losses and a decrease in the ability to get in foal during the year after an infective placentitis.

Scrutiny of the placenta in both normal and at-risk mares should be routine. The information obtained may be helpful in improving the survival rate of foals born alive and/or in preventing reproductive problems in the mare in the future.

INTRODUCTION

The integrity of the placenta, the structure formed when the fetal membranes make intimate contact with the uterine mucosa, is vital to the well-being of the developing fetus. The fetal side of the placenta, the chorioallantois (chorion), is the first of the fetal tissues to be exposed to any infectious agent that invades the uterus. Although the effects of viruses on the chorion are uncertain, bacteria and fungi are known to cause inflammatory lesions (placentitis/chorionitis) (Prickett 1967; Platt 1975). Since several fetal lesions are commonly associated with placentitis, an accurate diagnosis requires that the fetal membranes from aborted or sickly foals are examined carefully. Fortunately, in the United Kingdom veterinary surgeons and studfarm personnel are well aware of the importance of submitting the placenta as well as the fetus to the laboratory. Their efforts to do so are aided by the temperature climate, scarcity of predators, small paddock size, and intensive methods of management.

Pathology Unit, Animal Health Trust, P.O. Box 5, Snailwell Road, Newmarket, Suffolk CB8 7DW, England.

MATERIALS AND METHODS

The study includes the results of examinations of fetal membranes submitted alone (as when a foal had been born alive but abnormal) or in combination with other physical evidence in the case of an abortion, stillbirth, or neonatal death.

Routine methods. In the initial examination of the fetus or foal, samples were taken for virology, bacteriology, and histopathology. The fetal membranes were then examined, spread out on a large board. Since the mare has a diffuse type of placenta, the chorion is virtually a mirror image of the surface of the endometrium during pregnancy. The pregnant and nonpregnant horns and the body of the chorion were identified, and a search made for areas of chorionic thickening or discoloration and adherent mucoid exudate. Particular attention was given to the appearance of the folds of the cervical "star," which had been adjacent to the internal os of the cervix. Findings were recorded on a diagram of the chorion, together with comments on the amnion and umbilical cord. Selected sites, including a section of chorion across a cervical fold, were usually examined histologically, using hematoxylin and eosin stain. Bacteriology swabs were generally taken from abnormal areas on the villous surface and/or the cervical star. In addition to aerobic culture, swabs since 1977 have been plated on chocolate blood agar, with or without the addition of streptomycin, and incubated in a CO_2-enriched atmosphere at 37°C.

Special methods. When gross lesions suggested placentitis, swabs were also plated onto malt extract agar to isolate fungi. Direct smears of mucoid exudate were frequently inspected for fungal debris. Histological sections of suspected fungal lesions were stained with one of the standard methods for demonstrating fungi. During one breeding season, all placental swabs were cultured for mycoplasma species, and for two seasons they were screened for chlamydial organisms.

Interpretation. The significance of the cultures from the chorion depended on the proximity of the swab site to chorionic lesions; the profusion and purity of bacterial or fungal growth; the presence of fetal septicemia; evidence of infec-

Table 1A. Results of examination of 200 cases of placentitis during 1969-87

				Extent of infection[a] (postmortem cases only)			Fetal lesions	
Bacteria	Total no.	Premonitory signs	Placentitis evident macroscopically	Chorion only	Chorion & fetal stomach/lung	Chorion & fetal septicemia	Liver	Lung
β hemolytic streptococci	43	14/23	36/43	9	12	19	18/40	9/40
Strep. equisimilis	2	NR[b]	1/2	0	0	2	0/2	1/2
α hemolytic streptococci	2	NR	2/2	0	0	2	1/2	1/2
Micrococcus	1	NR	1/1	—	—	—	—	—
Staphylococcus	3	2/3	3/3	1	1	1	2/3	1/3
Taylorella equigenitalis	3	1/3	0/3	—	—	—	—	—
E. coli	17	6/12	10/16	1	5	10	5/15	3/15
Pseudomonas aeruginosa	7	1/4	5/7	0	0	6	1/6	3/6
Actinobacillus equuli	1	1/1	1/1	0	1	0	1/1	1/1
Klebsiella aerogenes	1	1/1	0/1	0	0	1	1/1	0/1
Enterobacter aerogens	2	1/1	0.2	0	0	2	1/2	0/2
Enterobacter agglomerans	3	1/2	2/3	3	0	0	1/3	1/3
Gemella haemolysans	1	NR	1/1	0	0	1	0/1	0/1
Mixed or uncertain	31	14/17	6/30	13	2	1	16/22	4/23

[a] Based on cultural results.
[b] NR = not recorded.

Table 1B. Results of examination of 200 cases of placentitis during 1969-87

				Extent of infection[a] (postmortem cases only)			Fetal lesions	
Fungi	Total no.	Premonitory signs	Placentitis evident macroscopically	Chorion only	Chorion & fetal stomach/lung	Chorion & fetal septicemia	Liver	Lung
Aspergillus fumigatus (or sp.) (37)	40	29/31	35/35	25	2	0	16/25	1/24
A. *terreus* (1)								
A. *flavus* (1)								
A. *ustus* (1)								
Absidia sp. (7)	14	7/10	14/14	9	2	0	10/12	4/12
Abs. ramosa (2)								
Abs. corymbifera (5)								
Mucor sp.	2	1/1	2/2	1	0	0	0/1	0/1
Thermomyces lanuginosus	1	1/1	1/1	—	—	—	—	—
Mixed fungal (no significant bacteria)								
Aspergillus sp. and Mucor sp.	6	3/3	4/4	3	1	0	0/2	0/3
Aspergillus sp. and Absidia sp.	3	2/3	3/3	1	1	0	1/2	0/2
Aspergillus and Candida	1	NR[b]	1/1	—	—	—	—	—
Aspergillus and *Rhizomucor pusillus*	1	—	1/1	—	—	—	—	—
Mixed fungal and bacterial	7	6/7	7/7	2	1	4[c]	3/6	3/6
Unidentified fungal	8	4/5	7/7	3	0	0	5/7	2/6

[a] Based on cultural results.
[b] NR = not recorded.
[c] Bacterial.

Table 2. Location and ease of recognition of areas of placentitis

Ease of recognition	Cervical star and variable amount of contiguous body	Distinct areas excluding cervical star		Other distinct areas in combination with cervical star		Uncertain site
Lesions not identified macroscopically ($N = 23$)	16	—		—		7
Lesions evident macroscopically ($N = 177$)	144	10		8		15
		Miliary	*(1)*	*Miliary*	*(1)*	
		One horn tip	*(3)*	*One horn tip*	*(1)*	
		One horn base	*(3)*	*Both horns*	*(6)*	
		Both horn bases	*(1)*			
		Midhorn	*(1)*			
		Body	*(1)*			

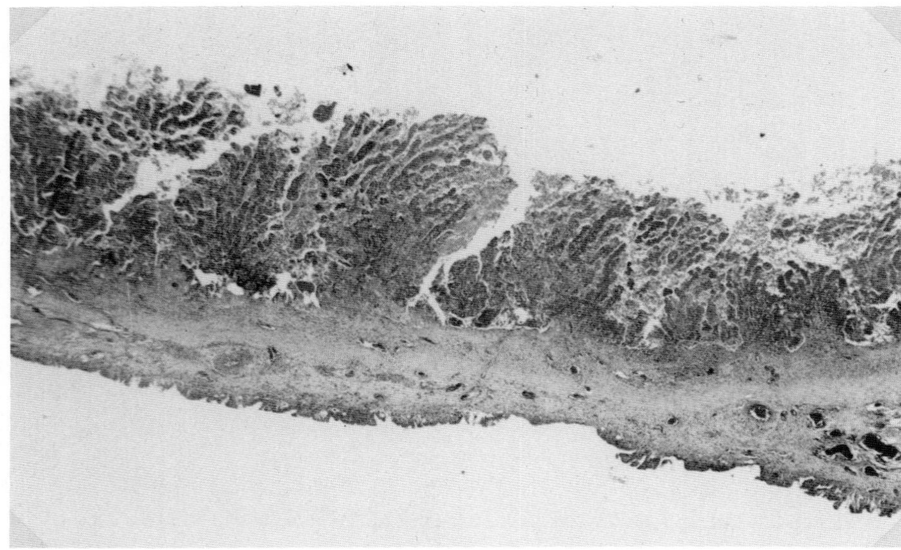

Fig. 1. Chronic chorionitis: villitis, stromal thickening, and allantoic hyperplasia (mag 40×, H&E).

tion of the amniotic fluid (such as organisms in the fetal stomach/lung); and the frequency of the isolate as an equine pathogen.

Blood samples were obtained from 24 cases of placentitis (200 days' gestation to term), either from the umbilical vein of the fresh placenta or from the fetus, and stored at −20°C. On 20 of the samples, serum albumin assays were performed by the bromocresol purple method (Blackmore, Henly & Mapp 1983) and IgG assays by immunoturbidimetry (Kent & Blackmore 1985). Six sera were tested for precipitating antibody to A. fumigatus and a Mucor species.

Thoroughbred breeding records were obtained from Wetherby's *General Stud Book*.

RESULTS

During the period under review there were 200 cases of gross and/or histological evidence of placentitis (gestation periods of 75 days to term). Only 13 of the mares were non-Thoroughbred. The ages ranged from three to 22 years, with many examples of placentitis in the first pregnancy.

All fetuses were negative for equid herpesvirus-1 (EHV-1). No mycoplasma or chlamydial organisms were isolated. *Beta hemolytic streptococci, E. coli,* and Aspergillus species together accounted for half the total infections (Table 1, A and B).

Effects on the fetal membranes. *Allantochorion.* In 88% of the cases, placentitis was recognized macroscopically, usually as a thickened area with discoloration of the villous surface, often with an overlying mucoid exudate. In all but 10 cases where the site of the infection was documented, the affected area included the region around the cervical star (Table 2). Some cases had a small area of cranial extension, but in others the infection involved most of the body of the chorion. Cranial spread appeared to be most pronounced among the ventral aspects of the chorion. In 12% of the cases, gross findings were absent or minimal (local congestion, edema, or discoloration), and the diagnosis was determined only by histological findings.

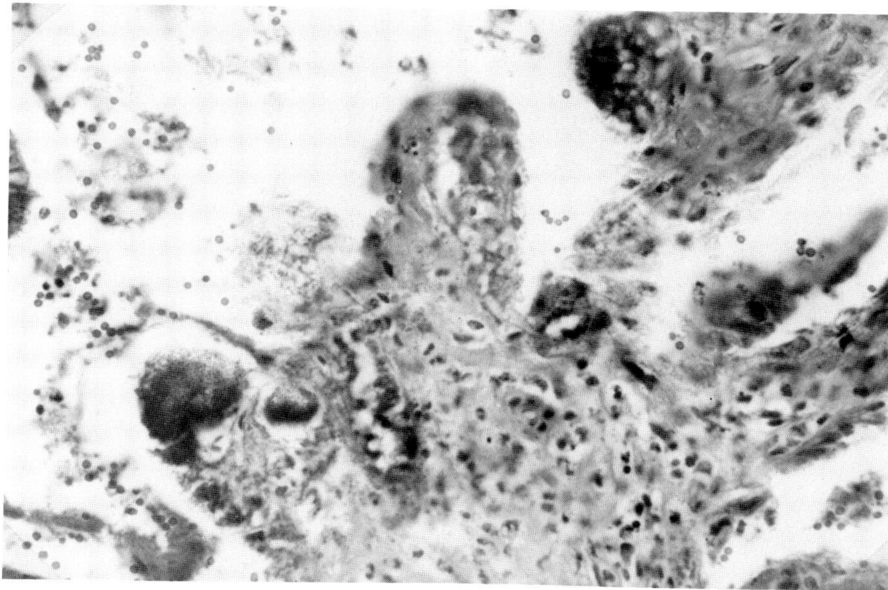

Fig. 2. Acute *E. coli* chorionitis: early neutrophil infiltration of villi and many bacterial colonies (mag 400 ×, H&E).

Histological results showed that most of the macroscopically evident cases were of a chronic nature. There was variable infiltrative villitis with fibroplasia and thickening of the underlying stroma (Fig. 1). Villus remnants were often covered by mucus and cellular exudate, possibly of endometrial origin, which suggested a localized endometrial separation for some time prior to parturition. Thrombosis, vasculitis, and necrosis were common, and the allantoic epithelium tended to be hyperplastic and/or cystic. Evidence of inflammation was observed within the remnants of the extra-embryonic coelom (EEC) (Whitwell & Jeffcott 1975). These often became obliterated by an accumulation of fibrin and inflammatory cells. Placentas from three mares with *Taylorella equigenitalis* infection had minor areas of discoloration at the chorionic cervical star at term. These were foci of low-grade subacute villitis, with invagination of inflammatory debris into the stroma of the chorion where *T. equigenitalis* was isolated.

In most cases in which histology was required to confirm the presence of placentitis, the lesion was of a recent, acute nature, with large numbers of bacteria visible within and on the surface of the chorion and within blood vessels (Fig. 2). Surface exudate was often minimal.

Three types of chorionic pathology may be confused macroscopically with infective placentitis. The first is a clearly defined zone of full-thickness chorionic necrosis at the cervical pole, which can cause abortion. It is associated with a long umbilical cord, probably the result of local ischemia (Whitwell 1975). If the fetus survives, granulation develops along the margin with healthy chorion. The second type includes a variable amount of brown discoloration and loss of villi beside the cervical folds. This is a common finding in chorions from normal-term foals. Histologically there is villus degeneration and atrophy, possibly secondary to placental separation. The third type is chorionic edema.

Allantoamnion. The incidence of lesions in the amnion was uncertain, as it was not always examined in detail and was often incomplete. Gross changes included congestion, petechiation, excessive tortuosity of vessels, edema, opacity, pallor, granularity, nodules, and adhesion of debris. The predilection site was the area close to the umbilical cord. Lesions were recognized as inflammatory only after histological assessment. Acute or chronic amnionitis was present in some bacterial or fungal infections, and microorganisms were seen in association with some lesions. Inflammatory changes affected the outer surface of the amnion in two cases of *T. equigenitalis* infection, and the inner surface and cord in cases of Pseudomonas and beta hemolytic streptococcal infection. On occasion changes appeared to originate within the amnion in the EEC. Small granulomas were seen in two cases of Absidia infection. Infarcts were not uncommon, delineated by a peripheral inflammatory response.

Effects on the fetus. In 14 of 17 cases with acute placental lesions, the fetus was septicemic when expelled (*E. coli*, six cases; *beta hemolytic streptococcus*, four; *Enterobacter aerogenes*, two; *Pseudomonas aerogenes*, one; and *Klebsiella pneumoniae*, one). Tissue autolysis progressed rapidly. In all cases of septicemia except one, the fetal stomach and blood contained the same organism. Septicemia was also present in a few fetuses with the more chronic placental infections, possibly as a terminal event. In most fungal infections the fetal tissues were sterile (Table 1). Extension of an infection along the fetomaternal junction caused placental separation and rendered the area functionally unavailable to the fetus. Probably for this reason, one of the commonest signs of chronic placental infection was fetal growth retardation—small thin fetuses with thin bones. A white granular deposit on the skin was another common finding, as well as meconium staining.

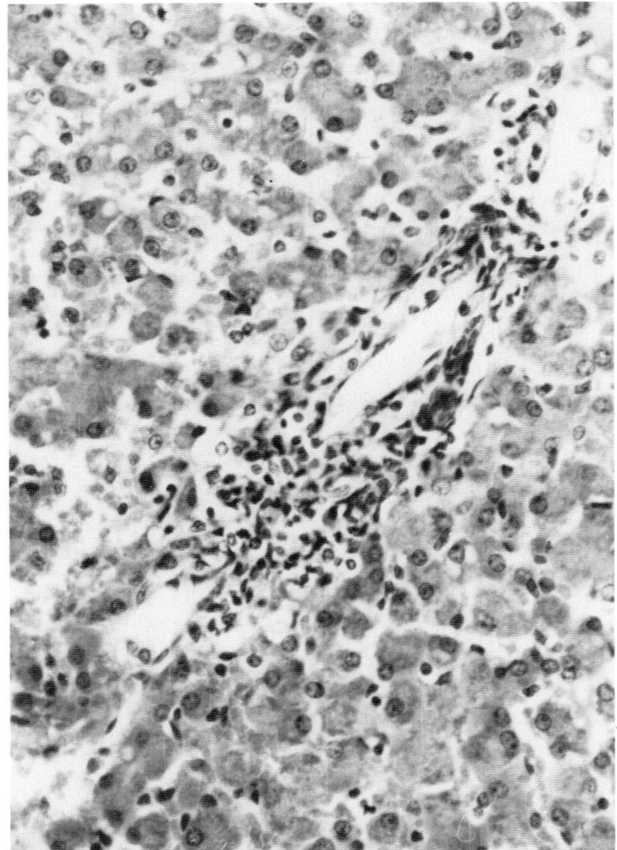

Fig. 3. Focal hepatic inflammatory lesion in a portal area: *A. fumigatus* placentitis (mag 375 ×, H&E).

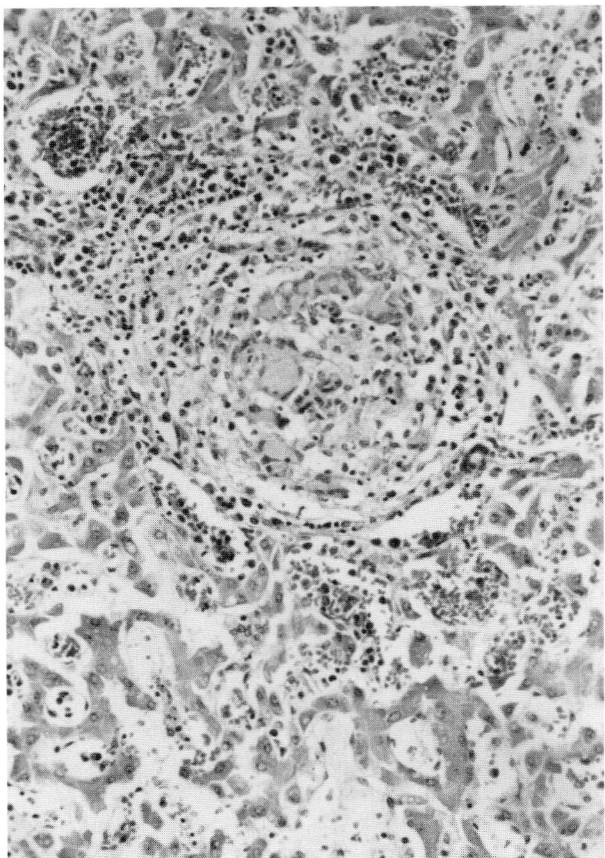

Fig. 4. Hepatic granuloma with giant cells in a fetus with chronic chorionitis (mag 175 ×, H&E).

From five months' gestation onward, small inflammatory foci were common in the liver of many fetuses with placentitis. The foci were present in both the parenchyma and in the portal areas (Fig. 3) and possibly resulted when antigenic material reached the liver via the umbilical vein. Several lesions also contained granulomas, giant cells, and sometimes fungal hyphae (Fig. 4). Aspergillus and Absidia infections had a high incidence of such lesions (Table 1). In chronic placental infections, the liver often appeared bronzed and there was hepatocyte vacuolation.

Bacteria were isolated from the lung in septicemic fetuses and from the lung and/or stomach even when the liver and heart were sterile. They had probably been inhaled or ingested from infected amniotic fluid (Table 1). A number of such fetuses had inflammatory lung changes (Fig. 5), and tracheitis was present in one acute Pseudomonas infection. In six of the chronic fungal infections (Absidia, 4 cases; Aspergillus, one case; unidentified fungus, one case), the lungs contained granulomas, usually evident as pale foci; one case had overlying pleural adhesions. Giant cells and fungal hypae were often seen histologically in the granulomas and also in amniotic nodules. More direct evidence of fetal ingestion of fungi was noted in two cases: fungi in the small intestine meconium, and a fungal granuloma (Absidia) in the wall of the colon. The latter fetus had a focus of epicarditis in the right ventricle, and a pericardial adhesion. In the three cases of *T. equigenitalis* chorionitis, the pregnancies continued to term and the foals showed no respiratory abnormality.

Some fetuses with chronic placentitis had small thymus glands. In a few cases of both acute and chronic placentitis, histological changes of mild or moderate degeneration and/or lymphoid depletion amounting to atrophy were recorded. Lymphoid hyperplasia was noted in the spleen in a few fungal infections.

Blood from 20 fetuses with placentitis had significantly lower serum albumin (mean 17.9 g/l, range 5.0-18.0) and higher IgG (mean 0.8 g/l, range 0.1-3.9) than normal foals' cord blood (albumin 26.7 g/l, range 18.0-35.0, $N = 23$; IgG ≤ 0.1 g/l, $N = 22$). The three highest values for IgG—3.9, 2.58 and 2.01 g/l—were found in fetuses whose dams had run milk for three months, three weeks, and four weeks, respectively, and in which a large area of chorion had become infected. Antibody to Aspergillus antigen was detected in fetal serum from a case of *A. fumigatus* placentitis, and a high titer was found in a case with a mixed bacterial and unidentified fungal infection. No antibody was detected in three other cases of *A. fumigatus* or one case of *A. terreus* infection. When two of the six sera submitted for serology were examined biochemically, a high *A. fumigatus* titer was found in the serum with 2.58 g/l IgG. All six sera were negative for Mucor species antibody.

Fourteen fetuses with chronic placentitis exhibited degrees of carpal flexion in one or both forelimbs, but in only one case was it associated with dystocia. The incidence was higher than that recorded in a survey of live Thoroughbred foals, of which 0.5% had "contracted legs" (Platt 1979).

Of the 32 fetuses born alive, 13 died or were euthanized within the first month. The 19 survivors, two of which had a gestation period of under 10 months, had mainly suffered fungal infections but also included the three *T. equigenitalis* cases. These three and one other were the only foals officially named.

Effects on the mare. *Premonitory signs*. Where records were available, continuous or intermittent antepartum clinical signs were present in 42/67 (63%) of cases of bacterial placentitis and 53/61 (86%) of fungal placentitis. The two commonest signs were premature lactation, sometimes with dripping of milk from the teats, and vaginal discharge. Other premonitory signs occasionally noted included pruritis of the perineum, abdominal discomfort, and estrous.

Vaginal discharges varied in amount from scanty to copious, and in quality from thin and watery to thick and creamy. Culture of the discharge usually revealed the same organism as was subsequently isolated from the area of placentitis. No vaginal discharge was seen in mares with placentitis at sites distant from the cervix. Vaginascopic examinations of discharging mares generally revealed signs of vaginitis and/or cervicitis, with the cervix closed or partly open. In the latter, part of the exudate probably came from the endometrium-chorion interface. In many mares the pregnancy continued for a period after the infection had entered the uterus, frequently long enough for the fetus to show growth retardation. The presence of an active infection of the posterior genital tract in pregnancy did not always indicate infection within the uterus. In a small number of mares with a discharge of many weeks' duration, examination of the chorion revealed only a very recent, acute chorionitis that had not spread beyond the folds of the cervical star, with no fetal growth retardation. A mare with *T. equigenitalis* vaginitis discharged for weeks but had a normal foal at term, and only a very small area of subacute chorionitis was found at the cervical star. In a pregnant mare found to have EHV-1 paresis and bladder paralysis, an ascending bacterial infection of the genital tract was considered secondary to vaginitis caused by urine pooling. Fetal death was caused by acute bacterial infection of the uterus and placentitis, not by virus infection.

A mare with placentitis affecting only the tip of one uterine horn had colic prior to aborting. Pain may have been caused by a secondary infective salpingitis, for a swelling was subsequently palpated adjacent to the ovary. Infective placentitis with an unusual distribution, widespread miliary foci, was found in the placenta of a mare that had suffered a severe undiagnosed systemic illness with purging nine days prior to aborting. *A. fumigatus* was isolated from and seen histologically in the chorionic lesions.

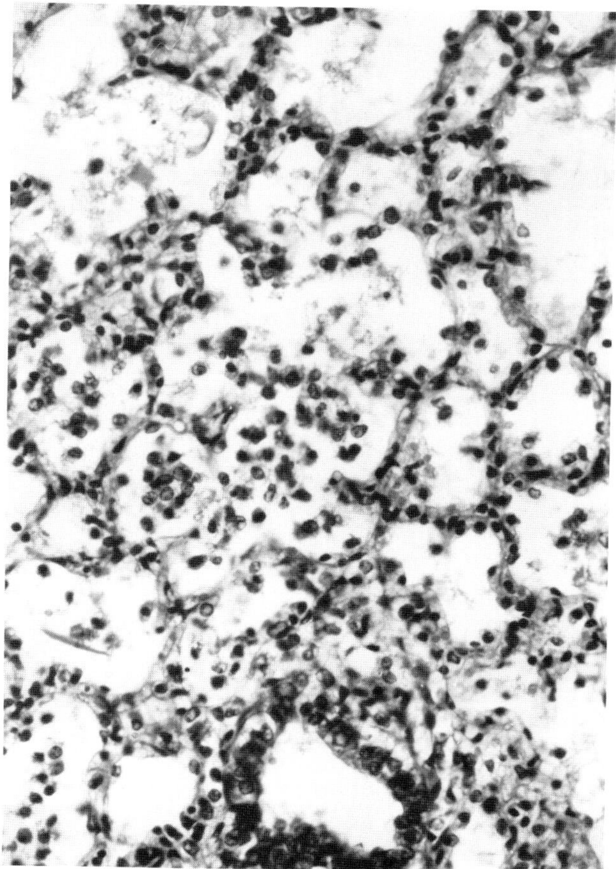

Fig. 5. Early fetal pneumonia from a case of streptococcal chorionitis (mag 400 ×, H&E).

Short-term effects. Among mares with placental infections, pregnancies terminated between 75 days' gestation and term. The bacterial infections tended to cause abortion throughout the period, whereas the fungal infections were more frequently carried to 10 months or longer. Examination of the uteri of two pregnant mares with placentitis, which died or were destroyed immediately after parturition, confirmed the presence of a severe, diffuse endometritis of areas corresponding to the areas of affected chorionitis. Groups of uterine glands were distended by inflammatory debris (Fig. 6). In many mares with marked inflammatory thickening and/or edema of the chorion at the cervical star, the chorion failed to rupture normally during second-stage labour and either it tore across the body or, occasionally, the fetus was expelled within the intact membranes. Dystocia was recorded five times, only once associated with fetal carpal flexion. Retention of fetal

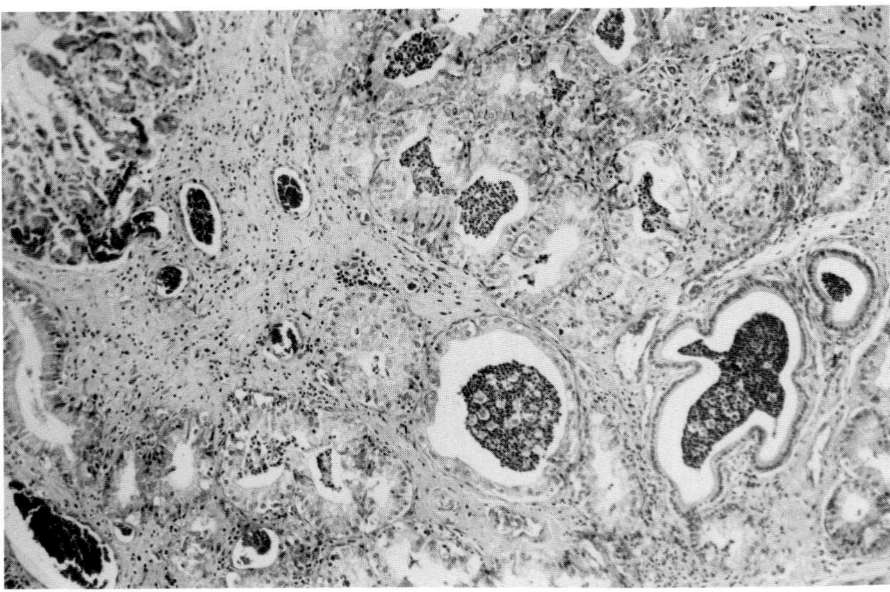

Fig. 6. Uterine glands contain inflammatory debris immediately after abortion due to infective placentitis (mag 400×, H&E).

membranes occurred occasionally, but apparently not with any greater frequency than is usual.

Deaths at one day and 16 days postpartum occurred in two mares that aborted following massive invasion of the uterus by *E. coli* or *Klebsiella aerogenes* capsule Type 1. In each mare the organism that had been isolated from a chronic vaginal discharge was the same one responsible for an acute ascending chorionitis and fetal septicemia. Postmortem findings were available only from the mare with Klebsiella infection. She had multiple endometrial abscesses, purulent arthritis, and endocarditis. Another mare with an acute *E. coli* chorionitis developed postparturient endometritis and acute laminitis, for which she was euthanized after one month. The presence of a small area of cervical chorionitis due to Aspergillus infection was considered an incidental finding in a pregnant mare that died from a cecal perforation. The foal was of normal size and its tissues were sterile.

Longer-term effects. Although there was no systematic follow-up, it was reported that some mares that were not treated remained infected for several weeks after parturition. A number of mares were said to have had previous abortions of a similar nature. Among the 200 pregnant mares in this study, infective placentitis had been diagnosed in 11 during more than one pregnancy—twice for nine of the mares and on three occasions for the other two. The interval between known infections ranged from one to eight years. In only one mare was the same organism implicated on two occasions (*Absidia ramosa*). In the case of 118 of the pregnancies, *General Stud Book* returns were available for both the year before and the year after placentitis was diagnosed (Table 3). The data showed an apparent increase in failure to conceive and in pregnancy losses following placentitis. However, the data also indicated that over half the affected mares were able to produce a live foal the following year. Approximately one in eight of the placentitis cases was entered as "no return" in the Stud Book.

DISCUSSION

This review confirmed the effects of placental infections on the fetus in terms of growth retardation, as well as documenting the nature of the fetal lesions. Low birth weight in placentitis cases was highlighted by Platt (1978), who compared the weights of foals aborted from equine rhinopneumonitis infection with those of fungal placentitis cases. There was an obvious flattening out of the growth curve in the placentitis cases. A lesion that was reported by Mahaffey and Adam (1964) in two cases of fungal placentitis—namely, adhesion of the amnion to the fetal head—was not encountered in the present series. The nature of the granular skin deposit in chronic placentitis cases has not yet been defined. The main problem in assessing the placenta was recognition of the very acute infections, which required a histological diagnosis: the foals were of normal size and it would be easy to overlook the placental lesion. Koterba (1983) suggested that fibrin deposits in the anterior chamber of the eye indicate adverse conditions in utero and probably fetal infection. This was not noted in the present series of foals, but would be worth checking routinely at autopsy. Both Prickett (1967) and Platt (1975) referred to a diffuse form of placentitis but gave few details that would indicate whether "diffuse" referred to placentitis of the entire chorionic surface, or to widespread multifocal infection.

In 1964 Mahaffey and Adam described several cases of fungal placentitis that they considered to have occurred early during pregnancy. Others suggested that the infections ascended via the cervix in the second half of gestation (Prickett 1967; Platt 1975). In the present study, 95% of the recorded sites of placentitis involved the cervical star, tending to sup-

Table 3. Studbook breeding records of 118 Thoroughbred mares in which infective placentitis was diagnosed

Studbook return	Year before placentitis	Year after placentitis	Difference
Live focal	91 (77%)	70 (59%)	− 18%
Fetus/foal loss	8 (7%)	20 (17%)	+ 10%
Barren	19 (16%)	28 (24%)	+ 8%

port the latter view. The cases were sporadic and occurred mainly in the second half of gestation. Swerczek (1980), describing outbreaks of placentitis occurring at 60 to 110 days' gestation, offered the plausible hypothesis that abortions were triggered by environmental factors that caused secondary ovulations, estrus, and cervical relaxation. This in turn allowed invasion of the uterus by bacteria. In early pregnancy, before the trophoblast has expanded into the body of the uterus, any infection passing into the uterus via the cervix might be expected to spread readily through the unoccupied parts of the uterine lumen (body and nonpregnant horn) and cause a diffuse endometritis. The likely effect on the expanding conceptus would be harmful, if not fatal. However, once the conceptus had expanded to fill the uterine body, an ascending cervical infection would be restricted to the cervical star by the physical presence of the chorion.

The range of organisms isolated from the placentitis cases in this review was very similar to those isolated from the reproductive tract of nonpregnant mares (Shin et al. 1979). It included not only ubiquitous contaminants but also organisms with the potential for contagious venereal infection (e.g., *T. equigenitalis, Klebsiella aerogenes* capsule Type 1, and *Pseudomonas aeruginosa*). Bacteria present in the amniotic fluid may colonize the sheath or clitoral fossa of the surviving foal. *T. equigenitalis* was isolated from the sheath of a colt foal for 105 days after birth (Powell & Whitwell 1979). It would be advisable to include these external sites when carrying out bacteriological screening of foals surviving after placental infections. Culturing the fetal lung and stomach is also recommended. Nakashiro and colleagues (1981) isolated *T. equigenitalis* from an eight-month fetus aborted by a mare with a clitoral fossa infection (the placenta was not examined). The potential role of anaerobic bacteria, leptospires, and protozoal infections in causing placental infections in mares remains to be investigated.

In most cases of cervical and other peripheral foci of placentitis. there was evidence of amnionitis and systemic spread of infection within the fetus, (i.e., granulomas in liver or lung). The peripheral foci may have resulted from secondary hematogenous spread of organisms (usually fungi) from the original cervical site. Of the 10 cases with no cervical site of placentitis, in only one were the lesions widespread and multifocal. The mare had recently had a severe illness, and it seems probable in this case that the route of infection was a maternal blood-borne infection. In the other nine cases, the route of infection remains a matter of conjecture. There may have been a deep-seated focus of uterine infection prior to conception, giving rise to a local chorionitis on the overlying chorion during pregnancy. Alternatively the lesions may have resulted from bacteremic episodes in the mare.

The intramembranous spread of infection via the EEC channels has not been previously recorded. The communicating channels within the fetal membranes are relics of membranogenesis and are readily seen histologically. In cases of placentitis with inflammatory exudate, organisms could often be identified within one or more of the EEC compartments (chorion, amnion, or infundibulum). This means of spread might explain the presence of amniotic lesions near the umbilical cord attachment.

The cause of the onset of parturition in the infected mares is uncertain. It cannot have been caused by death of the fetus, as many were alive at birth, nor by the placentitis having reached a critical area, since the area was not large in all cases. The association with premature lactation in some mares suggests a hormonal basis, possibly associated with placental separation over the affected areas, and uterine-generated endocrine disturbance.

The mare has an epitheliochorial placenta, and immune globulins are not normally transferred from dam to fetus during pregnancy. Globulins present in fetal serum are therefore likely to have been produced by the fetus itself. In the present study the IgG levels in foals and fetuses with placentitis were significantly higher than in normal foals. It would appear that infected fetuses (200 days to term) were immunocompetent and able to produce IgG in response to infection. The demonstration that two fetuses with elevated IgG values contained measurable specific *A. fumigatus* antibodies suggested that the IgG production was a response to this infection. Hartley (1983) also demonstrated an increase in IgG in sera from fetuses with placentitis. Future studies should seek simultaneous samples from the dams of infected fetuses to look for evidence of any possible leakage across the damaged placenta from the dam's circulation to the fetus. Reduced serum albumin in fetuses with placentitis might be the result of either exudation from the infected surface of the chorion, or reduced liver synthesis.

In the presence of infective placentitis, poor viability of foals born alive could be the result of several factors, including premature birth, chronic placental insufficiency due to reduced functional surface area of the placenta, the presence of infective organisms, and possibly toxins and tissue breakdown products within the fetoplacental unit. If the chorion fails to rupture normally at the cervical star during birth, severe hypoxia may occur, with meconium and microorganisms in the amniotic fluid being inhaled during parturition. The extent to which a foal is compromised by a placental infection also depends on the extent, the nature, and the duration of the infection, and its effect on colostral quality. The author would reinforce Koterba's suggestion (1983) that information from a placental examination could help to improve survival rates of such foals. Bacteriological examination of swabs from the area of infected placenta can help to determine suitable antibiotic treatment for the foal. There was ample evidence that successful treatment of a mare with a vaginal discharge could prevent penetration of bacteria into the uterus and subsequent abortion. The factors that predispose mares to vaginitis/cervicitis should be corrected to prevent reinfection. That EHV-1 paresis can predispose to bacterial placentitis was a surprising but not unpredictable finding.

Mares known to have had placentitis should receive prompt antibacterial treatment based on sensitivity testing, to hasten clearance of infection from the uterine mucosa. This should prevent the occasional mare from becoming systemically ill with a puerperal infection. Placental examination will also identify whether uterine infection occurred at sites around the fallopian tube entrances or at the base of the uterine horns, where implantation of the blastocyst is likely to occur in subsequent pregnancies.

Although many foals that have had placental infections survive the neonatal period, some cases require intensive therapy and the question of sentiment versus economics should be addressed. Platt (1979) published a survey of mortality and disorders in the Thoroughbred foal, including very low birth weight, below 90 lb, or "very small" size. Although precise details of the reason for the small size are not recorded, several cases were the result of fungal placentitis. Of 43 small single foals, 36 survived to over two years of age, but their performance was judged to be poor by comparison with foals of normal birth weight. Thirteen (30%) of the foals raced in the United Kingdom and Ireland as opposed to 60% of the total number of 1,045 followed.

This review of 200 cases highlights the importance of obtaining a thorough history of the mare during pregnancy and parturition, to identify at-risk mares. It is important to treat all mares with a vaginal discharge during pregnancy and to make a critical assessment of the fetal membranes of such mares to establish whether the cervical star is normal, including histological and bacteriological examination. At parturition the placenta of such mares should be examined to speed treatment of congenitally infected foals. It is good management practice for the stud groom to be instructed on how to check a placenta for macroscopic abnormalities as a routine procedure immediately a mare cleanses.

ACKNOWLEDGMENTS

I wish to thank past and present colleagues in the Pathology Unit of the Animal Health Trust for their contributions to the 1969-87 records on which this study was based. I should also like to thank Miss Joyce Kent of the AHT for carrying out the biochemical assays and Dr. J. Longbottom of the Cardiothoracic Unit of the University of London for performing the serological examinations.

REFERENCES

Blackmore, D.J.; Henley, M.I.; and Mapp, B.J. (1983) Colorimetric measurement of albumin in horse sera. *Equine Vet. J.* **15**, 373-74.

Hartley, W.J. (1983) Further observations on equine perinatal mortality in New South Wales. *Equine Practice, Diagnosis and Therapy* (Postgraduate Committee in Veteinary Science, University of Sydney), pp. 535-39.

Kent, J.E., and Blackmore, D.J. (1985) Measurement of IgG in equine blood by immunoturbidimetry and latex agglutination. *Equine Vet. J.* **17**, 125-29.

Koterba, A.M. (1983) Prenatal influences on neonatal survival in the foal. *Proc. 29th Ann. Conv. Am. Assoc. Equine Practnr.*, pp. 139-51.

Mahaffey, L.W., and Adam, N.M. (1964) Abortions associated with mycotic lesions of the placenta in mares. *J. Am. Vet. Med. Assoc.* **144**, 24-32.

Nakashiro, H.; Naruse, M.; Sugimoto, C.; Isayama, Y.; and Kuniyasu, C. (1981) Isolation of Haemophilus equigenitalis from an aborted equine foetus. *Natl. Inst. Anim. Health Q. (Jpn).* **21**, 184-85.

Platt, H. (1975) Infection of the horse fetus. *J. Reprod. Fert. Suppl.* **23**, 605-10.

———. (1978) Growth and maturity in the equine fetus. *J. R. Soc. Med.* **71**, 658-61.

———. (1979) A survey of perinatal mortality and disorders in the Thoroughbred. Animal Health Trust, Newmarket, England.

Powell, D.G., and Whitwell, K. (1979) The epidemiology of contagious equine metritis in England 1977-1978. *J. Reprod. Fert. Suppl.* **27**, 331-35.

Prickett, M.E. (1967) The pathology of the equine placenta and its effects on the fetus. *Proc. 13th Ann. Conv. Am. Assoc. Equine Practnr.*, pp. 201-16.

Shin, S.J.; Lein, D.H.; Aronson, A.L.; and Nusbaum, S.R. (1979) The bacteriological culture of equine uterine contents, in-vitro sensitivity of organisms isolated and interpretation. *J. Reprod. Fert. Suppl.* **27**, 307-15.

Swerczek, T.W. (1980) Early fetal death and infectious placental disease in the mare. *Proc. 26th Ann. Conv. Am. Assoc. Equine Practnr.*, pp. 173-79.

Whitwell, K. (1975) Morphology and pathology of the equine umbilical cord. *J. Reprod. Fertility Suppl.* **23**, 599-603.

Whitwell, K., and Jeffcott, L.B. (1975) Morphological studies on the foetal membranes of the normal foal at term. *Res. Vet. Sci.* **19**, 44-45.

The Influence of Estrogen and Progesterone on Antibody Synthesis by the Endometrium of the Mare

Elaine D. Watson

SUMMARY

The antibody response to intrauterine inoculation of *Streptococcus zooepidemicus* was measured in both serum and uterine secretions. Uterine infection stimulated an increase in local antibody titers, but there was no systemic response. Ovariectomized mares were treated with progesterone, estradiol, or oily vehicle for 14 days. On Day 7 of treatment, a suspension of *S. zooepidemicus* was infused into the mares' uteri. Seven days later, uterine secretions and endometrial biopsies were collected. A portion of the endometrial tissue was frozen for measurement of endogenous antibody content and another portion incubated for 24 hr to measure endometrial antibody synthesis. Compared with treatment with estradiol or oily vehicle, treatment of ovariectomized mares with progesterone tended to reduce titers of specific IgG and IgA in uterine secretions and titers of IgG and IgM in biopsy culture supernatant. However, rate of antibody synthesis was not affected by hormone treatment. Culture supernatants from endometrial tissue collected from mares during progesterone treatment were less effective at opsonizing *S. zooepidemicus* in vitro. Ovarian steroids appeared to influence the amount of endometrial antibody and the opsonizing capacity of biopsy culture supernatant.

INTRODUCTION

Uterine infection is a major factor contributing to infertility in Thoroughbred mares (Bain 1966). Although many different bacteria have been isolated from infected mares, *S. zooepidemicus* is the most prevalent (Shin et al. 1979; Wingfield Digby & Ricketts 1982).

Circulating concentrations of ovarian steroids have a profound influence on uterine resistance to infection. During periods of progesterone domination, the equine uterus is highly susceptible to establishment of infection by invading microorganisms, whereas under the influence of estrogen, or in mares that are ovariectomized, pathogens are rapidly eliminated (Ganjam et al. 1982; Watson et al. 1987a). Various factors such as decreased cervical drainage (Winter et al. 1960), defective function of systemic and uterine phagocytes (Ganjam et al. 1982; Watson, Stokes & Bourne 1987b), and reduced concentrations of bactericidal substances in genital secretions (Wira & Merritt 1977) may contribute to the increased uterine susceptibility observed in association with progesterone. However, bactericidal activity has been detected in equine uterine secretions during the progesterone phase of diestrus (Strzemienski, Do & Kenney 1984).

Specific deficiencies in the local humoral immune system of the uterus have been detected. Diestrous uterine secretions have a reduced ability to promote bacterial phagocytosis by neutrophils (Blue et al. 1982). This defect in opsonization was apparently not caused by a deficiency of C_{3b} in secretions of progesterone-treated mares (Watson et al. 1987a). The other humoral components notable in bacterial opsonization are immunoglobulins (Menzel, Jungfer & Gemsa 1978). Conflicting data are reported on the effect of ovarian steroids on immunoglobulins in uterine secretions (Asbury et al. 1980; Mitchell, Liu & Perryman 1982; Widders et al. 1985a). It is known that ovarian hormones do not influence the development of systemic antigen-specific antibody in the rat after intrauterine immunization (Lande 1986).

The present study was carried out in pony mares to measure the synthesis of specific antibody by endometrial tissue and the effect of ovarian steroids on antibody response.

MATERIALS AND METHODS

Experimental design. Four ovariectomized mares, with no evidence of inflammatory changes on histological examination of endometrial biopsies, were randomly assigned to receive one of three treatments. On any one occasion, therefore, the regime was different for each of three mares. On successive occasions, treatments were swapped, so that by the end of the experiment each mare had received all three. Treatment with ovarian steroids involved daily intramuscular injections for 14 days with progesterone (100 mg), estradiol benzoate (1 mg) or the oily vehicle arachis oil (Intervet Laboratories, Cambridge, UK). A period of two weeks elapsed between experiments. *S. zooepidemicus* (1×10^9) was infused on Day 7 of treatment into the uterus in 50-ml sterile phosphate-buffered saline (PBS; pH 7.3). Uterine washings (40 ml PBS) were collected via Foley catheters (24 FG) prior to infusion and on Day 14. The washings were centrifuged at $2000 \times g$ for 15 min at 4°C and the fluid was stored at −70°C. Before measurement of antibody titers, washings were concentrated 25× using Minicon-B con-

University of Bristol, School of Veterinary Science, Langford House, Langford, Bristol BS18 7DU, England. Present address: Section of Reproductive Studies, New Bolton Center, University of Pennsylvania, 382 W. Street Road, Kennett Square, Pennsylvania 19348.

centrating filters (Amicon, Surrey, UK) with an exclusion limit molecule weight of 15,000. On the same days as collections of washings, blood samples were taken from the jugular vein and stored at −20°C. An endometrial biopsy was collected on Day 14 and kept in ice-cold Hepes-buffered Hanks Balanced Salt Solution (HBSS, pH 7.3; Flow Industires, Irvine, UK).

Both endogenous antibody content and antibody synthesis by uterine tissue was measured by in vitro culture of endometrial tissue fragments. Antibody titers were measured in culture supernatants, uterine washings, and sera by enzyme-linked immunosorbent assay (ELISA).

Preparation of bacteria for intrauterine infusion. *S. zooepidemicus* was isolated from the uterus of a mare with acute endometritis. The bacteria were stored in aliquots (1 ml) at −70°C in 10% glycerol. On the day before infusion, an aliquot was thawed and inoculated into 60 ml of brain-heart infusion broth (BHIB) and incubated overnight at 37°C. To prepare the bacteria for infusion, the cells were washed twice in PBS and resuspended at 2×10^7/ml by calibration using a spectrophotometer.

Quantitation of specific antibody. Quantitation of specific antibody was performed as described by Widders and colleagues (1985b). After coating wells with antigen, six fivefold dilutions of uterine washings or culture supernatant, or 12 fivefold dilutions of serum, were added to each well. Positive (serum) and negative (PBS) standards were included in each assay. Alkaline phosphatase conjugates of IgG (prepared in the author's laboratory) were added to each well and the substrate (alkaline phosphatase conjugate; Sigma, Poole, UK) was added after a final wash. Color was allowed to develop and the plates were read on a Titertek Multiscan MC (Flow Laboratories, Irvine, UK) using the dual-wavelength mode at 405 and 494 nm.

Results were expressed as optical density at 1:25 dilution if all the sample in the experiment were analyzed in the same assay. Otherwise the titers were calculated relative to the positive standard and presented as sample titer/standard titer × 100%.

In preparing the reagents, the antigen, *S. zooepidemicus*, was the same strain as that used for intrauterine infusion. A colony from a blood agar plate was inoculated into BHIB and incubated for 24 hr at 37°C. The bacteria were then pelletted by centrifugation and washed three times in sterile PBS. After final resuspension in PBS, the bacteria were boiled in a water bath for 1 hr. The bacterial supernatant was collected after further centrifugation and used as the coating antigen in the ELISA.

Affinity-purified antisera against IgG and IgA were raised in sheep and were monospecific for their respective isotypes (Widders et al. 1984). Antiserum for equine IgM (Nordic Laboratories Ltd., Maidenhead, UK) was raised in rabbits, and its specificity was confirmed by immunodiffusion.

Biopsies were minced with a scalpel into approximately 2-mm pieces. The fragments were weighed and 120 mg were placed in 4-ml incubation medium (Hepes-buffered RPMI 1640, Flow Laboratories; penicillin/streptomycin 5,000 units/ml; L-glutamine 200 mM/liter; pH 7.3) and frozen at −20°C. This tissue was later assayed for antibody content. A further 300 mg of tissue was suspended in 10 ml medium and incubated at 37°C for 24 hr in an atmosphere of 95% O_2:5% CO_2. After 24 hr, the culture was frozen at −20°C. When the tissues were thawed prior to assay, the disruption of cells released the endogenous tissue antibody.

In vitro endometrial content and synthesis. Antibody production by endometrial tissue was measured by a modification of the technique described by Svennerholm and Holmgren (1977). The increase in titer over the 24-hr incubation period was used to assess de novo antibody synthesis.

Protein concentrations. Total protein was measured colorimetically in uterine washings using a Lancer Microprotein Rapid Stat kit (Clandon Scientific Ltd., Aldershot, UK).

Bactericidal assay. The bactericidal activity of neutrophils against *S. zooepidemicus* using biopsy-culture supernatants as opsonin was performed as described previously (Watson et al. 1987a). Culture supernatants were dialyzed overnight against PBS to remove the antibiotics. Bactericidal activity was calculated by counting colony-forming units (cfu) on blood agar plates that had been incubated overnight at 37°C and expressing the total as a percentage of cfu in tubes in which the opsonin was replaced by HBSS. In the control tubes, culture supernatant was present but the neutrophils had been replaced by HBSS.

Statistical analysis. Increases in antibody titer after in vitro culture were analyzed using a paired-t test. The effect of hormone on antibody synthesis was tested using an analysis of variance on the difference in titer in culture supernatant before and after incubation of the tissue. A figure of $P<0.05$ was considered significant.

RESULTS

Cultures of endometrial tissue synthesized significant amounts of specific IgG ($P<0.001$), IgM ($P<0.001$) and IgA ($P<0.02$). Figure 1 shows results from eight typical cultures demonstrating the increase in antibody levels between the 0-hr culture and the 24-hr culture.

Figure 2 shows the antibody titers in uterine washings collected from the four ovariectomized mares while they were receiving no hormonal treatment. Each line represents the titer before (left-hand side) and seven days after (right-hand side) infusion of *S. zooepidemicus*. There was a demonstrable increase in titer for each isotype in uterine washings collected postinfection. No response was detected in serum

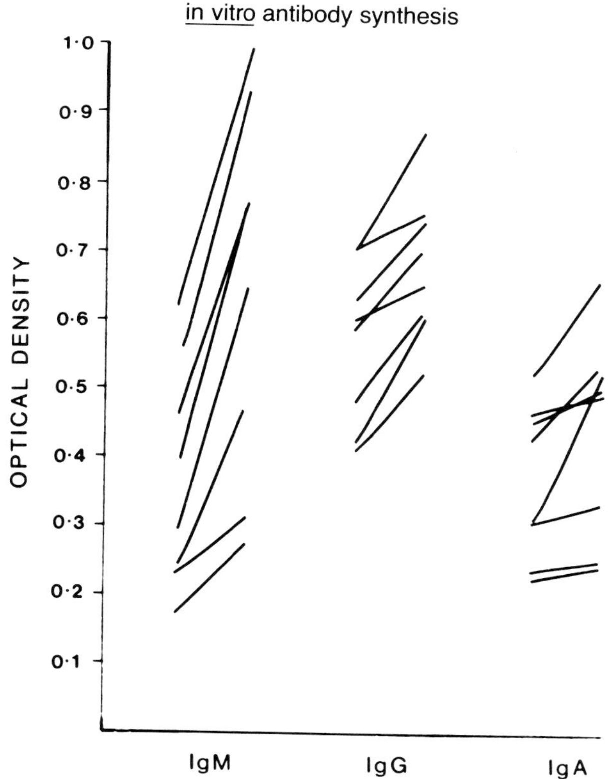

Fig. 1. Increase in antibody titer to *S. zooepidemicus* in culture supernatants of endometrial tissue after a 24-hr incubation.

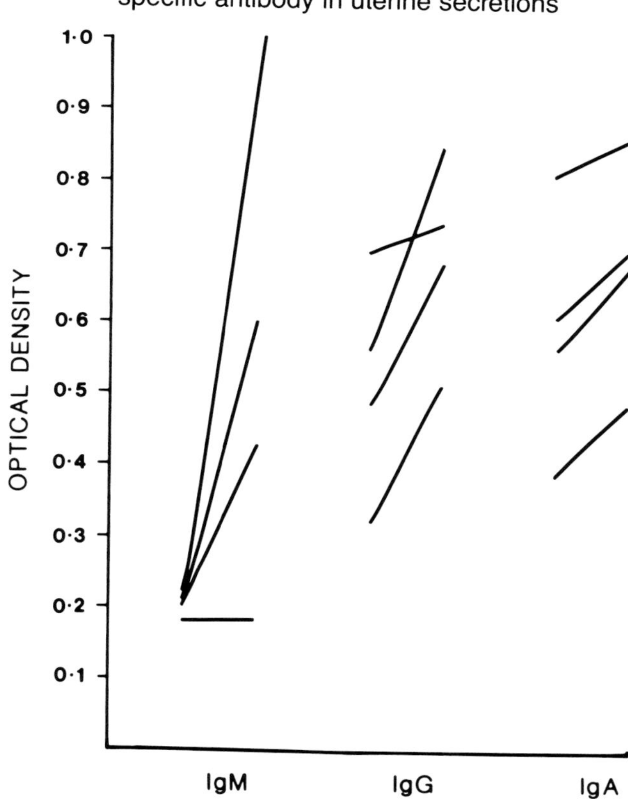

Fig. 2. Increase in titer of specific antibody in uterine washings prior to, and seven days after, intrauterine inoculation of *S. zooepidemicus*.

after intrauterine infection with the bacteria (data not shown).

Treatment with ovarian steroids did not have any effect on total titer of any of the isotypes in uterine washings after infection. However, when antibody titer was corrected relative to concentrations of total protein in washings, titers of specific IgG and IgA were lower during progesterone than estrogen treatment (Fig. 3).

Hormone treatment had no significant effect on antibody synthesis by endometrial explants. Therefore, subsequent results are those measured in the 24-hr tissue culture supernatants. In three of the four mares, progesterone treatment depressed levels of specific IgG and IgM (Fig. 4). However there was no obvious effect of steroid treatment on levels of IgA in culture supernatant.

When bacteria were opsonized with culture supernatant, omission of neutrophils resulted in 100% bacterial survival. In the presence of neutrophils, culture supernatants of biopsies from progesterone-treated mares were less effective at bacterial opsonization than culture supernatants of biopsies from estrogen-treated mares (Fig. 4).

Under the influence of progesterone, Mare D did not show depressed levels of IgG and IgM. Mare D also remained infected when treated with the oily vehicle whereas other mares remained infected at Day 7 only under the influence of progesterone.

DISCUSSION

The present study has demonstrated the ability of equine endometrial tissue to synthesize antibody in vitro, extending previous findings that the equine endometrium synthesized and secreted proteins when cultured in vitro (Buhi, Le Blanc & Hansen 1985). In rabbits and women the reproductive tissues have been reported to synthesize IgG and IgA (Bell & Wolf 1967; Lai a Fat, Suurmond & Van Furth 1973; Cowan, Buchan & Skinner 1982), and in cattle all three isotypes, including IgM, have been detected (Butler et al. 1971).

Intrauterine infection with *S. zooepidemicus* failed to produce a systemic response. In contrast, intrauterine immunization with killed *Taylorella equigenitalis* or dinitro-phenylated human serum albumin (DNP-HSA) stimulated a serum IgG titer (Widders et al. 1985a; Widders et al. 1986). Similarly, there were marked differences in local uterine response with each of these three antigens. Whereas *T. equigenitalis* stimulated a local IgA and IgM response, DNP-HSA induced a local IgG and IgA response, and *S. zooepidemicus* stimulated increases in titer of all three isotypes. It would appear, therefore, that there are differences in antigen handling within the tract.

By designing the experiment as a Latin Square, it was

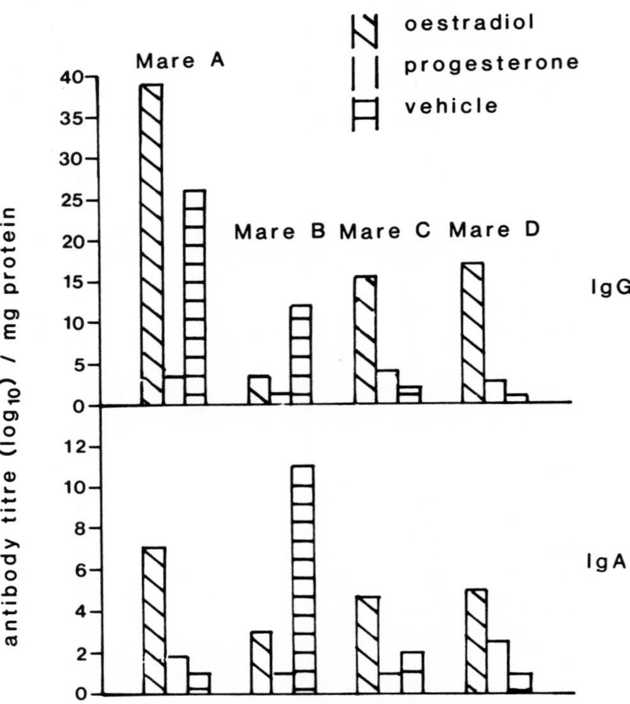

Fig. 3. Effect of ovarian hormones on antibody levels relative to total protein concentrations in uterine washings.

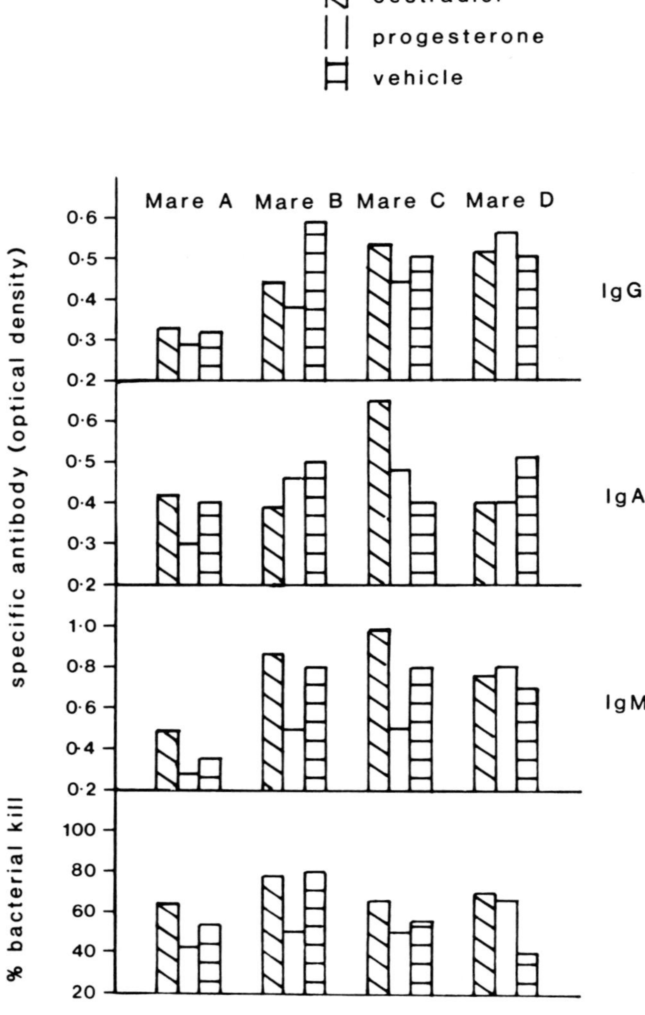

Fig. 4. Effect of ovarian hormones on postinfection antibody levels in 24-hr culture supernatant of endometrial tissue, and on the promotion of bactericidal activity of neutrophils in vitro by endometrial culture supernatant.

possible to use the same mares repeatedly. No carryover effect was apparent between treatments, indicating, perhaps, that the bacterium was a weak immunogen and induced poor immunological memory.

Progesterone treatment was associated with lower titers of IgG and IgM in culture supernatants and of all three isotypes in uterine washings. The lack of a demonstrable effect of hormone on synthesis of antibody by endometrial tissue in vitro is supported by results from immunohistological studies. These failed to demonstrate changes in numbers of endometrial plasma cells at different stages of the estrous cycle (Widders et al. 1985c). The findings suggest that in the mare, as in the rat (Sullivan & Wira 1984), the effect of hormones on local synthesis may not be as important as an active transfer of antibody from serum. It is also possible that the endometrial content of antibody varied as a secondary effect of hormones on vasodilation and vascular permeability in the endometrial tissue (Hawk, Brinsfield & Righer 1963).

In the present study, penicillin was incorporated in the medium to kill any *S. zooepidemicus* that may otherwise have bound to the available antibody, reducing the amount free to bind in both the ELISA and the bactericidal assay.

Bactericidal activity of neutrophils suspended in culture supernatant followed a trend similar to titers of IgG and IgM in the supernatant. When neutrophils were suspended in uterine washings from ovariectomized mares treated with ovarian steroids, progesterone treatment significantly decreased bactericidal activity (Watson et al. 1987a).

The activity of IgG and IgA in genital tract secretions has been investigated using cervico-vaginal mucus from cattle (Corbeil et al. 1974). Only IgG was found to be important in bacterial opsonization whereas both IgG and IgA were involved in immobilization of bacteria. The importance of IgG as an opsonin would explain the parallel trend between bactericidal activity and IgG titer in endometrial culture supernatant. Although IgM is an important opsonin in serum (Menzel et al. 1978), only a very small amount is present in uterine secretions (Asbury et al. 1980; Widders et al. 1984) and quantitatively, therefore, it may not hold a major role.

It is unlikely that the presence of hormones themselves had a direct influence on the bactericidal assay, as addition of 4 ng/ml of progesterone or 20 pg/ml of estradiol to an assay had no effect on neutrophil activity (Watson, unpublished results).

The reasons why Mare D reacted differently than the other mares remain obscure. It is possible that she may have been suffering from intercurrent subclinical infection that interfered with the normal immune response.

In conclusion, specific antibody was synthesized by the equine endometrium in vitro. Endogenous concentrations of specific IgG and IgM were modified by progesterone and may significantly influence susceptibility to endometritis during periods of high circulating concentrations of progesterone. The effect of ovarian hormones on antibody response to infection may be an important consideration in future development of vaccination regimes.

ACKNOWLEDGMENT

This study was supported by a grant from the Horserace Betting Levy Board.

REFERENCES

Asbury, A.C.; Halliwell, R.E.W.; Foster, A.W.; and Longino, S.J. (1980) Immunoglobulins in uterine secretions of mares with differing resistance to endometritis. *Theriogenology* **14**, 299-304.

Bain, A.M. (1966) The role of infection in infertility in the Thoroughbred mare. *Vet. Rec.* **78**, 168-73.

Bell, E.B., and Wolf, B. (1967) Antibody synthesis *in vitro* by the rabbit vagina against diphtheria toxoid. *Nature* **214**, 423-24.

Black, W.G.; Simon, J.; Kidder, H.E.; and Wiltbank, J.N. (1964) Bactericidal activity of the uterus in the rabbit and cow. *Am. J. Vet. Res.* **15**, 247-51.

Blue, M.G.; Brady, A.A.; Davidson, J.N.; and Kenney, R.M. (1982) Studies on the composition and antibacterial activity of uterine fluid from mares. *J. Reprod. Fert., Suppl.* **32**, 143-49.

Buhi, W.C.; Le Blanc, M.M.; and Hansen, P.J. (1985) Secretion of proteins by cultured endometrium from postpartum and cyclic mares (abstract). *J. Anim. Sci.* **61**, Suppl. 1, p. 388.

Butler, J.E.; Kiddy, C.A.; Maxwell, C.; Hylton, M.B.; and Asofsky, R. (1971) Synthesis of immunoglobulins by various tissues of the cow. *J. Dairy Sci.* **54**, 1323-24.

Corbeil, L.B.; Schurig, G.D.; Duncan, J.R.; Corbeil, R.R.; and Winter, A.J. (1974) Immunoglobulin classes and biological functions of Campylobacter (Vibrio) fetus antibodies in serum and cervicovaginal mucus. *Infect. Immun.* **10**, 422-29.

Cowan, M.E.; Buchan, A.; and Skinner, G.R.B. (1982) Synthesis of immunoglobulins by human endocervix in organ culture. *J. Exp. Pathol.* **63**, 125-32.

Ganjam, V.K.; McLeod, C.; Klesius, P.H.; Washburn, S.M.; Kwapien, R.K.; Brown, B.; and Fazeli, M.H. (1982) Effect of ovarian hormones on the phagocytic response of ovariectomized mares. *J. Reprod. Fert., Suppl.* **32**, 169-74.

Hawk, H.W.; Brinsfield, T.H.; and Righer, H.F. (1963) Control by ovarian hormones of vascular permeability in normal and experimentally infected sheep uteri. *J. Reprod. Fert.* **6**, 71-77.

Lai a Fat, R.F.M.; Suurmond, D.; and Van Furth, R. (1973) *In vitro* synthesis of immunoglobulins, secretory component and complement in normal and pathological skin and adjacent mucous membranes. *Clin. Exp. Immunol.* **14**, 377-95.

Lande, I.J.M. (1986) Systemic immunity developing from intrauterine antigen exposure in the nonpregnant rat. *J. Reprod. Immunol.* **9**, 57-66.

Menzel, J.; Jungfer, H.; and Gemsa, D. (1978) Amplification of the intracellular killing of Escherichia coli in human polymorphonuclear leukocytes by complement. In *Clinical Aspects of the Complement System.* Eds. W. Opferkuch, K. Rother, and D.R. Schultz. Georg Thieme, Stuttgart.

Mitchell, G.; Liu, I.K.M.; and Perryman, L.E. (1982) Preferential production and secretion of immunoglobulins by the equine endometrium—a mucosal immune system. *J. Reprod. Fert., Suppl.* **32**, 161-68.

Shin, S.J.; Lein, D.H.; Aronson, A.L.; and Nussbaum, S.R. (1979) The bacteriological culture of equine uterine contents, *in vitro* sensitivity of organisms isolated and interpretation. *J. Reprod. Fert., Suppl.* **27**, 307-15.

Strzemienski, P.J.; Do, D.; and Kenney, R.M. (1984) Antibacterial activity of mare uterine fluid. *Biol. Reprod.* **31**, 303-11.

Sullivan, D.A., and Wira, C.R. (1984) Hormonal regulation of immunoglobulins in the rat uterus: Uterine response to multiple estradiol treatments. *Endocrinology* **114**, 650-58.

Svennerholm, A.M., and Holmgren, J. (1977) Immunoglobulin and specific-antibody synthesis *in vitro* by enteral and non-enteral tissues after subcutaneous cholera immunization. *Infect. Immun.* **15**, 360-69.

Watson, E.D.; Stokes, C.R.; David, J.S.E.; and Bourne, F.J. (1987a) Effect of ovarian hormones on promotion of bactericidal activity by uterine secretions of ovariectomized mares. *J. Reprod. Fert.* **79**, 531-37.

Watson, E.D.; Stokes, C.R.; and Bourne, F.J. (1987b) Influence of administration of ovarian steroids on the function of neutrophils isolated from the blood and uterus of ovariectomized mares. *J. Endocrinol.* **112**, 443-48.

Widders, P.R.; Stokes, C.R.; David, J.S.E.; and Bourne, F.J. (1984) Quantitation of the immunoglobulins in reproductive tract secretions of the mare. *Res. Vet. Sci.* **37**, 324-30.

———. (1985a) Effect of cycle stage on immunoglobulin concentrations in reproductive tract secretions of the mare. *J. Reprod. Immunol.* **7**, 233-42.

———. (1985b) Specific antibody in the equine genital tract following systemic and local immunization. *Immunology* **54**, 763-69.

———. (1985c) Immunohistological studies of the local immune system in the reproductive tract of the mare. *Res. Vet. Sci.* **38**, 88-95.

———. (1986) Specific antibody in the equine genital tract following local immunization and challenge infection with contagious equine metritis organism (Taylorella equigenitalis). *Res. Vet. Sci.* **40**, 54-58.

Wingfield Digby, N.J.; and Ricketts, S.W. (1982) Results of concurrent bacteriological and cytological examinations of the endometrium of mares in routine stud farm practice 1978-1981. *J. Reprod. Fert.* **32**, 181-85.

Winter, A.J.; Broome, A.W.; McNutt, S.H.; and Casida, L.E. (1960) Variations in uterine response to experimental infection due to the hormonal state of the ovaries. 1. The role of cervical drainage, leukocyte numbers, and noncellular factors in uterine bactericidal activity. *Am. J. Vet. Res.* **21**, 668-74.

Wira, C.R., and Merritt, K. (1977) Effect of the estrous cycle, castration and pseudopregnancy on E. coli in the uterus and uterine secretions of the rat. *Biol. Reprod.* **17**, 519-22.

Vector-Borne Diseases

Quantifying the Role of Horse Flies as Vectors of Equine Infectious Anemia

Lane D. Foil, W.V. Adams, Jr., Jackie M. McManus, and Charles J. Issel

SUMMARY

In the mechanical transmission of EIAV by tabanids, the important variables are the clinical status and corresponding viremia of EIA antibody-positive horses, and the amount of blood transferred between the positive and negative horses. Horses with no clinical signs of EIA are usually less threatening as a source of infection than those exhibiting clinical signs; however, inapparently infected horses can be a source of infection. The physical distance between infected and susceptible animals, the total tabanid population, and the different tabanid species present influence the amount of blood transferred. The vector burden of the susceptible horses relative to that of infected horses can make a difference. The tabanid feeding occurrence of foals is lower than that of adults. The amount of blood that the horse fly species *T. fuscicostatus* transfers to a second host following an interrupted feeding is estimated at approximately 5 nl. Several management methods for reducing tabanid burden are suggested.

INTRODUCTION

Equine infectious anemia (EIA), a persistent viral disease of horses commonly referred to as swamp fever, is found worldwide in the family Equidae. EIA virus (EIAV) can produce a fatal, acute disease or a chronic infection in horses. The clinical signs are intermittent fever, depression, hemorrhage, progressive weakness, loss of weight, and swelling of the legs, brisket, and abdomen. However, probably more than 50% of EIAV-infected horses are inapparently infected: they harbor the virus for life but exhibit few or no overt signs of the disease (Issel et al. 1981).

Blood from persistently infected horses is the major source of EIAV for transmittion, transported either by man or by blood-feeding vectors. The hazards of owner- and/or veterinarian-induced infection should be reemphasized to minimize this type of transmission. (EIAV has been shown to remain infective on hypodermic needles for up to 96 hr; Williams et al. 1981.)

The mechanical transmission of pathogens by arthropods starts when the vector initiates feeding upon an infected animal. When feeding is interrupted, the vector transfers or flies to a susceptible animal, transporting the pathogen on or within the mouthparts. In feeding upon the susceptible animal, the vector inoculates the pathogen when the mouthparts are cleared or when the second feeding is initiated.

The study of the natural mechanical transmission of animal pathogenic agents is very complex. The pathogen titer within the vertebrate, the proximity of infected and susceptible hosts, the environmental stability of the pathogen upon the vector(s), and the types and relative populations of potential vectors are major variables that must be considered in field studies of mechanically transmitted diseases (Krinsky 1976; Foil 1983; Issel & Foil 1984). The mechanical transmission of EIAV by arthropods is generally accepted as a major factor in transmission of the EIA virus, which has not been shown to multiply in cells of living insects or to be maintained within populations of free-living insects (Shen et al. 1978). We consider tabanids (horse flies and deer flies) to be the primary mechanical vectors of EIAV in the United States. In addition to EIAV, tabanids have been reported to mechanically transmit more than 25 other animal pathogens (Krinsky 1976). Transmission of EIAV by a single horse fly has been reported (Hawkins et al. 1976), and there is a high prevalence of the infection in geographic areas with long vector seasons.

EIAV circulating titers can range from undetectable to greater than 10^6/ml; Table 1 provides a perspective on the number of insects required for transmission trials at the different levels of viremia. The circulating infectious titer of different retroviruses determines the types and number of vectors that are required to transfer the infection to susceptible hosts. Friend leukemia virus transmission by small numbers of mosquitoes and stable flies was demonstrated when viremia levels were about 10^9/ml (Fisher et al. 1973). Reports of the mechanical transmission of viruses by mosquitoes when the donor viremia reaches approximately 10^8 are not uncommon (for example, Hoch et al. 1985).

The next reference point is the horse with acute EIA with approximately CA 10^6 infectious doses per milliliter. Although mosquito transmission was reported once, no studies using present detection systems for EIA antibody have been

Departments of Entomology (Foil) and Veterinary Science (Adams, McManus, Issel), Louisiana Agricultural Experiment Station, Louisiana State University Agricultural Center, and Department of Veterinary Microbiology and Parasitology (Issel), School of Veterinary Medicine, Louisiana State University, Baton Rouge, Louisiana 70803. Approved for publication by the Director of the Louisiana Agricultural Experiment Station as paper No. 87-17-1460.

Table 1. Results of selected studies on retrovirus transmission by insects

Virus	Donor status	Donor infectious dose/ml	Mininum no. vectors for transmission species	Maximun no. vectors for negative trial species	References
Friend leukemia		$\leqq 10^{8.9}$	Mosquitoes (1) Stable flies (1)		Fisher et al., 1973
Equine infectious anemia	Febrile	$\sim 10^6$	Horse flies (1)		Hawkins et al., 1976
		$\sim 10^6$	Deer flies (6) Stable flies (52)		Foil et al., 1983
		$\geqq 10^5$	Mosquitoes (186)		Stein et al., 1943
				Mosquitoes (307)	Cupp and Kemen, 1980
Equine infectious anemia	Afebrile	—	Horse flies (3)	Horse flies (75)	Kemen et al., 1980
		$\sim 10^3$-10^6		Stable flies (234)	Cupp and Kemen, 1980
BLV	Persistent lymphocytosis	$\sim 10^{3.5}$	Horse flies (131)		Oshima et al., 1981
		$\sim 10^{3.5}$	Horse flies (50)		Foil et al., 1987a
				Horse flies (25)	
BLV	Normal	$\sim 10^{2.5}$		Horse flies (185)	Foil et al., 1987a
Equine infectious anemia	Inapparent	~ 1-10^3		Horse flies (25)	Issel et al. 1982

able to demonstrate this phenomenon. There has been a suggestion of an inhibitory factor associated with mosquito feeding (Williams et al. 1981). If this phenomenon does not exist, the transmission of virus from acute, febrile donors by mosquitoes could be demonstrated by a persistent researcher willing to test large enough groups of mosquitoes.

The next point in the scale is the EIAV donor that is afebrile but has a history of a clinical bout. The virus titer has been shown to fluctuate 1,000-fold within individual animals in periods of a few months (Issel et al. 1981). The viremia was not determined in the donors in two successful transmission trials (Kemen et al. 1978; Issel et al. 1982). Therefore, we can only comment that, as the circulating titer in afebrile donors approaches 10^6, the probability of vector transmission increases.

Bovine leukemia virus (BLV), the etiological agent of bovine leukemia, is a lymphocyte-associated retrovirus similar to the human T-lymphotropic viruses. BLV is associated with B cells rather than T cells. Epidemiological evidence has been presented to support a role for blood-feeding insects in horizontal transmission of BLV (Bech-Nielsen et al. 1978). Transmission of BLV by intact insects was demonstrated by Oshima and colleagues (1981) by transferring 131 to 140 tabanids (more than 90% *T. nipponicus*) from an infected cow with persistent lymphocytosis to two sheep. We have recently established that BLV can be transmitted by at least one fly in groups of 50 and 100 *T. fuscicostatus* when virus infectivity reaches $10^{3.5}$/ml (Foil et al. 1987a).

The final points in the table include donor status of EIAV and BLV for which there have not been successful insect transmission trials. We have initiated studies to determine the amount of blood meal residue on the mouthparts of potential vectors, for use in predicting the circumstances that would favor mechanical transmission. We project that in any group of 500 *T. fuscicostatus*, there would be at least one fly that would transfer BLV to a recipient from a donor that had a viremia of at least $10^{2.5}$. It should be kept in perspective that most retrovirus transmission trials have used limited numbers of animals because of physical and economic constraints. In most cases, these limitations impede our ability to describe the probability that a blood-feeding insect would mechanically transmit EIA when the titer of virus is lower than 10^6.

METHODS AND RESULTS

EIAV has been relatively easy to transmit by blood transfusion from agar gel immunodiffusion test-positive horses to susceptible ponies in experimental studies. In contrast, the virus has been transmitted with difficulty by vector feeding from horses that have been afebrile at the time of the transmission experiments, and then only from horses with a history of clinical EIA (Kemen et al. 1978; Issel et al. 1982). We have conducted an eight-year prospective study to examine the role of inapparently infected horses as sources of infection under field conditions, while monitoring tabanid populations associated with any EIAV transmission. The compiled results of this study are presented in Table 2.

The research sites for the prospective study were within 80 km of each other but were very different in respect to the physical parameters that affect horse fly burdens on horses. The Chackbay site, in LaFourche Parish in Louisiana, consisted of an 11-hectare (ha) pasture surrounded on three sides by a flooded hardwood forest. The horses were not allowed access to barns or sheds nor given enough space to escape

Table 2. Results of eight-year prospective study of transmission of EIAV when inapparent carriers were the infectious source

	Total no. at Chackbay, La.				Total no. at St. Gabriel, La.			
	1979	1980	1981	1982	1983	1984	1985	1986
Infected mares	5	11	22	15	6	13	17	11
Foals	5	8	6	15	7	12	17	11
Weaned	5	8	5	13	6	11	13	11
Seroconverted[a]	1	0	0	1	0	0	0	0
Sentinels	7	8	5	7	4	5 (9)[b]	2 (6)[b]	3 (7)[b]
Seroconverted	0	6	0	2	0	0	0	0
Stallions	1	1	1	1	1	1	1	1
Seroconverted	0	0	0	0	0	0	0	0

[a] Foal never seronegative when tested.

[b] Number in parentheses includes ponies maintained in contiguous pastures.

tabanid attack. The site at the St. Gabriel Research Station in Louisiana's Iberville Parish consisted of an 18-ha pasture more than 1,000 m from any wooded areas. The difference in horse fly populations between the two sites essentially represents the two extremes found in Louisiana. Foil has observed a landing rate of 50 tabanids in 6 min on one side of a tethered mare at the Chackbay site (a landing rate of 1,000 per hr). In contrast, horse flies are seldomly observed on the horses at St. Gabriel. The occurrence of tabanid feeding on one side of the horses was recorded from observations made from June to August at Chackbay in 1982 and at St. Gabriel in 1985. The counts were 297 flies in 139 observations at Chackbay and four flies in 84 observations at St. Gabriel. Mosquito populations were often high at both sites and stable fly populations were consistently low at both sites. The difference in transmission rates between the two sites was extreme (Table 2).

The titer of inapparent-carrier viremia varies among and within horses, arguing against attempts to establish two groups of inapparently infected horses that would be similar as a source of EIAV. We compared the two sites for transmission by following the same group at each site through a similar period of time.

The epizootic at Chackbay in 1980 was closely monitored. Eight AGID test–negative (NEG) sentinal mares were maintained in the 11-ha pasture in continual association with seven AGID-test-positive (POS) but inapparently infected mares (Foil et al. 1984). The rectal temperatures of six of the seven POS mares were monitored daily. (The seventh mare's disposition was not conducive to routine temperature monitoring). The AGID test was conducted on serum samples collected from the NEG sentinels every two weeks until 60 days after the first killing frost. Approximate date of EIAV field infection was calculated at 30 days prior to the first AGID-positive test reaction. Tabanid populations were monitored with canopy traps (Catts 1970) baited with dry ice as a CO_2 source. Trapping was done at least every two weeks, weather permitting.

Only four febrile episodes were recorded from 1440 daily observations of the six POS mares, and none of the febrile peaks was detected for more than one day. None of the POS mares developed any observable clinical signs compatible with EIA. Although the test-positive horses were inapparently infected, six of the eight test-negative horses became test-positive during one vector season (Table 2). Canopy trap surveillance revealed *Hybomitra lasiophthalma* as the only tabanid species present during two EIAV transmissions in March. A high population of *Tabanus lineola* was present during the remaining four virus transmissions, in July, September, and October (Fig. 1).

DISCUSSION

Total tabanid populations must be considered in EIAV field transmission studies, since many tabanid species have been

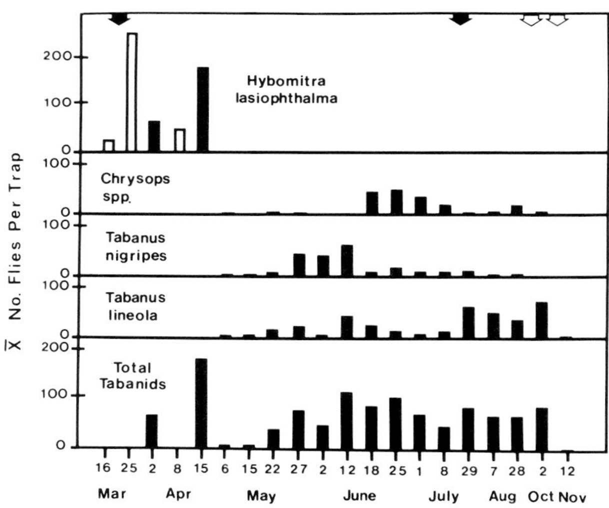

Fig. 1. Mean number of flies per canopy trap of the major tabanid species present at Chackbay during the 1980 equine infectious anemia field transmission study (closed bar). Number of traps per day ranged from two to four. *Hybomitra lasiophthalma* trap counts are supplemented by 1981 trapping results at the same location as the 1980 surveillance (open bar). Approximate date of EIA field infections in sentinel horses (arrows) was calculated at 30 days prior to the first AGID-positive test reaction (*solid arrows*, two horses infected; *open arrows*, one horse infected). (Reprinted, by permission of the editor, from the *Journal of Medical Entomology*, 1984).

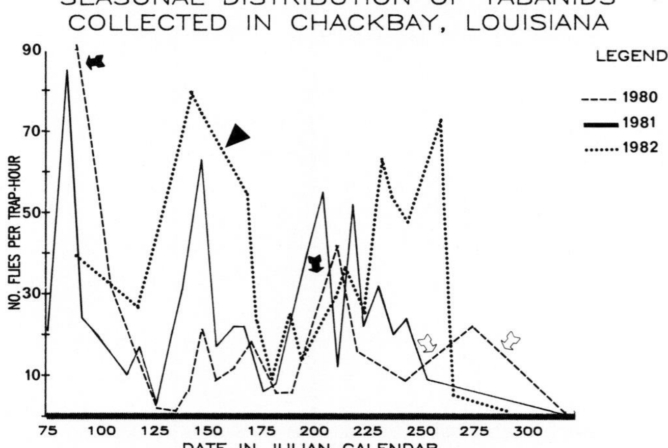

Fig. 2. A comparison of total tabanid population estimates by canopy trap surveillance at Chackbay during 1980-82. Dates of EIA infections in sentinel horses are approximate. *Solid arrows*, two horses infected in 1980; *open arrows*, one horse infected in 1980; *black wedge*, two horses infected in 1982.

shown to be capable of mechanically transmitting EIAV. Field EIAV transmission may, at times, result from the additive events of one or more flies of one or more species feeding first on a viremic horse and then on a susceptible horse. Total tabanid populations remained high throughout the Chackbay study (Fig. 2). Transmission was associated with all three peak activity periods in 1980 and one of the peak periods in 1982. However, there were periods of high tabanid activity during the three years when no transmission occurred. Therefore, EIAV field transmission was probably dependent upon many variables, including the level of viremia in infected horses, total tabanid populations, and feeding behavior of tabanid species present. Canopy trap surveillance contiguous to the pastures at St. Gabriel confirmed low tabanid activity, with less than two tabanids caught per hour from May to August in 1983 and 1984.

Our field study at Chackbay was closely followed for four years. During this time, eight of 27 negative sentinel horses contracted EIA. However, only two of 31 foals of POS mares contracted EIA. Protection of the other foals from EIA virus transmission may have been due to immunity afforded by maternal antibody or to the lesser vector burden incurred by foals (Issel et al. 1985).

The occurrence of tabanid feeding on mares and foals was compared. When mares and foals were observed freely moving within a pasture, foals had 2.43% (four flies in 77 observations) of the tabanid feeding occurrences of the mares (Foil et al. 1985). This difference in tabanid burden varied due to herd size, herd location, and tabanid species. Lower tabanid burden of foals was indicated as a practical protection against pathogenic agents mechanically transmitted by tabanids, such as EIAV.

However, lower foal vector burden cannot be considered an absolute protection, because a single fly transporting enough virus to escape the innate immune system and establish an infection is capable of transmitting EIA virus. This is supported by reports of foals contracting the disease during epizootics (Table 2). The titer of EIA virus in inapparently infected horses is extremely variable and although usually low, it can fluctuate dramatically. During febrile episodes, when viremia increases in pastured horses, the probability of transmission to horses, including foals, is increased. Therefore, pathogen titer must be taken into account when considering reduced tabanid burdens as a potentially protective mechanism for younger animals. The question of protection by colostral antibody has not been addressed appropriately but could also be an important factor.

The defensive behavior of foals, along with their relatively small size, was shown to account partially for their lower tabanid burden. When the mare was restricted to one spot while the foal remained free, the foal had only 1.4% of the mare's tabanid burden. However, when both dam and foal were tethered, the occurrence of tabanid feeding on the foal rose to 5.1% of the mare's tabanid burden, indicating that the difference in feeding was due partially to foals' defensive movements. The intensity of foals' evasive maneuvers when approached by flying insects is easily observed.

The defensive movements of horses can obviously influence the feeding behavior of flies. Since biological transmission of EIAV by insects has not been found, a fly completing a blood meal on a single host is not considered a potential vector. In the absence of studies to describe adequately the influence of host behavior on tabanid flight among horses, a few observations from the Louisiana study are in order. Most tabanids feeding upon tranquilized horses complete the blood meal, as is true with many older horses that have been exposed to heavy tabanid burdens for many years. Such animals can actually sleep through thousands of tabanid bites. It is probably during the acute stage of EIA that the infected horse ceases to resist tabanid feeding. Therefore, the early febrile periods of chronic and acute EIA may be the critical periods of vector transmission. A recent study on defensive movement causing dispersion of stable files supports this hypothesis (Warnes & Finlayson 1987). Older, infirm horses often separate themselves from the rest of the herd, which could have an influence on EIAV transmission.

Kemen and colleagues (1978), among others, observed that only if infected and susceptible horses were housed close together did transmission occur. They reported that susceptible horses separated by more than 100 m from infected horses were usually not infected. One of the most difficult tasks for regulatory personnel concerned with EIA is determining the minimum distance for separating AGID test-positive horses from susceptible horses if transmission of EIAV by insects is to be prevented. The amount of space required to inhibit mechanical transfer of pathogens by vectors is difficult to quantify because of the variety of blood-feeding vectors involved and the differences in physical environments where horses are kept. Most state regulatory agencies have been satisfied with the results of a specified segregation distance of 200 yards. Obviously, a 200-yd distance can be transversed rapidly by strong-flying tabanids or mosquitoes carried by strong winds, but studies that have demonstrated extreme flight capacity of tabanids have not taken into account the blood-feeding status of the vector. The completion of the blood meal effectively removes the vector from the transmission cycle of EIA virus. We maintain that the host-seeking activity of tabanids may take them far afield in search of a suitable host but that once blood-feeding activity begins, the vector will attempt to complete the blood meal on the original host or one nearby. The only critical study performed to evaluate the effect of spatial barriers on tabanid flight behavior among animals supports this position (Foil 1983).

Four horses, each accompanied by a researcher, were tethered in a pasture in a series of five square formations of varying side dimensions, with a north-south orientation. Each formation was more than 500 m distant from other horses. The side dimensions of the five squares were 3.1 m (10 ft), 4.6 m (15 ft), 9.1 m (30 ft), 18.3 m (60 ft), and 36.6 m (120 ft), respectively. The horses were rotated among the stations after each assay to prevent individual host attractiveness and site bias. Tabanids that had initiated feeding but were not visibly engorged were marked with nontoxic water-base paints on either the abdomen or thorax. This marking technique rarely disturbed the engorgement behavior of the flies. A different color of paint was used for each marking station.

To determine the probability of a repelled tabanid returning to the same horse or transferring to one of the other three tethered in the same square, flies were marked, trapped in plastic cups, and immediately released 0.31 m (1 ft) from the feeding site. Time of release and species were recorded. A complete inspection of the horse was then made to detect any marked flies. Marked flies feeding on the host were captured and eliminated from the experiment; time of capture, species, and color of marking were recorded. Each of the five squares was assayed at three times of day.

Of a total of 1157 flies that were marked, captured, and released, 602 (52%) were recaptured when they returned to one of the four horses in the formation. There was a proportional relationship between the number of tabanids returning to the original host and the distance between the horses. Additionally, there was a consistently higher attraction to the horses on adjacent corners of the square than to horses located at the longer, diagonal distance. During this entire study, 21% of the flies dispersed along the sides of the square compared with 8% along the diagonal, indicating a probable influence of distance. When the horses were tethered in a 36.6-m-square formation, 87.5% of the tabanids returned to the same host. Regression of the transformed percentages of tabanids returning to the original host on the distance between the horses revealed a linear relationship. Extrapolation from the linear regression indicated that approximately 99% of the horse flies would be expected to return to the original host when separated by as much as 49.3 m from other horses. This percentage undoubtedly would vary with different species of tabanids and in different environments. However, in our opinion a 200-yd separation reduces the potential for EIAV transmission by tabanids, even when keeping in mind the possibility of transmission of EIAV by a single fly.

The relative number of flies that would naturally leave a host before completing a blood meal is a factor in determining the spatial barriers to mechanical transmission. We have made some observations on what we refer to as feeding persistence—the tenacity with which different horse fly species pursue a single host until the blood meal is complete. Most of the laboratory transmissions of EIA have been done with very persistent tabanids. These horse fly species, in particular *Tabanus fuscicostatus*, feed readily when captured and brought into the laboratory, in contrast to most other tabanid species, which do not adapt well to captivity. Given the relative behaviors, many of the laboratory experiments that have been done with persistent-feeding tabanids simply demonstrate the potential of a virus being maintained on the mouthparts of tabanids long enough and at high enough titers for mechanical transmission to occur. In field situations, the less persistent horse fly species are probably the primary agents of mechanical transmission because, being more easily repelled by an infected animal, they more readily transfer to susceptible animals to complete the blood meal.

We compared the feeding persistence of different horse fly species in a previous study (Foil 1983) using four horses in a 9-m-square formation and a single color of marking paint for the feeders on each horse. Tabanids were marked and allowed to finish the blood meal on the original animal. The only flies captured were those that transferred from the original host to another in the formation. Of the 750 tabanids we marked, *Tabanus lineola* was by far the most plentiful species. Only 2% of 599 marked specimens of this species transferred to another host. Similarly, only 2.8% of the *Chrysops* spp. transferred from one host to another, while among the larger tabanids, 7.1% of the *Tabanus sulcifrons* and 12.3% of the *Tabanus petiolatus* transferred between hosts. It appeared that the larger the tabanid, the greater the potential for transferring between two animals.

We maintain that the two variables that contribute most to the transmission of viruses such as EIAV are the circulating titer of the agent and the amount of blood transferred among animals by the vector. We have initiated studies to determine blood meal residue on the mouthparts of potential vectors. These studies may be essential if the role of vectors in the epidemiology of mechanically transmitted diseases is to be evaluated when extensive transmission trials are not feasible. These studies have been greatly facilitated by an enzyme-linked immunosorbent assay (ELISA) modified from the techniques of Konishi and Yamanishi (1984), which they reported capable of detecting 7 nl of blood meal.

Horse flies, *Tabanus fuscicostatus*, were placed on a pony and allowed to feed until blood engorgement was obvious.

Table 3. Herd factors that influence the probability of mechanical transmission of equine infectious anemia by tabanids (horse flies and deer flies). Management strategies that are numbered are in order of preference.

Herd properties	Infection source	Location	Vector "attractiveness"
Examples	a. clinical status of individuals b. % infected	a. distance between negative and positive horses b. distance to vector source	a. Preference for susceptibles to be less attractive
Management strategies	1. test 2. remove all reactors 3. remove reactors with any history of clinical symptoms 4. isolate clinical cases	1. separate negative and positive by at least 200 yards 2. house during peak vector activity 3. allow free choice use of structures 4. Allow space for movement from wooded areas.	a. Frequent use of repellents; at least for susceptibles. b. foals have some natural protection.

The heads of the flies were severed from the thorax using fine forceps, and the mouthparts were removed from the head. Control mouthparts were included for all assays to ensure no background readings in the ELISA. All mouthparts were transferred in groups of 10 into 2-ml plastic screw-cap vials containing 1 ml buffered saline solution. Blood samples were obtained from the pony immediately before and after each feeding period for IgG quantitation.

The lower limits of the ELISA detection of IgG were between 1 and 7 nl whole blood for the pony used. Results of the ELISA detection of blood meal residue on mouthparts dissected immediately after feeding was approximately 10 nl with a standard deviation close to 5 nl (Foil et al. 1987b). If a 10% deposition of the residual blood meal during a second probe is taken as a minimum, the range of potential deposition would be between 10^{-6} and 10^{-5} ml. This estimate correlates well with actual transmission trials of EIAV by *T. fuscicostatus*. The results also fit well with our recent demonstration of BLV transmission.

The results of this study indicate that a model for the mechanical transmission of disease agents by arthropods can be established. We have initiated studies to estimate the blood meal residue on the mouthparts of other tabanid species. Many species of tabanids will not feed under laboratory conditions required for transmission studies with pathogenic agents. However, a relative scale of vector potential can be established under natural feeding conditions using blood meal components to estimate mouthpart residue. We have concentrated on tabanids because of their accepted importance as mechanical vectors, hoping to create a model for predicting field transmission scenarios. Ultimately, we hope these studies can be expanded to include other groups of arthropods and to examine the dynamics of blood meal residue deposition in the second host.

The properties of the herd that contribute to EIAV transmission by vectors are summarized in Table 3. Since there is no reservoir for EIAV outside of equids, testing and elimination of all reactors could ultimately result in eradication. Short of this, elimination of the sources of infection on the basis of clinical status—acute, chronic, or inapparent—can reduce the threat of epizootics.

There are no adequate control measures for tabanids, but a combination of herd management techniques can help (Foil & Foil 1986). A spatial barrier between positive and negative horses can reduce the probability of transmission, and the tabanid burden of the horses can be influenced by location, as demonstrated by our eight-year prospective study. The number of host-seeking tabanids decreases with distance from a wooded area (Sheppard & Wilson 1976). Given a large enough pasture, horses will move away from the wood's edge at peak tabanid activity. Since most tabanid species will not enter structures in pursuit of a blood meal, horses given free access to barns will seek shelter from tabanid attack. Reducing the tabanid burden of susceptible horses lowers the probability of infection. The use of repellents can help achieve this goal.

ACKNOWLEDGMENTS

The senior author would like to thank his research associates Mike Andis, Jay Bucholz, Greg Heath, Dave Stage, James Clower, Martin F. Klass, and Daniel Leprince and the many student workers whom they enslaved for their assistance. Debbie Woolf, Monique Ardoin, Audry Cashio, Royce Pierce, Kerney Sonnier of the 6th Louisiana District of Wildlife and Fisheries and his staff, Pat Lee, Rick Ramsey, Joanne Maki, Sharon Fagan, Michelle Brignac, Jim Higgins, and Hugh Keegan have all made notable contributions.

REFERENCES

Bech-Nielsen, S.; Piper, C.E.; and Ferrer, J.F. (1978) Natural mode of transmission of the bovine leukemia virus; role of bloodsucking insects. *Am. J. Vet. Res.* **39**, 1098.

Catts, E.P. (1970) A canopy trap for collecting Tabanidae. *Mosquito News* **30**, 472-74.

Cupp, E.Q., and Kemen, M.J. (1980) The role of stable flies and mosquitoes in the transmission of equine infectious anemia virus. *Proc. 84th Ann. Meet. US Anim. Health Assoc.*, pp. 362-67.

Fisher, R.G.; Lueck, D.H.; and Rehacek, J. (1973) Friend leukemia virus (FLV) activity in certain Arthropods III. Transmission Studies. *Neoplasma* **20**, 255-60.

Foil, L.D. (1983) A mark-recapture method for measuring effects of spatial separation of horses on tabanid (Diptera) movement between hosts. *J. Med. Entomol.* **20**, 301-5.

Foil, L.D., and Foil, C.S. (1986) Parasitic skin diseases of horses. In *Veterinary Clinics of North America, Equine*, pp. 425-59. Ed. R. Herd. W.B. Saunders, Philadelphia.

Foil, L.D.; Meek, C.L.; Adams, W.V.; and Issel, C.S. (1983) Mechanical transmission of equine infectious anemia virus by deer flies (*Chrysops flavidus*) and stable flies (*Stomoxys calcitrans*). *Am. J. Vet. Res.* **44**, 155-56.

Foil, L.D.; Adams, W.V.; Issel, C.J.; and Pierce, R. (1984) Tabanid (Diptera) populations associated with an equine infectious anemia outbreak in an inapparently infected herd of horses. *J. Med. Entomol.* **21**, 28-30.

Foil, L.D.; Stage, D.; Adams, W.V.; and Issel, C.J. (1985) Observations of tabanid feeding on mares and foals. *Am. J. Vet. Res.* **46**, 1111-13.

Foil, L.D.; Seger, C.L.; French, D.D.; Issel, C.J.; McManus, J.M.; and Ramsey, R.T. (1987a) The mechanical transmission of bovine leukemia virus by horse flies. *J. Med. Entomol.* **25,** 374-76.

Foil, L.D.; Adams, W.V., Jr.; McManus, J.M.; and Issel, C.J. (1987b) Estimation of the potential for mechanical transmission of pathogenic agents by *Tabanus fuscicostatus* (Diptera: Tabanidae). *J. Med. Entomol.* **24**, 613-16.

Hawkins, J.A.; Adams, W.V., Jr.; Wilson, B.H.; Issel, C.J.; and Roth, E.E. (1976) Transmission of equine infectious anemia virus by *Tabanus fuscicostatus*. *J. Am. Vet. Med. Assoc.* **168**, 63-64.

Hoch, A.L.; Gargan, T.P.; and Bailey, C.L. (1985) Mechanical transmission of rift valley fever virus by hematophagous Diptera. *Am. J. Trop. Med. Hyg.* **24**, 188-93.

Issel, C.J., and Foil, L.D. (1984) Studies on equine infectious anemia virus transmission by insects. *J. Am. Vet. Med. Ass.* **184**, 293-97.

Issel, C.J.; Adams, W.V., Jr.; Pierce, R.; McClure, J.J.; Foil, L.; Heath, K.; McClure, J.R.; and Meek, L. (1981) Observations of a band of horses inapparently infected with equine infectious anemia virus. *Livestock Producers Day Report*, Louisiana Agricultural Experiment Station Cooperative Extension Service Publication **22**, pp. 161-69.

Issel, C.J.; Adams, W.V.; Meek, L.; and Ochoa, R. (1982) Transmission of equine infectious anemia from horses without clinical signs of disease. *J. Am. Vet. Med. Assoc.* **180**, 272-75.

Issel, C.J.; Adams, W.V.; and Foil, L.D. (1985) Prospective study of the progeny of inapparent carriers of equine infectious anemia virus. *Am. J. Vet. Res.* **46**, 1114-16.

Kemen, M.J.; McClain, D.S.; and Matthysse, J.G. (1978) Role of horse flies in transmission of equine infectious anemia from carrier ponies. *J. Am. Vet. Med. Assoc.* **172**, 360-62.

Konishi, E., and Yamanishi, H. (1984) Estimation of blood meal size of *Aedes albopictus* (Diptera: Culicidae) using enzyme-linked immunosorbent assay. *J. Med. Entomol.* **21**, 506-13.

Krinsky, W.L. (1976) Animal disease agents transmitted by horse flies and deer flies (Diptera: Tabanidae). *J. Med. Entomol.* **13**, 225-75.

Oshima, K.; Okado, K.; Namakunai, S.; Yoneyama, Y.; Sato, S.; and Takahashi, K. (1981) Evidence on horizontal transmission of bovine leukemia virus due to blood-sucking tabanid flies. *Jpn. J. Vet. Sci.* **43**, 79.

Shen, D.T.; Gorham, J.R.; Jones, R.H.; and Crawford, T.B. (1978) Failure to propagate equine infectious anemia virus in mosquitoes and *Culicoides variipennis*. *Am. J. Vet. Res.* **39**, 875-76.

Sheppard, C., and Wilson, B.H. (1976) Flight range of Tabanidae in a Louisiana bottomland hardwood forest. *Environ. Entomol.* **5**, 752-54.

Stein, C.D.; Lotze, J.C.; and Mott, L.O. (1943) Evidence of transmission of inapparent (subclinical) form of equine infectious anemia by mosquitoes (*Psorophora columbine*) and by injection of the virus in extremely high dilution. *J. Am. Vet. Med. Assoc.* **102**, 163-69.

Warnes, M.L., and Finlayson, L.H. (1987) Effect of host behavior on host preference in *Stomoxys calcitrans*. *Med. Vet. Entomol.* **1**, 53-57.

Williams, D.L.; Issel, C.J.; Steelman, C.D.; Adams, W.V., Jr.; and Benton, C.V. (1981) Studies with equine infectious anemia virus: (1) Transmission attempts by mosquitoes; and (2) survival of virus on vector mouthparts, hypodermic needles, and in mosquito tissue culture. *Am. J. Vet. Res.* **42**, 1469-73.

Evolution of Equine Infectious Anemia Diagnostic Tests: Recognition of a Need for Detection of Anti-EIAV Glycoprotein Antibodies

Charles J. Issel, Paul M. Rwambo, and Ronald C. Montelaro

SUMMARY

Antibodies to equine infectious anemia virus (EIAV) were detected in horse serum samples by testing with agar gel immunodiffusion (AGID), competitive enzyme-linked immunosorbent assay (C-ELISA), and Western immunoblots. There was 100% agreement between tests on samples with unequivocal AGID test-positive results. On samples with equivocal AGID results or negative AGID test results (from a horse with a history of AGID test-positive reactions), the Western immunoblot procedure proved most sensitive, although seven of the eight samples in this category were also positive in C-ELISA.

Samples that were positive in Western immunoblots reacted with the two major glycoproteins (gp90 and gp45) as well as with the major core protein (p26) of prototype EIAV and two antigenic variants derived from it. This suggests the presence of conserved antigenic determinants of EIAV glycoproteins as well as the group-specific antigen p26. This study identified the need for the development of more sensitive diagnostic tests for detection of EIAV carriers.

INTRODUCTION

Equine infectious anemia (EIA) is a disease that has plagued the horse industry for years; the viral etiology was established in the early 1900s (Vallee & Carre 1904). We now realize that the lentivirus EIAV is a close relative of the human immunodeficiency virus (HIV) through genetic and antigenic analyses (Issel et al. 1988; Montagnier et al. 1984). The lentiviruses as a group induce persistent infections in their natural hosts and pose substantial challenges for immunogen development.

Control of EIA is currently based on the identification of EIAV carriers by detection of antibodies to EIAV in serologic tests, generally the AGID test or the C-ELISA test. Once a carrier is detected, its movement is limited by the imposition of quarantine. Many owners opt to euthanize or slaughter the EIAV carrier rather than to maintain it under the quarantine needed to prevent EIAV transmission. The focus of control efforts has been the carrier horse because chemical or mechanical control measures directed at the blood-feeding vectors of EIAV have not been effective in natural settings (Issel & Foil 1984). Conventional approaches to immunization for control of EIA have not succeeded or have been unacceptable. The antigenic drift or variation that is recognized in EIAV (Kono et al. 1973), which has recently been studied at the molecular level (Montelaro et al. 1984; Payne et al. 1984; Salinovich et al. 1986; Montelaro et al. 1986; Payne et al. 1987a; Hussain et al. 1987; Payne et al. 1987b), presents a major obstacle to immunization. There are two major justifications, however, for continuing the search. First, antigenic variation is common in lentiviruses, and discoveries in HIV immunogen development (where tremendous funds are being expended) may have immediate application in EIA control. The converse is also true and EIA therefore provides a useful animal model for research on acquired immuno deficiency syndrome (AIDS), linked to HIV. Second, although type-specific neutralizing antibodies to EIAV strains can be detected within 60 days of exposure, their absence in samples collected at the time when fever subsides and "recovery" occurs suggests that other immune factors are of importance in preventing virus spread and limiting disease. A full catalog of humoral and cell-mediated immune factors in response to EIAV infection is warranted, to identify protective responses that can be capitalized upon in devising novel immunogens.

This paper defines humoral responses to EIAV proteins in a diverse group of naturally infected horses, detected in AGID tests, C-ELISA tests, and Western immunoblots using antigens from three EIAV strains.

MATERIALS AND METHODS

Viruses. The cell culture-adapted Wyoming strain of EIAV (prototype) (Malmquist et al. 1973) was serially passaged in Shetland ponies (Orrego et al. 1982). The EIAV isolates 135/1 and 135/4 were recovered from acute-phase plasmas from a third-passage recipient (Pony 135) by endpoint dilution in fetal equine kidney (FEK) cells. The prototype EIAV and isolates 135/1 and 135/4 were propagated in FEK cell cultures and purified using previously described methods (Montelaro et al. 1982). Isolates 135/1 and 135/4 are structurally and serologically distinct as revealed by peptide map analysis of the envelope glycoproteins gp90 and gp45, and by cross-neutralization tests using convalescent sera (Rwambo

Departments of Veterinary Science (Issel) and Biochemistry (Montelaro), Louisiana Agricultural Experiment Station, Louisiana State University Agricultural Center, and Department of Veterinary Microbiology and Parasitology (Issel, Rwambo), School of Veterinary Medicine, Louisiana State University, Baton Rouge, Louisiana 70803. Approved for publication by the Director of the Louisiana Agricultural Experiment Station as Manuscript No. 88-64-2037.

et al. unpublished). The immunoreactivity of purified EIAV isolates and the prototype was evaluated in the Western immunoblot.

Serologic tests. The AGID test was conducted on samples using the approved protocol (Pearson & Coggins 1979) with USDA-approved, commercially available reagents (Pitman-Moore, Washington Crossing, N.J.). Results were read at 24 hr and interesting reactions were photographed for visual comparison. Samples that caused a deviation of the reference-positive serum line similar to observations made with the international reference serum, but that did not form a line of precipitation in common with the reference-positive serum, were judged as having weak positive reactions. Samples that led to a disagreement in the interpretation of the reaction by three trained individuals were regarded as equivocal. Those samples that formed a line of precipitation in common with the reference line were interpreted as positive. For comparison, all three serologic tests used international reference serum (IRS) for EIA (U.S. Department of Agriculture [USDA], Veterinary Services Laboratory, Ames, Iowa).

The C-ELISA test, a procedure recently approved by the USDA for EIA diagnosis (TechAmerica Corp., Kansas City, Kans.), was performed on all samples for comparative value. The positive C-ELISA result is defined by the manufacturer as having an intensity of color equal to or lower than that of the positive reference sample when judged by the naked eye. To compare the subjective AGID readings with more quantitative C-ELISA results, an optical density (O.D.) ratio of C-ELISA results was calculated and compiled on samples of interest. The O.D. of these samples was read at 410 nm on an automated ELISA plate reader (Dynatech Laboratories, McLean, Va.), and the ratio was calculated as the O.D. of the reference-positive sample divided by the O.D. of the test sample. The manufacturer's protocol was followed for evaluation of C-ELISA results on routine samples.

SDS-polyacrylamide gel electrophoresis (SDS-PAGE) and immunoblotting. EIAV proteins were separated on discontinuous (4% stacking gel), 7.5% to 20% gradient gels by SDS-PAGE under reducing conditions (Laemmli 1970). Before electrophoresis, purified EIAV was diluted 1:2 with sample buffer and boiled for 2 min. (The sample buffer was 100 mM Tris-HC1, pH 6.8, containing 138 mM SDS, 10% 2-mercaptoethanol, 10% glycerol, and 0.00125% bromophenol blue.) Samples were run at a concentration of 50µg of protein per lane at 16 mA/stacking gel and 24 mA/resolving gel for 5 hr.

The separated viral proteins were electroblotted to nitrocellulose membranes (0.45 µm) according to previously described methods (Burnette 1981) and blocked for nonspecific binding with 5% Blotto (bovine lacto transfer technique optimizer; Johnson et al. 1984) in Tris-buffered saline (TBS) (10 mM Tris-HC1, 0.9% NaC1, pH 7.4) for 2 hr at 37°C. All serum samples were diluted in TBS containing 1% Blotto,

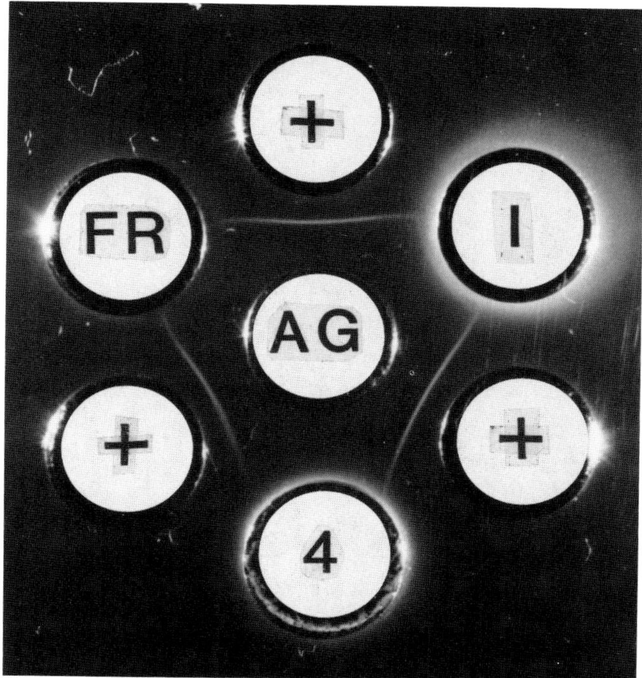

Fig. 1. Agar gel immunodiffusion test reactions of selected serum samples: + = reagent positive serum; *AG* = antigen; I = international reference serum; *FR* = Flicker; 4 = Mare 4, sample 10165.

and incubations and washes were done at 37°C with agitation. Membrane strips 0.5 cm wide were prepared and incubated for 2 hr with that sera (1:50), washed twice (10 min/wash) in TBS/0.05% Tween-20 (Sigma, St. Louis, Mo.) and incubated for 1 hr with peroxidase labeled rabbit antihorse IgG (1:3000; Miles-Yeda Ltd., Israel). After two washes (10 min in TBS/0.05% Tween-20 and 10 min in TBS), bound antibody was detected with 4-chloro-1-napthol (Bio-Rad, Richmond, Calif.).

Horses. Blood samples were collected from bands of horses in south-central Louisiana and south Florida. Serum harvested from the blood in evacuated glass collection tubes was stored in sterile 1-dram glass vials at −20°C until tested. The horses sampled in Florida were from a quarantined farm with 89 EIA test-positive and six test-negative horses. The six negative horses had been comingled with the positive horses for periods ranging from six months to eight years.

Samples from horses in Louisiana were selected from research horses that had been donated to Louisiana State University after they were found to be AGID test-positive. One horse, Flicker, has been the subject of an extensive study (Issel & Adams 1982). The sample selected from Flicker was uniformly interpreted as a weak positive reaction. Mare 4, from which two samples were tested (10126 and 10165), has been observed for over two years. The AGID test–reaction of this mare's serum was positive earlier in the two-year period, but samples collected within the past six months have given negative or equivocal AGID reactions (Fig. 1).

Table 1. Correlation of C-ELISA and Western immunoblot results with intensity of reaction in AGID test for equine infectious anemia

Source of horse serum samples	AGID reaction	No. of samples tested	No. of positive results			
			C-ELISA	Western immunoblot[a]		
				gp90	gp45	p26
Louisiana	Negative	2	1	2	2	2
	Equivocal	3	3	3	2	2
	Weak positive	10	10	10	10	10
Florida	Negative	6	0	0	0	0
	Equivocal	3	3	3	3	3
	Weak positive	28	28	28	28	28
	Positive	22	22	22	22	22

[a] Samples were tested at a 1:50 dilution against the prototype cell-adapted strain of EIAV.

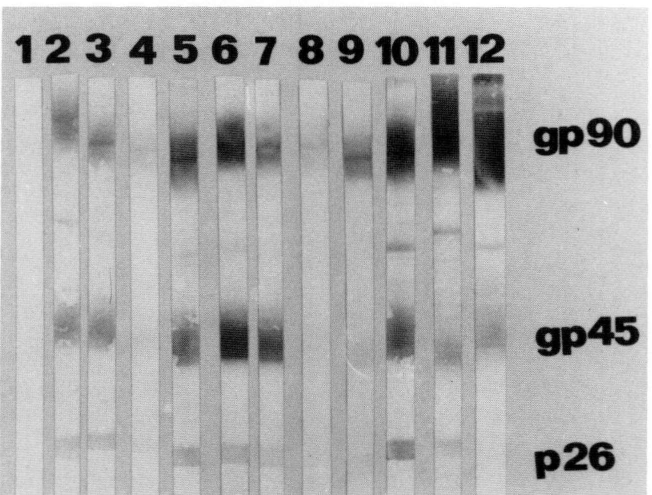

Fig. 2. Western immunoblot profiles of selected serum samples against the prototype cell-adapted strain of EIAV are shown in Lanes 1-10. The reactivity of one serum sample is compared in terms of prototype (*Lane 10*) isolate 135/1 (*Lane 11*), and isolate 135/4 (*Lane 12*). Serum samples, *Lanes 1-12*, are as follows: *1*, reference EIA-negative horse serum; *2*, international reference serum; *3*, 10165; *4*, Flicker; *5*, FLA 253; *6*, Mare 51; *7*, Mare 40; *8*, Stallion 6; *9*, 10126; and *10-12*, FLA 191.

RESULTS

All serum samples were tested by AGID and C-ELISA. The results of both procedures were negative for the six horses from Florida that had an AGID test–negative history, and these horses had no detectable activity against EIAV proteins in Western immunoblots (Table 1). There was complete agreement of AGID and C-ELISA results for groups of samples with weak-positive and positive AGID results. Ten of those samples from Louisiana and 50 from Florida were further tested in Western immunoblots (Table 1). It was necessary to dilute the samples fiftyfold to eliminate background staining in Western immunoblots. All 60 samples produced detectable reactions against gp90, gp45, and p26 of prototype EIAV. The same 50 positive samples from Florida were also tested against isolates 135/1 and 135/4 in Western immunoblots. All 50 samples recognized the gp90, gp45, and p26 of both antigenic variants but with variable intensity of staining. For example, sample FLA 191 recognized with equal intensity the gp90 and gp45 of prototype, 135/1, and 135/4, but had at least four times lower detectable staining against p26 of 135/4 when compared with prototype (Fig. 2, Lanes 10-12).

All six samples with equivocal AGID reactions gave positive results in C-ELISA (Table 1), and in Western immunoblots all six of them recognized gp90; five of the six also reacted with gp45 and p26. The Stallion 6 sample failed to recognize gp45 and p26 at the 1:50 dilution used (Table 2; Fig. 2, Lane 8).

Two samples (10126 and 10165) from Mare 4, which had a history of AGID test-positive reactions, were interpreted as AGID test-negative. Although one of these samples (10126) gave a negative C-ELISA result (Table 2), both samples from this mare recognized gp90, gp45, and p26 of prototype EIAV in Western immunoblots (Table 2; Fig. 2, Lanes 3 and 9).

The AGID reaction of the international reference serum (IRS) was compared with those of Flicker and Mare 4 (Fig. 1). The IRS was also compared in C-ELISA and Western immunoblot procedures with samples demonstrating different intensities of AGID reactions (Table 2). Although the IRS and the sample for Flicker had similar AGID reactions, their C-ELISA and Western immunoblot reactions differed considerably. Comparable Western immunoblot reactions were noted with IRS and a negative AGID sample (10165) collected from Mare 4.

DISCUSSION

Tremendous strides have been made in controlling the spread of EIA through the AGID test. As the test requires the presence of relatively large quantities of antigen and antibody to produce a visible line of precipitation, and as some horses produce IgG(T) which can interfere with precipitation reac-

Table 2. Comparison of reactions of selected serum samples in three serologic tests for equine infectious anemia

Sample	AGID reaction	C-ELISA O.D. ratio[a]	Western immunoblot reactions[b]		
			gp90	gp45	p26
Mare 4-10126	Negative	0.7	+ +	+	+
10165	Negative	1.3	+ + +	+ + +	+ +
Stallion 6	Equivocal	1.4	+	−	−
C-ELISA reference positive	Equivocal	1.0	−	+ +	+
Flicker	Weak positive	1.1	+	+	+
International reference	Weak positive	4.7	+ + +	+ + +	+ +
FLA 233	Positive	6.1	+ + +	+ + +	+ +

[a] Calculated as the ratio of the O.D. reading of the positive reference divided by that of the test sample.
[b] A 1:50 dilution of test serum was used; intensity of reactions was graded from + (barely visible) to + + + (strong).

tions (McGuire 1977), more sensitive procedures should be considered if the AGID test fails to detect EIAV-seropositive horses.

This study found excellent agreement among the three serologic tests for detection of anti-EIAV antibodies in samples with AGID test reactions equal in intensity to or stronger than the international reference serum. We estimate that more than half of qualified trained personnel would interpret as negative those AGID reactions that were assigned "equivocal" status in this report. This estimate is based on interpretations by our laboratory personnel and on the results of test samples sent to approved diagnostic laboratories (Pearson & Knowles 1984). If we assume that 50% of the equivocal samples would be assigned a negative AGID test report, then four horses from the group of 103 tested with a history of AGID test-positive reactions would have escaped detection at the time of sampling if only the AGID test had been used. The C-ELISA reference-positive reagent serum appeared to have less EIAV antibody than the IRS as measured qualitatively and quantitatively in all three serologic procedures. A higher percentage of samples with low quantities of EIAV antibodies seem to have been detected with the C-ELISA test. Only one sample (Mare 4, sample 10126) in the group of four false negatives escaped detection in C-ELISA. Anti-EIAV activity was detected in that sample, but a negative result was reported because the color of the reaction was slightly greater than that in the reference-positive sample (an O.D. ratio of 0.7). In contrast, samples negative on all three serologic tests had O.D. ratios which ranged from 0.29 to 0.48 ($x = 0.39$). These could be clearly differentiated from the reference-positive sample with the naked eye.

Antibodies to EIAV proteins were detected in Western immunoblots in all horses with a history of AGID test-positive reaction(s). Apparently, either the antibodies were cross-reactive or they recognized conserved determinants of EIAV proteins, as they reacted with similar intensity to the variant glycoproteins of two antigenic variants of EIAV. We have previously recognized the role of EIAV glycoproteins gp90 and gp45 as major antigens that stimulate a disproportionate share of antibodies in reference to their mass in the virion (Montelaro et al. 1984). Recently we have documented the presence of highly conserved epitopes in both of the extremely mutable glycoproteins gp90 and gp45 (Hussain et al. 1987). The inclusion of conserved epitopes of these potent EIAV antigens should be considered in future diagnostics for EIA.

Until recently, the AGID test and the horse inoculation test have been the only two approved diagnostic tools for EIA. Several horses with positive or equivocal AGID test reactions have been removed from quarantine because of negative horse inoculation test results (J. Pearson, U.S. Veterinary Services Laboratory, Ames, Iowa; personal communication). It appears that some horses infected with EIAV limit virus multiplication to such an extent that only at rare intervals can virus be isolated from the blood (Coggins & Kemen 1976; Issel & Adams 1982). Other reports document the presence of EIAV in cells collected from seronegative horses (McConnell et al. 1983; Toma 1980). The use of more sensitive diagnostics, both for anti-EIAV antibodies and perhaps for proviral DNA in circulating leukocytes, could help clarify the true status of such animals and improve our control program for this disease.

ACKNOWLEDGMENTS

The authors wish to recognize the cooperation of the dedicated owners and caretakers of horses at the J&W Ranch in Sunshine, Florida, and personnel of the Florida Department of Agriculture and Consumer Services, Divisions of Animal Industry, Fort Lauderdale, Florida, especially Dr. John E. Bryant and Jimmie Cangemie. The authors also thank W.V. Adams, Jackie McManus, and Sue Hagius for excellent technical assistance and Emily Longnecker for superb word processing and editing skills.

REFERENCES

Burnette, W.N. (1981) "Western blotting" electrophoretic transfer of proteins from sodium dodecylsulfate-polyacrylamide gels to unmodified nitrocellulose and radiographic detection with antibody and radioiodinated protein A. *Analyt. Biochem.* **112**, 195-203.

Coggins, L., and Kemen, M.J. (1976) Inapparent carriers of equine infectious anemia (EIA) virus. *Proc. 4th Int. Conf. Equine Infect. Dis.*, pp. 14-22.

Hussain, K.A., Issel, C.J., Schnorr, K.L., Rwambo, P.M., and Montelaro, R.C. (1987) Antigenic analysis of equine infectious anemia virus (EIAV) variants using monoclonal antibodies: epitopes of glycoprotein 90 (gp90) of EIAV stimulate neutralizing antibodies. *J. Virol.* **61**, 2956-61.

Issel, C.J., and Adams, W.V., Jr. (1982) Detection of equine infectious anemia virus in a horse with an equivocal agar gel immunodiffusion test reaction. *J. Am. Vet. Med. Assoc.* **180**, 276-78.

Issel, C.J., and Foil, L.D. (1984) Studies on equine infectious anemia virus transmission by insects. *J. Am. Vet. Med. Assoc.* **184**, 293-97.

Issel, C.J.; Rushlow, K.; Foil, L.D.; and Montelaro, R.C. (1988) A perspective on equine infectious anemia with an emphasis on vector transmission and genetic analysis. *Vet. Micro. Supp. on Animal Retroviruses*. In press.

Johnson, D.A.; Gautsch, J.W.; Sprotsman, J.R.; and Elder, J.H. (1984) Improved technique utilizing nonfat dry milk for analysis of proteins and nucleic acids transferred to nitrocellulose. *Gene Analyt. Techn.* **1**, 3-8.

Kono, Y.; Kobayasi, K.; and Fukunaga, Y. (1973) Antigenic drift of equine infectious anemia virus in chronically infected horses. *Arch. Virol.* **41**, 1-10.

Laemmli, U.K. (1970) Cleavage of structural proteins during the assembly of the head of bacteriophage T4. *Nature* **227**, 680-85.

Malmquist, W.A.; Barnett, D.; and Becvar, C.S. (1973) Production of equine infectious anemia antigen in a persistently infected cell line. *Arch. Virol.* **42**, 361-70.

McConnell, S.; Katada, M.; and Darnton, S.M. (1983) Occult equine infectious anemia in an immunosuppressed serologically negative mare. *Equine Practice* **5**, 32-39.

McGuire, T.C. (1977) Immunoglobulin G subclass [IgG and IgG(T)] interaction with the p26 group spcific antigen of equine infectious anemia virus: Immunodiffusion and complement-fixation reactions. *Am. J. Vet. Res.* **38**, 655-58.

Montagnier. L.; Dauguet, C.; Azler, C.; Chamaret, S.; Gruest, J.; Nugeyre, M.T.; Rey, F.; Barré-Sinousi, F.; and Chermann, J.C. (1984) A new type of retrovirus isolated from patients presenting with lymphadenopathy and aquired immune deficiency syndrome: Structural and antigenic relatedness with EIA virus. *Ann. Virol. Inst. Pasteur* **135E**, 119-34.

Montelaro, R.C.; Lohrey, N.; Parekh, B.; Blakeney, E.W.; and Issel, C.J. (1982) Isolation and comparative biochemical properties of the major internal polypeptides of equine infectious anemia virus. *J. Virol.* **42**, 1029-38.

Montelaro, R.C.; Issel, C.J.; Payne, S.; and Salinovich, O. (1986) Antigenic variation during persistent infections by equine infectious anemia virus. In *Antigenic Variation in Infectious Diseases*, pp. 41-56. Eds. T.H. Birkback and C.W. Penn. IRL Press, Oxford.

Montelaro, R.C.; Parekh, B.; Orrego, A.; and Issel, C.J. (1984) Antigenic variation during persistent infection by equine infectious anemia virus, a retrovirus. *J. Biol. Chem.* **259**, 10539-44.

Montelaro, R.C.; West, M.; and Issel, C.J. (1984) Antigenic reactivity of the major glycoprotein of equine infectious anemia virus, a retrovirus. *Virology.* **136**, 368-74.

Nishimura, M., and Nakajima, H. (1984) Structural proteins of equine infectious anemia virus and their antigenic activity. *Am. J. Vet. Res.* **45**, 5-10.

Orrego, A.; Issel, C.J.; Montelaro, R.C.; and Adams, W.V., Jr. (1982) Virulence and *in vitro* growth of a cell-adapted strain of equine infectious anemia virus after serial passage in ponies. *Am. J. Vet. Res.* **430**, 1556-60.

Payne, S.; Parekh, B.; Montelaro, R.C.; and Issel, C.J. (1984) Genomic alterations associated with persistent infections by equine infectious anemia virus, a retrovirus. *J. Gen. Virol.* **65**, 1395-99.

Payne, S.L.; Fang, F.; Liu, C.; Dhruva, B.R.; Rwambo, P.; Issel, C.J.; and Montelaro, R.C. (1987a) Antigenic variation and lentivirus persistence: Variations in envelope gene sequences during EIAV infection resemble changes reported for sequential isolates of HIV. *Virology.* **161,** 321-31.

Payne, S.L.; Salinovich, O.; Nauman, S.M.; Issel, C.J.; and Montelaro, R.C. (1987b) Course and extent of variation of equine infectious anemia virus during parallel persistent infections. *J. Virology* **61**, 1266-70.

Pearson, J.E., and Coggins, L. (1979) Protocol for the immunodiffusion (Coggins) test for equine infectious anemia. *Proc. Am. Assoc. Vet. Lab. Diag.* **22**, 449-62.

Pearson, J.E., and Knowles, R.C. (1984) Standardization of the equine infectious anemia immunodiffusion test and its application to the control of the disease in the United States. *J. Am. Vet. Med. Assoc.* **184**, 298-301.

Rwambo, P.M.; Issel, C.J.; Adams, W.V., Jr.; Hussain, K.A.; and Montelaro, R.C. Equine infectious anemia virus (EIAV): Humoral responses and antigenic variation during persistent infection in ponies. Submitted for publication.

Salinovich, O.; Payne, S.L.; Montelaro, R.C.; Hussain, K.A.; Issel, C.J.; and Schnorr, K.L. (1986) The rapid emergence of novel antigenic and structural variants of equine infectious anemia virus during persistent infection. *J. Virology* **57**, 71-80.

Toma, B. (1980) Persistent negative serologic reaction in a mare infected with equine infectious anemia virus. *Rec. Med. Vet.* **156**, 55-63.

Vallee, H., and Carre, H. (1904) Sur la natur infectieuse de l'anemie du cheval. *C.R. Acad. Sci.* **139**, 331-33.

Studies on Passive Immunity and the Vaccination of Foals against Eastern Equine Encephalitis in Florida

E. Paul J. Gibbs, Julia H. Wilson, and Ben P. All III

SUMMARY

To determine the decay of passive immunity to eastern equine encephalitis (EEE) virus in foals from vaccinated dams and the potential interference with vaccination, 67 foals of various breeds on five widely separated farms in Florida were serologically monitored from birth to 12 months of age.

Foals on four of the farms were inoculated with a commercial inactivated vaccine at three, four, and ten months of age and were tested serologically when they were one day old, then monthly. Prior to vaccination, the serum antibody titer to EEE virus, as assessed by the hemagglutination inhibition test, diminished progressively; by three months the majority of foals had antibody titers less than 10. Regression analysis of a group of 16 foals left unvaccinated on one of the farms indicated a half-life of 33 days for colostral antibody EEE virus. Colostrally derived HI antibody titers of less than 10 did not appear to interfere with vaccination of foals at three months. At four months, prior to the second vaccination, all foals had detectable antibodies to EEE virus. At 10 months of age, before the third vaccination, the antibody titers of 48% of the foals had fallen to less than 20. Titers after vaccination at 10 months were generally higher than those following vaccination at four months. Vaccination of foals against EEE in high-risk areas, such as Florida, is recommended at three, four, and six months of age and biannually thereafter.

INTRODUCTION

Eastern equine encephalitis is caused by an arthropod-borne virus within the family Togaviridae and is maintained in endemic areas in a cycle involving wild birds and mosquitoes. In the United States, the virus causes disease in horses principally in those states bordering the Atlantic Ocean and the Gulf of Mexico. Outbreaks of EEE in horses have also occurred on islands in the Caribbean, and an antigenic variant of EEE virus exists in South America. Both the North American and South American variants of EEE virus can produce encephalitis in humans. The importance of the virus as a pathogen of humans and horses is reflected by the availability of several excellent reviews on the history of the disease, the causative virus, and the differentiation of EEE from western and Venezuelan equine encephalitis (WEE and VEE) (Gibbs 1975; Monath 1979; Hayes 1981; Walton 1981).

Eastern equine encephalitis has been recognized since the turn of the century in Florida, where the virus is considered endemic. Bigler and his colleagues (1976) reviewed the records of EEE in horses and humans in Florida from 1955 to 1974 and concluded that, whereas the virus was a significant cause of equine mortality each year, disease was only sporadic in humans. Although analysis of the data revealed that the disease had been recorded in every month of the year, the majority of the cases of EEE occurred in the summer months, when mosquito activity is high.

An increased incidence of laboratory-confirmed cases (319) of EEE in Florida in 1982-83 was suspected to be only partly reflective of the number of equine deaths throughout the state. A survey of veterinarians in equine practice in Florida confirmed this suspicion and indicated that approximately 17% of the cases of EEE had occurred in horses vaccinated within the preceding seven to twelve months and 5% in horses vaccinated within the previous six months (Wilson et al. 1986). Reflecting the field data, there was an increase in the number of horses submitted to the College of Veterinary Medicine, University of Florida because they were suspected of having EEE during this period. Further, many of the horses referred to the college had a history of previous vaccination, supporting the view of many practitioners that current vaccination programs for EEE in Florida were not fully effective. The greatest concern was foal vaccination, because the majority of cases in vaccinated horses affected animals less than two years old, and the year-round occurrence of the disease dictates vaccination of foals as soon as passive immunity wanes.

An experiment was designed to study the efficacy of one of the commonly used commercial EEE vaccines. The principal objective was to document the decay of passive immunity to EEE virus in foals and, through serological monitoring, to relate it to current vaccination practices advocated for foals in Florida. The program was designed to cover one foaling season at each of five horse farms in widely separated areas in Florida. Mosquito species and populations were studied concurrently at each site.

MATERIALS AND METHODS

Study sites. Of the five study sites (Fig. 1), Farm 1 was located near Tallahassee in an area of well-drained soil and mixed woodland. The owners bred Appaloosa and Arabian horses. Farm 2 housed the research herd of the College of Veterinary Medicine, a mixture of ponies and horses on

College of Veterinary Medicine, University of Florida, Gainesville, Florida 32610.

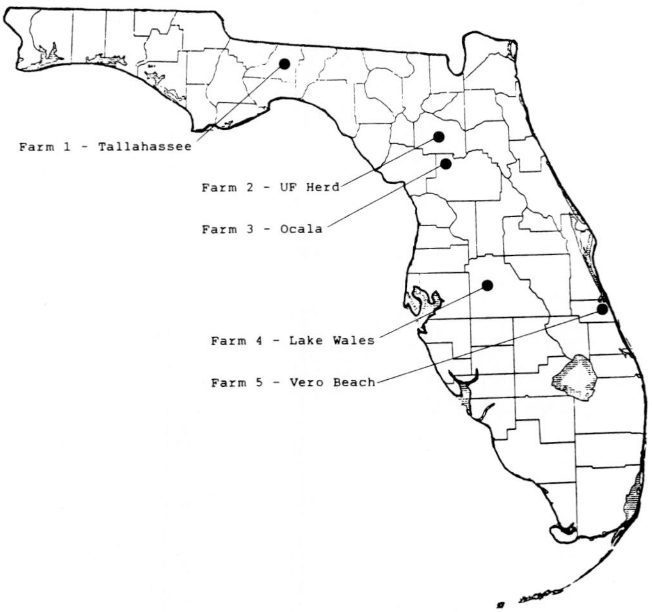

Fig. 1. Geographic locations of horse farms in Florida used in vaccination studies in monitoring for EEE.

Table 1. History of foals used in studies on vaccination against eastern equine encephalitis

Location in Florida	No. of foals at beginning of study	Foals lost to study	No. of foals available after 12 mo.
Farm 1	12	1 died shortly after birth; 11 sold when weaned	0
Farm 2	16 (not vaccinated)	1 died at 3 weeks of age; 6 sold when weaned	9
Farm 3	18	4 sold when weaned	14
Farm 4	11	1 died at 7 months of age; 7 sold when weaned	3
Farm 5	10	9 sold when weaned	1
Totals	67	40	27

pastures close to a large swamp. On Farm 3, an Arabian breeding operation near Ocala, most of the land drained well, but at the beginning of the study there were areas of wet woodlands and swamps. In 1983-84, three young vaccinated horses had died of EEE on this farm. Farm 4, 12 miles west of Lake Wales in central Florida, was well-drained land near a large lake where the owners bred and raced Quarter Horses. Farm 5 was on the outskirts of Vero Beach, approximately 8 miles inland on poorly draining soil near areas of pine woodland. The owners bred and showed palominos and Quarter Horses. The veterinarian on each farm cooperated fully with the study.

Vaccination and monitoring. At each location, at least 10 pregnant mares were entered in the study. Each had been vaccinated previously but was revaccinated approximately three weeks before the anticipated date of parturition. Samples of colostrum and serum were collected from each mare within 12 hr of foaling. The protocol called for bleeding the foals when one day old and monthly thereafter only during calendar year 1985, or until lost to the study (Table 1), but it was possible to follow some foals for a longer period. After the youngest of the foals at each study site had reached four months of age, they were bled as a group on the first Monday of each month.

With the exception of the foals at the College of Veterinary Medicine, which were left unvaccinated to provide comparative data on the decline of passive immunity, all available foals were vaccinated at three, four, and ten months of age with one dose of an inactivated EEE/WEE vaccine (Encephaloid, Fort Dodge Laboratories, Fort Dodge, Iowa). The vaccine contained virus propagated in cell culture, inactivated with formalin, and combined with aluminum phosphate as the adjuvant.

Laboratory procedures. Antibody titers to EEE virus were determined using a hemagglutination inhibition (HI) test (Clarke & Casals 1958) with standardized reagents supplied by the U.S. Centers for Disease Control, Atlanta, Georgia. The serum neutralization test used BHK 21 cell cultures and incorporated approximately 100 tissue-culture infective doses ($TCID_{50}$) of EEE virus and doubling dilutions of sera (Parker et al. 1975). All sera were also examined in parallel for HI antibodies to WEE, VEE, and St. Louis encephalitis viruses. Fat and cell debris was removed from the colostrum samples by centrifugation before examination in the HI test.

RESULTS

Passive immunity of the foal. The mares, which were vaccinated approximately three weeks prior to foaling, generally had a serum HI antibody titer to EEE virus of 40 to 160 at parturition. The colostral samples had similar values, and the serum titer in the foal at one day of age closely reflected the colostral titer. Thus by analogy, the serum titer of the mare was found to be an indicator of the titer of the passive immunity acquired by the foal.

The titer of colostral-derived antibody in foals diminished progressively. At two months of age, 23% of all foals in the study had antibody titers of less than 10 by the HI test. By the time of the first vaccination (three months), 50% (20/40) of the foals on Farms 1, 3, 4, and 5, had antibody titers of less

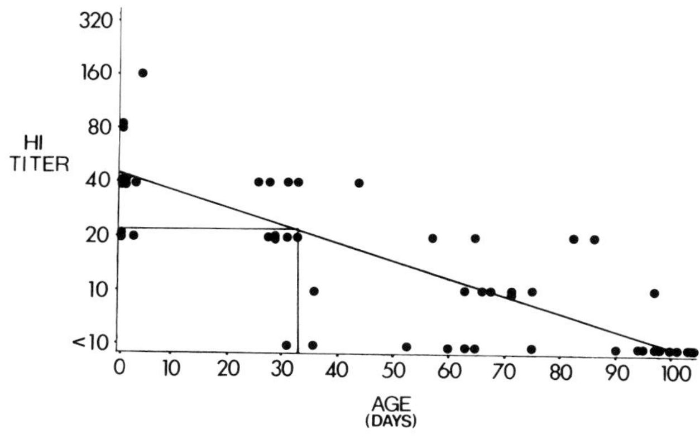

Fig. 2. Scattergram of diminishing HI antibody titers to EEE in sera of foals from vaccinated dams on Farm 2 at various intervals after parturition: N = 52; b_o = 42.952 (y - intercept); b_i = 0.449 (slope of the regression line); half-life = 33 days.

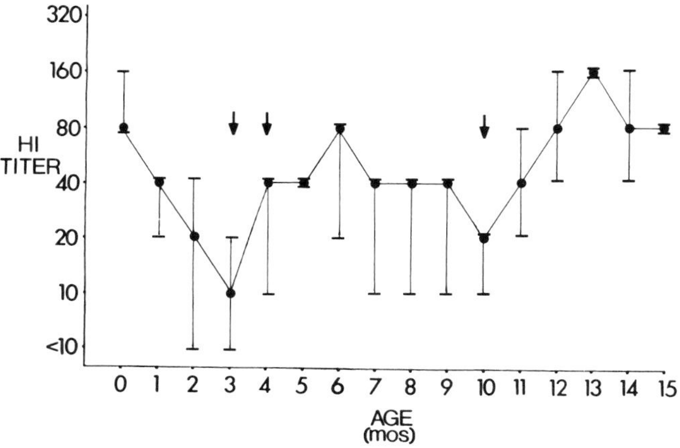

Fig. 3. Mode hemagglutination inhibition titers to EEE virus in foals vaccinated at 3, 4, and 10 months of age.

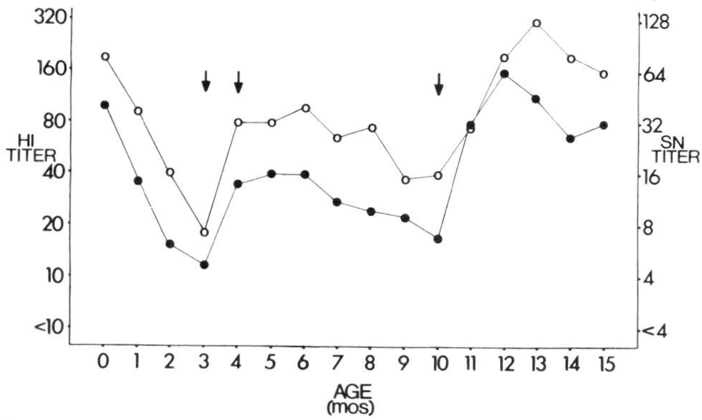

Fig. 4. Mean virus neutralization and HI titers in sera of foals on Farm 4 vaccinated against EEE virus at 3, 4, and 10 months of age.

than 10. Regression analysis of the data for the 16 foals that were left unvaccinated on Farm 2 indicated a half-life of 33 days for colostral antibody to EEE virus (Fig. 2).

Response to vaccination. Colostrally derived HI antibody titers of less than 10 did not appear to interfere with vaccination of foals at three months. Ninety-three percent (28/30) of such foals demonstrated a serological rise in titer. Seventy percent (7/10) of foals with titers greater than 20 did not show a rise in titer. At four months, prior to the second vaccination, all vaccinated foals had detectable antibodies although some of them (3/42; 7%) had a titer of only 10.

Administration of the second dose of vaccine did not necessarily induce a detectable rise in antibodies, but the majority of foals in the study, (38/42; 90%), maintained, or attained, an antibody titer of greater than 40.

Before the third vaccination, at 10 months of age, the antibody titers of nearly half of the remaining foals (13/27; 48%) had fallen to less than 20. The mode of the HI antibody titer for the entire group was 20 to 10 months. Vaccination at 10 months resulted in an anamnestic response. At 11 months, titers were generally higher (mode 80 for 11/26, or 42%) than following the four-month vaccination (mode 40 for 24/42 or 57%). The data for Farm 4 are summarized in Figure 3.

Neutralization antibody titers to EEE virus paralleled the HI titers (Fig. 4). HI antibody to WEE virus followed a trend similar to that for EEE virus.

DISCUSSION

The literature on the vaccination of horses against EEE and WEE is replete with remarks that comparatively little is known about either the protection provided by vaccination or the response of horses to inactivated vaccines (Byrne 1969; Gutekunst 1969; Ferguson, Reeves & Hardy 1979; Eisner & Nusbaum 1979). Despite these reservations, the safety and efficacy of the vaccines have seldom been doubted (Gutekunst 1969). While experience in Florida indicates that vaccination of horses two years of age or older will provide protection, the recent history of EEE cases in young vaccinated horses challenged this broad assumption. This study focused on the practice of foal vaccination, the cause of most concern to clinicians. The vaccination program adopted for this study was based upon one most frequently used by practitioners in Florida (Wilson et al. 1986). The AVMA Council on Biologic and Therepeutic Agents (1984) recommends vaccination at three months, to be repeated in one to two months.

In general, the vaccination program was successfully established and the monitoring maintained on each of the farms. Nevertheless, many foals were at times moved from the study sites to allow their dams to be bred; for example, several mares from Farm 3 were taken to Kentucky or Ohio. Despite the goodwill and cooperation of the owners and the veterinarians on the farms to which the mares had been sent, a

Table 2. Current recommendations for vaccination against EEE in Florida

Adults	Start with 2 doses 3-4 weeks apart. Revaccinate every 6 months (March-Aug. or Feb.-July).
Broodmares	Schedule spring revaccination 3-4 weeks prior to foaling.
Foals	Determine success of passive transfer. Vaccinate at 3, 4, and 6 months; then every 6 months.

complete monthly collection of serum from every foal in the study was not possible.

No clinical cases of EEE occurred on any of the farms during the study; indeed the reported incidence of EEE throughout Florida was lower than normal in 1985 (35 laboratory-confirmed cases). For legal reasons, no foals could be left unvaccinated on the privately owned farms to indicate subclinical infections. Since past experience indicates that infection with EEE virus causes a higher HI antibody titer than vaccination, and since no foal developed an antibody titer in excess of 160, our interpretation was that subclinical infection of the foals did not occur during the study.

In this study, foals were monitored over a longer period than previously (Eisner & Nusbaum 1979; Ferguson, Reeves & Hardy 1979). Several of the foals that responded to vaccination at three or four months demonstrated a decline in detectable antibody at seven or eight months. This may explain why cases of EEE can occur in vaccinated young horses. Although low levels of detectable antibody cannot be equated with susceptibility, it is prudent to regard such foals as vulnerable to infection until proven otherwise. Designing a suitable vaccine schedule then becomes difficult. To paraphrase Eisner and Nusbaum (1979), it would appear that vaccination before six months of age fails to immunize many foals, leaving them susceptible to encephalitis at an inopportune time. In spite of studies indicating that detectable passive immunity in the foal declines to insignificant levels by four months of age (Jeffcott 1974), foals of this age may not respond adequately to vaccination. On the other hand, when vaccination takes place only after six months, some foals may be unprotected at an early age if the dam provides little or no antibody at foaling.

Interference from persisting colostral immunity may not be the explanation for the poor response of foals to vaccination. When used as an inactivant, formalin is known to selectively denature different epitopes of respiratory syncytial virus (Murphy et al. 1986). Other unpublished studies in this laboratory have established that, in contrast to natural infection, formalin-inactivated EEE vaccines do not elicit a detectable IgM response in foals. Further, we suspect a state of immune tolerance may be induced when formalin-inactivated EEE vaccines are administered to the foal shortly after birth (a practice reported by 10% of veterinarians in Florida; Wilson et al. 1986). Whether these observations have any relevance to the cases of EEE seen in vaccinated horses in Florida is unknown.

There is no question that additional studies on experimental infections of vaccinated foals are needed to develop improved vaccination programs for EEE. However, pragmatism dictates that a vaccination program for foals in Florida be advocated now. The program outlined in Table 2 is the one presently recommended.

ACKNOWLEDGMENTS

We would like to acknowledge the support of the owners and veterinarians of the horses in this study; the enthusiasm of Drs. I. Barineau, R. Bloomer, F. Ryland, T. Schotman, and R. Banks ensured its success. We would also like to thank the American Veterinary Medical Association and Dr. John Schnackel of Fort Dodge Laboratories for their support of this project.

REFERENCES

American Veterinary Medical Association Council on Biologic and Therapeutic Agents (1984) Recommendation. *J. Am. Vet. Med. Assoc.* **185,** 32-34.

Bigler, W.J.; Lassing, E.B.; Buff, E.E.; Prather, E.C.; Beck, E.C.; and Hoff, G.L. (1976) Endemic eastern equine encephalomyelitis in Florida: a twenty-year analysis, 1955-1974. *Am. J. Trop. Med. Hyg.* **23,** 884-90.

Byrne, R.J. (1969) Immunity against eastern and western equine encephalomyelitis viruses. *J. Am. Vet. Med. Assoc.* **155,** 364-68.

Clarke, D.H., and Casals, J. (1958) Techniques for hemagglutination and hemagglutination-inhibition with arthropod-borne viruses. *Am. J. Trop. Med. Hyg.* **7,** 561-62.

Eisner, R.J., and Nusbaum, S.R. (1979) A study to determine the optimum time for vaccination of foals against eastern and western encephalitis viruses. *Proc. 22nd Ann. Meet. Am. Assoc. Vet. Lab. Diagn.*, pp. 435-48.

Ferguson, J.A.; Reeves, W.C.; and Hardy, J.L. (1979) Studies on immunity to alphaviruses in foals. *Am. J. Vet. Res.* **40,** 5-10.

Gibbs, E.P.J. (1975) Equine viral encephalitis. *Equine Vet. J.* **8,** 66-71.

Gutekunst, D.E. (1969) Immunity to bivalent tissue culture origin equine encephalomyelitis vaccine. *J. Am. Vet. Med. Assoc.* **155,** 368-74.

Hayes, R.O. (1981) Eastern and western encephalitis. In *CRC Handbook Series in Zoonoses*, Section B: Viral Zoonoses, pp. 29-57. Eds. J. H. Steele and G.W. Beran. CRC Press, Boca Raton, Fla.

Jeffcott, L.B. (1974) Studies on passive immunity in the foal. *J. Comp. Path,* **84,** 93-101.

Monath, T.P. (1979) Arthropod-borne encephalitides in the Americas. *Bull. Wld. Hlth. Org.* **57,** 513-33.

Murphy, B.R.; Alling, D.W.; Snyder, M.H.; Walsh, E.E.; Prince, G.A.; Chanock, V.G.H.; Rodriquez, W.J.; Kim, H.W.; Graham, B.S.; and Wright, P.F. (1986) Effect of age and preexisting antibody on serum antibody response of infants and children to the F and G glycoproteins during respiratory syncytial virus infection. *J. Clin. Microbiol.* **24(5)**, 894-98.

Parker, J.; Herniman, K.A.J.; Gibbs, E.P.J.; and Sellers, R.F. (1975) An experimental inactivated vaccine against bluetongue. *Vet. Rec.* **96,** 284-87.

Walton, T.E. (1981) Venezuelan, eastern and western encephalomyelitis. In *Virus Diseases of Food Animals,* Vol. 2, pp. 587-625. Ed. E.P.J. Gibbs. Academic Press, London.

Wilson, J.H.; Rubin, H.L.; Lane, T.J.; Gibbs, E.P.J. (1986) A survey of eastern equine encephalomyelitis in Florida horses: prevalence, economic impact, and management practices, 1982-83. *Prev. Vet. Med.* **4,** 261-71.

Evaluation of a Vaccine for Equine Monocytic Ehrlichiosis (Potomac Horse Fever)

Miodrag Ristic, Cynthia J. Holland, and Thomas E. Goetz

SUMMARY

A commercially produced *Ehrlichia risticii* vaccine, intended for protection of horses against equine monocytic ehrlichiosis (EME, Commonly known as Potomac horse fever), has been evaluated in a series of four experiments of vaccination and artificial-challenge exposure. In the first two experiments the vaccine was administered subcutaneously and in the last two, intramuscularly, each time in the lateral cervical region. A local reaction at the site of inoculation was usually noted when the vaccine was administered subcutaneously but not so with the intramuscular route. All vaccinated and control ponies were challenge-exposed by intravenous inoculation of 2.5×10^8 cell-free *E. risticii* at four weeks following the second vaccine dose. The protection criteria included days and degrees of fever, depression, and diarrhea, and number of days of anorexia. Postvaccinal and postchallenge immune responses were measured by the indirect fluorescent antibody (IFA) test.

Based on the above criteria, the average protection conferred to subcutaneously inoculated animals in Experiments 1 and 2 was 77.8%. The combined estimated average protection in intramuscularly inoculated ponies in Experiments 3 and 4 was also 77.8%. All control ponies developed clinical EME. Two of these ponies died and one was enthanized while in a comatose state. Consequently, there was a complete absence of "protection" in control animals in all four experiments. In general, clinical manifestations observed in vaccinated ponies were slight to moderate and of a relatively short course as compared with clinical signs of the majority of control ponies, which were greatly augmented and of longer duration.

The IFA titers were detectable at eight to 12 days following the first vaccine dose and increased significantly after the booster dose. After challenge exposure, vaccinated ponies showed an anamnestic antibody response, indicating the establishment of immunologic memory.

Under the conditions of the experiments and the protection criteria set forth, the vaccine appears to be safe and effective for use in the field.

Departments of Veterinary Pathobiology (Ristic, Holland) and Veterinary Clinical Medicine (Goetz), College of Veterinary Medicine, University of Illinois, Urbana, Illinois 61801.

INTRODUCTION

EME has been recognized as an infectious disease of horses and ponies only since 1979 (Knowles et al. 1983). Clinical signs often associated with the disease are highly variable and may include any combination of the following: fever 102°-107°F), depression, anorexia, leukopenia followed by leukocytosis, mild to severe colic, mild to profuse ("pipestream") diarrhea, and laminitis (Whitlock et al. 1984). The mortality rate of affected horses has been reported to be as high as 30%.

In 1984 the etiologic agent was isolated from the blood monocytes of an experimentally infected pony and determined to be a new rickettsia of the genus *Ehrlichia* (Holland et al. 1985a). The development of a method for continuous in vitro propagation of the agent, *Ehrlichia risticii* (Holland et al. 1985b), provided for enough antigen to develop an IFA test for confirmatory serodiagnosis of EME (Ristic 1986). Since clinical signs and pathologic manifestations of EME are highly variable and often confused with other equine diseases, such as acute salmonellosis, the IFA test has proven to be an extremely valuable tool in confirmatory diagnosis of the disease. While EME was first recognized in Montgomery County, Maryland, it now appears to be well established throughout the country. The IFA test has, thus far, aided in the confirmed clinical diagnosis of EME in 29 states representing all regions of the United States and the province of Ontario, Canada (Fig. 1). Although it has not yet been confirmed, EME is suspected to occur in other countries as well. While the identity of the vector responsible for transmission of EME is still unknown, it is of interest to note the geographic correlation between states in which EME has been found and the incidence of *Dermacentor variabilis*, the American dog tick (Fig. 1). A significant prevalence of subclinical infections has been suggested based upon a recent serologic survey of horses in Illinois with no previous history of EME. Results of the survey revealed that approximately 24% of 1,400 horses sampled had antibodies reactive against *E. risticii* (Goetz et al. 1986).

Historically, rickettsial vaccines have been found more effective in experimental animals than in the humans for whom they were intended. Early chicken embryo–derived vaccines for *Rickettsia rickettsii* and *R. prowazeki* containing egg protein contaminants were not protective. More recent human studies with cell culture-derived *R. rickettsii* vaccine showed only partial protection against Rocky Mountain spotted fever, but the vaccine did serve to ameliorate the illness when it occurred (Clements et al. 1983).

Until now, no vaccines have been developed for any of the diseases caused by agents of the genus *Ehrlichia*, such as canine ehrlichiosis, caused by *E. canis*, and equine ehrlichiosis, caused by *E. equi*. Similar to *E. ristícii*, *E. canis* is a monocytic invader whereas *E. equi* has a predilection for blood neutrophils (Ristic & Huxsoll 1984).

Studies on protective immunity with members of the genus *Ehrlichia* have been limited to *E. canis* and *E. equi*. Infection-immunity seems to be a functional protective mechanism in infections with *E. canis*, while conclusive evidence of sterile immunity has been demonstrated in horses recovered from experimentally induced infections with *E. equi* (Nyindo et al. 1978). Studies with *E. canis* demonstrated that the maximal destruction of this organism depends on the interaction between humoral and cellular immune responses (Lewis & Ristic 1978; Lewis, Hill & Ristic 1978). Researchers have suggested that the induction of cell-mediated immunity (CMI) to other rickettsiae in humans may be the most important correlate of protection against intracellular rickettsial infection (Clements et al. 1983; Shirai et al. 1976). Among other factors, the ability to induce CMI depends on the choice of the adjuvant. In humans, the choice is basically limited to aluminum hydroxide (Clements et al. 1983). On the other hand, the choice of adjuvants for use in animals is much broader, which may explain why immunization with rickettsial vaccines is more successful in animals than in humans.

In a series of studies on protective immunity to *E. risticii*, it was established that recovery from an infection results in resistance to clinical disease when subsequently challenged (Whitlock et al. 1985; Ristic et al. 1987). All efforts to culture the organism from the blood and solid tissues (for example, spleen, bone marrow, liver, and colonic or mesenteric lymph nodes) of clinically recovered horses have failed (Ristic et al. 1987). These findings led to the preliminary conclusion that the protective immunity against EME is of the sterile type. Consequently, development of immunoprophylactic methods was deemed possible.

The purpose of this study was to evaluate the safety and efficacy of a commercially produced *E. risticii* vaccine.

Distribution of *Dermacentor variabilis* and *Ehrlichia risticii* in the United States

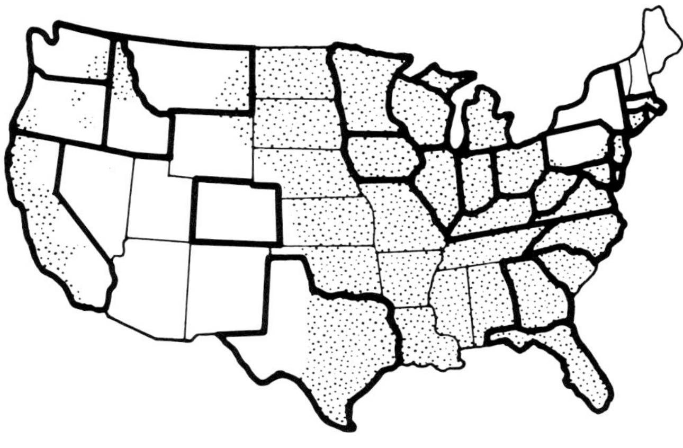

Fig. 1. Distribution of EME in continental United States. Note close geographic correlation between distribution of disease and incidence of *Dermacentor variabilis*, the American dog tick.

MATERIALS AND METHODS

Vaccine. The vaccine P.H.F.-Vax (Schering Animal Health, Elkorne, Neb.) is an inactivated, adjuvant-fortified suspension of cell-free *E. risticii*. The recommended use of the vaccine is two 1-ml initial doses given intramuscularly at 21-day intervals, followed by an annual booster dose.

Experimental animals and vaccination procedures. In all four vaccination experiments, ponies of various breeds and ages and both sexes were used. Before each experiment, each animal received anthelmintic treatment and was vaccinated against influenza, strangles, and rhinopneumonitis. In addition, each pony was proven negative for antibodies to *E. risticii* using the IFA test. The ponies were kept outdoors prior to challenge, and indoors in climate-controlled insect-proof isolation units following challenge. All animals were fed a diet of grass/alfalfa hay and grain (Omolene; Purina Feeds, St. Louis, Mo.) An automatic water supply was available outside and in each stall. The 40 ponies were divided among experiments as follows: Experiment 1, five ponies; Experiment 2, eight; Experiment 3, twelve; Experiment 4, fifteen ponies. Vaccinated ponies received two 1-ml doses at 21-day intervals. In the first two experiments, the vaccine was administered subcutaneously, while in the last two it was administered intramuscularly. Inoculation in both routes utilized the lateral cervical region. Following vaccination, animals were observed daily for any adverse effects, including fever and local tissue reactions.

Challenge and protection criteria. In all four experiments, animals were challenged at approximately four weeks following the second vaccine dose. Challenge consisted of an intravenous inoculation of 2.5×10^8 cell-free *E. risticii* that were propagated in primary canine blood monocytes (Holland et al. 1985a). Following challenge, all animals were observed twice daily for 30 days for any clinical signs of disease. The protection criteria included days and degrees of fever, depression, and diarrhea, and number of days of anorexia. The degrees of depression and diarrhea were graded as follows:

Depression: 1+ = reduced activity; 2+ = listless attitude; 3+ = total lack of alertness; 4+ = comatose.

Table 1. Vaccine trial 1: Clinical responses following challenge of vaccinated and nonvaccinated (control) ponies

Animal ID No.	IFA titer at challenge[a]	Response (D = No. of days postchallenge)				Protection
		Fever	Depression	Anorexia	Diarrhea	
Vaccinated						
86	1:2560	102 (D6); 102.2 (D7)	None	None	None	Yes
87	1:1280	102 (D13)	2+(D19-21)	None	2+ (D19-21)	No
88	1:10	102.4 (D6); 102 (D10)	None	None	None	Yes
Control						
19	<1:10	102-106 (D11-16)	3+(D10-16)	(D11-16)	3+(D13) 4+(D14-16)	No (comatose D16; euthanized)
68	<1:10	102 (D8); 102-104 (D10-15)	3+ (D10-20) 2+ (D21-22)	(D10-19)	3+ (D12-19)	No

[a] <1:10 = negative at a baseline dilution of 1:10.

Diarrhea: 1+ = soft, moist stool; 2+ = cowpie; 3+ = green running diarrhea; 4+ = pipestream (brownish water). Experiments were terminated at one month following challenge.

Serology. Two weeks before vaccination and throughout the postvaccination and postchallenge periods, serum samples were collected twice weekly from vaccinated and control animals for examination in the IFA test. The organism used for the IFA test was propagated in the continuous murine macrophage cell line P388D1 at 37°C in an atmosphere of 5% CO_2 in air. The procedure used to prepare *E. risticii* antigen for the IFA test has been described (Ristic et al. 1986). Beginning at a predetermined baseline dilution of 1:10, serial twofold dilutions of the test sera were made in 0.15-M phosphate-buffered saline (PBS). Fluorescein-conjugated rabbit antihorse immunoglobulin G was obtained commercially (Cooper Diagnostics, West Chester, Pennsylvania).

RESULTS

Experiment 1. The first experiment, the smallest of the four, utilized three vaccinated and two control ponies (Table 1). At approximately 24 hours following subcutaneous administration of the vaccine, all three vaccinated ponies showed slight swelling at the inoculation site, approximately 2cm in diameter. The swelling gradually disappeared over three to six days. Within nine days following the primary vaccine dose, all three ponies showed antibodies to *E. risticii* as demonstrated by the IFA test. The maximum titer after the first vaccine dose was 1:320; after the second dose, 1:2560.

Following challenge, all three vaccinated ponies showed transitory fever (102°-102.4°F), limited to one or two days. Pony 87 showed 2+ degree of depression and diarrhea on Days 19-21 postchallenge (p.c.) and was not considered to be protected. The remaining two vaccinates, 86 and 88, remained clinically healthy throughout the postchallenge study period.

The two control ponies, 19 and 68, had persistent fever for at least five days beginning on Days 11 and 10, respectively. The temperature range for Pony 19 was 102°-106°F and for Pony 68, 102°–104°F. Similarly, both ponies showed persistent depression, anorexia, and diarrhea ranging between 3+ and 4+. Pony 19 became comatose and was euthanized on Day 16 p.c. Pony 68 showed clinical recovery on day 22 p.c. Accordingly, in Experiment 1, two out of three (67%) of the vaccinated ponies were clinically protected from challenge exposure to *E. risticii*, whereas a complete absence of protection was noted in the two control ponies.

Experiment 2. Six ponies were vaccinated and two served as nonvaccinated controls (Table 2). No adverse clinical changes were observed in any of the vaccinated ponies with the exception of a local reaction (swelling) at the site of injection, as described in the previous experiment. Following the first vaccination, all recipients seroconverted for *E. risticii* antibodies by Day 11 postinjection (p.i.), with ponies 214 and 220 becoming positive by Day 8 p.i. Maximum average IFA titers of 1:320 and 1:640 were recorded on Days 15 and 13 following the first and the second vaccine dose, respectively. Titers of individual ponies at the time of challenge are shown in Table 2.

Pony 216 developed a mild case of EME, but none of the remaining five vaccinates showed any clinical abnormalities other than a slight transitory increase in temperature (101.7°-102.8°F) between Days 10 and 18 p.c. Throughout the 30-day p.c. study period, all of the five ponies maintained a bright and alert attitude and a normal appetite, and no signs of abnormal feces were observed. Pony 216 remained clinically normal until Day 18 p.c., at which time a temperature of 102°F was recorded. On Day 20 p.c., Pony 216 was afebrile but developed severe diarrhea (3+ to 4+), which lasted two days, followed by soft feces (1+) for three days. However, this pony showed no signs of anorexia and only mild depression on Days 20-21.

On day 12 p.c., both control ponies, 211 and 218, developed fevers—102°F and 102.4°F, respectively—which subsided by Day 13. No other abnormalities were observed in

Table 2. Vaccine trial 2: Clinical responses following challenge of vaccinated and nonvaccinated (control) ponies

Animal ID No.	IFA titer at challenge[a]	Response (D = No. of days postchallenge)				Protection
		Fever	Depression	Anorexia	Diarrhea	
Vaccinated						
214	1:640	102.6(D10); 101.7(D11)	None	None	None	Yes
216	1:20	103.2(D10); 102(D18)	2+(D20, 21)	None	3+(D20,21) 1+(D22-24)	No
217	1:320	102(D11); 102(D15)	None	None	None	Yes
219	1:40	102(D15)	None	None	None	Yes
220	1:640	102.8(D11); 102.7(D15)	None	None	None	Yes
221	1:160	102.2(D11); 101.8(D15)	None	None	None	Yes
Control						
211	<1:10	102(D6);102(D12); 102-102.5(D15-19)	3+(D16-21); 2+(D22-25)	(D16-24)	2+(D19-21)	No
218	<1:10	102(D8); 102(D11); 102.4(D12); 104.6(D15); 103.8-104(D16-19)	3+(D15-23); 2+(D24-30);	(D15-31)	3+(D16-17) 4+(D18-24) 3+(D25-29) 2+(D30)	No

[a] <1:10 = negative at a baseline dilution of 1:10.

Table 3. Vaccine trial 3: Clinical responses following challenge of vaccinated and nonvaccinated (control) ponies

Animal ID No.	IFA titer at challenge[a]	Response (D = No. of days postchallenge)				Protection
		Fever	Depression	Anorexia	Diarrhea	
Vaccinated						
46	1:10240	102-104(D11-13)	None	None	None	Yes
188	1:10240	102-102.6(D13-15)	None	None	None	Yes
189	1:1280	102(D15-17)	None	None	None	Yes
208	1:5120	102.4(D11)	1+(D19-20)	(D18-19)	3+(D19-21)	No
223	1:320	None	None	None	None	Yes
225	1:10240	None	None	None	None	Yes
231	1:5120	None	None	None	None	Yes
239	1:640	102(D19)	3+(D19-20); 2+(D21-22)	(D19-22)	3+(D20-22)	No
Control						
206	<1:10	102-104.2(D15-24)	2+(D14); 3+(D15-19)	(D16-19)	None	No
207	<1:10	102-103.2(D13-18)	2+(D14-20); 1+(D21)	(D15-20)	2+(D19-20)	No
226	<1:10	102-103.6(D15-22)	2+(D15-16); 3+(D17-21); 4+(D22)	(D15-22)	4+(D17-22)	No (died D22)
242	<1:10	102.2-103.5(D14-17)	1+(D15); 3+(D16-22); 4+(D23)	(D15-23)	4+(D17-23)	No (comatose D23; euthanized)

[a] <1:10 = negative at a baseline dilution of 1:10.

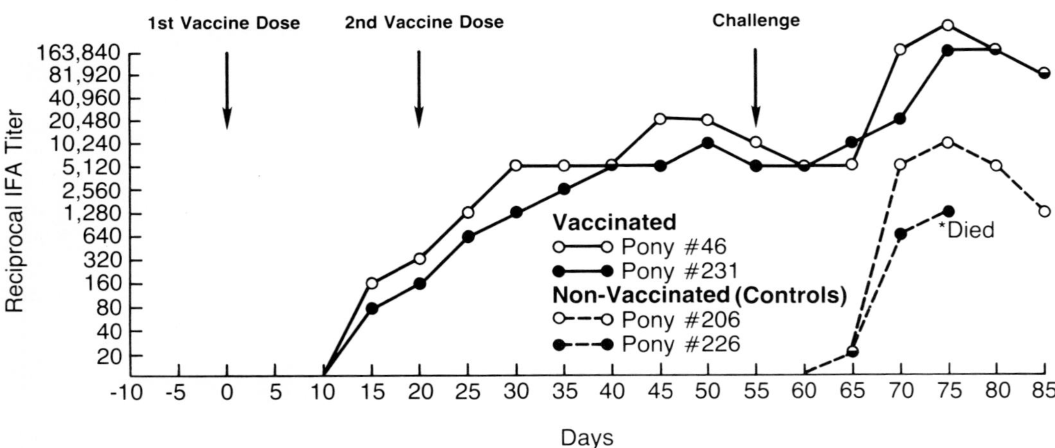

Fig. 2. Representative patterns of serologic response of two vaccinated and two control ponies in Experiment 3.

these two ponies until Day 15, when both began to show clinical signs of EME. On this day, a second increase in temperature (102°F) was noted in Pony 211. By Day 16 p.c., 211 became depressed and experienced 3+ anorexia and mild colic, with no fecal output. By Day 19 the temperature returned to normal but the pony remained depressed, with 2+ anorexia and 2+ diarrhea. This pony recovered uneventfully by Day 25 p.c. Seroconversion in the IFA test was first observed on Day 9 at a titer of 1:20, with a maximum IFA titer of 1:10,240 being recorded on Day 29.

Pony 218 remained clinically normal until Day 15 p.c., when this pony experienced fever (104.6°F), depression, anorexia (3+), and mild to moderate colic. On Day 16, its status was febrile (104°F), severely depressed, weak, and anorexic (4+). At this time, Pony 218 developed 3+ diarrhea, which became 4+ in character (profuse brown water) by Day 18. The pony became too weak to stand and spent most of the time lying down. Severe dehydration was evident, along with signs of hemoconcentration, marked increase in respiration (greater than 100/min), and a decrease in blood pressure. By Day 26, Pony 218 began to show gradual clinical improvement and recovered by Day 34. A positive IFA response was first recorded on Day 13 p.c. (1:40), reaching a maximum titer of 1:10,240 by Day 29.

Experiment 3. In this experiment, utilizing eight vaccinated and four control ponies (Table 3), no adverse clinical changes were observed following vaccination via the intramuscular route. All vaccinated ponies demonstrated seroconversion for antibodies to *E. risticii* by Day 13 after the first injection. Maximum antibody titers prior to the second injection ranged from 1:160 to 1:2560. Significantly higher IFA titers were recorded in each of the eight vaccinated ponies following the second dose. At the time of challenge, antibody titers of vaccinated ponies ranged from 1:320 to 1:10,240. All four control ponies remained clinically healthy and serologically negative throughout the prechallenge study period.

Following challenge, three ponies of the vaccinated group (223, 225, and 231) showed no clinical signs of any kind, including fever. Three other ponies (46, 188, and 189) developed a mild to moderate degree of fever following challenge for three-day periods, as follows: No. 46, 102°-104°F on Days 11-13; No. 188, 102°-102.6°F, Days 13-15: and No. 189, 102°F, Days 15-17. However, no other clinical signs of EME were observed. These six ponies were considered protected. The remaining two ponies vaccinated, 208 and 239, were not considered protected from challenge. Although the maximum temperature of vaccinated Pony 208 was only 102.4° (Day 11), this animal experienced anorexia on Days 18-19, 1+ depression on days 19-20, and 3+ diarrhea on Days 19-21 p.c. Similarly, Pony 239 showed an increased temperature of 102°F (Day 19), depression (Days 19-22), anorexia (Days 19-22), and 3+ diarrhea (Days 20-22).

An interesting pattern of serologic response following challenge of the above vaccinated ponies was an accelerated anamnestic reaction preceded by an early decrease in IFA titers (Fig. 2).

Following challenge, all control ponies developed clinical signs of EME beginning on Days 13-15 p.c. Pony 206 developed fever (102°-104°F, Days 15-24), depression (Days 14-19), and anorexia (Days 16-19). However, this pony showed no signs of diarrhea. Pony 207 experienced a similar pattern of fever, depression, and anorexia but also developed 2+ diarrhea on Days 19-20 p.c. The other two control ponies, 226 and 242, became severely affected by EME. Pony 226 developed fever (102°-103.6°F, Days 15-22), 2+ to 4+ depression (Days 15-22), anorexia (Days 15-22), and 4+ diarrhea (Days 17-22). This pony died on Day 22 p.c. Pony 242 developed fever (102.2°-103.5°F, Days 14-17), 1+ to 4+ depression (Days 15-23), anorexia (Days 15-23) and 4+ diarrhea (Days 17-23). This pony became comatose on Day 23 and was euthanized for humane reasons, as death was inevitable.

All control ponies became seropositive for antibodies to

Table 4. Vaccine trial 4: Clinical responses following challenge of vaccinated and nonvaccinated (control) ponies

Animal ID No.	IFA titer at challenge[a]	Response (D = No. of days postchallenge)				Protection
		Fever	Depression	Anorexia	Diarrhea	
Vaccinated						
271	1:1280	102.8(D8)	None	None	None	Yes
275	1:10240	102.2(D7)	None	None	None	Yes
279	1:5120	102.4(D7)	None	None	None	Yes
297	1:5120	None	None	None	None	Yes
301	1:640	103.4(D7); 102(D13)	None	None	None	Yes
302	1:640	102.4(D7); 102.8(D8); 102(D29)	2+(D29-30)	(D29-30)	2+(D29-30)	No
306	1:5120	None	None	None	None	Yes
307	1:1280	None	None	None	None	Yes
309	1:640	102.3(D7); 103.8(D16)	1+(D17); 1+(D25-28)	(D17; D26-29)	1+(D29)	No
311[a]	1:1280	102(D7)	None	None	None	Yes
Control						
300	<1:10[b]	102.0-103.8 (D7-14)	1+(D10,14-15) 3+(D16-17)	D14-17	None	No
308	<1:10	103.4(D7); 102.8(D8) 103.2(D13); 102.2(D14-15)	1+(D10); 2+(D13-14); 3+(D15-17); 1+(D18-20)	D13-19	2+(D13); 3+(D14-17); 2+(D18); 1+(D19-20)	No
310	<1:10	102.1(D4); 102.8(D9-8); 103.4(D9); 102.2(D10); 103.6(D13); 102.0(D15-16)	1+(D13-14)	D13,15-16	1+(D13); 2+(D14-18)	No
328	<1:10	102.7(D7); 102.6(D13)	2+(D15); 3+(D16-18); 2+(D19-20); 3+(D21); 2+(D22-25); 1+(D26-27)	D15-21, 24; 26	3+(D15-27) 2+(D28-30)	No
330	<1:10	102.6-104.2(D1-5); 102.6(D7); 102.0-104.6(D9-11); 102.0-104.0(D14-16)	2+(D15-16); 3+(D17-18); 1+(D19-20); 2+(D21); 1+(D22-25)	D15-23	3+(D19-20); 2+(D21-27); 1+(D28-30)	No

[a] Delivered full-term health foal Day 28 postchallenge.
[b] <1:10 = negative at a baseline dilution of 1:10.

E. risticii by Day 10 p.c. Maximum IFA titers ranged from 1:2560 to 1:10,240. These values were considerably lower than those for the vaccinated ponies, which ranged from a low peak of 1:80,920 (Pony 239) to a maximum IFA peak of 1:655,360 (Pony 46).

Based on established criteria, 75% protection was demonstrated among the eight vaccinated ponies and 0% protection among the controls.

Experiment 4. In this last and largest experiment (Table 4), there were 10 vaccinated and five control ponies. As in Experiment 3, no changes were visible at the site of the intramuscularly administered vaccine. All vaccinated ponies seroconverted by Day 12 following the first vaccine dose. Maximum antibody titers in these ponies prior to the second dose ranged from 1:80 to 1:1280. Following the second vaccine dose, the IFA titers increased to a range of 1:1280 to 1:20,480. Titers of individual vaccinated ponies recorded at the time of challenge are given in Table 4. All control ponies remained negative in the IFA test throughout the postvaccination period.

Most vaccinated ponies showed a transitory fever on Day 7 p.c. In no instance did the fever persist for more than two consecutive days. No sign of depression, anorexia, or diarrhea was noted in eight of the vaccinated ponies. The remaining two, 302 and 309, experienced slight depression and anorexia and mild diarrhea.

Of special interest among the eight fully protected animals

was No. 311. It was obvious at the time of challenge that this pony was in foal, but the stage of gestation was not known. On Day 28 postchallenge she delivered a full-term, healthy foal.

All five control ponies developed clinical signs of EME. Persistent fever was common for most of them. While the majority of ponies began the febrile phase after the first postchallenge week, Pony 330 showed fever as early as Day 1 p.c. Depression and anorexia were common in all five controls. Only one, Pony 300, showed no signs of diarrhea, while the remaining four developed various degrees of rather persistent diarrhea. As a result of the clinical manifestations, all controls lost considerable body weight and were easily distinguishable from vaccinated ponies, which maintained their condition throughout the experiment.

The protection rate among vaccinated ponies was 80% and among control ponies, 0%.

DISCUSSION

Under the conditions of the experiments and the protection criteria set forth, the vaccine for EME appears to be safe and effective. The primary reason for resorting to the intramusuclar route of inoculation in Experiments 3 and 4 was to avoid any local reaction, usually noted when the vaccine was administered subcutaneously. The intramuscular route fully accomplished its purpose, leaving no evidence of local tissue change or soreness—i.e., swelling and induration at the site of inoculation—in any of the vaccinated ponies.

Transitory fever, as noted in most vaccinated ponies following challenge exposure, was believed to be immunologically mediated, arising when vaccination-generated immune elements interacted with the massive influx of the intravenously administered challenge. Thus, unless the fever persisted beyond three consecutive days, only anorexia, depression, and diarrhea were considered in determining the presence or absence of protection, since all control ponies developed various combinations of these three clinical signs. The three criteria were followed very strictly. For example, even a single day of anorexia in a vaccinated pony ruled out protection. On this basis, the average protection conferred on subcutaneously inoculated ponies in Experiments 1 and 2 was 77.8%. A combined estimated average protection in intramuscularly inoculated ponies in Experiments 3 and 4 was also 77.8%. There was a complete absence of "protection" in the control ponies of all four experiments. The clinical manifestations of the disease among controls varied to a great degree. The variations ranged from a short duration of fever, anorexia, and depression but no diarrhea, to a long course (more than two weeks) of full clinical disease, including severe diarrhea followed by recovery or death. One must conclude that the susceptibility to artificial infection with *E. risticii* differs greatly among individual ponies. This conclusion agrees with our earlier observations under laboratory and field conditions.

At the time of the original isolation of *E. risticii* in the fall of 1984 (Holland et al. 1985a), we inoculated one pony and one horse each by intravenous administration of 50 ml of whole blood derived from a horse acutely affected with EME. Although inoculum from the same source was administered to both animals, only the pony developed clinical EME. However, the horse, too, showed serologic evidence of infection (Ristic et al. 1986).

Similar observations were made during a seroepidemiologic study in an endemic area of Maryland. On a farm there with a history of EME, six horses converted from a seronegative to a seropositive status during the summer of 1985. Two of the horses died with clinical signs of EME and two others experienced a mild form of the disease, but there was no clinical evidence of EME in the remaining two. The data is further substantiated by the results of a serologic survey of healthy horses in Illinois discussed earlier (Goetz et al. 1986). This pattern of clinical inconsistency after challenge exposure—ranging from asymptomatic to severe clinical disease and death—is not unique for EME; it has been well documented in other infectious diseases caused by leukocytic and erythrocytic rickettsial agents (Ristic 1980; Keefe, et al. 1982).

Another point that demands some consideration is the relationship between the challenge dose in these studies and the one that horses may be exposed to under field conditions. One does not propose that a suspected vector would instantaneously deliver a dose of the organism at the level of 2.5×10^8. Nevertheless, acutely affected animals are readily seen in endemic areas of natural exposure, attesting to a fulminating form of the disease that may end in mortality. Given this, the experimental data generated in this study indicate the value of the vaccine. A more valid estimation as to its efficacy should be forthcoming after two to three years of experience in the field.

In this study, all ponies were challenge-exposed approximately four weeks after the second vaccine dose. Accordingly, the duration of protection imparted by this vaccine cannot be answered by the results of this study. Humoral antibody responses peak at approximately three weeks following the second dose and then gradually decline. There was also an indication of an anamnestic antibody response following challenge of vaccinated ponies, indicating the establishment of immunologic memory. Long-term protection studies with the vaccine, however, will be needed to establish the actual duration of protection.

Among more recent studies on EME is the finding that the pathogenesis of this disease in a pregnant mare can include the transmission of *E. risticii* from the infected dam to the fetus (Dawson et al. 1987). Vaccinated animal No. 311 in the fourth experiment was apparently in the final month of gestation at the time of challenge. The pony remained clinically healthy throughout Day 28 postchallenge, when she delivered a healthy foal. Since an appropriate control was not available among nonvaccinated animals, it would not be proper at this time to suggest that vaccination of pregnant mares prevents fetal infection upon challenge exposure. Only studies specifically aimed at pregnant animals can determine the efficacy of the vaccine in protecting pregnant mares and their offspring against EME.

Only two years ago, EME was considered to be limited to a small sector in the eastern portion of the United States (Knowles et al. 1983). However, since the discovery of the etiologic agent and the development of serodiagnostic methods, the disease has now been recognized in all regions of the country. The impact of this newly recognized disease on the equine population of this country and possibly abroad is difficult to estimate at this time. Nevertheless, the availability of this first vaccine for prevention of EME, coupled with established serodiagnostic and therapeutic means, should provide the equine industry with a strong degree of safety and comfort when threatened by EME.

REFERENCES

Clements, M.L; Wisseman, C.L., Jr.; Woodward, T.E.; Fiset, P.; Dumier, J.S.; McNamee, W.; Black, R.E.; Rooney, J.; Hughes, T.P.; and Levine, N.M. (1983) Reactogenicity, immunogenicity, and efficacy of a chick embryo cell-derived vaccine for Rocky Mountain spotted fever. *J. Infect. Dis.* **148**, 922-30.

Dawson, J.; Ristic, M.; Holland, C.J.; Whitlock, R.; and Sessions, J.E. (1987) Isolation of *Ehrlichia risticii,* the causative agent of Potomac horse fever, from the fetus of an experimentally infected mare. *Vet. Rec.* **121,** 232.

Goetz, T.E.; Johnson, P.J.; Ristic, M.; Holland, C.J.; and Dawson, J. (1986) The serologic incidence of equine monocytic ehrlichiosis (synonym—Potomac horse fever) in selected areas of Illinois: A preliminary report. *Proc. 67th Ann. Conf. Res. Workers Anim. Dis.*, p. 62.

Holland, C.J.; Ristic, M.; Cole, A.I.; Johnson, P.; Baker, G.; and Goetz, T.E. (1985a) Isolation, experimental transmission, and characterization of causative agent of Potomac horse fever. *Science* **227,** 522-24.

Holland, C.J.; Weiss, F.; Burgdorfer, W.; Cole, A.I.; and Kakoma, I. (1985b) *Ehrlichia risticii* sp. nov.: etiological agent of equine monocytic ehrlichiosis (synonym, Potomac horse fever). *Int. J. Syst. Bacteriol.* **35,** 524-26.

Keefe, T.J.; Holland, C.J.; Salyer, P.A.; and Ristic, M. (1982) Distribution of *Ehrlichia canis* among military working dogs in the world and selected civilian dogs in the United States. *J. Am. Vet. Med. Assoc.* **181,** 236-38.

Knowles, R.C.; Anderson, D.W.; Shipley, W.D.; Whitlock, R.H.; Perry, B.D.; and Davidson, J.P. (1983) Acute equine diarrhea syndrome (AEDS): a preliminary report. *Proc. 29th Ann. Conv. Am. Assoc. Equine Practnr.* pp. 353-57.

Lewis, G.E., Jr., and Ristic, M. (1978) Effect of canine immune serum on the growth of *Ehrlichia canis. Am. J. Vet. Res.* **39,** 77-82.

Lewis, G.E., Jr.; Hill, S.L.; and Ristic, M. (1978) Effect of canine immune serum on the growth of *Ehrlichia canis* within nonimmune canine macrophages. *Am. J. Vet. Res.* **39,** 71-76.

Nyindo, M.B.A.; Ristic, M.; Lewis, G.E., Jr.; Huxsoll, D.L.; and Stephenson, E.H. (1978) Immune response of ponies to experimental infection with *Ehrlichia equi. Am. J. Vet. Res.* **39,** 15-18.

Ristic, M. (1980) Anaplasmosis. In *Bovine Medicine and Surgery,* Vol. 1, pp. 324-48. Ed. H.E. Amstutz. American Veterinary Publications, Santa Barbara, Calif.

Ristic, M., and Huxsoll, D.L. (1984) *Ehrlichieae. Bergey's Manual of Systematic Bacteriology*, Vol. 1, pp. 704-9. Ed. N.R. Krieg. Williams & Wilkens, Baltimore, Md.

Ristic, M.; Holland, C.J.; Dawson, J.E.; Sessions, J.; and Palmer, J. (1986) Diagnosis of equine monocytic ehrlichiosis (Potomac horse fever) by indirect immunofluorescence. *J. Am. Vet. Med. Assoc.*, **189,** 39-46.

Ristic, M.; Dawson, J.; Holland, C.J.; and Jenny, A. (1987) Susceptibility of dogs to *Ehrlichia risticii,* causative agent of Potomac horse fever. *Am. J. Vet. Res.* In press.

Shirai, A.; Cantazzro, P.J.; Phillips, S.M.; and Osterman, J.V. (1976) Host defenses in experimental scrub typhus: role of cellular immunity in heterologous protection. *Infect. Immun.* **14,** 39-46.

Whitlock, R.H.; Palmer, J.E.; Benson, C.E.; Acland, H.M.; Jenny, A.L.; and Ristic, M. (1984) Potomac horse fever: clinical characteristics and diagnostic features. *Proc. 27th Ann. Meet. Am. Assoc. Vet. Lab. Diagn.*, pp. 103-24.

Whitlock, R.H.; Perry, B.; Jenny, A.; Palmer, J.; Ristic, M.; Schmidtmann, E.; Holland, C.; Sessions, J.; Robl, M.; Rikihisa, Y.; Benson, C., Dutta, S.; and Meinersmann, R. (1985) Potomac horse fever: Update and research priorities. *Proc. 89th Ann. Meet. U.S. Anim. Health Assoc.*

Isolation of *Ehrlichia risticii* from the Fetus of a Mare with Potomac Horse Fever

Jacqueline E. Dawson, Miodrag Ristic, Cynthia J. Holland, Robert H. Whitlock, and Jean E. Sessions

SUMMARY

A mare experimentally infected with culture-derived *Ehrlichia risticii*, the causative agent of Potomac horse fever (PHF), developed clinical PHF and later recovered. Upon necropsy, four months after infection, it was determined that the mare had been in foal. *E. risticii* was isolated, in culture, from the spleen, bone marrow, and mesenteric and colonic lymph nodes of the fetus. This finding, along with an earlier observation that a precolostrum serum sample from a foal born to a PHF-affected mare contained *E. risticii* antibodies, strongly suggests that this organism may induce in utero infection. In another case, when a mare had clinical PHF at approximately two months' gestation, the fetus was naturally aborted at 10¾ months of gestation and proved to be serologically positive for antibodies to *E. risticii*. Other possible causes for the abortion were differentially excluded. These data are discussed in the context of a possible link between PHF and some cases of abortion.

INTRODUCTION

PHF was first recognized as a disease of equidae in Maryland in 1979 (Knowles et al 1983). In 1984, the isolation of *E. risticii*, the causative agent of PHF, was shortly followed by the development of a culture system suitable for continuous in vitro propagation of this agent (Holland et al. 1985a; Holland et al 1985b). Antigens generated by this method were then used for the development of an indirect fluorescent antibody (IFA) test for the detection of antibodies in horses affected by PHF (Ristic et al. 1986). By use of this test in conjunction with clinical signs, the disease has currently been diagnosed in 30 states of the United States and in the province of Ontario, Canada.

PHF has recently been confirmed in Alabama, Colorado, Massachusetts, Montana, Tennessee, and Wyoming. The disease is often characterized by fever, anorexia, depression, leukopenia, colic, and mild to severe diarrhea (Whitlock et al. 1984). However, an asymptomatic form of the disease has also been documented (Ristic et al. 1986).

Dawson, Ristic, Holland: Department of Veterinary Pathobiology, College of Veterinary Medicine, University of Illinois, Urbana, Illinois 61801. Whitlock: New Bolton Center, University of Pennsylvania, Kennett Square, Pennsylvania 19348. Sessions: Glenvilah Veterinary Clinic, Potomac, Maryland 20854.

Clinical observations (Sessions, unpublished data) indicate that abortions in some mares affected by PHF may be linked to fetal infection with *E. risticii*. Recently we experimentally infected a mare with *E. risticii* during the third month of gestation. In addition, a serological investigation was conducted on 10 foals born to dams with a history of PHF. We now report our observations on experimentally induced and naturally acquired PHF in pregnant mares and relate these data to the possible role of *E. risticii* in some abortion cases.

MATERIAL AND METHODS

Precolostral serum samples were collected from 10 foals born to mares with a known history of PHF. *E. risticii* antigen slides were prepared as described previously (Holland et al. 1985a). Beginning at a baseline dilution of 1:10, the IFA test was conducted to determine whether the sera of these foals contained *E. risticii* antibodies generated in utero. In addition, two of these foals, as well as their dams, were followed serologically for one year.

In a subsequent experiment, a pony was intravenously inoculated with a 1-ml suspension of 2.85×10^7 *E. risticii*. Four months after infection the mare was euthanized and necropsied. At necropsy, it was revealed that the mare had been approximately seven months pregnant. Tissue specimens were taken aseptically from both the dam and the fetus. These tissues included the spleen, liver, bone marrow, and mesenteric and colonic lymph nodes.

One gram of each of these tissues was ground in a tissue homogenizer containing 5 ml of culture medium. After manual homogenization, the suspension was allowed to sediment at room temperature.

One milliliter of each of the cell suspensions was added to primary canine monocyte cultures established 48 hr previously. The above cell cultures were propagated in 25-cm^2 tissue culture flasks at 37°C in Medium 199, 1% L-glutamine, and 20% heat-inactivated normal canine serum. Each culture was examined biweekly for evidence of infection with *E. risticii* using the Giemsa method (Nyindo et al. 1971).

Finally, a fetus aborted by a mare subsequent to naturally acquired PHF was subjected to gross and histopathologic examination, and various tissue specimens were collected for bacteriologic and serologic evaluation. Serologic tests were conducted for the following: equine rhinopneumonitis—di-

Table 1. Sequential indirect fluorescent antibody titers[a] of sera from two dams with a known history of PHF and from their foals.

		Months after foal's birth											
Precolostrum		1	2	3	4	5	6	7	8	9	10	11	12
Foal 1	40	80	160	320	160	160	640	1280	160	40	20	40	20
Dam 1	—	40	40	80	80	80	160	80	160	160	320	640	320
Foal 2	N[b]	80	80	40	20	10	10	10	N	N	N	N	N
Dam 2	—	40	80	160	320	640	1280	2560	2560	2560	640	1280	640

Note: Dam and foal samples were tested in parallel for direct comparison of titers.
[a] Reciprocal of dilution.
[b] N = no reaction at serum dilution of 1:10.

rect fluorescent antibody (FA) test, leptospirosis—microscopic agglutination lysis test, and PHF—indirect fluorescent antibody (IFA) test.

RESULTS

Of the 10 foals serologically tested for precolostral antibodies, one had a titer of 1:40. The remaining nine foals were serologically negative. However, the remaining nine foals promptly developed *E. risticii* antibody titers following consumption of colostrum.

Two foals and their dams were monitored serologically for one year. The sequential IFA titers on Foal 1, which had a precolostral positive IFA response, and Foal 2, which was serologically negative prior to ingestion of colostrum, are shown in Table 1. The foal with precolostral *E. risticii* antibodies at a titer of 1:40 continued to show a rise in titer to a peak of 1:1280 at seven months. In contrast, the foal that acquired colostral *E. risticii* antibodies peaked quite rapidly at 1:80 at one month of age. Thereafter this foal's titer continued to decline and was negative after seven months.

Comparative examination of antibody titers from the foals and their dams showed that, at birth, Foal 1 and Dam 1 each had the same titer, 1:40. At three months the foal's titer was 1:320 while the dam's titer was 1:80. At seven months of age, the foal attained a peak titer of 1:1280 while the dam remained at 1:80 (Table 1). A significant difference in antibody titers between the foal with passively acquired antibodies (Foal 2) and its dam was observed. While the foal's antibody titer peaked at 1:80 in its first month and the foal then became seronegative after seven months, the dam's titer peaked at 1:2560 seven months after foaling (Table 1).

The pregnant mare that was experimentally inoculated with culture-derived *E. risticii* developed clinical PHF and then recovered. Approximately four months after infection the mare was euthanized and tissue specimens were collected from both the mare and her seven month fetus for *E. risticii* isolation studies. The organism was isolated in the cultures from the fetal bone marrow, spleen, and mesenteric and colonic lymph nodes. The organism was not detected in cultures inoculated with the fetal liver homogenate. It is interesting to note that the organism was not isolated from any of the corresponding tissues obtained from the dam.

Gross pathological examination of the aborted fetus of a mare previously affected as a natural case of PHF revealed partially aerated lungs, froth in the trachea, and hemorrhage in the shoulder joint. The placenta was found to be entire, but the amnion showed infarcts and calcified plaques.

Histopathologic changes in the tissues collected from the fetus were not remarkable. No pathogenic bacteria were isolated from the lung, liver, or stomach of the fetus, or from the dam's placenta.

The fetus was serologically negative for equine rhinopneumonitis and leptospirosis. A serum sample collected from this fetus, however, was seropositive for antibodies to *E. risticii* at a titer of 1:320. Serum obtained from the dam at abortion was serologically positive at a titer of 1:2560.

DISCUSSION

Potomac horse fever affects thousands of horses across the United States every year. In many cases, mortality occurs despite chemotherapeutic intervention. This report reveals another threat to the equine industry: the danger to the unborn foal.

Of the 10 foals born to PHF-affected mares, one had an *E. risticii* antibody titer prior to the consumption of colostrum, indicating the existence of specific antibodies generated in utero. The remaining foals were serologically negative at birth but developed antibody titers promptly after the consumption of colostrum, indicating the presence of passively acquired antibodies.

It is evident from serologic data presented in Table 1 that a foal delivered by a PHF-affected mare may not only acquire *E. risticii* antibodies by passive transfer from the dam but also by direct fetal synthesis of antibodies, possibly in response to an in utero infection. These data indicate a need for serologic examination of both the foal and the dam to further elucidate the role of *E. risticii* in the pathogensis of PHF.

The recovery of *E. risticii* from the fetus of an experimentally infected mare, and the finding of specific *E. risticii* antibodies in an aborted fetus from a field case, may relate to the occurrence of abortions in mares affected by PHF. We have received a number of field reports on this subject. There are many causes of equine abortion, and in a large percentage of cases the cause is eventually determined. However, for a significant number of equine abortions, the etiologic agent remains undetermined. We believe that PHF may account for some of these unresolved cases. Accordingly, we strongly recommend a systematic experimental and clinical investigation into the role of PHF in equine abortion.

ACKNOWLEDGMENTS

We are indebted to A. Wayne Roberts, Livestock Disease Diagnostic Center, and David Powell, Department of Veterinary Science, University of Kentucky, for providing pathology reports and blood samples from the mare and her aborted fetus. The technical assistance of Dr. Indra Abeygunawardena, Department of Pathobiology, University of Illinois, and Dr. Richard Meinersmann, New Bolton Center, University of Pennsylvania, is sincerely appreciated. The editorial comments of Dr. Ibulaimu Kakoma are greatly appreciated.

REFERENCES

Holland, C.J.; Ristic, M.; Cole, A.I.; Johnson, P.; Baker, G.; and Goetz, T. (1985a) Isolation, experimental transmission, and characterization of causative agent of Potomac horse fever. *Science* **227,** 522-24.

Holland, C.J.; Weiss, E.; Burgdorfer, W.; Cole, A.I.; and Kakoma, I. (1985b) *Ehrlichia risticii* sp. nov.: Etiologic agent of equine monocytic ehrlichiosis (synonym, Potomac horse fever). *Int. J. Syst. Bacteriol.* **35,** 524-26.

Knowles, R.C.; Anderson, D.W.; Shipley, W.D.; Whitlock, R.H.; Perry, B.D.; and Davidson, J.P. (1983) Acute equine diarrhea syndrome (AEDS): A preliminary report. *Proc. 29th Ann. Conv. Am. Assoc. Equine Practnr.* pp. 353-57.

Nyindo, M.B.A.; Ristic, M.; Huxsoll, D.L.; and Smith, A.R. (1971) Tropical canine pancytopenia: *In vitro* cultivation of the causative agent—*Ehrlichia canis. Am. J. Vet. Res.* **32,** 1651-58.

Ristic, M.; Holland, C.J.; Dawson, J.E.; Sessions, J.E.; and Palmer, J.E. (1986) Diagnosis of equine monocytic ehrlichiosis (Potomac horse fever) by indirect immunofluorescence. *J. Am. Vet. Med. Assoc.* **189,** 39-46.

Whitlock, R.H.; Palmer, J.E.; Benson, C.E.; Acland, H.M.; Jenny, A.L.; and Ristic, M. (1984) Potomac horse fever: clinical characteristics and diagnostic features. *27th Ann. Proc., Am. Assoc. Vet. Lab. Diagnosticians* pp. 103-24.

Foal Mortality Associated with Natural Infection of Pregnant Mares with *Borrelia burgdorferi*

Elizabeth C. Burgess, Annette Gendron-Fitzpatrick, and Mark Mattison

SUMMARY

Borrelia burgdorferi infection in horses has been shown to cause arthritis, lameness, and panuveitis. Infection of pregnant humans has been associated with abortions and infant mortality. This report is on the effect of *B. burgdorferi* infection on seven naturally infected pregnant mares and one stallion from a breeding herd located in an area of Wisconsin where Lyme disease is endemic. The horses were tested for *B. burgdorferi* antibodies over the period from August 1985 through January 1987. All eight horses had antibodies during this time. In 1986 two of the mares aborted or resorbed their fetuses, three foals died within days, and two mares each had a live foal that survived, one of which was euthanized at one year of age due to neurologic disease. Two of the three dead foals had tubular nephrosis of the kidney, and *B. burgdorferi* was isolated from the kidneys of both and the brain of one. The colostrum of the mare with the euthanized yearling foal had a *B. burgdorferi* antibody titer of 1:256. These findings show that *B. burgdorferi* can cause in utero infections in foals and is associated with foal mortality.

INTRODUCTION

Borreliosis (a spirochetal infection caused by *Borrelia burgdorferi*) was first reported in horses in 1986 as causing arthritis, panuveitis, salpingitis, and endometritis (Burgess, Gillette & Pickett 1987). Horses from Connecticut and Massachusetts have been shown to have antibodies to *B. burgdorferi* (Marcus et al. 1985). *B. burgdorferi* is transmitted primarily by ixodid ticks (Steere, Broderick & Malawista 1978), but nonarthropod contact transmission has also been shown in dogs (Burgess 1986). Transplacental transmission of *B. burgdorferi* has been demonstrated in humans, associated with abortions, infant deaths, and possible heart defects (Macdonald 1986). The objective of this study was to determine if transplacental transmission of *B. burgdorferi* occurs in horses.

MATERIALS AND METHODS

Horses. The eight Appaloosa horses examined were from a breeding herd near La Crosse, Wis. This herd was chosen because of reproductive problems (abortions, resorptions) in 1985 and because it was located in an endemic area for borreliosis. The seven mares were hand-bred and were then turned out in paddocks next to a wooded area. Mares were palpated for pregnancy on Days 25 and 40 postbreeding. Mares positive by palpation were serum-tested for pregnancy between 30 and 90 days.

Blood samples. Blood samples were drawn from the jugular vein on October 10, 1985, from the stallion and on the dates shown in Table 1 from the mares. Blood was drawn into tubes with no anticoagulant and allowed to clot. The tubes were sent chilled to Madison, Wisconsin, and serum was drawn off for antibody testing. Blood was also collected in citrated blood tubes for culturing and sent chilled to Madison. Sera from the foals and their dams were sent to the Wisconsin Animal Health Laboratory for serum neutralization testing for equine rhinopneumonitis.

Indirect immunofluorescent antibody test (IFA). Sera collected from the horses was tested upon arrival by the IFA test for antibodies to *B. burgdorferi* using standard techniques (Burgess et al. 1986). The IFA endpoint was the highest serum dilution to show distinct fluorescence of the spirochetes. Serum was stored at −20°C after testing.

B. burgdorferi isolation. Whole blood (0.1 ml) from each sample was placed in 7-ml tubes of BSK 11 medium (Johnson et al. 1984) and incubated at 34°C. A drop of medium from each tube was placed on a slide and examined for the presence of spirochetes by dark-field microscopy. This was done biweekly for six weeks. Any spirochetes found were placed on a slide, incubated overnight at 37°C, and then tested by immunofluorescence using a monoclonal antibody (H5532) followed by a fluorescein isothiocynate (FITC) conjugated antimouse serum to ensure identification.

Foals. Blood, urine, heart, liver, brain, and kidney samples were taken from most foals. Samples were sent chilled on ice to Madison. Because of the long distances between the farm, the attending veterinarian (Mattison), and the laboratory (Burgess), we attempted to take tissues from which *B. burgdorferi* could best be isolated. We did not attempt to sample all tissues. Blood and urine samples (0.1 ml) were placed in BSK 11 medium for spirochete isolation. Formalin-fixed tissue samples from each foal were paraffin-embedded, and

University of Wisconsin–School of Veterinary Medicine, 2015 Linden Drive West, Madison, Wisconsin 53706.

Table 1. ***Borrelia burgdorferi*** **antibody titers and reproductive performance in seven Appaloosa mares naturally infected with *B. burgdorferi***

Mare	Age, yrs.	Date sampled	Antibody titer[a]	Reproductive outcome
A	13	8-22-85	128	Open—no '85 foal
		3-23-86	1024	Twin foals, No. 2 & 3, born 3-18-86; both died within days
		6-12-86	512	Sold mare
B	6	8-22-85	Negative	Unknown
		3-23-86	1024	Open
		6-12-86	512	Sold mare
C	8	8-22-85	Negative	Live foal born 2-21-85
		3-23-86	1024	Live foal born 2-27-86
		6-12-86	512	In foal
D	2	8-22-85	Negative	Unknown
		3-23-86	256 colostrum, negative blood	Live foal No. 4 born 4-25-86[b]
		6-12-86	Negative	Aborted twins at 9 mo., 2-5-87
E	9	8-22-85	Negative	Aborted
		3-23-86	Negative	Open
		10-21-86	1024	Sold mare
F	13	8-22-85	128	Unknown
		3-23-86	Negative	Open
		10-21-86	512	Sold mare
G	6	3-23-86	1024	Foal No. 1 born 1-31-86
		6-12-86	1024	In foal
		10-21-86	512	Aborted 103 days

[a] Indirect immunofluorescent antibody titer given as the highest twofold dilution of serum showing fluorescence of the spirochetes. A titer of 128 or above is considered positive.

[b] Foal was euthanized as a yearling with neurologic signs.

7-μm sections were cut, deparaffinized, mounted on slides, and stained with hematoxylin and eosin. In addition, a duplicate set of 7-μm sections were cut, deparaffinized, and stained with monoclonal antibody for *B. burgdorferi* as described above. Another part of each tissue sample was triturated with 2 ml of BSK 11 medium in tenbrock tissue grinders, and 0.1 ml of the material was inoculated into BSK 11 medium for spirochete isolation.

RESULTS

Serology. The results of the *B. burgdorferi* antibody testing are shown in Table 1. All of the mares and the stallion had antibodies to *B. burgdorferi* on at least one occasion during the test period. Serum neutralization tests for equine rhinopneumonitis on serum from Foals 1-4 and their dams were negative.

Foals. Of the seven mares successfully bred in 1985, Mares B, E, and F resorbed or aborted their fetuses, G had a foal that never stood (1), Mare A bore live twins that did not survive beyond six days after birth (Foals 2, 3) and Mares C and D had live foals, one of which (No. 4) was euthanized as a yearling in 1987.

Necropsy. *Foal 1.* The foal was found dead next to the placenta. The lungs were inflated, indicating the foal had been born alive. Three days prior the foal had been palpated in the normal fetal position and was alive. No histologic lesions were seen in the heart or brain, but the kidney had diffuse patchy hypercellular glomeruli and vacuolation of the tubular epithelium in the medulla and cortex. Cortical tubules showed prominent necrosis with loss of nuclei and epithelial sloughing (Fig. 1). *B. burgdorferi* was isolated from the kidney. Serum from the foal was negative for *B. burgdorferi* antibodies and spirochetes. The mare had a *B. burgdorferi* antibody titer of 1:1024.

Foal 2: The first twin was euthanized with pentobarbital at two days of age. It had been weak and unable to stand or nurse. Histologic examination of the heart revealed a small focus of subendocardial hemorrhage and multiple foci of linear hypercellularity within the myocardium. The liver had diffuse congestion. The splenic follicles appeared active and plasma cells were noted in the pulp. The brain had multifocal hemorrhages. The kidney was congested with vacuolated tubular epithelium. *B. burgdorferi* was isolated from the kidney and the brain. *B. burgdorferi* was demonstrated in the glomeruli by immunofluorescence. The foal had a *B. burgdorferi* antibody titer of 1:128 and the mare a titer of 1:1024.

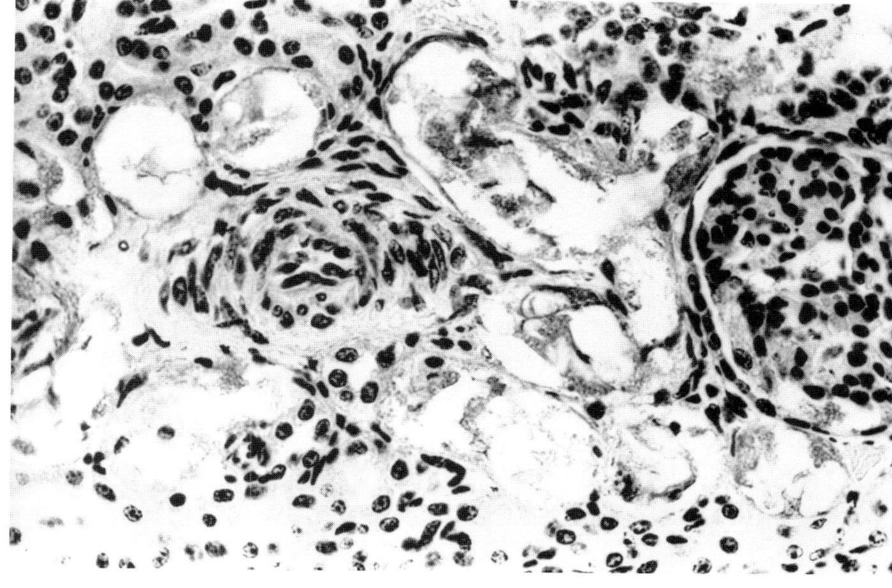

Fig. 1. The kidney in Foal 1 reveals acute necrosis of the renal tubular epithelium (7-μm section stained with mag. 40 × hematoxylin and eosin).

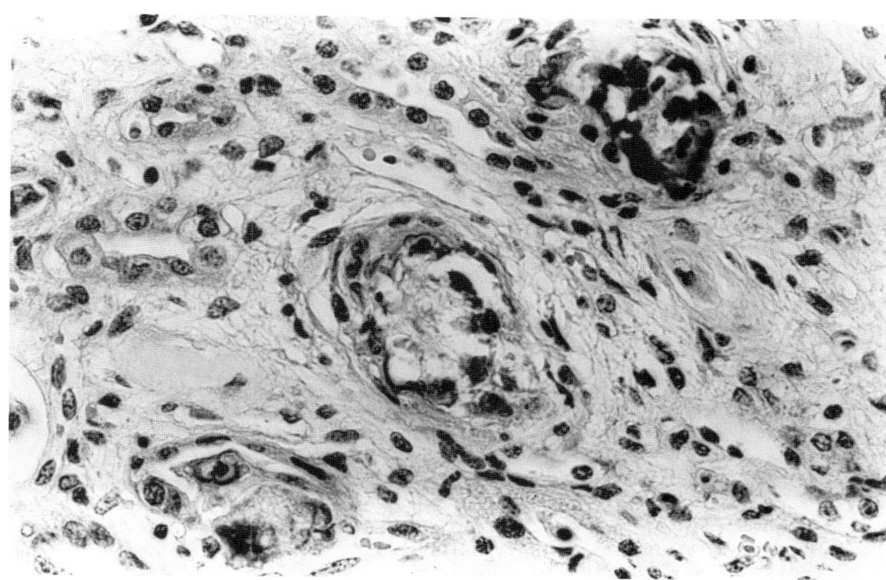

Fig. 2. The renal tubules of Foal 4 show chronic tubular damage with resulting calcification and bizarre epithelial regeneration (7-μm section stained with mag. 40 × hematoxylin and eosin).

No *B. burgdorferi* were cultured from the foal's urine. No pathogenic organisms were found on culture of the liver on blood agar and eosin methylene blue agar.

Foal 3. The second twin foal was unable to stand to nurse and was bottle-fed the mare's milk. On Day 4 it became weaker and was given gentamicin 100 mg IM, and a blood transfusion of 1 pint of the mare's blood and 100 ml of lactated Ringer's solution. The foal died at six days of age. The thoracic and abdominal cavities contained a serosanguinous fluid. No lesions were seen on histologic examination of the heart, brain, spleen, or liver. The kidney showed vacuolated tubular epithelium and minimal epithelial sloughing.

Foal 4. This foal was healthy when born. The mare's colostrum had a *B. burgdorferi* antibody titer of 1:256, but the serum was negative. At six months of age the foal started having difficulty stepping up with the hind legs. It became progressively worse and in March 1987 was euthanized, when it could no longer stand and spinal meningitis was suspected. Unfortunately, due to the difficulty of performing a necropsy on the farm and the distance between farm and the laboratory, only the blood, liver, and kidney were saved. The liver showed hydropic degeneration of the hepatocytes as well as scattered small foci of mixed mononuclear cells. The kidney contained numerous foci of mineralization within the tubules. Tubules both with and without mineralization had vacuolation of the tubular epithelium, cellular debris in the lamina, and eosinophilic casts (Fig. 2). There were multiple foci of tubular loss and interstitial lymphoplasmocytic cellular infiltration. These lesions suggest a chronic sequela of the more acute lesions seen in the younger foals. *B. burg-*

dorferi was isolated from both the kidney and liver. The serum *B. burgdorferi* titer was 1:1024.

The stallion on the farm had a periodic lameness migrating from front to rear legs. Mare A had a nonspecific lameness for three weeks after foaling, and another mare was lame for two weeks prior to foaling. Four of the mares, A, B, E, and F, were not kept for breeding in 1986; of the remaining three, Mares D and G aborted, and Mare C was in foal (Table 1).

DISCUSSION

This study shows that *B. burgdorferi* can cause in utero infections in horses and can be associated with foal mortality. The kidney lesions in the foals that died soon after birth and in the yearling contributed to the deaths of the animals. The lesions were attributed to *B. burgdorferi* infection, as *B. burgdorferi* was isolated from the kidneys of three of the four animals and spirochetes were identified in the kidneys on histologic sections. A previously reported pony with *B. burgdorferi* infection had glomerulonephritis (Burgess et al. 1986). *B. burgdorferi* was demonstrated in the proximal convoluted tubules of the kidney and in the spleen of a premature human infant of woman positive for *B. burgdorferi* antibody (Schlesinger et al. 1985). These findings give evidence that *B. burgdorferi* causes tubular damage of the kidneys. Another closely related *Borrelia* of cattle, *B. coriaceus,* is the cause of epizootic bovine abortion that occurs when the infected vector tick *Ornithodorus coriaceus* feeds on pregnant cows. This disease is characterized by late-term abortions and birth of weak calves at term. Early lesions are most commonly seen in the lung, thymus, and lymph nodes and consist of lymphocytic and mononuclear proliferation. Later changes include necrotizing foci in the lymph nodes and spleen, vasculitis, and meningitis (Kennedy et al. 1986). These findings indicate that in the future the lymph nodes, lungs, and thymus should be examined when foals are suspected of dying of *B. burgdorferi* infection.

The demonstration of antibodies in the serum of Foal 2 and the isolation of spirochetes from Foal 1 suggest infection took place in utero. There is no transplacental transfer of antibodies in the horse (Tizard 1982) and Foal 2 received no colostrum, indicating that the antibodies were made by the foal. Foal 1 lived for no more than a few hours and did not have time to acquire the infection after birth. The yearling colt could have acquired *B. burgdorferi* after birth from a tick bite in the fall of 1986. However, the chronicity of the kidney lesions and the similarity to those seen in the foals strongly support a nonfatal fetal infection. We cannot say that the neurologic signs were caused by *B. burgdorferi* infection but borreliosis encephalitis has been reported in a horse (Burgess 1987).

The only signs of infection in the adult horses were stiffness and lameness. It is interesting that the mares developed the lameness within three weeks of foaling. Of 19 women naturally exposed to *B. burgdorferi* during their pregnancy, 10 also developed arthralgia or arthritis (Markowitz et al. 1986).

The *B. burgdorferi* antibody titers of three of the mares, A, F, and G, remained positive (128 or above) for the entire period studied. Mare D did not have a serum antibody titer, but did have antibodies in the colostrum. This might indicate a localized infection in the mammary gland. Mare F had a positive antibody titer that became negative and then positive again over a 14-month period. It is possible that, like Mare D, she had a localized infection of the uterus. We cannot say the resorptions and abortions were caused by *B. burgdorferi* infection but suggest they were related to it.

This herd of horses had only one viable offspring by the end of one year from the breedings in 1985. These findings suggest that *B. burgdorferi* infection in a breeding herd of horses must be considered as a cause of reproductive failure, especially in endemic areas where reinfections can readily occur.

REFERENCES

Burgess, E.C. (1986) Experimental inoculation of dogs with *Borrelia burgdorferi*. *Zbl. Bakt. Hyg.* **263,** 49-54.

Burgess, E.C., and Mattison, M. (1987) Encephalitis in a Wisconsin horse: association with *Borrelia burgdorferi* infection. *J. Am. Vet. Med. Assoc.* **191,** 1457-58.

Burgess, E.C.; Amundson, T.E.; Davis, J.P.; Kaslow, R.A.; and Edelman, R. (1986) Experimental inoculation of *Peromyscus sp.* with *Borrelia burgdorferi:* evidence of contact transmission. *Am. J. Trop. Med. Hyg.* **35,** 359-63.

Burgess, E.C.; Gillette, D.; and Pickett, J.P. (1986). Arthritis and panuveitis as manifestations of *Borrelia burgdorferi* infection in a Wisconsin pony. *J. Am. Vet. Med. Assoc.*, 1340-42.

Johnson, S.E.; Klein, G.C.; Schmid, G.P.; Bowen, J.C.; Feeley, S.C.; and Schulze, T. (1984) Lyme disease: a selective medium for isolation of the suspected etiologic agent, a spirochete. *J. Clin. Microbiol.* **19,** 81-82.

Kennedy, P.C.; Casaro, A.P.; Kimsey, P.B.; Bon Durant, R.H.; Bushnell, R.B.; and Mitchell, G.F. (1983) Epizootic bovine abortion: histogenesis of the fetal lesions. *Am. J. Vet. Res.* **44,**, 1040-48.

McDonald, A.B. (1986) Human fetal borreliosis, toxemia of pregnancy and fetal death. *Zbl. Bakt. Hyg.* **263,** 189-200.

Marcus, L.C.; Patterson, M.M.; Gillifan, R.E.; and Urband, P.H. (1985) Antibodies to *Borrelia burgdorferi* in New England horses. *Am. J. Vet. Res.* **46,** 2570-71.

Markowitz, L.E.; Steere, A.C.; Benach, J.L.; Slade, J.D.; and Broome, C.V. (1986) Lyme disease during pregnancy. *J. Am. Vet. Med. Ass.* **255,** 3394-96.

Schlesinger, P.A.; Duray, P.H.; Burke, S.A.; Steere, A.C.; and Stillman, M.J. (1985). Maternal fetal transmission of the Lyme disease spirochete *Borrelia burgdorferi*. *Ann. Intern. Med.* **103,** 67-68.

Steere, A.C.; Broderick, T.F.; and Malawista, S.E. (1978) Erythema chronicum migrans and Lyme arthritis: epidemiologic evidence for a tick vector. *Am. J. Epidemiol.* **108**, 312-21.

Tizard, I. (1982) Immunization in the fetus and newborn animal. In: *Introduction to Veterinary Immunology*, 2d ed., W.B. Saunders, Philadelphia.

Gastrointestinal Infections

A Plasmid Profile Study of *Salmonella typhimurium* Strains Isolated from Horses in Japan

Gihei Sato, Yuji Nakaoka, Saori Marufuji, Naotaka Ishiguro, and Morikazu Shinagawa

SUMMARY

Plasmid profiles were investigated on *Salmonella typhimurium* strains isolated from horses and their environment on 47 farms in three districts of Hokkaido from 1976 to 1985, and the profiles were compared with those of organisms from calf salmonellosis in the same district, to investigate possible epidemiological relationships of salmonellosis between horses and cattle.

Three types of plasmid profiles (A, C, and D) were found in equine strains, and two of them (A and C) were distributed among equine and bovine strains in two districts. The most prevalent A type profile consisted of 60-, 5.0-, and 3.9-magadalton (Md) plasmids. The 60-Md plasmid, either conjugative or nonconjugative, controlled resistance to streptomycin (Sm), sulfadimethoxine (Su), tetracycline (Tc), and kanamycin (Km); the 5.0-Md plasmid controlled ampicillin (Ap) resistance; and 3.9-Md plasmid controlled Su resistance. The A type profile strains indicated almost uniform biovars (26e and 26b) (Duguid et al. 1975) and multiresistance [ApSmSuTc(Km)].

Although the frequency of conjugative R plasmid differed in the type A strains from horses (28.9%) and cattle (1.4%), genetic and molecular studies of plasmid DNAs of the A type and C type profile revealed similarity between *S. typhimurium* strains from both animal species. This indicates that *S. typhimurium* strains from both horses and cattle were closely correlated. The results suggest that one source of equine salmonellosis was calf salmonellosis, previously prevalent in Hokkaido.

INTRODUCTION

Gibbons (1980) pointed out that by the 1950s the incidence and significance of *Salmonella abortus-equi* had declined virtually to the point of extinction, while *S. typhimurium* isolates from horses in the United States and Britain have shown a progressive increase. In Japan a similar tendency has been observed. Since an outbreak of *S. typhimurium* infection among horses on a farm in eastern Hokkaido in 1976, there have been endemic outbreaks among horses in various districts of Hokkaido (Sato et al. 1984). In 1981, the infection was found mainly in foals, especially in the Hidaka district, where many Thoroughbred farms are located. The infection occurred there endemically or sporadically until 1985.

Plasmid profiles identified by agarose gel electrophoresis have recently been used as an epidemiological marker in human and animal salmonellosis (Riley & Cohen 1982; Taylor et al. 1982; Taylor et al. 1982; Benzanson et al. 1983; Yataya et al. 1983). Plasmid profile analysis is a valuable tool in epidemiological investigations of the disease (Riley & Cohen 1982; Taylor et al. 1982) and is estimated to be at least as specific as phage typing in the classification of *S. typhimurium* (Holmberg et al. 1984). From the viewpoint of disease control and the role of animal salmonellosis in public health, epidemiological studies of equine salmonellosis are needed. However, such studies using plasmid profile analysis are few in number (Sato et al. 1984; Ikeda & Hirsh 1985; Nakamura et al. 1986; Rumschlag & Boyce 1987).

In this study, we investigated *S. typhimurium* strains isolated from horses and cattle in the same districts in Hokkaido to better define the epidemiology of salmonellosis. The relation of the plasmid profile to the biovar and antibiotic resistance pattern of the strains was also investigated.

MATERIALS AND METHODS

Salmonella strains. A total of 230 *S. typhimurium* strains, 132 were from horses and 98 from cattle, were investigated (Table 1). These strains were isolated from diseased or healthy animals and from the environments on various farms in three districts of Hokkaido. On some of the farms, Salmonella strains were isolated in two or three successive years and kept on Dorset's egg slopes.

Bacterial strains and plasmids. A derivative of *Escherichia coli* K-12 strain, SG11 (recA-mutant of Rif^r *E. coli* C600 *thi, thr, leu, lac*) (Ishiguro & Sato 1984) was used for genetic experiments with plasmids. *E. coli* V517 (Macrina et al. 1978), a multiple plasmid–containing strain, was used as a source of molecular weight standards (35.8, 4.8, 3.7, 3.4, 2.6, 2.0, 1.8, and 1.4 Md) for electrophoresis of intact plasmids. Other plasmids of the molecular weight standards were RA1 (86 Md), R27 (112), R478 (166), TP 114 (41), R621a (65), and R6k (26). pOH44, used for mobilization testing of R plasmids, was an F plasmid obtained by transposition of Cm-marked IS*3411* from pOH24 to pED100 (Ishiguro & Sato 1984).

Department of Veterinary Public Health, Obihiro University of Agriculture and Veterinary Medicine, Obihiro, Hokkaido 080, Japan.

Table 1. Isolation of *S. typhimurium* from horses and cattle in Hokkaido, 1976-85

Source	Location	Number of strains (number of farms)								Total
		1976	1977	1980	1981	1982	1983	1984	1985	
Horse	Tokachi	12(1)	3(1)	—	—	—	—	—	—	15(1)
	Kushiro	—	—	12(3)	—	—	—	—	—	12(3)
	Hidaka	—	—	—	29(15)	38(20)	19(10)	18(4)	1	105(43)
	Total									132(47)
Cattle	Tokachi	—	—	—	9[a]	—	—	—	—	9
	Kushiro	—	—	7(3)	14(1)	—	—	—	—	21(4)
	Hidaka	—	—	—	15(2)	—	—	44(9)	9(2)	68(10)
	Total									98(15)

[a] Isolated at a slaughterhouse.

Media. Nutrient broths were penassay broth (PAB, Difco) and L-broth (Lennox 1955). Heart infusion (HI) agar, deoxycholate hydrogen sulfide-lactose (DHL) agar, and Simmons citrate agar (Eiken) were the basic media for selection (Ishiguro et al. 1980). HI agar and Mueller Hinton (MH) agar were used for antibiotic sensitivity testing.

Biotyping. Biotyping was done by the method of Duguid et al. (1975).

Antibiotic sensitivity. Antibiotic sensitivity testing was performed by the agar dilution method (Ishiguro et al. 1980). Antimicrobial agents were used in the following amounts (µg/ml): ampicillin (Ap), 25; streptomycin (Sm), 12.5; tetracycline (Tc), 25; kanamycin (Km), 25; chloramphenicol (Cm), 25; nalidixic acid (Na), 25; furatrizine (Ft), 6.3; gentamicin (Gm), 12.5; rifampin (Rif), 25; and colistine (Cl), 12.5^{U}/ml. Resistance to sulfadimethoxine (Su, 800 µg/ml) and trimethoprim (Tp, 25 µg/ml) was determined on MH agar.

Conjugation. Resistance transfer experiments by broth mating were done as previously described (Ishiguro et al. 1980). *E. coli* SG11 was the recipient in the experiment.

Mobilization. Mobilization tests were done by the method of Tanabe (1986). An autotransferring F plasmid pOH44 was used for the test. SG11 carrying the pOH44 (donor I) and *Salmonella* strains with nontransferable resistance determinants (recipient I) were incubated together in PAB for 4 hr at 37°C with gentle shaking, and the mixture was plated on Simmons citrate agar containing Cm. When *Salmonella* colony with Cm-resistance was obtained, the second mating was carried out in a similar way between the *Salmonella* colony obtained (donor II) and SG11 (recipient II). The transconjugants were selected on HI agar containing Rif and a suitable antibiotic. When any antibiotic resistance except Cm-resistance was transferred to the final recipient, plasmid DNA of the transconjugant was examined by electrophoresis to confirm mobilization of plasmids. For Cm-resistant *Salmonella* strains, this mobilization test could not be applied.

Plasmid profile analysis. Plasmid DNAs for screening of plasmid profiles were prepared by the method of Kado and Liu (1981). Purified plasmid DNA was prepared by the method of Portnoy and Falkow (1981), and Clewell and Helinski (1969), with some modifications. Agarose gel electrophoresis was done as described by Niida and colleagues (1983). DNA samples were applied to a horizontal 0.8% agarose gel in TBE-buffer (50 mM Tris-HC1, 50 mM boric acid, 2.5 mM sodium EDTA, 0.5 µg/ml EtBr, pH8.3) and electrophoresed for 6 hr at 80 V. Appropriate plasmids used as the molecular weight standards were coelectrophoresed.

Plasmid transformation. Purified plasmid DNA or single-plasmid DNA isolated from agarose gels was used for transformation, essentially as described by Cohen and colleagues (1973).

Restriction enzyme digestion. Purified plasmid DNA or single-plasmid DNA isolated from agarose gel was digested with restriction endonuclease EcoRI or PstI (Takara-shizo, Japan) for 6 hr at 37°C under the conditions specified by the manufacturer. DNA fragments were sized by comparing their migration distance in 0.8% agarose gel with HindIII-cleaved λ phage fragments as molecular weight standards.

Southern hybridization. Plasmid DNAs fractionated by agarose gel electrophoresis were transferred from the gel to a nitrocellulose filter by the method of Southern (1975). PstI digested plasmid DNA isolated from a *S. typhimurium* strain was labeled with ^{32}P and used for the probe.

RESULTS

Classification of plasmid profiles. Out of 230 strains tested, six types (A, BI, BII, C, D, and E) of plasmid profiles were found among 228 strains, (131 from horses and 97 from cattle) (Table 2). The remaining two strains from horses and cattle were untypable. The profile of each type is shown in Figure 1. Among the 230 strains tested, only 12 from horses in Tokachi district in 1976 (Table 1) were antibiotic-sensitive; they were classified as type D. Types A, C, and D were found

Table 2. Classification of plasmid profile in 230 *S. typhimurium* strains isolated from horses and cattle in Hokkaido

		Number of Strains[b]							
		Hidaka		Kushiro		Tokachi		Total	
Type[a]	Plasmid profile (Md)	H	C	H	C	H	C	H	C
A	60, 5.0, 3.9	102	42	12	21	—	8	114	71
BI	60, (40)[c], 5.0, 3.9, 3.2, 2.2	—	5	—	—	—	—	—	5
BII	60, 5.0, 3.9, 2.0	—	1	—	—	—	—	—	1
C	(120)[c], 60, 3.7 2.4	2	19	—	—	—	—	2	19
D	60, (36)[c], 1.4	—	—	—	—	15	—	15	—
E	2.2, 2.0	—	—	—	—	—	1	—	1
Untypable		1	1	—	—	—	—	1	1

[a] Year of isolation: type A, 1980-85; BI, 1984; BII, 1985; C, 1984-85; D, 1976-77; E, 1981.
[b] H, horse; C, cattle.
[c] Irregular occurrence.

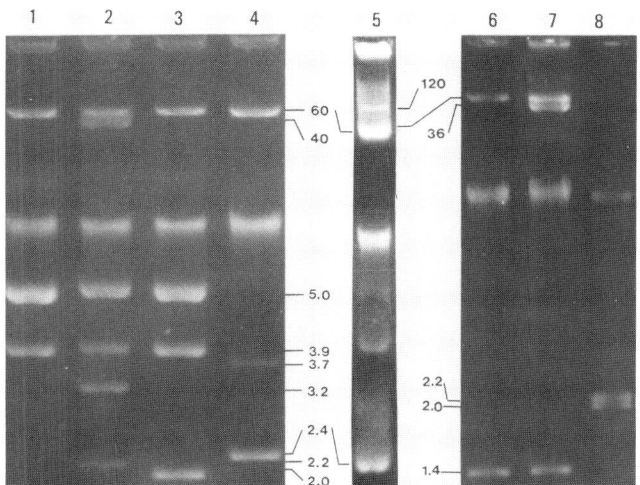

Fig. 1. Agarose gel electrophoresis of plasmid DNAs isolated from plasmid profile types A, BI, BII, C, D, and E: *Lane 1*, type A (60, 5.0, and 3.9 Md); *Lane 2*, type BI (60, 40, 5.0, 3.9, 3.2, and 2.2 Md); *Lane 3*, type BII (60, 5.0, 3.9, and 2.0 Md); *Lane 4*, type C (60, 3.7, and 2.4 Md); *Lane 5*, type C (120, 60, 3.7, and 2.4 Md); *Lane 6*, type D (60 and 1.4 Md); *Lane 7*, type D (60, 36, and 1.4 Md); *Lane 8*, type E (2.2 and 2.0 Md).

in horse strains. Types A, BI, BII, C, and E were found in bovine strains. In both animals, type A strain was the most prevalent, accounting for 114 (87.0%) of 131 typable horse strains and 71 (73.2%) of 97 typable bovine strains. Type A strains were isolated from horses at the highest frequency from 1980 to 1984; only two type C strains were isolated from horses in 1984 and 1985; type D strains were isolated in 1976 and 1977 only in Tokachi district. Isolation frequency of type A strains from cattle was 88.9% to 100% in 1980, 1981, and 1985, but decreased to 45.4% in 1984, when strains of type C (43.2%) and type BI (11.4%) were isolated in Hidaka district.

Characteristics of plasmids. Plasmids of each profile were characterized by conjugation, mobilization, transformation, restriction enzyme analysis, or hybridization.

Of 114 equine type A strains, 33 (28.9%) transferred their resistance to SG11 by conjugation (strains 1814, 2140, and 2313 in Table 3). On the other hand, only one (1.4%) of 71 bovine strains showed resistance transfer (strain 1841 in Table 4). These transferable resistances (SmTcKm, SmSuTcKm, and SmTcCm) were carried by 60-Md plasmid (Tables 3 and 4). Moreover, 21 (60%) of 35 strains not carrying conjugative R plasmids isolated from horses in Hidaka district and Kushiro district mobilized resistance by the F plasmid (pOH44) (strain 2216 in Table 3). The same mobilization was observed in seven (58.3%) of 12 strains not carrying conjugative R plasmids isolated from cattle in Hidaka district (strain 2432 in Table 4). The mobilization was observed only in type A strains. These R plasmids mobilized were 60-Md and conferred SmTc resistance (Tables 3 and 4). Type A strains had conjugative or nonconjugative 60-Md plasmid conferring multiresistance, 5.0-Md plasmid conferring Ap resistance, and 3.9-Md plasmid conferring Su resistance.

In the conjugation experiment with type A strains, Ap resistance was transferred at high frequency singly or together with other resistance determinants to the recipient. However, in a portion of the strains tested, only the Ap resistance was not transmitted by the secondary mating using transconjugants obtained. Moreover, in the incompatibility test, a great part of the conjugative R plasmids carrying multiple resistance determinants, other than Ap resistance, were classified as Iα of incompatibility group, but Ap resistance determinant in all cases coexisted with known Iα reference plasmid, suggesting that Ap resistance would be controlled by another plasmid (data not shown). The transconjugants obtained by the primary mating from 34 strains, including the 33 strains carrying conjugative R plasmids, were examined for plasmid pattern and antibiotic resistance pattern (Table 5). The transconjugants obtained from four representative strains indicated three patterns of antibiotic resistance (strain 1809 not carrying conjugative R plasmid transferred only Ap resistance). Since transformation experiments indicated that Ap resistance was encoded by 5.0-Md plasmid (Tables 3 and 4), these data revealed that there were two kinds of 60-Md conjugative plasmids: one was cryptic and the other conferred multiresistance that mobilized the

Table 3. Characteristics of plasmids carried by *S. typhimurium* strains isolated from horses

Strain	Year of isolation	Plasmid profile type	Resistance pattern	Plasmid (Md)	Detection procedure for plasmid	Resistance determinant of plasmid
1814	1981	A	ApSmSuTcKmCl	60	Conjugation	SmTcKm
				60	Conjugation	—
				5.0	Transformation	Ap
				3.9	Transformation	Su
2140	1982	A	ApSmSuTcKm	60	Conjugation	SmSuTcKm
				5.0	Transformation	Ap
				3.9	Transformation	Su
2216	1983	A	ApSmSuTcNa	60	Mobilization	SmTc
				5.0	Transformation	Ap
				3.9	Transformation	Su
2313	1984	A	ApSmSuTcCmNa	60	Conjugation	SmTcCm
				60	Conjugation	—
				5.0	Transformation	Ap
				3.9	Transformation	Su
2504	1985	C	ApSmSuTcKmCmNa	60	Nonconjugative[a]	(?)
				3.7	Transformation	Su
				2.4	Undetectable[b]	—
1177	1977	D	ApSmSuTcCm	60	Conjugation	ApSuTcCm
				36	Undetectable[b]	—
				1.4	Undetectable[b]	—

[a] Mobilization test could not be performed because of absence of appropriate resistance marker for selection.
[b] Transformant could not be obtained.

Table 4. Characteristics of plasmids carried by *S. typhimurium* strains isolated from cattle

Strain	Year of isolation	Plasmid profile type	Resistance pattern	Plasmid (Md)	Detection procedure for plasmid	Resistance determinant of plasmid
1841	1980	A	ApSmSuTcKm	60	Conjugation	SmTcKm
				5.0	Transformation	Ap
				3.9	Transformation	Su
2432	1984	A	ApSmSuTcNa	60	Mobilization	SmTc
				5.0	Transformation	Ap
				3.9	Transformation	Su
2402	1984	BI	ApSmSuTcCmTpNaCl	60	Nonconjugative[a]	(?)
				40	Conjugation	SmCmTp
				5.0	Transformation	Ap
				3.9	Transformation	Su
				3.2	Undetectable[b]	—
				2.2	Undetectable[b]	—
2511	1985	BII	ApSmSuTcNa	60	Nonconjugative[c]	(?)
				5.0	Transformation	Ap
				3.9	Transformation	Su
				2.0	Undetectable[b]	—
2421	1984	C	ApSmSuTcKmCm	120	Conjugation[d]	ApSmSuTcKmCm
				60	Nonconjugative[a]	(?)
				3.7	Transformation	Su
				2.4	Undetectable[b]	—

[a] Mobilization test could not be performed because of absence of appropriate resistance marker.
[b] Transformant could not be obtained.
[c] Was not mobilized.
[d] Temperature-sensitive R plasmid.

Table 5. Resistance pattern and plasmid pattern of transconjugants to which Ap resistance was transferred from equine *S. typhimurium* with type A plasmid Profile

S. typhimurium strain	Year of isolation	Resistance pattern	Resistance pattern of transconjugant	Plasmid pattern of transconjugant (Md)
1809	1981	ApSmSuTcKmCl	Ap	60, 5.0
1814	1981	ApSmSuTcKmCl	Ap	60, 5.0
			ApSmTcKm	60, 5.0
			SmTcKm	60
2221	1983	ApSmSuTcNa	Ap	60, 5.0
			ApSmTc	60, 5.0
			SmTc	60
2313	1984	ApSmSuTcCmNa	Ap	60, 5.0
			ApSmTcCm	60, 5.0
			SmTcCm	60

5.0-Md plasmid. This type of mobilization was restricted to the type A horse strains isolated in Hidaka district. However, the restriction patterns of three 60-Md plasmids—cryptic, conjugative, and nonconjugative R plasmids—with EcoRI were similar to each other (data not shown). Further study is needed to characterize the cryptic 60-Md plasmids.

Representative 14 type A strains isolated from horses and cattle during 1981-85 were analysed by hybridization testing to ascertain extent of the homology of 5.0- or 3.9-Md plasmids among different *S. typhimurium* strains. Either ^{32}P-labeled PstI-digested 5.0- or 3.9-Md plasmid from a representative type A strain was used as a probe. The 5.0- and 3.9-Md plasmids of all type A strains tested hybridized strongly with the probes of 5.0- and 3.9-Md plasmids, respectively, indicating that the 5.0- and 3.9-Md plasmids had much homology among type A strains (data not shown).

Type BI strains were isolated from cattle and only one had a conjugative 40-Md plasmid conferring SmCmTp resistance (strain 2402, Table 4). In types BI and BII strains, 60-Md plasmids could not be characterized, nor did 3.2-Md and 2.2-Md plasmids in type BI and 2.0-Md plasmid in type BII give any transformants. However, similar restriction patterns were observed for the 60-Md R plasmids of type A strains and the unidentified 60-Md plasmids of types BI and BII strains with EcoRI. Moreover, 5.0-Md plasmid conferring Ap resistance and 3.9-Md plasmid with Su determinant of BI and BII showed sequence homology with 5.0- and 3.9-Md plasmids of the strains of type A, respectively, by the hybridization test (data not shown). These results suggested that types BI and BII must have been generated by the addition of other plasmids to type A plasmid profile.

Of the 21 type C strains isolated from horses and cattle in 1984 and 1985, one strain derived from a horse and 14 from cattle transferred the whole resistance pattern (ApSmSu-TcKmCm). These resistance determinants were coded by 120-Md plasmids. The 60-Md plasmids of type C strains could not be evaulated for their biological properties (Tables 3 and 4). However, transformation experiments indicated that 3.7-Md plasmid in type C strains conferred Su resistance. No transformant with 2.4-Md plasmid of type C strains was obtained. EcoRI digestion patterns indicated no homology between 60-Md plasmid from type A strains and from type C strains (data not shown). This indicates that type C plasmids had no relationship to other types.

Type D strains were isolated from horses in 1976 and 1977 in Tokachi district. Two of 15 strains had a conjugative 60-Md plasmid (Table 3). Neither transconjugants nor transformants carrying 36-Md or 1.4-Md plasmids were detected.

One type E strain from cattle was found in 1981. Transformation testing failed to characterize 2.2- and 2.0-Md plasmids of the strain.

Correlation between plasmid profile, biovar, and antibiotic resistance. Of 132 equine *S. typhimurium* strains, 120 (90.1%) were resistant to one or more antibiotics, and 12 strains isolated in 1976 in Tokachi district were sensitive. A total of 11 resistance patterns were found. All 98 bovine strains tested were antibiotic-resistant and indicated 17 resistance patterns. Analysis of the data indicated that strains with resistance patterns of ApSmSuTcKm and ApSmSuTc, with or without Cl and/or Na resistance, were prevalent in horses and cattle during 1980-85. Eight resistance patterns were found among 113 (99.1%) of 114 type A horse strains. Seven resistance patterns were observed among 68 (95.8%) of 71 type A bovine strains (Table 6). The relationship between antibiotic resistance pattern and types BI, BII, C, D, and E of plasmid profile is shown in Table 7.

One hundred and thirty-two *S. typhimurium* strains from horses were divided into four primary biovars (1, 5, 9, and 26) and 13 full biovars. Primary biovar 26 was detected most frequently. Of all biovar 26 strains, 26e was the most frequent from 1980 to 1983. Biovar 26b was isolated at a relatively high frequency in 1983 and 1984. Among bovine strains, five primary biovars (1, 5, 10, 26, and 28) and 13 full biovars were found. Biovar 26e was detected most frequently in 1984 and 1985. Among type A strains from horses and cattle, biovars 26e and 26b were prevalent (Table 6). The relationship of other plasmid profile types to antibiotic resistance

Table 6. Biovar and antibiotic resistance pattern of plasmid profile type A strains

	Number of strains in each biovar									
Horses	9i	26a	26b	26be	26bei	26e	26ef	26eh	26ei	Total
ApSmSuTcKmCmNa	—	—	2	—	—	—	—	—	—	2
ApSmSuTcCm(Na)[a]	—	—	7	—	—	—	—	—	—	7
ApSmSuTcNa	—	1	11	—	—	7	—	—	—	19
ApSmSuTcKm(Cl)[a]	3	3	—	8	1	33	2	—	—	50
ApSmSuTc(Cl)[a]	—	3	—	3	—	26	1	1	1	35
Total	3	7	20	11	1	66	3	1	1	113
Cattle	1a	10b	26a	26b	26be	26bf	26e	26ef	28b	Total
ApSmSuTcCmNa	1	—	—	—	—	—	—	—	—	1
ApSmSuTcNa(Cl)[a]	—	1	2	18	—	4	—	—	1	26
ApSmSuTcKm(Cl)[a]	—	—	—	—	5	—	18	—	—	23
ApSmSuTc(Cl)[a]	—	—	—	—	—	—	14	4	—	18
Total	1	1	2	18	5	4	32	4	1	68

Note: Type A strains were 05^{-}.
[a] With or without resistance.

Table 7. Biovar and antibiotic resistance pattern of *S. typhimurium* strains of plasmid profile types BI, BII, C, D, and E

Type of plasmid profile	Source	Biovar	Antibiotic resistance pattern	Year of isolation	05 antigen
BI	Cattle	26b	ApSmSuTcCmNaClTp, ApSmSuTcNa(Cl)[a]	1984	−
BII	Cattle	26b	ApSmSuTcNa	1985	−
C	Horses	1dh, 5bd	ApSmSuTcKmCmNa	1984-85	+
	Cattle	5bd, 5d	ApSmSuTcKmCmNa, ApSmSuTcCmNa	1984	+
D	Horses	1a	sensitive	1976	−
		1b	ApSmSuTcCm, SmSuCm, sensitive	1976-77	−
E	Cattle	1bd	SmSuTc	1981	+

[a] With or without resistance.

pattern and biovar is shown in Table 7. Type A strains from horses and cattle were closely related to primary biovar 26 and multiresistance.

DISCUSSION

In Hokkaido area where *S. typhimurium* infection occurred among horses during 1976-85, calf salmonellosis had prevailed since 1970 (Makino et al. 1981; Tanabe 1986). The results of this study indicated that among the plasmid profile types A, C, and D found in horse strains, types A and C were common to bovine strains. Type A strains were the most prevalent in both species of animals. Tanabe (1986) detected four types of plasmid profiles among bovine *S. typhimurium* strains isolated in Tokachi district during 1975-85. He indicated that one of the four types containing three R plasmids (60 Md, 5.0 Md, and 3.9 Md) appeared in 1979 and it was then the most prevalent in the district. This type was identical with the type A of plasmid profile in our study. Nakamura et al. (1986) concluded that when *S. typhimurium* strains isolated from animals reared in limited areas exhibit identical or similar plasmid patterns, they are derived from the same source. In our study, no type A *S. typhimurium* strain was isolated from horses until 1980. Only type D strains had been isolated from horses in 1976 and 1977. Type A *S. typhimurium* strains were isolated for the first time from horses and cattle in 1980 in Kushiro district and in 1981 in Hidaka district adjoining Tokachi ditrict. These data suggest that one of the infection sources of equine salmonellosis was calf salmonellosis, which had been prevalent in Hokkaido. However, the mechanism of transmission of *S. typhimurium* from cattle to horses remains unresolved.

Although type A of plasmid profile was found most frequently among *S. typhimurium* strains from horses and cattle, there was a difference in the frequency of conjugative 60-Md R plasmid in the type A strains from horses (28.9%) and cattle (1.4%). Moreover, about one-third of type A strains isolated from horses in Hidaka district carried a conjugative, cryptic 60-Md plasmid coexisting with the conjugative 60-Md R plasmid. It has been reported that R plasmids may have been introduced by conjugation or deleted independently of the presence of other plasmids (Nakamura et al. 1986), and that a plasmid encoding multiresistance in *Serratia* was transferred to a variety of other genera of bacteria by conjugation in vivo (Tompkins et al. 1980). Therefore, it is presumed that the transferability of nonconjugative 60-Md R plasmid and the addition of conjugative cryptic 60-Md plasmid to type A plasmid profile may have emerged after introduction of *Salmonella* from cattle to a horse population. Further study is needed to clarify the reason why the cryptic 60 Md plasmid emerged in type A strains.

In this study, almost all *S. typhimurium* strains, even antibiotic-sensitive strains (type D), carried 60-Md plasmids. It is probable that the plasmids are virulence-associated (Helmuth et al. 1985).

This study indicated that the most prevalent type A strains had a close relationship to primary biovar 26, especially 26e and 26b, in both horses and cattle. Type C strains belonged to primary biovar 5 and type D strains to the biovar 1. Barker (1986) emphasized that biotyping should be considered as ancillary to either phage typing or plasmid analysis to determine the relatedness or unrelatedness of *S. typhimurium* isolates.

In the present study, all the tested strains recently isolated from horses and cattle were multiresistant and, in addition to large plasmids conferring multiresistance, small plasmids coding Ap or Su resistance (5.0- and 3.9-Md plasmids in types A, BI, and BII; 3.7-Md plasmid in type C) were found. This seems to be related to the spread of antibiotic resistance in *Salmonella* organisms. Mobilization may play a role for transmitting the resistance. A conjugative cryptic plasmid or conjugative R plasmid may mobilize the small R plasmids to other bacteria.

It has been reported that plasmid pattern analysis was useful in understanding the epidemiology of equine salmonellosis with *S. krefeld*, *S. saintpaul*, and *S. muenchen* (Ikeda & Hirsh 1985; Rumschlag & Boyce 1987). Four *Salmonella* serovars other than *S. typhimurium* were isolated from diseased or healthy horses and their environment in Hokkaido during 1982-85 (unpublished data): *S. paratyphi-B*, d-tartrate^{+} *S. java*, *S. infantis*, *S. isangi*, and *S. london*. About one-third of the strains were antibiotic-sensitive. Except for a multiresistant *S. london* strain with the same plasmid profile as the type A in *S. typhimurium*, only a few of the strains had very simple plasmid profiles.

ACKNOWLEDGMENTS

We are grateful to Drs. I. Yamaguchi, T. Asai, H. Kato, S. Honma, N. Nagase, T. Yasui, and K. Hirose, Livestock Hygiene Service Centers, Hokkaido Prefectural Government, and Drs. H. Senba and H. Ohishi, Hidaka Agricultural Aid Association, for the supply of *Salmonella* strains. We also thank Dr. M. Kamada and Dr. Y. Akiyama, Equine Research Institute, Tokyo, for advice. This study was supported by a grant-in-aid from the Equine Research Institute, Japan Racing Association.

REFERENCES

Barker, R.M. (1986) Tracing *Salmonella typhimurium* infections. *J. Hyg. Camb.* **96**, 1-4.

Bezanson, G.S.; Khakhria, R.; and Pagnutti, D. (1983) Plasmid profiles of value in differentiating *Salmonella muenster. J. Clin. Microbiol.* **17**, 1159-90.

Clewell, D.B., and Helinski, D.R. (1969) Supercoiled circular DNA-protein complex in *Escherichia coli*: purification and induced conversion to an open circular DNA form. *Proc. Natl. Acad. Sci. USA* **62**, 1159-66.

Cohen, S.N.; Chang, A.C.Y.; Boyer, H.W.; and Helling, R.B. (1973) Construction of biologically functional bacterial plasmid in vitro. *Proc. Natl. Acad. Sci. USA* **70**, 3240-44.

Duguid, J.P.; Anderson, E.S.; Alfredsson, G.A.; Barker, R.; and Old, D.C. (1975) A new biotyping scheme for *Salmonella typhimurium* and its phylogenetic significance. *J. Med. Microbiol.* **8**, 149-66.

Gibbons, D.F. (1980) Equine salmonellosis: A review. *Vet. Rec.* **106**, 356-59.

Helmuth, R.; Stephan, R.; Bunge, C.; Hoog, B.; Steinbeck, A.; and Bulling, E. (1985) Epidemiology of virulence-associated plasmids and outer membrane protein patterns within seven common *Salmonella* serotypes. *Infect. Immun.* **48**, 175-82.

Holmberg, S.D.; Wachsmuth, I.K.; Hickman-Brenner, F.W.; and Cohen, M.L. (1984) Comparison of plasmid profile analysis, phage typing, and antimicrobial susceptibility testing in characterizing *Salmonella typhimurium* isolated from outbreaks. *J. Clin. Microbiol.* **19**, 100-104.

Ikeda, J.S., and Hirsh, D.W. (1985) Common plasmid encoding resistance to ampicillin, chloramphenicol, gentamicin, and trimethoprim-sulfadiazine in two serotypes of *Salmonella* isolated during an outbreak of equine salmonellosis. *Am. J. Vet Res.* **46**, 769-73.

Ishiguro, N., and Sato, G. (1984) Spontaneous deletion of citrate-utilizing ability promoted by insertion sequences. *J. Bacteriol.* **160**, 642-50.

Ishiguro, N.; Makino, S.; Sato, G.; and Hashimoto, K. (1980)) Antibiotic resistance and genetic properties of R plasmids in *Salmonella* isolates of swine origin in Japan. *Am. J. Vet. Res.* **41**, 46-50.

Kado, C.I., and Liu, S.-T. (1981) Rapid procedure for detection and isolation of large and small plasmids, *J. Bacteriol.* **145**, 1365-73.

Lennox, E.S. (1955) Transduction of linked genetic characters of the host by bacteriophage P1. *Virology* **1**, 190-206.

Macrina, F.L.; Kopecko, D.J.; Jones, K.R.; Ayers, D.J.; and McCowen, S.M. (1978) A multiple plasmid-containing *Escherichia coli* strain: convenient source of size reference plasmid molecules. *Plasmid* **1**, 417-20.

Makino, S.; Ishiguro, N.; Sato, G.; and Seno, N. (1981) Change of drug resistance patterns and genetic properties of R plasmids in *Salmonella typhimurium* of bovine origin isolated from 1970 to 1979 in northern Japan. *J. Hyg., Camb.* **87**, 257-69.

Nakamura, M.; Sato, S.; Ohya, T.; Suzuki, S.; and Ikeda, S. (1986) Plasmid profile analysis in epidemiological studies of animal *Salmonella typhimurium* infection in Japan. *J. Clin. Microbiol.* **23**, 360-65.

Niida, M.; Ishiguro, N.; Shinagawa, M.; and Sato, G. (1983) Genetic and molecular characterization of conjugative R plasmids detected in *Salmonella* strains isolated from humans and feral pigeons in the same district. *Jpn. J. Vet. Sci.* **45**, 647-58.

Portnoy, D.A., and Falkow, S. (1981) Virulence-associated plasmids from *Yersinia enterocolitica* and *Yersinia pestis. J. Bacteriol.* **148**, 877-93.

Riley, L.W., and Cohen, M.L. (1982) Plasmid profiles and *Salmonella* epidemiology. *Lancet* **i**, 573.

Rumschlag, H.S., and Boyce, J.R. (1987) Plasmid profile analysis of salmonellae in a large-animal hospital. *Vet. Microbiol.* **13**, 301-11.

Sato, G.; Nakaoka, Y.; Ishiguro, N.; Ohishi, H.; Senba, H.; Kato, H.; Honma, S.; and Nagase, N. (1984) Plasmid profiles of *Salmonella typhimurium* var. *copenhagen* strains isolated from horses. *Bull. Equine Res. Inst.* **21**, 105-9.

Southern, E.M. (1975) Detection of specific sequences among DNA fragments separated by gel electrophoresis. *J. Mol. Biol.* **98**, 503-17.

Tanabe, M. (1986) A plasmid profile study of multiresistant *Salmonella typhimurium* isolated from calves in Tokachi district from 1975 to 1985. Master's thesis, Obihiro University of Agriculture and Veterinary Medicine.

Taylor, D.E.; Levine, J.G.; and Kouvelos, K.L. (1982) Incidence of plasmid DNA in *Salmonella* strains isolated from clinical sources in Ontario, Canada, during 1979 and 1980. *Can. J. Microbiol.* **28**, 1150-57.

Taylor, D.N.; Wachsmuth, I.K.; Schangkuan, Y.-H.; Schmidt, E.V.; Barrett, T.J.; Schrader, J.S.; Scherach, C.S.; McGee, H.B.; Feldman, R.A.; and Brenner, D.J. (1982) Salmonellosis associated with marijuana—A multistate outbreak traced by plasmid fingerprinting. *N. Engl. J. Med.* **306**, 1249-53.

Tompkins, L.S.; Plorde, J.J.; and Falkow, S. (1980) Molecular analysis of R-factors from multiresistant nosocomial isolates. *J. Infect. Dis.* **141**, 625-36.

Yataya, K.; Terakado, N.; and Hashimoto, K. (1983) Epizootiological observation from plasmid DNA on *Salmonella typhimurium* infection in a human infant and calves. *J. Jpn. Vet. Med. Assoc.* **36**, 274-77.

An Epidemiological Investigation of Equine Salmonellosis in Central Kentucky during 1985 and 1986

David G. Powell, Michael Donahue, K. Ferris, Meta Osborne, and Roberta Dwyer

SUMMARY

A total of 157 cases of salmonella infection among horses in central Kentucky during 1985 and 1986 were studied retrospectively. Depending on the clinical, bacteriological, and postmortem findings, cases were defined as mild or severe. The majority of cases occurred among foals during the first six months of each year. Salmonellae were isolated primarily from fecal samples, but also from a variety of tissues and anatomical sites during postmortem examination. Although a number of serotypes were identified *S. saint-paul* was predominant in both years, and plasmid typing confirmed that the majority of *S. saint-paul* isolates belonged to a single plasmid type. Two-thirds of the salmonella isolates were obtained shortly after horses were admitted to a medical or surgical facility. Relatively few multiple cases of salmonellosis occurred on any single farm, and no farm had multiple cases in both years. The strains of *S. saint-paul* isolated during the study were highly resistant to antibiotics.

INTRODUCTION

Outbreaks of enteric disease among horses in Kentucky have been attributed to salmonella infection at intervals during the last 50 years. The first, described by Edwards (1934), was caused by *S. typhimurium*. Bryans, Fallon & Shephard (1961) reported further outbreaks caused by the same serotype during 1959 and 1960. The emergence of *S. agona* as an equine pathogen between 1980 and 1984 was first described by Donahue (1986). Over the years, the incidence of salmonella infection in horses has increased not only in the United States (Smith 1981) but also in other countries, including Britain (Gibbons 1980), Japan (Sato et al. 1984), and Australia (Roberts & O'Boyle 1981). As a consequence, fecal samples are routinely examined for salmonella as a possible cause of clinical disease or asymptomatic infection. The effect of environmental and stress factors in predisposing horses to salmonella infection has been extensively discussed (Gibbons 1980; Smith et al. 1978, Hird, Pappaioanou & Smith 1984). Among the many salmonella serotypes isolated from horses, antibiotic-resistant strains have been described (Ikeda & Hirsh 1985; Donahue 1986). Several recent reports of animal salmonellosis in the United States have examined the role of veterinary hospitals in facilitating dissemination of the infection (Ikeda et al. 1986; Carter et al. 1986; Rumschlag & Boyce 1987). Along with these primarily descriptive case studies, a case control study by Hird and colleagues (1986) identified some of the factors that expose the hospitalized horse to the risk of salmonellosis.

Although plasmid profile analysis is a valuable epidemiological tool in cases of salmonellosis, it has been used to only a limited degree to investigate outbreaks in the horse (Sato et al. 1984; Ikeda & Hirsh 1985; Rumschlag & Boyce 1987).

The present study used plasmid profile analysis to examine the distribution of clinical salmonellosis within the equine population of central Kentucky during 1985 and 1986, as well as investigating the antimicrobial susceptibility pattern of some of the strains isolated.

Powell, Donahue, Osborne, Dwyer: Department of Veterinary Science, University of Kentucky, Lexington, Kentucky 40546. Ferris: National Veterinary Services Laboratories, Ames, Iowa 50010. Published as paper No. 88-4-22 with the approval of the Director, Kentucky Agricultural Experiment Station.

MATERIALS AND METHODS

Field samples. Salmonellae were cultured from several sources, the majority from fecal samples of clinical cases of enteritis submitted by veterinary practitioners to either the Livestock Disease Diagnostic Center (LDDC) in Lexington, Kentucky, or to private veterinary diagnostic laboratories in the vicinity. Other isolates came from tissues obtained at necropsy when fatalities were submitted to the LDDC. Clinical histories were available in the majority of cases, as well as postmortem findings from the fatalities.

For the purpose of this study, salmonellosis was categorized as either mild or severe. In a mild case, salmonellae were isolated from a fecal sample in association with signs of intestinal disease, usually manifest as diarrhea. A severe case was defined as one in which salmonellae were isolated from a fecal sample or from the small or large intestine and from other sites in the body, while clinical and/or postmortem evidence also indicated septicemia.

Culture testing procedures. Salmonellae were isolated by inoculating fecal and tissue swabs onto blood agar and eosin-methylene blue agar (EMB) plates. In respect of intestinal or fecal specimens, a swab was also inoculated onto a Hektoen enteric agar (HEA) plate and into a tube of selenite broth. After overnight incubation at 37°C, a subculture of the selenite broth was inoculated onto EMB and HEA plates. The agar plates were examined for bacterial colonies with culture characteristics of salmonella (lactose-negative on EMB, and

Table 1. Distribution of cases from which Salmonellae were isolated, in terms of age, clinical severity and mortality, and time of year

Year	Age	Clinical severity (mortality[a])		Time of year	
		Mild	Severe	1st half	2nd half
1985	Less than 1 year	26(0)	28(16)	42	12
	More than 1 year	14(0)	7(4)	7	14
1986	Less than 1 year	25(0)	23(19)	41	7
	More than 1 year	18(0)	12(9)	16	14

Note: Excludes four animals of indeterminate age.
[a] Number of fatalities attributable to Salmonella.

Table 2. Serotypes of Salmonellae isolated from horses in central Kentucky during 1985 and 1986

Serotype	1985	1986
S. agona	4	—
S. anatum	1	2
S. cerro	—	3
S. infantis	4	5
S. javiana	—	1
S. johannesburg	—	1
S. montevideo	—	1
S. muenchen	—	5
S. muenster	—	1
S. ohio	—	1
S. oranienburg	—	1
S. schwarzengrund	—	2
S. saint-paul	61	47
S. thomasville	1	—
S. thompson	—	4
S. typhimurium	4	3
S. typhimurium (var. copenhagen)	—	1
Group B (untyped)	4	—

Table 3. Major serotypes of Salmonellae isolated from horses in central Kentucky 1981-86

	1981	1982	1983	1984	1985	1986
S. agona	26	28	21	18	4	—
S. saint-paul	—	1	1	6	61	47
S. typhimurium	18	8	16	10	4	3
S. typhimurium var. copenhagen	21	32	3	30	—	1

lactose-negative and hydrogen sulfide–positive on HEA) after 24 and 48 hr incubation. The biochemical reactivity of isolates was determined using conventional bacteriological media or a miniaturized system (API 20E; Analytical Products, Plainview, N.Y.). The identity of cultures giving biochemical reactions consistent with those for salmonella was confirmed by slide agglutination using specific O-grouping antiserum. All isolates were sent to the National Veterinary Services Laboratories (NVSL) in Ames, Iowa, for serotyping. Plasmid profile analysis was performed at the NVSL by Kathleen Ferris using a modification of the agarose gel electrophoresis method of Kado and Lui (1981).

The antimicrobial susceptibilities of the *S. saint-paul* strains were determined using the Kirby-Bauer single disk susceptibility test (Bauer et al. 1966). The disks (Difco Laboratories, Detroit, Mich.) used were ampicillin, amikacin, carbenicillin, cephalothin, chloromycetin, erythromycin, gentamicin, kanamycin, neomycin, furadantin, penicillin G, polymyxin B, streptomycin, tetracycline, trimethoprim/sulphadiazine (Tribrissen), and triple sulfonamides (sulfa drugs).

RESULTS

Of the 157 cases of salmonellosis diagnosed during 1985 and 1986, 102 occurred in horses less than one year of age and 51 cases among adult animals, while in 4 cases the age was not recorded (Table 1). Eighty-three cases were defined as mild, with no mortality, and 70 as severe, with mortality occurring in 48 cases. Two-thirds of the cases occurred during the first six months of each year, the majority being horses less than one year of age. Salmonellae were isolated only from fecal samples in mild cases. In severe cases, salmonellae were isolated from the intestinal tract without exception, as well as from the liver, joint cavities, lung, chest cavity, lymph nodes, blood, or abscesses in various parts of the body.

During the study 17 different serotypes were identified (Table 2). Of the 157 isolates, 108 were *S. saint-paul* and 65 of them were isolated from animals under one year of age. During 1986, 15 different serotypes were identified, with *S. saint-paul* comprising the majority: 47 of 78. The other 14 serotypes were represented by 31 isolates, 15 of them from horses over one year of age.

From the equine samples submitted to the LDDC between 1981 and 1986, the predominant serotype isolated was *S. agona* during 1981-84 and *S. saint-paul* in 1985-86 (Table 3). *Salmonella typhimurium* and *S. typhimurium var. copenhagen* were also isolated in significant numbers between 1981 and 1984.

In plasmid typing of 105 isolates of *S. saint-paul*, nine different plasmid types were identified (Table 4); plasmid type 1 accounted for 64 of 105 isolates, evenly distributed between mild and severe cases.

The majority of cases, 90, were identified at a medical facility when sick horses, usually foals with diarrhea, were admitted for intensive care (Table 5). Following admission, fecal samples were obtained daily over a period of several

Table 4. Distribution of *Salmonella saint-paul* plasmid types according to severity of clinical disease, 1985-86

	1985		1986	
Plasmid type	Mild	Severe	Mild	Severe
I	15	14	17	18
II	5	8	3	—
III	1	2	1	1
IV	—	1	—	—
V	4	2	3	3
VI	—	3	—	—
VII	1	—	—	—
VIII	—	—	—	—
IX	2	—	—	—
X	—	—	—	1

Note: Three isolates were not typed.

Table 5. Types of establishments where Salmonellae isolated from horses, 1985-86

Year	Horse farm	Medical facility	Surgical facility
1985	14	55	4
1986	36	35	7
Totals	50	90	11

Note: No record for six isolates.

days, resulting in a large number of isolations of salmonellae.

The incidence of multiple cases (two or more) was greatest on Farm B, which had seven cases during 1985 (Table 6). While most of the outbreaks were attributable to *S. saint-paul*, more than one serotype was isolated during an outbreak on Farms C and F.

All plasmid types of the *S. saint-paul* isolates were sensitive to amikacin, cephalothin, furadantin, and polymixin B, but resistant to ampicillin, carbenicillin, chloromycetin, erythromycin, penicillin, and sulfa drugs. The sensitivity pattern varied, depending on plasmid type, for neomycin, kanamycin, tetracycline, streptomycin, gentamicin, and Tribrissen (Table 7). The predominant plasmid type 1 was sensitive to tetracycline and streptomycin but resistant to neomycin, kanamycin, gentamicin, and Tribrissen.

DISCUSSION

The data presented in this study were derived from a large but concentrated population of horses that was well served by veterinarians specializing in equine practice, supported by good laboratory and postmortem facilities. Through the cooperation of many people working in various disciplines, access to case histories, laboratory findings, and postmortem reports was readily available. However, this study, being retrospective in nature, suffers from certain inevitable deficiencies. The relevant data were extracted from a large body of information, some of it imprecise, making interpretation difficult on occasion. Cases of salmonellosis categorized as mild could not be differentiated in terms of nosocomial infection, disease resulting directly from the presence of salmonellae, and disease related to other organisms in the gastrointestinal system. Severe cases could be more precisely defined, on the basis of clinical, bacteriological, and in many cases postmortem data.

The majority of mild and severe cases occurred among animals less than one year of age, a finding consistent with earlier reports that young, "stressed" foals are at risk for salmonella infection (Gibbons 1980; Smith 1981). However, as many as one-third of the cases occurred among clinically ill or asymptomatic adult horses. Among the older animals, the variety of serotypes was greater than among animals of less than a year, which were predominantly associated with *S. saint-paul*. This finding supports the hypothesis that the adult animal acts as a reservoir of salmonellae within the equine population. The high incidence of cases among foals during the first six months of the year reflects their high-risk status following birth during the months of February, March, April, and May.

In many of the severe cases, salmonellae were isolated from several anatomical sites in addition to the gastroin-

Table 6. Horse farms with multiple isolations of Salmonellae

	Farm	Serotype and plasmid		No. of cases
1985	A	S. saint-paul	I	5
	B	S. saint-paul	I	1
			II	6
	C	S. typhimurium		1
		S. infantis		1
		S. saint-paul	II	1
	D	S. saint-paul	V	2
	E	S. saint-paul	I	4
	F	S. infantis		1
		S. saint-paul	I	1
1986	G	S. infantis		3
	H	S. saint-paul	I	5
	I	S. saint-paul	I	2
	J	S. saint-paul	I	1
			III	1

Note: Serotypes isolated either on farm or after admittance to clinic.

Table 7. Antibiotic sensitivity pattern of *Salmonella saint-paul* in terms of plasmid type, 1985-86 samples

	Plasmid type								
	I-65	II-16	III-5	IV-1	V-12	VI-3	VII-1	IX-2	X-1
Neomycin	R/S	R	S	R	R	R	S	R	R
Kanamycin	R	R	R	R	R	R	S	R	R
Tetracycline	S	R	S	R	R/S	S	S	R	S
Streptomycin	S	R/S	S	R	R/S	S	S	R	S
Gentamicin	I/R	S	I	S	S	S	S	S	S
Tribrissen	R	R	R	S	R	S	S	R	S

Note: S = sensitive; I = Intermediate; R = resistant.

testinal tract. The isolation from the joint and chest cavities demonstrates the ability of salmonellae to cause a bacteremia in both foals and adult animals. The suggestion that some serotypes of salmonella are nonpathogenic and rarely cause clinical disease in the horse (Smith et al. 1978) was not substantiated in this study. The comment by Gibbons (1980) that "horses when exposed to salmonellae in sufficient numbers regardless of serotype or phage type behave in disease terms like other species," would seem to be more accurate.

A considerable variety of salmonella serotypes were isolated from horses in central Kentucky during 1985-86, although *S. saint-paul* was by far the most numerous. The extensive use of feed supplements containing bone and other meals has been suggested (Gibons 1980) as one of the means by which animals are exposed to the various serotypes. Sampling of feeds, however, was not performed in this study. *Salmonella saint-paul* is not a common serotype in animals, although it was associated with an outbreak of salmonellosis among horses in a veterinary teaching hospital in California during 1981-82 (Ikeda & Hirsh 1985), and has also been isolated from turkeys (Ferris, Murphy & Blackburn 1986) and from humans (U.S. Centers for Disease Control, 1983). The two-year time period of this study was very short in terms of observing the prevalence of salmonella within a population, but results over the more extended period 1981-86 indicated a cyclical pattern for prevalence of the major serotypes. A similar pattern was observed by Ikeda and colleagues (1986) and Carter and colleagues (1986), in their studies of salmonella serotypes isolated from small and large animals, including horses, admitted to a veterinary teaching hospital between 1971 and 1983. The predominance of a single serotype at any one time suggests the possibility of a single focus for the dissemination of salmonella within the population. The fact that the majority of *S. saint-paul* isolates during 1985 and 1986 were plasmid type 1 would support this suggestion. Approximately two-thirds of the isolates came from horses admitted to a medical or surgical facility, reflecting the intensive bacteriological screening of horses at the time of admission and throughout their stay. The role that veterinary clinics and veterinary teaching hospitals play in the dissemination of salmonellosis is well recognized, as discussed by Hird and colleagues (1986). They observed that in a veterinary teaching hospital, the risk of salmonella isolations from feces was greater for horses treated with antibiotics and intubated with nasogastric tubes after admission because of colic than for horses that were not subject to any of these three conditions. When salmonella is isolated from a hospitalized horse, it is difficult to determine whether it represents nosocomial infection or activation of latent infection. Since horses admitted to a medical or surgical facility are invariably "under stress" for a variety of reasons, they are necessarily at greater risk of acquiring infection and developing clinical salmonellosis. Stressors identified in the present study included weakness and prematurity in foals, transportation, intercurrent disease, antibiotic therapy, and traumatic injury. Environmental sampling was not undertaken during this study, but the preponderance of *S. saint-paul* plasmid type 1 is circumstantial evidence that nosocomial infections may have played some part in the dissemination of salmonellosis.

Bearing in mind the large and concentrated nature of the equine population of central Kentucky, the number of multiple cases occurring on any single farm was low, suggesting that the overall standard of farm management and hygiene was satisfactory. No outbreaks of salmonellosis recurred on any single farm, which suggests that precautions following an outbreak were successful. On several farms that were the site of an outbreak in 1985, an autogenous salmonella bacterin had been administered to mares just prior to foaling in 1986.

A considerable variety of antimicrobial drugs, singly and in combination, are used to treat cases of gastrointestinal disease in horses, especialy young foals. Donahue (1986) reported the isolation of antibiotic-resistant *S. agona* from horses in Kentucky between 1980 and 1984, and strains of *S. saint-paul* isolated from horses in California during 1981-82 had multiple antibiotic resistances (Ikeda & Hirsh 1985). Given this, it is not surprising that a high degree of antibiotic resistance was observed among the strains of *S. saint-paul* isolated during this study. Multiple resistance significantly reduces the efficacy of antimicrobial drugs and may have been a factor in the high mortality rate for severe cases reported in this study. The emergence of multiple-resistant strains of bacteria is usually due to resistance plasmids (R-plasmids) that can transfer to other strains, serotypes, species, and even genera of bacteria. Evidence of transfer between serotypes was reported in the recent salmonellosis outbreak among horses in California (Ikeda & Hirsh 1985). It is recognized that resistance plasmids may be shared extensively between animal and human bacteria, and that spread of multiple-resistant strains of salmonella between animals and humans can give rise to serious human illness (Holmberg et al. 1984). These reports and the findings of this study emphasize the need for the judicious use of antibiotics to treat gastrointestinal disease of horses, especially young foals.

ACKNOWLEDGMENTS

We would like to express our considerable appreciation to the many people who contributed to this study: to the equine practitioners of central Kentucky and their hospital staff, who provided case records; to the pathologists at the Livestock Disease Diagnostic Center, Lexington, Kentucky, for access to postmortem records; and to the bacteriologists at the several private diagnostic laboratories in Lexington who provided cultures of salmonellae isolated from specimens submitted to them.

The study was funded in part by Lloyds of London, Brokers and Underwriters, and their Kentucky agents, to whom we express our thanks.

REFERENCES

Bauer, A.W.; Kirby, W.M.; Sherris, J.C.; and Turck, M. (1966) Antibiotic susceptibility testing by a standardized single disk method. *Am. J. Clin. Path.* **45**, 493-96.

Bryans, J.T.; Fallon, E.H.; and Shephard, B.P. (1961) Equine salmonellosis. *Cornell Vet.* **51**, 467-77.

Carter, J.D.; Hird, D.W.; Farver, T.B.; and Hjerpe, C.A. (1986) Salmonellosis in hospitalized horses: Seasonality and case fatality rates. *J. Am. Vet. Med. Assoc.* **188**, 163-67.

Centers for Disease Control (1983) Human salmonella isolates—United States 1982. *Morbidity and Mortality Weekly Report* **32**, 598-600.

Donahue, J.M. (1986) Emergence of antibiotic-resistant *S. agona* in horses in Kentucky, *J. Am. Vet. Med. Assoc.* **188**, 592-94.

Edwards, P.R. (1934) Salmonella aertyrke in colitis of foals. *J. Infect. Dis.* **54**, 85-90.

Ferris, K.; Murphy, C.D.; and Blackburn, B.O. (1986) Salmonella serotypes from animals and related sources reported during fiscal year 1985. *Proc. 19th Ann. Meet. U.S. Anim. Health Assoc.*, pp. 381-96.

Gibbons, D.J. (1980) Equine salmonellosis: A review. *Vet. Rec.* **106**, 356-59.

Hird, D.W.; Pappaioanou, M.; and Smith, B.P. (1984) Case control study of risk factors associated with isolation of *Salmonella saintpaul* in hospitalized horses. *Am. J. Epidemiol.* **120**, 852-64.

Hird, D.W.; Casebolt, D.B.; Carter, J.D.; Pappaioanou, M.; and Hjerpe, C.A. (1986). Risk factor of salmonellosis in hospitalized horses. *J. Am. Vet. Med. Assoc.* **188**, 173-77.

Holmberg, S.D.; Osterholm, M.T.; Senger, K.A.; and Cohen, M.L. (1984) Drug resistant salmonella from animals fed antimicrobials. *N. Engl. J. Med.* **311**, 617-22.

Ikeda, J.W., and Hirsch, D.C. (1985) Common plasmid encoding resistance to ampicillin, chloromycetin, gentamicin and trimethoprim-sulfadazine in two serotypes of salmonella isolated during an outbreak of equine salmonellosis. *Am. J. Vet. Res.* **46**, 769-73.

Ikeda, J.W.; Hirsh, D.C.; Jang, S.S.; and Biberstein, E.L. (1986) Characteristics of salmonella isolated from animals at the veterinary medical teaching hospital. *Am. J. Vet. Res.* **47**, 232-35.

Kado, C.I., and Liu, S.T. (1981) Rapid procedure for detection and isolation of large and small plasmids. *J. Bacteriol.* **145**, 1365-73.

Roberts, M.C., and O'Boyle, D.A. (1981) The prevalence and epizootiology of salmonellosis among groups of horses in south-east Queensland. *Aust. Vet. J.* **57**, 27-35.

Rumschlag, H.S., and Boyce, J.R. (1987) Plasmid profile analysis of salmonella in a large-animal hospital. *Vet. Microbiol.* **13**, 301-11.

Sato, G.; Nakaoka, Y.; Ishiguro, N.; Ohishi, H.; Senba, H.; Kato, H.; Honma, S.; and Nagase, N. (1984) Plasmid profiles of *Salmonella typhimurium var. copenhagen* strains isolated from horses. *Bull. Equine Res. Inst.* **21**, 105-9.

Smith, B.P. (1981) Equine salmonellosis: A contemporary review. *Equine Vet. J.* **13**, 147-51.

Smith, B.P.; Reina-Guerra, M.; and Hardy, A.J. (1978) Prevalence and epizootiology of equine salmonellosis. *J. Am. Vet. Med. Assoc.* **172**, 353-56.

Association of *Clostridium difficile* with Foal Diarrhea

Robert L. Jones, Robert K. Shideler, and Gary L. Cockerell

SUMMARY

Routine microbiological examinations of feces from a group of diarrheic foals were performed in an attempt to identify the cause of severe watery diarrhea at three to five days of age. Commonly expected bacterial and viral agents were not identified. *Clostridium difficile* was isolated from the feces of 27 of 43 diarrheic foals (63%) by use of selective media, but was not isolated from the feces of 18 normal foals without diarrhea nor from 62 adult horses. Isolates of *C. difficile* produced both toxins A (enterotoxin) and B (cytotoxin). Cytotoxin was detected in the feces from 28 of 43 diarrheic foals (65%) by an in vitro cytotoxin neutralization test.

Lesions in the intestines of foals that died varied from localized damage of villus tips with destruction of the basement membrane, progressing to sloughing of the epithelium from the villi with subepithelial edema of the villi, and eventually to massive necrosis of the villi with hemorrhage.

Administration of *C. difficile* by nasogastric tube to foals induced diarrhea within 8 hr in one foal, the deaths of two foals within 20 hr, and lesions ranging from loss of epithelium from tips of villi to diffuse loss of epithelium, shortened denuded villi, and necrosis of villi.

We thus fulfilled Koch's postulates by experimentally producing diarrhea and lesions in foals that were similar to naturally occurring diarrhea associated with *C. difficile*.

The finding of *C. difficile* and its toxin in association with diarrhea in foals and the experimental reproduction of the disease add another to the list of infectious agents that may cause foal diarrhea. The origination of cases from widely separated areas indicates that this disease problem may be widespread.

INTRODUCTION

Clostridia are sporadically associated with gastrointestinal disease in horses. Hemorrhagic necrotizing enterocolitis in foals has been associated with *C. perfringens* (Dickie, Klinkerman & Petrie 1978; Howard-Martin et al. 1986; Mason & Robinson 1938; Montgomery & Rowlands 1937; Niilo & Chalmers 1982; Pearson et al. 1986; Sims et al. 1985), with *C. sordelli* (Hibbs et al. 1977), and with unidentified causes (Cudd & Pauly 1987; White et al. 1987). Diarrhea and enteritis following experimental clostridial infection in horses was reported by Wierup (1977).

Diagnostic Laboratory (Jones) and Departments of Clinical Sciences (Shideler) and Pathology (Cockerell), College of Veterinary Medicine and Biomedical Sciences, Colorado State University, Fort Collins, Colorado 80523.

Recently, *C. difficile* has been isolated from foals with hemorrhagic necrotizing enterocolitis (Jones et al. 1987a); it has been found in the feces of foals that experienced diarrhea but not in unaffected foals (Jones, Adney & Shideler, 1987b).

In the infrequent cases when *C. difficile* has been isolated from adult horses (Hafiz & Oakley, 1976; Ehrich et al. 1984), it was not associated with diarrhea (Harbour 1985). *C. difficile* was first identified in 1978 as the cause of pseudomembranous colitis in humans (Bartlett et al. 1978), where it is commonly found in conjunction with antibiotic-associated colitis and diarrhea (George 1984). Infection with *C. difficile* also causes colitis in hamsters, mice, guinea pigs, and rabbits (Silva 1979).

The purpose of this study was to characterize the clinical features of *C. difficile* infection of foals and to produce infection in foals experimentally.

MATERIALS AND METHODS

Foals. A breeding farm housing 56 mares with foals and 36 pregnant mares was the source of foals with naturally occurring diarrhea. Fecal specimens were collected from the rectum of foals on the breeding farm during a four-week period, from foals at two days of age and daily thereafter from foals with diarrhea.

For experimental studies, pregnant mares were purchased and housed in individual pens. When a foal was delivered, it was fitted with a mask as soon as possible, to prevent colostrum consumption, and was fed artificial milk replacer.

Microbiological methods. Feces were inoculated into tetrathionate broth (BBL Microbiology Systems, Cockeysville, Md.) and onto Hektoen enteric agar plates for attempted isolation of *Salmonella* sp.; Campylobacter agar plates and Campylobacter thioglycollate medium for attempted isolation of *Campylobacter* sp.; and *Clostridium difficile* agar plates, also known as cycloserine-cefoxitin-fructose agar (CCFA), for attempted isolation of *C. difficile* (Allen 1985; George et al. 1979). Trypticase soy agar plates with 5% sheep's blood and MacConkey II agar plates were also inoculated with feces to detect changes in aerobic bacterial fecal flora. Bacterial isolates were identified by standard methods (Allen 1985; Koneman et al. 1983). Fecal specimens collected within the first two days of diarrhea were examined for viruses by negative contrast-staining electron microscopy

(England & Reed 1980). Fecal filtrates were tested for *C. difficile* cytotoxin using a commercial tissue culture cytotoxicity neutralization kit (Nachamkin, Lotz-Nolan & Skalina 1986; Wu & Gersch 1986; Bartels Immunodiagnostic Supplies, Bellevue, Wash.).

Inoculation procedure. *C. difficile* was isolated from naturally occurring cases of hemorrhagic necrotizing enterocolitis in foals. Isolated bacterial colonies were picked from blood agar and inoculated into 10 ml of brain-heart infusion (BHI) broth and incubated anaerobically for 4 hr at 37°C. The 10-ml culture was then added to 50 ml of BHI broth and incubated anaerobically for 18 hr at 37°C. The viable colony-forming unit (cfu) count of the inoculum was determined by triplicate spread plate count and cytotoxicity was verified. The 50-ml inoculum was administered to each foal by nasogastric tube. The tube was flushed with 100 ml of 1.0 M $NaHCO_3$. The foals were checked at 8-hr intervals post-inoculation for depression, fever, diarrhea, and the presence of blood or mucus in the feces.

Culture dialysate was prepared as a source of crude toxin by the method of Lyerly and colleagues (1985).

Tissue collection and processing. Foals were euthanized and two segments each of the duodenum, upper and lower jejunum, ileum, large colon, and small colon were collected. One segment from each site was inflated with buffered formalin and fixed for histological examination of H&E stained sections. The other segment was used for microbiological examination as described above for feces.

RESULTS

Clinical features of naturally occurring disease. Intestinal infection of foals by *C. difficile* presented one of two clinical syndromes: fatal hemorrhagic necrotizing enterocolitis, or severe watery diarrhea.

Newborn foals (less than three days) that subsequently died of hemorrhagic necrotizing enterocolitis, presented clinical evidence of acute, severe enteritis; either severe diarrhea or colic. The foals died or were found dead within 24 hr after the onset of signs of illness. The small intestine was the most severely affected organ, either diffusely or segmentally, with necrosis of the mucosa and watery, red-to-black-colored contents. The enteritis was characterized by coagulative necrosis of the villi with desquamation of lining epithelium, hemorrhage, and subepithelial edema. The villar crypts were intact, with minimal inflammatory response. Massive numbers of large, rod-shaped, Gram-positive bacteria were seen colonizing the surfaces of denuded villi and in the lumen. Mild to severe necrotizing colitis was observed, indicating that the infection probably developed first in the small intestine and descended along the intestinal tract. If the foal survived the illness long enough, severe watery diarrhea containing blood was observed. *C. difficile* was isolated in large numbers from the intestinal contents of the foals. Cytotoxin was identified in specimens from two foals, and the isolates from each foal produced cytotoxins when grown in broth.

Foals with hemorrhagic necrotizing enteritis came from three farms in Colorado and one in New Mexico.

Foals older than three days at the onset of clinical signs usually developed a severe, watery diarrhea, and some of them required intravenous fluid therapy to correct dehydration. The foals excreted yellow, watery feces with a very foul odor that contained mucus and occasional flecks of blood. Most foals did not become anorectic, although they were slightly depressed, during the course of the diarrhea. The symptomatic treatment was oral electrolyte fluids and activated charcoal powder adsorbent. Antimicrobial treatment with trimethoprim-sulfamethoxazole or metronidazole did not seem to alter the course of the diarrhea, which ranged from five days to more than two weeks. *C. difficile* was isolated from 27 of 43 diarrheic foals and cytotoxin was detected in feces from 28 diarrheic foals on the farm where the original outbreak of disease occurred. Foals continued to shed *C. difficile* and toxin in feces for five to seven days. *Campylobacter* and *Salmonella* spp. were not isolated from any of the diarrheic specimens. Rotaviruses were observed in the diarrheic feces of nine foals, six of them being *C. difficile*-positive and the other three *C. difficile*-negative. In five of the six foals infected with both *C. difficile* and rotavirus, the onset of diarrhea occurred at three to five days of age. The other rotavirus-infected foals were seven to 14 days old.

C. difficile and cytotoxin were detected in feces from 12 of 20 foals that did not have diarrhea at two days of age. Eleven of these foals developed diarrhea when three to nine days old, whereas only three of 18 foals without *C. difficile* infection developed diarrhea within the next week. The frequency of diarrhea in foals that were positive for *C. difficile* on their second day was significantly greater than for those foals that were not shedding *C. difficile* ($P < 0.002$, Fisher's exact test; Daniel 1978).

Gross lesions were not evident in the intestinal tract of foals that died as a result of severe diarrhea. However, viewed microscopically, the severity of lesions ranged from localized loss of epithelium from villus tips with subepithelial edema, progressing to sloughing of epithelium and edema of the villi, and eventually to necrosis of the villi and hemorrhage.

Experimental production of disease. In the experimental production of disease in foals (Table 1), culture dialysate (crude toxin) was administered by nasogastric tube to a two-week-old foal that was euthanized 24 hr later for examination of the intestinal tract. The foal had not developed diarrhea, and no excessive fluid was present in the intestines. Grossly, the intestines appeared to be normal. Microscopic changes in the small intestine consisted of localized damage of villus tips with sloughing of epithelium from the tips of villi and subepithelial edema of the villi.

Table 1. Results of administration of *C. difficile* preparations to foals by nasogastric tube

Foal no.	Age (days)	Serum IgG (mg%)	Dosage	Lesions	Outcome
1	14	45	*C. difficile* crude toxin (100 ml)	Localized loss of epithelium from villous tips; subepithelial edema in small intestine.	Toxin not detected at necropsy.
2	4	140	*C. difficile* (9.9×10^9 cfu)	Diffuse edema of villi; loss of epithelium in small intestine.	Severe, watery diarrhea; *C. difficile* present in large intestine.
3	1	1700	*C. difficile* (1.68×10^8 cfu)	Subepithelial edema; limited loss of epithelium in small intestine.	No diarrhea; *C. difficile* and cytotoxin present in large intestine.
4	1	3000	*C. difficile* (3.37×10^8 cfu)	Mild subepithelial edema in small intestine.	No diarrhea; *C. difficile* and cytotoxin present in large intestine.
5	1	40	*C. difficile* (8.67×10^8 cfu)	Necrosis, degeneration, and loss of epithelium at tips of villi; subepithelial edema in small intestine.	Died 20 hr postinoculation; hemorrhage into lumen of intestine; *C. difficile* and cytotoxin present in large intestine.
6	1	0	*C. difficile* (4.25×10^{10} cfu)	Denuded and shortened villi in small intestine; superficial loss of epithelium in large intestine.	Died 15 hr postinoculation; *C. difficile* and cytotoxin present in large intestine.

Foal 2 was inoculated with 9.9×10^9 viable *C. difficile*. Severe, watery diarrhea was observed 8 hr postinoculation, and at 18 hr the foal was euthanized for necropsy. Diffuse mucosal edema was present throughout the small intestine, with localized damage to the tips of villi and some loss of epithelium. Four foals (Nos. 3-6) did not develop diarrhea within 24 hr postinoculation; Foals 5 and 6 died within that time. Foals 3 and 4 had nursed and received large amounts of passively transferred immunoglobulin (Table 1). Microscopic lesions in the small intestines of these foals were similar to those observed in Foal 1 and less severe than in Foal 2. Foals 5 and 6, which had been deprived of colostrum, both died within 20 hr postinoculation with *C. difficile*. There was a uniform loss of epithelium over the villi, with shortening of villi and some subepithelial edema in the upper small intestine. Similar morphologic changes were less severe in the lower small intestine, and superficial loss of epithelium was observed in the large intestine of Foal 6. The morphologic changes observed in Foals 5 and 6 were the most severe of the group of experimental foals. There was a remarkable absence of inflammation in the enteric lesions in these foals.

C. difficile was recovered from the large intestine of foals inoculated with viable bacteria, and cytotoxin was demonstrated in the same specimens. Cytotoxin was not demonstrated in specimens from the foal that received culture filtrate.

DISCUSSION

The association of *C. difficile* and its cytotoxin with diarrhea in foals has recently been reported (Jones et al. 1987b). The severity of diarrhea and its early onset and high incidence suggested an infectious etiology for most cases. Common infectious causes of foal diarrhea were not consistently identified. Some diarrheic foals were shedding rotaviruses, which typically cause mild diarrhea (Tzipori, Chandler & Smith 1983). A synergistic infection with rotaviruses and *C. difficile* may have occurred in some of the foals.

Isolates from naturally occurring cases of disease were used in this study to experimentally produce infection. The clinical signs, lesions, and presence of the organism and its cytotoxin were similar to findings in the natural disease process. Thus, we have fulfilled Koch's postulates in establishing *C. difficile* as a possible cause of enteritis and diarrhea in foals.

The manifestation of *C. difficile*-induced disease in humans ranges from mild diarrhea to severe disease with leukocytosis, severe abdominal pain (colic), profuse diarrhea (increased mucus and blood), and hemorrhagic necrotizing enteritis (George 1984). Most strains of *C. difficile*, like those we have isolated from foals, produce two toxins, A and B (Jones et al. 1987b). Toxin A, an enterotoxin, causes hemorrhagic fluid accumulation in the ileum of rabbits, with detachment of the epithelial cells (Mitchell et al. 1986). In addition, toxin A seems to exert a long-term effect on the mucosa, increasing the susceptibility to damage by small amounts of toxin A itself and also acting synergistically with toxin B, a cytotoxin, to cause intestinal pathology (Lyerly et al. 1985). Toxin A may also increase the permeability of intestinal mucosa, magnifying the susceptibility to other microbial toxins and diseases (Wilkins et al. 1985). Toxin B exacerbates the hemorrhagic necrotizing response to toxin A in hamsters and mice (Lyerly et al. 1985).

Mitchell and colleagues (1986) have shown that toxin A

induces morphological changes in rabbit ileum before the onset of fluid accumulation. Damage progresses from being localized on the villus tips to eventual destruction of villi and gross hemorrhage. Toxin A also induces extensive extravasation of plasma proteins. These data suggest that fluid accumulation in rabbit ileal loops is initially induced by the cytopathic effect on toxin A on enterocytes, and later to its effects on the vasculature of the villi.

The susceptibility of the equine intestinal mucosa to the effects of *C. difficile* toxins is not known. However, the series of lesions that we have observed in natural and experimental disease in foals are similar to the lesions described in rabbit intestinal loops (Mitchell et al. 1986). Based on the mechanism of action of *C. difficile* toxins in experimental animals (Stephen & Pietrowski 1986) and the pathogenesis of infection in human adults (Chang 1985), we propose the following pathogenesis of disease in foals. *C. difficile* readily establishes itself in the intestine of the young foal, which has not yet become colonized with a stable flora as microbial competition. As a spore-forming organism, *C. difficile* can survive in the environment as a reservoir of infection for the susceptible foal, and the coprophagic nature of foals would enhance transmission of the infection. Foals younger than three days probably are more susceptible to rapid overgrowth by *C. difficile*, as observed in focal lesions. Massive hemorrhagic, necrotizing enteritis without a history of diarrhea may be due to the production of very large quantities of toxins that are quickly lethal when absorbed.

As the foal develops a more stable flora, it becomes more resistant to rapid overgrowth of the intestine by *C. difficile*. Lower numbers of organisms in a limited number of foci in the intestine may produce sublethal quantities of toxins that cause ultrastructural, microscopic lesions leading to diarrhea, as observed in Foal 2 and foals naturally infected at two days that subsequently developed diarrhea. The persistence of diarrhea may be explained by continued toxin production, reinfection with small numbers of toxigenic organisms, or secondary infection of damaged intestinal epithelium by other enteropathogens.

This proposed pathogenesis is consistent with the findings in experimentally inoculated foals. Morphologic changes were observed in the small intestine of Foal 1 after it received crude toxin; toxin could not be recovered at necropsy (24 hr postinoculation); and diarrhea did not develop. The amount of toxin administered induced changes similar to those described in rabbits (Mitchell et al. 1986) and was consumed in the process. Complete absorption of toxin A occurs within 6 hr in rabbits (Mitchell et al. 1987).

When foals were inoculated with viable organisms in addition to toxin, continued production of toxin was possible. Foals 3 and 4, which had received colostrum, were protected from the systemic lethal effects of toxin, but its superficial activity resulted in morphologic changes in the intestinal epithelium. Further analysis is necessary to determine whether toxin-neutralizing antibodies were present in the colostrum. Toxin-neutralizing antiserum has shown such a partial protective effect in rabbits (Stephen & Pietrowski 1986).

Foals 5 and 6, which received no passive immunity, were apparently much more susceptible to the toxins. The greater morphologic change in the mucosa, especially in Foal 6 which received a larger inoculum, was lethal. The few extra days in the age of Foal 2 when inoculated may have given it an advantage in terms of intestinal flora, or in susceptibility and permeability of the mucosa to *C. difficile* toxins. This foal developed severe, watery diarrhea typical of the diarrhea naturally occurring in older foals.

The mechanism of action of *C. difficile* toxins in these foals is not known, but the series of morphological changes seem to begin with subepithelial edema in the villi, leading to sloughing of the epithelium. This process appears to be a peracute reaction, with minimal necrosis and lack of a recognizable inflammatory response. Additional studies and controls are needed to more clearly define the significance of lesions found in these studies and to identify the active toxin of *C. difficile* and the specific mechanism of action in foals.

ACKNOWLEDGMENTS

We thank Karen Baucus, Dale Davis, Bill Adney, and Marcia Davis for technical assistance.

Financial assistance was provided in part by the U.S. Department of Agriculture Animal Health and Disease, through the College of Veterinary Medicine and Biomedical Sciences, Colorado State University.

REFERENCES

Allen, S.D. (1985) Clostridium. In *Manual of Clinical Microbiology*, 4th ed., pp. 434-49. Eds. E.H. Lennette, A. Balows, W.J. Hausler, Jr., and H.J. Shadomy. American Society for Microbiology, Washington, D.C.

Bartlett, J.G.; Chang, T.W.; Gurwith, M.; Gorbach, S.L.; and Onderdonk, A.B. (1978) Antibiotic-associated pseudomembranous colitis due to toxin-producing clostridia. *N. Engl. J. Med.* **298**, 531-34.

Chang, T.W. (1985) Antibiotic-associated injury to the gut. In *Gastroenterology*, 4th ed., pp. 2583-92. Ed. J.E. Berk. W.B. Saunders, Philadelphia.

Cudd, T.A., and Pauly, T.H. (1987) Necrotizing enterocolitis in two equine neonates. *Comp. Contin. Educ. Pract. Vet.* **9**, 88-96.

Daniel, W.W. (1978) *Applied Nonparametric Statistics*, pp. 110-14. Houghton Mifflin, Boston.

Dickie, C.W.; Klinkerman, D.L.; and Petrie, R.J. (1978) Enterotoxemia in two foals. *J. Am. Vet. Med. Assoc.* **173**, 306-7.

Ehrich, M.; Perry, B.D.; Troutt, H.F.; Dellers, R.W.; and Magnusson, R.A. (1984) Acute diarrhea in horses of the Potomac River area: examination for clostridial toxins. *J. Am. Vet. Med. Assoc.* **185**, 433-35.

England, J.J., and Reed, D.E. (1980) Negative contrast electron microscopic techniques for diagnosis of viruses of veterinary importance. *Cornell Vet.* **70**, 125-36.

George, W.L. (1984) Antimicrobial agent-associated colitis and diarrhea: historical background and clinical aspects. *Rev. Infect. Dis. Suppl.* **6**, 208-13.

George, W.L.; Sutter, V.L.; Citron, D.; and Finegold, S.W. (1979) Selective and differential medium for isolation of *Clostridium difficile*. *J. Clin. Microbiol.* **9**, 214-19.

Hafiz, S., and Oakley, C.L. (1976) *Clostridium difficile:* isolation and characteristics. *J. Med. Microbiol.* **9**, 129-37.

Harbour, D.A. (1985) Infectious diarrhoea in foals. *Equine Vet. J.* **17**, 262-64.

Hibbs, C.M.; Johnson, D.R.; Reynolds, K.; and Harrington, Jr., R. (1977) *Clostridium sordellii* isolated from foals. *Vet. Med.* **72**, 256-58.

Howard-Martin, M.; Morton, R.J.; Qualls, Jr., C.W.; and MacAllister, C.G. (1986) *Clostridium perfringens* type C enterotoxemia in a newborn foal. *J. Am. Vet. Med. Assoc.* **189**, 564-65.

Jones, R.L.; Adney, W.S.; Alexander, A.F.; Shideler, R.K.; and Traub-Dargatz, J.L. (1987a). Hemorrhagic necrotizing enterocolitis associated with *Clostridium difficile* in four foals. *J. Am. Vet. Med. Assoc.* **193,** 76-79.

Jones, R.L.; Adney, W.S.; and Shideler, R.K. (1987b) Isolation of *Clostridium difficile* and detection of cytotoxin in the feces of diarrheic foals in the absence of antimicrobial treatment. *J. Clin. Microbiol.* **25**, 1225-27.

Koneman, E.W.; Allen, S.D.; Dowell, Jr., V.R.; and Sommers, H.M. (1983) *Color atlas and textbook of diagnostic microbiology.* 2d ed. J.B. Lippincott, Philadelphia.

Lyerly, D.M.; Saum, K.E.; McDonald, D.K.; and Wilkins, T.D. (1985) Effects of *Clostridium difficile* toxins given intragastrically to animals. *Infect. Immun.* **47**, 349-52.

Mason, J.H., and Robinson, E.M. (1938) The isolation of Cl welchii, type B, from foals affected with dysentery. *Onderstepoort J. Vet. Sci.* **11**, 333-37.

Mitchell, T.J.; Ketley, J.M.; Haslam, S.C.; Stephen, J.; Burdon, D.W.; Candy, D.C.A.; and Daniel, R. (1986) Effect of toxin A and B of *Clostridium difficile* on rabbit ileum and colon. *Gut* **27**, 78-85.

Mitchell, T.J.; Ketley, J.M.; Burdon, D.W.; Candy, D.C.A.; and Stephen, J. (1987). Biological mode of action of *Clostridium difficile* toxin A: a novel enterotoxin. *J. Med. Microbiol.* **23**, 211-19.

Montgomery, R.F., and Rowlands, W.T. (1937) "Lamb dysentery" in a foal. *Vet. Rec.* **49**, 398-99.

Niilo, L., and Chalmers, G.A. (1982). Hemorrhagic enterotoxemia caused by *Clostridium perfringens* type C in a foal. *Can. Vet. J.* **23**, 299-301.

Nachamkin, I.; Lotz-Nolan, L.; and Skalina, D. (1986) Evaluation of a commercial cytotoxicity assay for detection of *Clostridium difficile* toxin. *J. Clin. Microbiol.* **23**, 954-55.

Pearson, E.G.; Hedstrom, O.R.; Sonn, R.; and Wedam, J. (1986) Hemorrhagic enteritis caused by *Clostridium perfringens* type C in a foal. *J. Am. Vet. Med. Assoc.* **188**, 1309-10.

Silva, Jr., J. (1979) Animal models of antibiotic-induced colitis. In *Microbiology—1979*, pp. 258-63. Ed. D. Schlessinger. American Society for Microbiology, Washington, D.C.

Sims, L.D.; Tzipori, S., Hazard, G.H., and Carroll, C.L. (1985) Hemorrhagic necrotizing enteritis in foals associated with *Clostridium perfringens*. *Aust. Vet. J.* **62**, 194-96.

Stephen, J., and Pietrowski, R.A. (1986) *Bacterial toxins*, 2d ed., pp. 88-93. American Society for Microbiology, Washington, D.C.

Tzipori, S.; Chandler, D.; and Smith, M. (1983) The clinical manifestation and pathogenesis of enteritis associated with rotavirus and enterotoxigenic *Escherichia coli* infections in domestic animals. *Prog. Fd. Nutr. Sci.* **7**, 193-205.

White, N.A.; Tyler, D.E.; Blackwell, R.B. and Allen, D. (1987) Hemorrhagic fibrinonecrotic duodenitis-proximal jejunitis in horses: 20 cases (1977-1984). *J. Am. Vet. Med. Assoc.* **190**, 311-15.

Wierup, M. (1977) Equine intestinal clostridiosis. *Acta Vet. Scand.* (suppl.) **62**.

Wilkins, T.D.; Krivan, H.; Stiles, B.; Carman, R.; and Lyerly, D. (1985) Clostridial toxins active locally in the gastrointestinal tract. In *Microbial Toxins and Diarrhoeal Diseases*, (Ciba Found. Symp. 112), pp. 230-41. Pitman, London.

Wu, T.C., and Gersch, S.M. (1986) Evaluation of a commercial kit for the routine detection of *Clostridium difficile* cytotoxin by tissue culture. *J. Clin. Microbiol.* **23**, 792-93.

Infectivity and Immunity Studies in Foals with Cell Culture-Propagated Equine Rotaviruses

William P. Higgins, James H. Gillespie, Emery I. Schiff, Nancy N. Pennow, and Michael J. Tanneberger

SUMMARY

The objectives were to determine whether cell culture-propagated equine rotavirus (ERV) alone can infect and/or produce clinical disease in neonatal or young foals; to assess the immune response of foals to infections with ERV; and to better understand the epizootiology of ERV. Twelve pony mares were maintained in isolation units prior to foaling. All foals nursed, acquiring essentially the same serum neutralization (SN) titers that their dams had. At two to 12 days of age, 10 foals were inoculated by nasogastric tube with $10^{2.6}$ to $10^{8.6}$ $TCID_{50}$ of one of two cell culture-propagated ERV strains that had been determined to be serotypically distinct in reciprocal SN tests. Seven of the ten foals exhibited diarrhea and shed ERV for up to 11 days postinoculation, as did two foals that were first inoculated at 30 and 34 days of age, respectively. Of the nine foals that exhibited diarrhea, six had a significant rise in SN titer to the strain of ERV to which they were first exposed. Two of the three foals remained clinically normal and exhibited a significant rise in SN titer to the homologous ERV. Eight mares developed an increase in SN antibody titers to ERV, indicating that they had acquired subclinical infections from their foals. Essentially all the foals were resistant to clinical reinfection with both the homologous and the heterologous ERV strains.

It was concluded that susceptible foals can become infected with cell culture-propagated ERV, exhibiting diarrhea and other clinical signs of ERV disease. There was no correlation between serum antibody titer and susceptibility to clinical ERV infection. The cross-protection between heterologous ERV strains may indicate that only a monovalent ERV vaccine need be developed. Asymptomatic infections play a significant role in the epizootiology of ERV disease.

INTRODUCTION

Rotaviruses were first observed in foal diarrheal feces in 1975 (Flewett, Bryden & Davis 1975). Since this original report, much has been published to substantiate that rotavirus is a significant foal pathogen (Conner & Darlington 1980; Kanitz 1976; Mitchell 1982; Scrutchfield et al. 1979; Strickland et al. 1982; Tzipori & Walker 1978).

New York State College of Veterinary Medicine, Cornell University, Ithaca, New York 14853. Present address, Higgins: P.O. Box 290, Centreville, MD 21617.

The prevalence of rotavirus antibody has been demonstrated to be essentially 100% in adult horses (Conner & Darlington 1980; Pearson et al. 1982). However, only a small percentage of foals have rotavirus antibody (Imagawa et al. 1982). The majority of rotaviruses isolated to date, classified as group A rotaviruses, possess a common inner capsid nonneutralizing antigen (Nicolas et al. 1984). Although the common antigen does not elicit neutralizing antibody, it does facilitate the detection of most rotaviruses since heterologous antiserum can be used in assays for strains of rotavirus for which there is no homologous antibody (Woode et al. 1976).

The source of ERV in an outbreak of infection is not easily defined. Some reports have implicated recently imported foals that were in the incubation stage of rotaviral disease. (Conner & Darlington 1980). Mild or asymptomatic rotaviral infections in adult horses are suspected of a role in the spread of equine rotaviral disease (Scrutchfield et al. 1979). Experimentally, asymptomatic infections have been produced in foals (Tzipori et al. 1982). It has also been suggested that some adult horses may be persistently infected carriers of ERV (Conner et al. 1983).

Another possible source of ERV is the environment itself. Rotaviruses are quite stable and have been reported to remain viable for up to nine months at room temperature (Keswick et al. 1983; Moe & Shirley 1982; Woode 1978).

Published reports indicate that there are at least two ERV serotypes (Hoshino et al. 1983a, b). Although the incidence of rotaviral disease has been shown to be significant and of economic importance in foals, no vaccine is available for immunization of foals and horses.

MATERIALS AND METHODS

Experimental animals. Mixed-breed pregnant pony mares designated A through L, ranging in age from two to more than 12 years, were maintained as part of a closed herd in pasture. Before being placed in an individual isolation unit, at least two weeks prior to foaling, each mare was cleaned and disinfected with a 10% solution of Clorox (Clorox Company, Oakland, Calif.).

Although mares were closely monitored, the foalings were unattended. All foals nursed within a few hours of birth. Navels were disinfected and enemas were administered to foals soon after birth. The body temperature of each mare and foal was determined twice daily. Daily fecal samples and

Table 1. Age of foals (in days) when inoculated with equine rotavirus (ERV)

	Cell culture[a]				Fecal suspension[b]	
Foal	FI13, passage 8		FI14, passage 4 or 5		FI13	FI14
A	2[c]	21	29	37	—	54
B	2[c]	15	23	31	—	48
C	12[c]	30	43	51	—	59
D	25	31	2[c]	17	39	—
E	4	19	27	35	—	43
F	30	37	2[c]	18	44	—
G	12	22	29	37	—	43
H	23	30	2[c]	16	37	—
I	26	33	2[c]	13[c]	40	—
J	23	29	4	15	37	—
K	—	—	—	—	45	30[c]
L	—	—	—	—	34[c]	48

[a] $TCID_{50}$ of cell culture–adapted virus was calculated to range from $10^{2.6}$ to $10^{8.6}$ using Karber method after virus had been titrated in cell culture.

[b] $TCID_{50}$ of virus contained in fecal suspension, no longer adapted to cell culture, was estimated from FA examination of cell culture titrations to range from $10^{7.7}$ to $10^{9.9}$.

[c] Foal exhibited diarrhea 1-4 days postinoculation.

semiweekly serum samples were collected from each mare and foal. During these studies, no foal received medical treatment.

Foal inoculation. Foals were inoculated with two serotypically distinct strains of ERV designated FI13 and FI14, which had been isolated during separate outbreaks of foal diarrhea in New York State during 1980 (Table 1). FI14 is a serotype 3 rotavirus (Hoshino et al. 1987), while FI13 (EID4) (Gillespie et al. 1984) belongs to neither serotype 3 nor serotype 5 (M.E. Conner, personal communication).

Rotaviruses were propagated in an established cell line of fetal rhesus monkey kidney cells (MA104; M.A. Bioproducts, Walkersville, Maryland) as previously described (Gillespie et al. 1984).

Foals A through J were inoculated four times with cell culture-propagated ERV (FI13 or FI14). Foals C and G were administered virus-free cell culture control fluid containing MA104 cells at two days of age. At 12 days of age they were inoculated with FI13 cell culture–propagated ERV. Foals K and L were first inoculated at 30 days (FI14) and 34 days (FI13) of age, respectively, with fecal suspensions containing ERV. To prepare the suspensions, rotavirus-containing feces of foals infected with cell culture–propagated ERV were diluted in phosphate-buffered saline (PBS). The fecal suspensions were also used for the final inoculation of the 12 foals involved in these studies.

For 4 hr before and 1 hr after each foal was inoculated, its dam's udder was covered with a modified Tamm bovine udder support (Franksville Specialty Co., Franksville, Wis.).

Between $10^{2.6}$ and $10^{8.6}$ $TCID_{50}$ of rotavirus were contained in each 25-ml to 35-ml cell culture fluid inoculum. Cell culture-propagated ERV inocula were prepared by freeze-thawing three times 75-cm^2 flasks that exhibited 70% to 80% cytopathic effect (CPE) after being infected with FI13 passage 7 or FI14 passage 3 or 4. Fecal suspensions contained approximately $10^{7.7}$ to $10^{9.9}$ $TCID_{50}$ of ERV. All inocula were administered via a sterile foal nasogastric tube (Portex Ltd., Hythe Kent, England). Viral and cell culture control fluid inocula were preceded by 50 ml of sterile 7.5% $NaHCO_3$ solution and followed by 25 ml of sterile PBS. All solutions were deposited in the nasogastric tube via a sterile 60-cc syringe with a catheter tip (Monoject, Division of Sherwood Medical, St. Louis, Mo.). Viral cultures and suspensions were at room temperature when administered. Sodium bicarbonate and PBS were warmed to 37°C before administration.

During these studies, diarrhea was defined as the passage of three or more loose bowel movements within a 24-hr period (Barron-Romero et al. 1985; Santosham et al. 1985; Stibon et al. 1985).

Enzyme-linked immunosorbent assay (ELISA). Each fecal sample collected (20% suspension in PBS) was subjected to an ELISA test for the detection of rotavirus antigen (Grauballe et al. 1981). Antibodies (Dako Patts, Copenhagen) used in the ELISA test were: rabbit antirotavirus (human) immunoglobulin fraction (code B218); peroxidase conjugated rabbit antirotavirus (human) immunoglobulin fraction (code 219); immunoglobulin fraction of normal rabbit serum (code X904), which served as a negative control serum.

Electron microscopy (EM). Forty-five fecal samples were subjected to examination on a Philips EM 201 electron microscope using standard techniques (Flewett 1978).

Serum neutralization test in MA104 cell culture. Serum neutralization tests with minor modification were run in 24-well plates as previously described (Hoshino et al. 1982). Serial twofold dilutions of the sera (previously heat-inactivated at 56°C for 30 min) were made in Falcon 2054 clear plastic tubes with caps (Falcon, Div. Becton, Dickinson and Co., Oxnard, Calif.) containing maintenance media (Eagle's minimal essential medium with antibiotic-antimycotic). Serum dilutions ranged from 1:5 to 1:2560. Stocks of ERV (FI13 passage 8 and FI14 passage 6) were propagated in MA104 cell cultures for use in serum neutralization tests. One milliliter of stock equine rotavirus was pretreated with 20 µg/ml of Trypsin XI Lot No. 128C-8015 (Sigma Chemical, St. Louis, Mo.) for 60 min at 37°C, after which it was diluted 1:500 in maintenance media. To each tube containing 0.5 ml of diluted serum, 0.5 ml of diluted stock virus was added, resulting in a final dilution of 1:1000 for the stock virus. The final dilutions of the stock viruses FI13 and FI14 contained

Table 2. Clinical signs exhibited by pony foals after initial inoculation with equine rotavirus

Foal	Days postinoculation					ELISA positive for rotavirus
	Diarrhea	Malodorous feces	Depression	Anorexia	Fever	
A	3-5	3-7	3-5	—	—	3-7
B	2-5	2-5	2-5	—	—	2-6
C	2-5	2-7	2-4	2-4	—	1-8
D	4-5	4-7	4-6	4-6	—	4-9
E	—	—	—	—	—	7
F	1-2	1-4	1	1	—	1-11
G	—	1	—	—	—	—
H	1-9	1-9	3-5	3-5	—	1-11
I	1-4	1-4	—	—	—	3-5
J	—	4	—	—	—	—
K	1-5	1-2	1-2	—	—	1-8
L	1-3	1-4	1-2	1-2	—	1-8

approximately $10^{2.2}$ and $10^{2.7}$ $TCID_{50}$ per ml, respectively. While each tube containing virus and serum was incubated at 37°C for 60 min, 24-well plates containing confluent MA104 cell monolayers were washed three times with maintenance media. Of each of the 10 dilutions of serum-virus mixture, 0.2 ml was deposited onto the MA104 cell monolayers in two of the wells; 0.2 ml of the 1:500-diluted stock virus was deposited into two other wells, and 0.1 ml of maintenance media was deposited into the remaining two wells, which served as cell controls. Inocula were allowed to adsorb onto MA104 cell monolayers for 60 min at 37°C. The contents of each well were then aspirated using a sterile Pasteur pipette connected to a vacuum bottle. The plates were then washed once with maintenance media. To each well was added 1 ml of serum-free maintenance media containing 1 μg/ml trypsin. Each plate was placed into a Kapak/Scotch Pak heat-sealable pouch (Kapak Corp., St. Louis Park, Minn.) and allowed to incubate at 47°C for five days. Plates were read on an inverted microscope using the 4× objective. Endpoints were determined to be the wells containing no visible CPE. The neutralizing titer was expressed as the reciprocal of the highest serum dilution that exhibited no CPE. Sera from each mare and her foal were tested together in the same SN test.

Fluorescent antibody (FA) staining of MA104 cells. Two hundred fecal samples from 12 foals and 133 fecal samples from nine mares, obtained both before and after foal rotavirus inoculation, were inoculated onto MA104 cell monolayers as previously described (Gillespie et al. 1984).

Approximately seven days after inoculation, MA104 cell monolayers were fixed in acetone in preparation for indirect fluorescent antibody (FA) staining using standard techniques (Hoshino et al. 1982). Anti-FI13 hyperimmune chicken serum was followed by an FITC conjugated chicken IgG antibody (Miles Laboratories, Naperville, Ill.). Both infected and uninfected control cells were stained and examined by an epifluorescence microscope at 125× magnification.

RESULTS

Upon initial inoculation with cell culture–propagated equine rotavirus, seven of 10 foals exhibited signs of clinical diarrhea, which persisted from 12 hr to 10 days (Table 2). The onset of diarrhea occurred one to four days postinoculation. Diarrheal feces were formless, mostly liquid, malodorous (a distinct odor best described as that of fermenting milk), and uncontrollable. Foals E, G, and J exhibited no signs of diarrhea. Foals G and J both passed distinctly malodorous feces on Day 1 and Day 4, respectively, after first inoculation. In the case of foals K and L, first inoculated at 30 and 34 days of age, respectively, with fecal suspensions containing FI13 and FI14, diarrhea persisted for five days and three days, respectively, after initial inoculation.

Foal I, which exhibited only mild signs of diarrhea on Days 1-4 after the initial inoculation, was reinoculated with the same serotype of ERV (FI14) 13 days later. The second episode of diarrhea started 7 hr after reinoculation and persisted for 10 days in Foal I. No bacterial pathogens were detected nor parasite ova observed. No other foal exhibited signs of diarrhea on reinoculation. Although inoculated three more times, Foal I at no time exhibited further signs of clinical rotaviral disease.

Foals A, B, C, D, F, H, K, and L were depressed after the first rotaviral inoculation, and Foals C, D, F, H, and L were also anorectic. No foal registered a fever during these studies. Sunken eyes were seen only in Foal C, which developed dehydration two to five days after its first inoculation with ERV, coincident with severe clinical diarrhea. No mare exhibited any clinical signs of rotaviral disease during these studies.

ELISA tests. Rotavirus antigen could be detected by ELISA tests in the feces of all foals that exhibited diarrhea. In general, feces first tested positive for rotavirus concurrent with the appearance of diarrhea and continued to be ELISA-positive for one to 10 days after diarrhea had subsided.

Table 3. Acute and convalescent serum neutralization (SN) titers of infected pony foals and their dams to two-tissue culture–adapted equine rotavirus strains

		FI13				FI14			
Foal (F) or Mare (M)	Initial viral inoculum	≥Fourfold rise in titer by serum neutralization test	SN titer Preinoc.	SN titer Postinoc.	Days when SN titer increased	≥Fourfold rise in titer by serum neutralization test	SN titer Preinoc.	SN titer Postinoc.	Days when SN titer increased
F-A	FI13	+	40	160	29-44	+	10	40	29-44
M-A		+	40	320	<9	+	10	40	<28
F-B	FI13	+	10	80	23-35	–	10	10	—
M-B		+	20	160	7-14	+	10	40	<20
F-E	FI13	+	10-20	320-640	15-31	–	20	40-80	31-46
M-E		–	80	80	—	–	80	80	—
F-C	FI13	+	40	160	30-46	–	20	40	30-46
M-C		+	80	640	7	+	40	320	<30
F-D	FI14	–	80	160	31-46	–	80	80	—
M-D		–	40	80	<19	–	80-160	320	<19
F-J	FI14	–	20	40-80	31-3	–	<5	10	<31
M-J		–	40	80	<17	–	5	10	<33
F-G	FI13	+	10	40-80	17	–	5-10	20	17
M-G		+	20	320-640	10	–	20	40	15
F-F	FI14	+	5-10	20-40	16-28	+	20	160	16-28
M-F		+	5	40-80	<16	+	20	160-320	<16
F-I	FI14	–	40	40	—	+	10-20	20-40	26-47
M-I		–	40	40	—	–	10	20	<13
F-H	FI14	–	40	20	—	+	40	160	21-35
M-H		–	20	40	<21	+	20	80	21-35
F-L	FI13	+	10-20	160	11-26	–	5-10	10	11-26
M-L		+	40	320	<14	+	40	160	<14
F-K	FI14	–	20	20	—	–	10-20	10-20	—
M-K		+	80	640	6-15	+	20	160-320	<15

Of the three foals that did not exhibit diarrhea at any time, Foal E was weakly ELISA-positive on Day 7 postinoculation. When an MA104 cell culture was inoculated with a fecal sample from Foal E, fluorescent antibody staining was positive for rotavirus antigen.

Although Foal A had no clinical signs of illness after challenge with the fecal suspension containing FI14 (fifth inoculation), its feces were positive for rotavirus in ELISA testing on Days 2 and 3 after this final inoculation. Foal I, which experienced diarrhea and other signs of rotaviral disease after the first and second inoculations with FI14, was ELISA-positive after both inoculations. Fecal samples obtained three to five days after the first inoculation and one to two days after the second were positive for rotavirus. With the exception of Foals A and I, no foal was ELISA-positive for rotavirus after any inoculation beyond the first one.

None of the mares exhibited any signs of illness during these studies, but three of them were briefly ELISA-positive for rotavirus after their foals were inoculated for the first time: Mare C on Days 3 and 4 after the first foal inoculation, Mare F on Day 8, and Mare L on Days 7 and 10.

Fluorescent antibody test of MA104 cell cultures. Eighteen of the 200 foal fecal samples tested positive for rotavirus antigen when they were inoculated onto MA104 cell cultures and subjected to FA staining. The majority of positive samples had been collected one to eight days after first inoculation. No samples from Foal I or Foal D were positive. Foals E and H were positive on Days 10 and 14, respectively, after first inoculation. Samples from Foal A on Days 2 and 3 after its final inoculation were positive on FA examination.

Samples from four mares (G, K, B, and F) were positive for rotavirus antigen by FA examination on Days 3, 6, 10, and 14, respectively, after the first foal inoculation.

All fecal samples obtained from mares and foals prior to the first foal inoculation were negative when subjected to FA staining of MA104 cell cultures. All samples collected and tested after the final inoculation were negative by FA examination with the exception of two positive tests of Foal A, on Days 2 and 3.

Electron microscopy (EM). The 45 fecal samples subjected to EM examination showed an excellent correlation with the

ELISA results. Only samples that were positive by ELISA were positive by EM examination, although some ELISA-positive samples tested negative by EM examination. All fecal samples negative by ELISA were also EM-negative.

Serum neutralization test. Foal rotaviral SN titers to both FI13 and FI14 at the time of the first inoculation ranged from <5 to 80 (Table 3). With the exception of Foal E, each foal passively acquired serum antibody titers that were within a twofold dilution factor of its dam's titers. Foal E acquired serum antibody titers that were approximately 25% of its dam's.

Of the nine foals that experienced diarrhea, six (A, B, C, F, H, and L) had a fourfold or greater rise in SN titer to the strain of equine rotavirus to which they were first exposed. The SN titer of Foals D, I, and K did not rise significantly (≥ fourfold).

Of the three foals that did not show diarrhea, Foals E and G both had a significant rise in SN titer to FI13, the first strain of ERV to which they were exposed. For Foal J, there was no like increase in SN titer to either ERV strain.

Of the eight foals that exhibited a significant rise in SN titer to the first-exposure strain of ERV, two foals (A and F) also reacted significantly to the second inoculation strain.

After their foals were first inoculated, eight of the 12 mares (A, B, C, F, G, H, K, L) exhibited a significant increase in SN titer to the first strain of ERV, and six of these mares had a similar reaction to the second strain.

On average, it took between 25 and 35 days for the foals to exhibit a rise in SN titer to ERV. For the mares, the average was 9 to 12 days after their foals' inoculation with ERV.

No mare had a meaningful increase in SN titer to ERV while it was housed in the isolation unit prior to foaling, a period which ranged from 10 to 57 days, with an average of 30 days. Nor was there an increase in titer of Mares K and L or their offspring until the two foals were inoculated, at 30 or 34 days of age. After that, SN titer rose significantly for both Mares K and L.

DISCUSSION

The clinical signs of the foals that received cell culture–propagated ERV were indistinguishable from those of the foals inoculated with fecal suspensions containing ERV, and were comparable in all nine cases to clinical signs reported during field outbreaks of ERV diseases.

Fever is usually, though not always, exhibited by foals with rotaviral disease in the field (Scrutchfield et al. 1979; Strickland et al. 1982; Tzipori et al. 1978). No foal in these studies registered a fever following inoculation with ERV. Perhaps secondary bacterial infection, which is more likely to occur under field conditions, determines whether or not an infected foal is febrile.

Field cases of rotaviral diarrhea last two to 12 days (Conner & Darlington 1980; Kanitz 1976; Strickland et al. 1982; Tzipori & Walker 1978). The rotaviral diarrhea observed during these studies which first appeared one to four days after inoculation, persisted for two to ten days. In most cases, the other clinical signs of rotaviral disease—malodorous feces, depression, and anorexia—appeared at the same time as diarrhea and often subsided before the diarrhea resolved. There were no cases of chronic diarrhea, as have been reported from the field (Scrutchfield et al. 1979).

The foals in these studies developed no serious complications, such as severe dehydration (Conner & Darlington 1980; Studdert et al 1978), intussusception (Strickland et al. 1982; Studdert et al. 1978), or gastric ulceration (Merritt 1985). All 12 foals inoculated with ERV survived and were in good condition some nine months after the studies had been completed.

Rotavirus shedding patterns observed during these studies agree with those reported in the literature for humans and mice (Blackwell, Tennant & Ward 1966; Eydelloth et al. 1984; Kapikian et al. 1983; Stals, Wlather & Bruggeman 1984).

Only Foal I exhibited signs of rotaviral disease upon inoculation subsequent to the first challenge. Serological results indicate that Foal I did not mount a systemic immunological response to either ERV strain, making it susceptible to reinfection.

Foal A exhibited clinical signs after its first inoculation with FI13, and shed rotavirus on Days 2 and 3 after its final inoculation with the fecal suspension containing FI14. Reports of rotaviral infections in human infants indicate that while rotavirus infection will usually protect an infant from serious rotaviral disease upon reexposure soon afterwards, it may not prevent reinfection from occurring (Bishop et al. 1983; Yamaguchi et al. 1985). Kanitz (1976) reported that a foal was resistant to reinfection with homologous ERV two months after it had first been infected, at four days of age—the only published experiment to examine the duration of rotaviral immunity in the foal.

Since inoculations 2 through 5 were performed in close succession, it is possible that nonspecific immune factors such as interferon made the foals refractory to reinfection with ERV (Tzipori, Makin & Smith, 1980). Maternal antibody obtained by these nursing foals through their dams' milk may also have contributed to their resistance to reinfection, as the majority of mares became asymptomatically infected after the first inoculation of the foals.

There appeared to be no correlation between serum antibody titer and susceptibility to disease. Foals J and G had serum antibody titers of <5 and <10, respectively, to the rotavirus of the first inoculation, yet they had barely perceptible signs of rotaviral disease (malodorous feces). Foal E, which was free of any signs of clinical rotaviral disease during these studies, had an SN titer of 10-20 on the day it was inoculated and shed virus on only one day. For the nine foals that had clinical signs, the antibody titer ranged from 10 to 80 at the time of first inoculation. Other reports have suggested that serum antibody titers are not good indicators of resistance to rotaviral disease (Estes, Palmer & Obijeski 1983; Kapikian & Chanock 1985; Wenman et al. 1979).

Two foals, A and F, exhibited a heterotypic rise in serum antibody titer following a reinoculation, suggesting reinfection with heterologous rotavirus. Foal A shed detectable rotavirus on Days 2 and 3 after final inoculation with the fecal suspension containing FI14.

Detection of ERV in the feces of three mares within seven days after initial inoculation of their foals was the first evidence that mares could become asymptomatically infected. Fluorescent antibody staining confirmed that mares were shedding rotavirus in their feces, but since they practiced coprophagy at times in the isolation units, it was possible that the mares were merely passing ERV ingested with the foal feces. Serology gave a definitive answer: eight of the 12 mares had more than a fourfold increase in homologous SN titer to the first strain of ERV with which their foals had been inoculated. For six of the mares, there was also a significant rise in SN titer to the second ERV strain.

All of the mares involved in these studies had previously been exposed to ERV, and it has been reported that an animal's antibody response "broadens" after sequential infection with rotaviruses (Hodes 1980; Holmes 1979). In such cases, rabbits with preexisting antibody to rabbit rotavirus produced antibody to both simian rotavirus and the "O" rotaviral agent after inoculation with either (Holmes 1979; Malherbe & Strickland-Cholmley 1967), while rabbits with no preexisting rotaviral antibody produced only monospecific antibody (Holmes 1979; Lecatsas 1972). The serological results of this study indicated that the majority of mares became infected with ERV after foal inoculation.

It was also concluded from this study that ERV alone can produce clinical disease in foals and that challenge is successful using cell culture–propagated ERV, which is more easily manipulated than rotaviral fecal filtrates.

An epizootiological model for ERV can be proposed, based on the asymptomatic infection of eight mares and two foals, according to serological results. Asymptomatic horses would shed rotavirus, which can survive for months in the environment (Keswick et al. 1983; Moe & Shirley 1982; Woods 1978), and horses would periodically become asymptomatically reinfected as their immunity wanes. The successive contamination of the environment would serve to infect susceptible foals. This study yielded no evidence to support the theory that the reservoir of ERV between outbreaks is a persistently infected adult carrier that is asymptomatic.

Postinoculation SN titers above 80 appeared to be correlated with resistance to rotavirus infection. Whether an elevated SN titer directly confers rotaviral immunity on a foal or merely reflects the local intestinal status of an immune foal was not determined. While some foals became reinfected when inoculated with the heterotypic ERV strain, no foal became clinically ill. This result, coupled with the once-only occurrence of clinical rotaviral disease in foals under field conditions, may be interpreted to indicate that only a monovalent ERV vaccine is needed.

REFERENCES

Barron-Romero, B.L.; Barreda-Gonzalez, J.; Doval-Ugalde, R.; Zermeno-Eguializ, J.; and Huertoa-Pena, M. (1985) Asymptomatic rotavirus infections in day care centers. *J. Clin. Microbiol.* **22,** 116-18.

Bishop, R.F.; Barnes, G.L.; Cipriani, E.; and Lund, J.S. (1983) Clinical immunity after neonatal rotavirus infection. A prospective study in young children. *N. Eng. J. Med.* **309,** 72-76.

Blackwell, J.H.; Tennant, R.W.; and Ward, T.G. (1966) Serological studies with an agent of epizootic diarrhea of infant mice. *Natl. Cancer Inst. Monograph* **20,** 63-66.

Conner, M.E., and Darlington, R.W. (1980) Rotavirus infection in foals. *Am. J. Vet. Res.* **41,** 1699-1703.

Conner, M.E.; Gillespie, J.H.; Schiff, E.I.; and Frey, M.S. (1983) Detection of rotavirus in horses with and without diarrhea by electron microscopy and Rotazyme test. *Cornell Vet.* **73,** 280-87.

Estes, M.K.; Palmer, E.L.; and Obijeski, J.F. (1983) Rotaviruses: A review. *Curr. Top. Microbiol. Immunol.* **105,** 123-84.

Eydelloth, R.S.; Vonderfecht, S.L.; Sheridan, J.F.; Enders, L.D.; and Yolken, R.H. (1984) Kinetics of viral replication and local and systemic immune responses in experimental rotavirus infection. *J. Virol.* **50,** 947-50.

Flewett, T.H. (1978) Electron microscopy in the diagnosis of infection diarrhea. *J. Am. Vet. Med. Assoc.* **173,** 538-43.

Flewett, T.H.; Bryden, A.S.; and Davis H.A. (1975) Virus diarrhea in foals and other animals. *Vet. Rec.* **96,** 477.

Gillespie, J.; Kalica, A.; Conner, M.; Schiff, E.; Barr, M.; Holmes, D.; and Frey, M. (1984) The isolation, propagation and characterization of tissue-cultured equine rotaviruses. *Vet. Micro.* **9,** 1-14.

Grauballe, P.C.; Vestergaard, B.F.; Meyling, A.; and Garner, J. (1981) Optimized enzyme-linked immunosorbent assay for detection of human and bovine rotavirus in stools: Comparison with electron microscopy, immunoelectro-osmophoresis and fluorescent antibody techniques. *J. Med. Virol.* **7,** 29-40

Hodes, H.L. (1980) Gastroenteritis with special reference to rotavirus. *Adv. Pediatr.* **27,** 195-245.

Holmes, I.H. (1979) Viral gastroenteritis. *Prog. Med. Virol.* **25,** 1-36.

Hoshino, Y.; Wyatt, R.G.; Scott, F.W.; and Apple, M.J. (1982) Isolation and characterization of a canine rotavirus. *Arch. Virology.* **72,** 113-25.

Hoshino, Y.; Wyatt, R.G.; Greenberg, H.B.; Kalica, A.R.; Flores, J.; and Kapikian, A.Z. (1983a) Isolation and characterization of an equine rotavirus. *J Clin. Microbiol.* **18,** 585-91.

———. (1983b) Isolation, propagation and characterization of a second equine rotavirus serotype. *Infect. Immun.* **41,** 1031-37.

Hoshino, Y.; Gorzinglia, M.; Valdesuso, J.; Askaa, J.; Glass, R.I.; and Kapikian, A.Z. (1987) An equine rotavirus (FI-14 strain) which bears both subgroup I and subgroup II specificities on its VP6. *Virology* **157,** 488-96.

Imagawa, H.; Hirasaw, K.; Akiyama, Y.; and Omori, T. (1982) A sero-epizootiological survey on rotavirus infection in foals. *Jpn. J. Vet. Sci.* **44,** 819-21.

Kanitz, C. L. (1976) Identification of an equine rotavirus as a cause of neonatal foal diarrhea. *22d Proc. Am. Assoc. Equine Practnr.* 155-65.

Kapikian, A.Z., and Chanock, R.M. (1985) Rotaviruses. In *Virology*, Chapter 37, pp. 863-906. Ed. B.N. Fields. Raven Press, New York.

Kapikian, A.Z.; Wyatt, R.G.; Levine, M.M.; Yolken, R.H.; Van Kirk, D.H.; Dolin, R.; Greenberg, H.B.; and Chanock, R.M. (1983) Oral administration of human rotavirus to volunteers: Induction of illness and correlates of resistance. *J. Infect. Dis.* **147,** 95-106.

Keswick, B.H.; Pickering, L.K.; DuPont, H.L.; and Woodward, W.E. (1983) Survival and detection of rotaviruses on environmental surfaces in day care centers. *Appl. Environ. Microbiol.* **46,** 813-16.

Lecatsas, G. (1972) Electron microscopic and serological studies on simian virus SA11 and the "related" O agent. *Onderstepoort. J. Vet. Res.* **39,** 133-38.

Malherbe, H.H., and Strickland-Cholmley, M. (1967) Simian virus SA11 and the related O agent. *Arch. Virusforch.* **22,** 235-45.

Merritt, A.M. (1985) Gastroduodenal ulcer disease. *Equine Vet. Data* **6,** 200-2.

Mitchell, W.C. (1982) Rotaviral diarrhea in foals. *Mod. Vet. Prac.* **63,** 896.

Moe, K., and Shirley, J.A. (1982) The effects of relative humidity and temperature on the survival of human rotavirus in feces. *Arch. Virol.* **72,** 179-86.

Nicolas, J.C.; Pothier, P.; Cohen, J.; Lourenco, M.H.; Thompson, R.; Guimband P.; Chenon, A.; Dauvergna, M.; and Bricout, F. (1984) Survey of human rotavirus propagation as studied by electrophoresis of genomic RNA. *J. Infect. Dis.* **149,** 688-93.

Pearson, N.J.; Fulton, R.W.; Issel, C.J.; and Springer, W.I. (1982) Prevalence of rotavirus in chickens and horses in Louisiana U.S.A. *Vet. Rec.* **110,** 58-59.

Santosham, M.; Yolken, R.H.; Wyatt, R.G.; Bertrando, R.; Black, R.E.; Spira, W.M.; and Sack, R.B. (1985) Epidemiology of rotavirus diarrhea in a prospectively monitored American Indian population. *J. Infect. Dis.* **152,** 778-83.

Scrutchfield, W.L.; Eugster, A.K.; Abel, H.; and Ward, J.E. (1979) Rotavirus infections in foals. *25th Proc. of Am. Assoc. Equine Practnr.*, 217-23.

Stals, F.; Wlather, F.J.; and Bruggeman, C.A. (1984) Faecal and pharyngeal shedding of rotavirus and rotavirus IgA in children with diarrhea. *J. Med. Virol.* **14,** 333-39.

Stibon, M.; Lecerf, A.; Garin, Y.; and Ivanoff, B. (1985) Rotavirus prevalence and relationships with climatological factors in Gabon, Africa. *J. Med. Virol.* **16,** 177-82.

Strickland, K.L.; Lenihan, P.; O'Connor, M.G.; and Condon, J.C. (1982) Diarrhea in foals associated with rotavirus. *Vet. Rec.* **111,** 421.

Studdert, M.J.; Mason, R.W.; and Patten, B.E. (1978) Rotavirus diarrhea in foals. *Aust. Vet. J.* **54,** 363-64.

Tzipori, S., and Walker, M. (1978) Isolation of rotavirus from foals with diarrhea. *Aust. J. Exp. Biol. Med. Sci.* **56,** 453-57.

Tzipori, S.R.; Makin, T.J.; and Smith, M.L. (1980) The clinical response of gnotobiotic calves, pigs and lambs to inoculation with human, calf, pig and foal rotavirus isolates. *Aust. J. Exp. Biol. Med. Sci.* **58,** 309-18.

Tzipori, S.; Makin, T.; Smith, M.; and Krautil, F. (1982) Enteritis in foals induced by rotavirus and entero toxigenic *Escherichia coli*. *Aust. Vet. J.* **58,** 20-23.

Wenman, W.M.; Hinde, D.; Feltman, S.; and Gurwith, M. (1979) Rotavirus infections in adults. *N. Eng. J. Med.* **301,** 303-6.

Woode, G.N. (1978) Epizootiology of bovine rotavirus infection. *Vet. Rec.* **103,** 44-46.

Woode, G.N.; Bridges, J.C.; Jones, J.M.; Flewett, T.H.; Bryden, A.S.; Davies, H.A.; and White, G.B.B. (1976) Morphological and antigenic relationship between viruses (rotaviruses) from acute gastroenteritis of children, calves, piglets, mice and foals. *Infect. Immun.* **14,** 804-10.

Yamaguchi, H.; Inouye, S.; Yamauchi, M.; Morishima, T.; Malsuno, S.; Isomura, S.; and Suzuki, S. (1985) Anamnestic response in fecal IgA antibody production after rotaviral infection of infants. *J. Infect. Dis.* **152,** 389-400.

General

Mechanism of Anemia in Equine Infectious Anemia: Virus and Complement-Mediated Lysis and Phagocytosis of Horse Erythrocytes

Hiroshi Sentsui and Yuji Kono

SUMMARY

Horse erythrocytes (RBCs) treated with equine infectious anemia (EIA) virus hemagglutinin were found to be lysed after incubation with fresh horse or guinea pig serum at 37°C. Direct immunofluorescence testing revealed adsorption of the complement on the surface of the RBCs. Calcium and magnesium ions were necessary for hemolysis to take place. Antibody against EIA virus enhanced the virus-induced complement-mediated hemolysis. These observations indicated that the classical pathway of complement activation was responsible for this virus-induced hemolysis. When EIA virus-adsorbed RBCs were incubated with fresh horse serum at low temperature to prevent hemolysis, these complement-coated RBCs were phagocytized by cultivated horse leukocytes. Addition of antiserum showed a slightly suppressing but no enhancing effect on the phagocytosis. Phagocytosis thus seemed to be caused by recognition of the third complement component (C3) on the affected RBCs with the C3-receptor carrying phagocytes, but not by the recognition of immunoglobulin. These results suggest that the interaction of RBCs with EIA virus and complement attachments play important roles in the induction of the anemia and the production of sideroleukocytes in EIA virus-infected horses.

INTRODUCTION

Equine infections anemia is characterized by repeated febrile relapses accompanied by anemia and an increase of virus in circulating blood (Ishii 1963; Kono 1969). Several mechanisms have been proposed for the pathogenesis of anemia. Virus multiplication in the bone marrow, spleen, lymph nodes, and other visceral organs, resulted in reduced hematopoiesis (Kono, Kobayashi & Fukunaga 1971a; McGuire, Crawford & Henson 1971; McGuire, Henson & Quist 1969a; Yamamoto & Konno 1967). The life span of erthyrocytes of infected horses was shortened to a considerable extent in and around the febrile stage (McGuire, Henson & Quist 1969b; Obara & Nakajima 1961). The presence of complement-coated RBCs, active deposition of complement in the glomeruli, and a depression in circulating complement levels were observed in infected horses (McGuire, Henson & Bueger 1969; Perryman et al. 1971). On the other hand, EIA virus was found to possess a hemagglutinin (HA) to horse RBCs and to coexist with hemagglutination inhibition (HI) antibody in infected horse serum (Sentsui & Kono 1981a, b). These observations indicate that the virus or virus antibody complex is attached to horse RBCs in the circulation, and direct and indirect complement-mediated anemia is induced in EIA. In this report, the mechanism of anemia in the EIA virus-infected horse was examined using in vitro experimental systems.

National Institute of Animal Health, Kannondai 3-1-1, Tsukuba-shi, Ibaraki, 305, Japan.

MATERIALS AND METHODS

Virus antigen. The Wyoming strain of EIA virus (Kono, Kobayashi & Fukunaga 1971b) propagated on horse leukocyte cultures was used during this experiment. The culture fluid, concentrated by centrifugation to 1/25 the original volume (Sentsui & Kono 1978), was mixed with ethyl ether for 10 min with occasional shaking. Water phase was collected and mixed with 1/20 volume of concanavalin A-conjugated Sepharose 4 B (Pharmacia Fine Chemical, Sweden) for 18 hr at 4°C. The Con-A Sepharose 4 B was washed three times with phosphate-buffered saline (PBS) solution. Virus components combined with Con-A Sepharose 4 B were released in PBS with 1/4 the original volume containing 0.2 M α-methyl mannoside. The α-methyl mannoside was removed from the virus solution by dialysis in PBS. The partially purified virus components, which had an HA titer of 16-32, were used as virus antigen. The control was normal horse leukocyte cultures handled under identical conditions.

HA activity was determined by mixing each serial twofold dilution of virus antigen in 0.05 ml with an equal volume of 0.5% RBC suspension (Sentsui & Kono 1981a). The reciprocal of the highest dilution of antigen showing complete hemagglutination was considered to be the HA titer.

Erythrocytes and fresh sera as complement. Erythrocytes obtained from heparinized blood from the jugular vein of horses were washed three times with PBS and used within 12 hr.

Fresh sera were obtained from healthy guinea pigs and a healthy horse, from which the RBCs were collected. Blood was kept at 37°C for 30 min. The sera were separated from the blood clot and stored at − 80° C until use. The guinea pig serum was mixed with 1/10 volume of washed, packed horse RBCs for 20 min in icewater to remove hemagglutinin against horse RBCs before use.

Antisera. Antiserum to the Wyoming strain was obtained from a horse 49 days after experimental inoculation. The serum had a virus neutralization titer of 64 and an HI titer of 128 against the homologous strain. Nonspecific hemagglutinin inhibitor and isohemagglutinin in the serum had been removed before use by adsorption with kaolin and packed horse RBCs (Sentsui & Kono 1981b).

In preparing antisera to horse complement, zymosan (40 mg) was added to 40 ml of fresh horse serum, incubated at 37° C for 1 hr, and washed six times each with 40 ml of PBS. The washed complement conjugate zymosan was suspended in 2 ml of PBS and emulsified in an equal volume of Freund's complete adjuvant. Each rabbit was injected intramuscularly with 1 ml of the emulsion with adjuvant, four times at 10–day intervals. The immunological specificity of the antisera, obtained from these rabbits seven days after the last injection, was examined by immunoelectrophoresis. The immune rabbit sera (antihorse complement rabbit sera) were mixed and conjugated with fluorescein isothiocyanate (FITC).

Horse leukocyte culture. Horse leukocytes in the plasma, sedimented by low-speed centrifugation, were suspended in a 0.83% solution of ammonium chloride (NH_4C1) and incubated at room temperature for 5 min to lyse contaminating RBCs. The leukocytes were washed twice with a Hanks' solution, suspended in a medium consisting of 50% Eagle's minimal essential medium (MEM), 40% bovine serum, and 10% horse serum, and cultivated in glass bottles at 37° C for 24 hr.

The leukocytes were employed for virus propagation, the medium in culture bottles was replaced with fresh medium of the same composition and inoculated with viral fluid. The culture fluid was harvested when the cytopathic effect was maximum.

When employed for phagocytosis assay, the bottles were washed gently with PBS to remove nonadherent cells. Next, PBS containing 0.02% disodium ethylenediaminetetraacetatic acid (EDTA) was added to the bottles, and kept at 37° C for 5 min. Adherent cells released from the glass were collected, washed with Eagle's MEM and suspended at a concentration of 5×10^6 cells/ml in an assay medium that consisted of 95% Eagle's MEM and 5% inactivated horse serum. The serum was obtained from a healthy horse from which the RBCs, leukocytes, and fresh serum as complement were collected. The leukocyte suspension in the amount of 0.5 ml was added to each well (16 mm in diameter) of a 24-well multidish plate (FB-16-24-TC) Linbro, Hamden, Conn.), incubated at 37°C for 2 hr in a CO_2 incubator and used for the phagocytosis assay.

Hemolytic reaction. A suspension of 2% horse RBC in 0.2 ml of PBS was added to each diluted virus antigen in 0.2 ml of PBS and incubated for 2 hr at room temperature. The RBC suspension mixed with the virus antigen was centrifuged at 500 × g for 10 min. After removing the supernatant, sedimented RBCs were suspended in 0.6 ml of fresh horse serum or diluted fresh guinea pig serum. After incubation at 37°C for 2 hr, nonlysed cells were sedimented by centrifugation. The degree of hemolysis was determined by detecting hemoglobin in the supernatant in each tube by extinction measurements at a wavelength of 540 nm, using a digital double-beam programmable multiwavelength spectrophotometer (UVIDEC-1M; Nihon Bunkou Co., Japan). Percentage of hemolysis was calculated from a standard curve drawn from completely lysed RBCs of different concentrations.

Assay of phagocytosis of radiolabeled RBCs. Approximately 5×10^8 of RBCs were suspended in 0.2 ml PBS containing 200 μCi of $^{51}Cr\text{-}Na_2CrO^4$ and kept at 37°C for 2 hr with occasional shaking. The ^{51} Cr-labeled RBCs were suspended in 0.2 ml of various concentrations of virus antigen and kept for 2 hr at 37°C with occasional shaking. The treated RBCs were suspended in 5 ml of fresh horse serum and further kept for 30 min in an icewater bath. These RBCs were washed twice with Eagle's MEM and suspended in the assay medium at a concentration of 1×10^8 cells/ml. Controls were treated RBCs suspended in inactivated horse serum. The RBC suspension, 0.1 ml, was added to the leukocyte cultures in the wells (16 mm in diameter), and the leukocyte cultures were placed for 2 hr in a CO_2 incubator at 37°C. The medium was then aspirated from each well, and 0.5 ml of a 0.83% NH_4C1 solution was added and kept at room temperature for 5 min to lyse the RBCs that were not phagocytized. After removal of the NH_4Cl solution, each well was washed twice with 1 ml of PBS and the solution was replaced with 0.5 ml of a 0.1% Triton X-100 solution. After standing at room temperature for 15 min, the cells were further disrupted by pipetting and transferred to a vial for determination of the radioactivity in a gamma counter (Beckman Gamma 5500 Counting System; Beckman Instruments Inc., Fullerton, Calif.). The ratio of phagocytized RBCs was calculated by dividing the radioactivity of cultivated leukocytes by the radioactivity of RBCs added, then multiplying by 100.

Effect of antibody on hemolysis and phagocytosis. To investigate the effects of antibody on hemolysis, each 0.2 ml of 2% horse RBC suspension of PBS, virus antigen, and antiserum that showed an HI titer of 32 was mixed in a glass tube (1.3 × 10 cm). In the first tube, RBCs and virus antigen were mixed and kept at 37°C for 2 hr; after the same procedure with the second tube, the antiserum was added. In the third tube, the virus antigen and antiserum were first mixed and kept at 37° C for 2 hr, and the RBCs then added. In the fourth tube, RBCs, virus antigen, and antiserum were mixed simultaneously, then kept at 37°C for 2 hr. All the tubes were then further incubated for 2 hr at 37°C, centrifuged at 500 × g for 5 min, and the supernatant was removed. Sedimented RBCs in each tube were suspended in 0.6 ml of PBS containing 4 units of guinea pig complement and incubated for 2 hr at 37°C. Supernatant of each tube was tested for the intensity of hemolysis by the detection of hemoglobin.

To investigate the effects of antibody on phagocytosis, virus antigen (2 or ½ HA titer), antiserum (64 HI titer), and a quantity of 1 × 10^8 RBCs were mixed in the glass tubes in the same four sequences. The volumes used were 0.2 ml each of virus antigen and antiserum. All the tubes were kept at 37°C for 2 hr and maintained in an icewater bath for 30 min, and 5 ml of fresh horse serum or inactivated horse serum was added to each. The RBCs were washed twice with Eagle's MEM and suspended in the assay medium at a concentration of 1 × 10^8/ml. These RBC suspensions (0.1 ml) were overlaid on 2.5 × 10^6 of cultivated horse leukocytes.

Hemolysis under divalent cation-chelating agent. Ethylene-glycol-bis-(β-aminoethyl ether(N, N'-tetraacetic acid (EGTA), and EDTA, the divalent cation-chelating agents (Schmid & Reilley 1957) were used to analyze the calcium (Ca)- and magnesium (Mg)-ion dependency of the lysis of horse RBCs treated with EIA virus. A volume of 0.2 ml of a 2% suspension of horse RBCs treated with 4 HA units of virus antigen was mixed with 0.1 ml of 1.5 mM EDTA and EGTA, 0.1 ml of $CaCl_2$ or $MgCl_2$ at different concentrations; 0.2 ml of 4 units of guinea pig complement were added and the mixture was incubated at 37°C for 2 hr. The supernatant of each sample was tested for the intensity of hemolysis by detection of hemoglobin. As a control, a classical complement activation system was tested with sensitized sheep RBCs.

Detection of complement on RBCs by immunofluorescence. Horse RBCs treated with 4 HA units of virus antigen were kept in fresh horse serum for 30 min in ice water, washed twice with PBS, and then suspended in FITC-conjugated antihorse complement rabbit serum for 30 min in ice water. Controls were horse RBCs treated with the antigen and then incubated with inactivated horse serum or fresh horse serum containing 0.25 mM EDTA, as well as horse RBCs treated with the control preparation from normal horse leukocyte cultures and then incubated with fresh horse serum. The RBCs were washed twice with PBS, resuspended in PBS and reread with a fluorescence microscope (Photomicroscope III; Carl Zeiss, West Germany).

Observation of phagocytosis by light microscopy. Observation of phagocytosis by light microscopy was performed using leukocytes cultivated in glass petri dishes. After each procedure, the cells were dipped into distilled water for 5 sec to lyse the RBCs that were not ingested and washed with PBS. The cells on the petri dishes were further released by adding PBS containing 0.02% EDTA, suspended in horse serum, and dried as smears on slide glasses. The cells were fixed with methyl alcohol and stained with giemsa or hematoxylin and eosin.

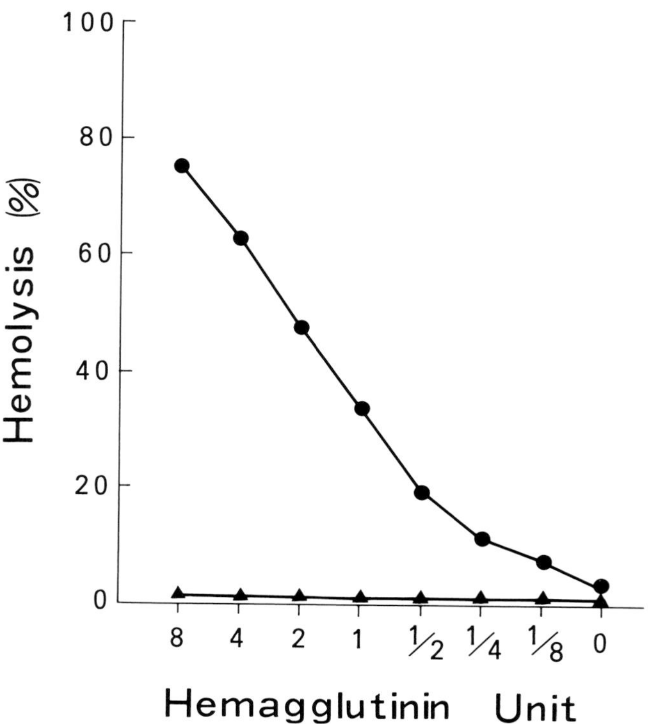

Fig. 1. Lysis of horse RBC treated with various concentrations of EIA virus antigen; treated horse RBCs were incubated with 4 units of guinea pig complement (*circles*) or inactivated complement (*triangles*) at 37°C for 2 hr.

RESULTS

Lysis of horse RBCs. Horse RBCs treated with 4 HA units of virus antigen exhibited about 20% lysis after a 2-hr incubation at 37°C when they were suspended in undiluted fresh horse serum. The hemolysis developed markedly in the presence of fresh guinea pig serum. The degree of hemolysis increased with the concentration of the guinea pig complement after a 2-hr incubation at 37°C. However, more than 8 units of guinea pig complement induced the lysis of normal horse RBCs. The intensity of hemolysis with various concentrations of virus antigen after a 2-hr incubation at 37°C with 4 units of guinea pig complement is shown in Figure 1. The percentage of hemolysis increased with the increase in the HA titer of the treated virus antigen.

Effect of antibody to hemolysis. Even when using antigen that had lost its hemagglutinating activity beforehand by being mixed with the antiserum, hemolysis was induced, though to a somewhat lesser extent.

Table 1. Effect of HI antibody on hemolysis

Treatments of horse RBCs (2 hr at 37°C)		Degree of hemolysis (%) of horse RBCs treated with EIA virus antigen					
		No. of HA units					
First	Second[a]	4	2	1	1/2	1/4	1/8
RBCs[b] and virus antigen[c]	PBS	63.15	48.87	33.90	19.54	11.49	7.93
RBCs and virus antigen	Antiserum[d]	84.71	76.37	64.36	45.74	24.53	12.24
Virus antigen and antiserum	RBCs	45.86	29.53	17.01	10.11	6.66	5.34
Virus antigen, antiserum and RBCs		52.98	38.79	25.34	15.40	8.73	7.01

[a] After second incubation, treated RBCs were incubated at 37°C for 2 hr in 5 ml of PBS containing 4 units of guinea pig complement.
[b] 2% horse RBC suspension (0.2 ml).
[c] EIA virus antigen (0.2 ml) with different HA titer.
[d] Antiserum (0.2 ml) having an HI titer of 32.

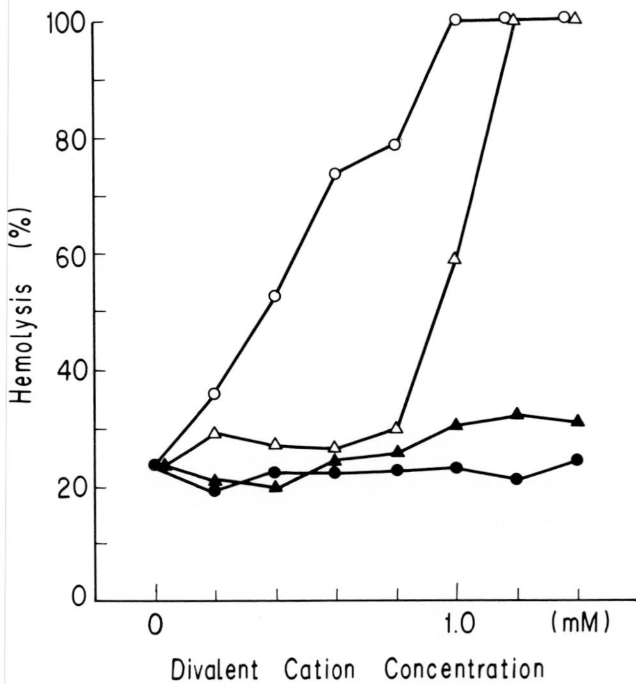

Fig. 2. Effects of Ca (*open triangles*) and Mg (*solid triangles*) ions on lysis of horse RBCs treated with EIA virus antigen; treated RBCs were suspended in PBS containing 4 units of guinea pig complement, 0.25 mM EGTA, and various concentrations of divalent cation, and then incubated at 37°C for 2 hr. As controls effects of Ca (*open circles*) and Mg (*solid circles*) ions on lysis of sensitized sheep RBCs were observed under the same conditions.

On the other hand, the addition of antiserum to virus antigen-treated RBCs enhanced the hemolysis, to a greater degree when RBCs were treated with less than 1 HA unit of virus antigen. However, when the EIA virus and antibody were mixed with RBCs simultaneously, the hemolysis was less efficient (Table 1).

Requirement of calcium ions on hemolysis. Calcium ions restored a capacity equivalent to 4 units of guinea pig complement containing 0.25 mM EGTA in the hemolysis of horse RBCs treated with the virus antigen, as well as that of sensitized sheep RBCs. The hemolysis of both RBCs was enhanced with the increase of the concentration of Ca ions. However, Mg ions did not increase the hemolysis under the same condition (Fig. 2).

Mg or Ca ions did not restore the capacity equivalent to 4 units of guinea pig complement with 0.25 mM EDTA when the concentration of Mg or Ca ions increased to 2.0 mM.

Complement attachment on the surface of RBCs. Horse RBCs treated with virus antigen and fresh horse serum were stained with FITC-conjugated antihorse complement rabbit serum (Fig. 3). Membrane immunofluorescence was not observed when RBCs were treated with inactivated horse serum or fresh horse serum containing EDTA.

Phagocytosis of horse RBCs. As horse RBCs sensitized with virus antigen and then treated with fresh horse serum were overlaid onto leukocyte cultures, the RBCs were actively phagocytized by cultivated leukocytes. Based on several preliminary experiments, conditions for the phagocytosis assays were determined to be suitable when the suspension (0.1 ml) containing 1×10^7 of horse RBCs treated with fresh horse serum was added to 2.5×10^6 of the leukocytes obtained from a 1-day culture, followed by incubation at 37°C for 2 hr.

Phagocytosis was observed in the RBC sensitized with a quantity as small as 1/16 HA unit of virus antigen, and it reached a maximum when the RBCs were sensitized with 8 HA units. No significant phagocytic activity was observed when the RBCs treated with inactivated horse serum were overlaid on cultivated leukocytes (Fig. 4).

Effect of antibody on phagocytosis. The addition of antiserum to virus antigen-treated RBCs slightly suppressed but had no enhancing effect on phagocytosis. Erythrocytes that were mixed simultaneously with virus antigen and antiserum and then treated with fresh horse serum were also phagocytized. Phagocytosis occurred even when fresh horse serum was added to RBCs treated with virus antigen that had been inhibited beforehand by antiserum. However, treat-

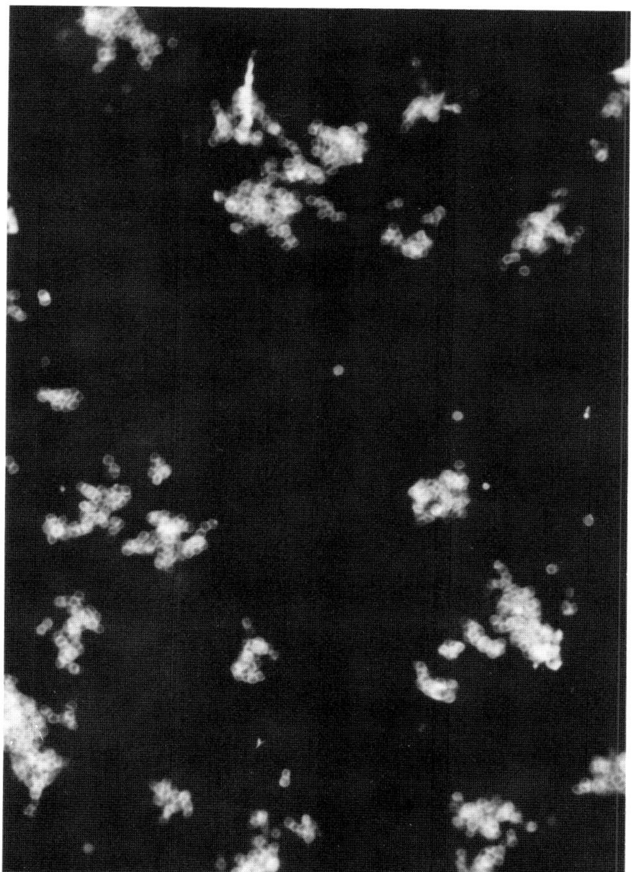

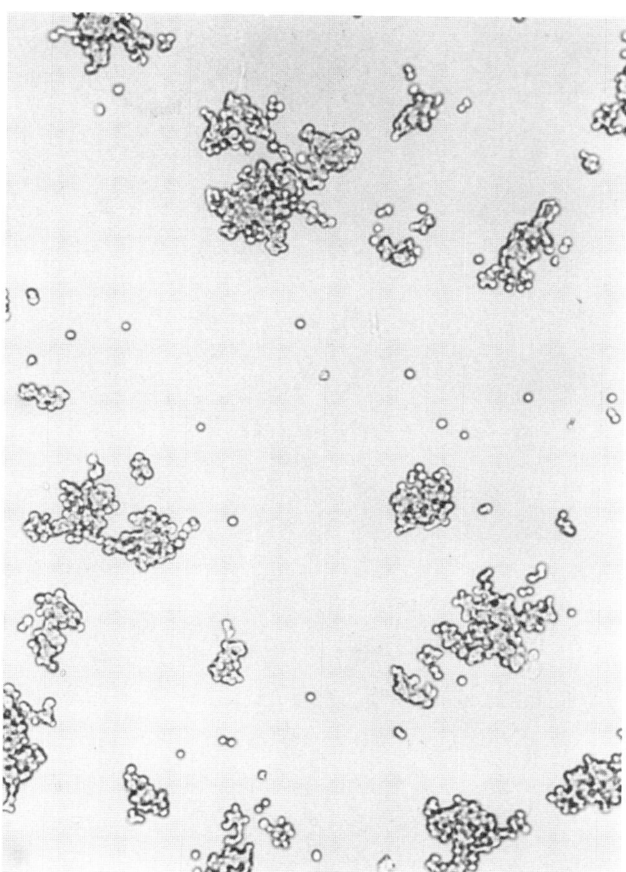

Fig. 3. Adsorption of complement onto horse RBCs treated with 4 units of EIA virus antigen; treated RBCs were mixed with fresh horse serum, kept in icewater, then stained with FITC-conjugated antihorse complement rabbit serum. *Left*, fluorescence microscopy; *right*, light microscopy.

ments with antiserum appeared to slightly decrease the ratio of phagocytosis (Table 2).

Observation of phagocytosis by light microscopy. Leukocytes released and collected from glass bottles after 24-hr cultivation consisted primarily of mononuclear macrophage-like cells and a small number of polymorphonuclear granulocytes. Most of the phagocytized RBCs were found in macrophage-like cells, while others were ingested in polymorphonuclear cells (Fig. 5).

Table 2. Effect of antibody on phagocytosis

Treatments of horse RBCs (2 hr at 37°C)[a]		Ratio of phagocytized RBCs treated with HA (%)	
First	Second	2 U	1/2 U
RBCs[b] and virus antigen[c]	PBS	6.16	4.81
RBCs and virus antigen	Antiserum[d]	6.05	3.64
Virus antigen and antiserum	RBCs	5.22	2.56
Virus antigen, antiserum and RBCs		5.92	3.14

[a] After treatments, RBCs were suspended in fresh horse serum and 1×10^7 of RBCs were overlaid on 2.5×10^6 of leukocytes.

[b] Horse RBCs (1×10^8)

[c] EIA virus antigen (0.2 ml) with 2-HA titer.

[d] Antiserum (0.2 ml) having an HI titer of 64.

DISCUSSION

Horse RBCs treated with EIA virus antigen were lysed in fresh serum. Direct immunofluorescence testing revealed adsorption of complement factors on the surface of RBCs, indicating that the RBCs had activated the complement and induced hemolysis. Since hemolysis increased when antiserum was added to the virus antigen-attached RBCs and since both Ca and Mg ions were necessary for hemolysis, activation of complement was considered to be enhanced by

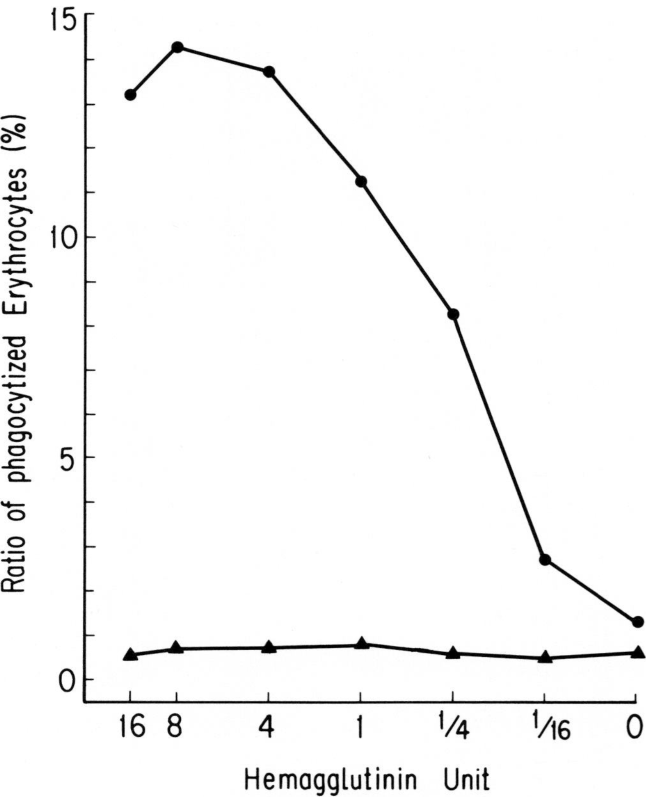

Fig. 4. Ratio of phagocytized RBCs treated with various concentrations of EIA virus antigen; treated RBCs were mixed with fresh (*circles*) or inactivated (*triangles*) horse serum, kept for 30 min in an icewater bath, and 1×10^7 of the RBCs were then overlaid onto 2.5×10^6 of cultivated leukocytes.

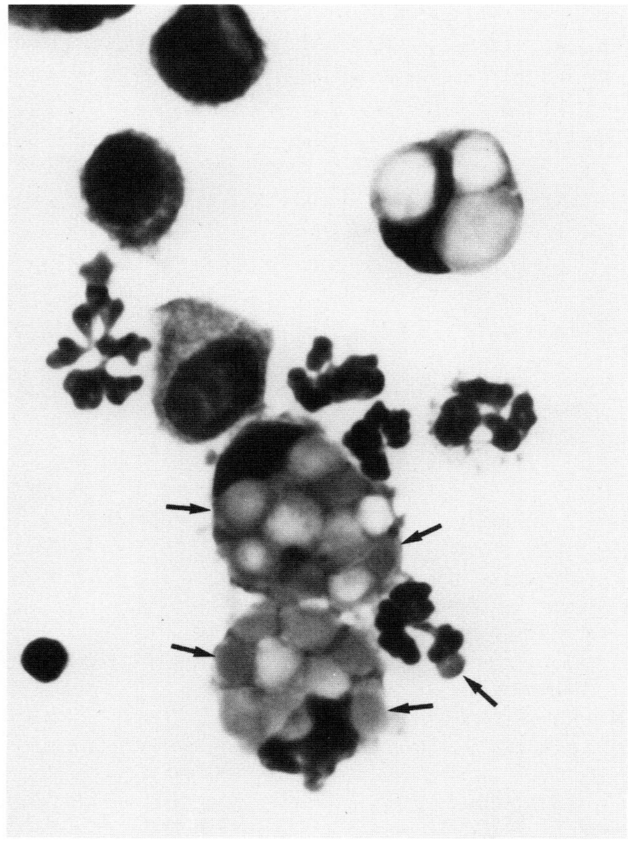

Fig. 5. Smears of cultivated leukocytes that phagocytized horse RBCs (*arrows*) treated with EIA virus antigen and fresh horse serum (giemsa staining).

antigen-antibody complex through the classical pathway. It is not clear why the virus antigen, which lost the HA activity after incubation with the antibody, still maintained the hemolytic activity. One possibility is that hemagglutinin has multiple sites that bind to RBCs, some of which were not covered completely with antibodies. Another possibility is that the virus antigen was firmly bound to RBCs but was bound to the antibody in a reversible manner. When the antigen dissociated from the antibodies, it became bound to the RBCs, possibly modifying the cell surface components and activating complement. Some substances, including a special protein complex, are known to activate complement without antibody via the classical pathway. It is thus possible that the EIA virus glycoprotein and horse RBC surface protein complex activate complement in the same way.

Horse RBCs treated with EIA virus antigen were ingested by cultivated leukocytes after treatment with fresh horse serum. The antiserum treatment had no enhancing effect on phagocytosis. Phagocytosis was judged to be associated primarily with the presence of complement on the RBCs and of C3 receptors on the leukocytes. It is not known why the addition of antiserum to the virus antigen-bound RBCs did not induce them to be phagocytized by cultivated leukocytes even though macrophages and polymorphonuclear cells have receptors for immunoglobulin (Banks & McGuire 1975; Shurin & Stossel 1978). It remains to be determined whether the hemagglutinins that bind to RBCs can keep their antigencity to combine with HI antibody.

Some reports have suggested the existence of complement-mediated hemolysis in EIA although the mechanisms of complement attachment on RBCs is not elucidated (Issel & Coggins 1979; McGuire & Crawford 1979). Present in vitro experimental systems may help explain the pathogenesis of the anemia. The fact that RBCs with virus attached were lysed by complement activation seems to be closely associated with the mechanism of anemia. However, in vivo, many factors inhibit the activation of serial complement components in the classical or alternative pathway (Brown & Frank 1981). Activation of the first component of complement seldom leads to lysis of RBCs. It is possible, however, that the binding of the virus component or complement to the RBC surface may induce anemia indirectly. The complement attachment may modify the RBC surface configuration and promote osmotic fragility, or leukocytes that have C3 receptors may phagocytize modified RBCs. Since the cultivated leukocytes were able to phagocytize RBCs sensitized with a quantity of hemagglutinin too small to induce agglutination, the participation of these cells in the phagocytic process seems to be one of the leading mechanisms causing anemia and promoting formation of sideroleukocytes in horses infected with the EIA virus. Direct erythrocyte lysis by complement and phagocytosis of the C3-coated cells by macrophages and polymorphonuclear cells seem to play important roles in the pathogenesis of anemia in EIA.

REFERENCES

Banks, K.L., and McGuire, T.C. (1975) Surface receptors on neutrophiles and monocytes from immunodeficient and normal horses. *Immunology* **28,** 581-88.

Brown, E.J., and Frank, M.M. (1981) Complement activation. *Immunol. Today* **2,** 129-34.

Ishii, S. (1963) Equine infectious anemia or swamp fever. *Adv. Vet. Sci. Comp. Med.* **8,** 263-98.

Issel, C.J., and Coggins, L. (1979) Equine infectious anemia: Current knowledge. *J. Am. Vet. Med. Assoc.* **174,** 727-33.

Kono, Y. (1969) Viremia and immunological responses in horses infected with equine infectious anemia virus. *Natl. Inst. Anim. Health Q. (Jpn.)* **9,** 1-9.

Kono, Y.; Kobayashi, K.; and Fukunaga, Y. (1971a) Distribution of equine infectious anemia virus in horses infected with the virus. *Natl. Inst. Anim. Health Q.* (Jpn.) **11,** 11-20.

———. (1971b) Serological comparison among various strains of equine infectious anemia virus. *Arch. Ges. Virusforsch.* **34,** 202-8.

McGuire, T.C., and Crawford, T.B. (1979) Immunology of a persistent retrovirus infection—Equine infectious anemia. *Adv. Vet. Sci. Comp. Med.* **23,** 137-59.

McGuire, T.C.; Crawford, T.B.; and Henson, J.B. (1971) Immunofluorescent localization of equine infectious anemia virus in tissue. *Am. J. Pathol.* **62,** 283-92.

McGuire, T.C.; Henson, J.B.; and Bueger, D. (1969) Complement (C3)-coated red blood cells following infection with the virus of equine infectious anemia. *J. Immunol.* **103,** 293-99.

McGuire, T.C.; Henson, J.B.; and Quist, S.E. (1969a) Impaired bone marrow response in equine infectious anemia. *Am. J. Vet. Res.* **30,** 2099-2104.

———. (1969b) Viral induced hemolysis in equine infectious anemia. *Am. J. Vet. Res.* **30,** 2091-97.

Obara, J., and Nakajima, H. (1961) Life-span of ^{51}Cr-labeled erythrocytes in equine infectious anemia. *Jpn. J. Vet. Sci.* **23,** 207-10.

Perryman, L.E.; McGuire, T.C.; Banks, K.L.; and Henson, J.B. (1971) Decreased C3 levels in a chronic virus infection: Equine infectious anemia. *J. Immunol.* **106,** 1074-78.

Schmid, R.W., and Reilley, C.N. (1957) New complexon for titration of calcium in the presence of magnesium. *Analyt. Chem.* **29,** 264-68.

Sentsui, H., and Kono, Y. (1978) Preparation of hemagglutinating antigen of equine infectious anemia virus from infected equine leukocyte cultures. *Natl. Inst. Anim. Health Q. (Jpn.)* **18,** 39-40.

———. (1981a) Hemagglutination by several strains of equine infectious anemia virus. *Arch. Virol.* **67,** 75-84.

———. (1981b) Hemagglutination-inhibition tests with different strains of equine infectious anemia virus. *Am. J. Vet. Res.* **42,** 1949-52.

Shurin, S.B., and Stossel, T.P. (1978) Complement (C3)-activated phagocytosis by lung macrophages. *J. Immunol.* **120,** 1305-12.

Yamamoto, H., and Konno, S. (1967) Pathological studies on bone marrow in equine infectious anemia. I. Macroscopical finding on whole longitudinal sections of bone marrow. *Natl. Inst. Anim. Health Q. (Jpn)* **7,** 40-53.

A Seven-Year Serological Study of Viral Agents Causing Respiratory Infection with Pyrexia among Racehorses in Japan

Takeo Sugiura, Tomio Matsumura, Hiroshi Imagawa, and Yoshio Fukunaga

SUMMARY

A serological study at two training centers from 1980 to 1986 found that a total of 4,142 horses developed pyrexia. Of the total, 3,102 were tested for equid herpesvirus-1 (EHV-1), equine rhinovirus type 1 (ERhV-1), rotavirus, and equine adenovirus (EAdV). The results indicated that 738 (23.7%) horses seroconverted: 543 to EHV-1, 102 to ERhV-1, 69 to rotavirus, and 24 to EAdV.

Racehorses that developed pyrexia but did not seroconvert to EHV-1, ERhV-1, rotavirus, and EAdV were examined serologically for evidence of antibody to *Chlamydia psittaci* (*C. psi.*), reovirus, equid herpesvirus-2 (EHV-2), and parainfluenza virus type 3 (PI-3). In testing of paired sera from 800 horses, eight horses showed seroconversion to *C. psi.* and one to reovirus. No horses sampled had seroconverted to EHV-2 and none had antibody to PI-3.

INTRODUCTION

Numerous serological studies have recently focused on infectious agents associated with respiratory disease among racehorses from Canada (Sherman et al. 1979; Sturm, Lang & Mitchell 1980), the United States, (Conner et al. 1984; Keman, Frank & Babish 1985), and Great Britain (Powell et al. 1978; Burrows et al. 1982).

In Japan a large-scale epizootic of influenza at the end of 1971 (Kono et al. 1972) caused racing to be canceled for several months. The spread of Getah virus infection at the Miho Training Center also interfered with racing during 1978 (Fukunaga et al. 1981; Kamada et al. 1980; Sentsui & Kono 1980).

The Japan Racing Association operates two training centers (TCs), at each of which approximately 2,000 racehorses are accommodated and trained. Although such concentrated facilities are convenient, they inevitably harbor a great risk of an epizootic.

Accordingly, all the racehorses at the TCs are inoculated against equine influenza, Japanese encephalitis (JE), and Getah virus. Horses with pyrexia or signs of respiratory disease are subjected to serological examination for EHV-1, ERhV-1, and EAdV, which are recognized causes of respiratory infection, as well as testing for rotavirus.

Epizootic Research Station, Equine Research Institute, Japan Racing Association, 1400-4, Shiba, Kokubinji-Machi, Shimotsuga-gun, Tochigi 329-04, Japan.

MATERIALS AND METHODS

Horses. The Ritto TC is in Shiga Prefecture, in the western part of Japan, and the Miho TC in Ibaraki Prefecture, in the east. Racehorses are transported from the TC for each race meeting except during the months of July and August, when horses stay at the local racetracks. The turnover at each TC is about 200 to 400 horses per month.

All horses including recent arrivals are vaccinated annually against Getah virus and JE in May and June and against equine influenza in October.

Serum samples. A serum sample was obtained from each horse exhibiting pyrexia exceeding 38.5°C, followed by a convalescent in two weeks' time.

Serological tests. During 1980-86, paired samples from 3,102 horses were examined for EHV-1, ERhV-1, EAdV, and rotavirus. Paired samples selected at random that did not show seroconversion to EHV-1, ERhV-1, EAdV, or rotavirus were tested for *C. psi.*, EHV-2, reovirus, and PI-3.

Complement fixation (CF) test. Antigen was prepared from the HH-1 strain of EHV-1 (T. Shimizu, National Institute of Animal Health—NIAH), EHV-2 (Y. Kono, NIAH), the T-1 strain of EAdV-1 (W. H. McCollum, University of Kentucky), and neonatal calf diarrhea virus, the Lincoln strain of rotavirus (M. Kodama, NIAH). In preparation, the infected culture fluid and cell debris of RK-13, MDCK, or MA-104 cells were concentrated by polyethylene glycol No. 6000 at 10% (w/w) and sodium chloride at 3% (w/w) and treated with ultrasonication. The resulting product was centrifuged at $6{,}000 \times g$ for 30 min. The supernatant was used as antigen. Antigens of *C. psi.* and reovirus type 3 were obtained commercially (Denka Sieken Co. Ltd., Tokyo).

The comparative CF test was conducted by the CH_{50} method developed by the U.S. Centers for Disease Control, Atlanta, Georgia, as modified by Inoue (1978). The modified method uses 0.05 ml of 5 units of guinea pig complement, 0.025 ml of 4 units of antigen, 0.025 ml of a serum sample from which serial twofold dilutions were prepared, and 0.05 ml of 1.7% sensitized sheep red blood cells. The antibody titer was expressed as the reciprocal of the highest dilution that inhibited hemolysis greater than 50%.

Virus neutralization (VN) test. Antibody against the NM-11 strain of ERhV-1 (W. H. McCollum, University of

Table 1. Monthly distribution of pyrexia among horses at Ritto and Miho Training Centers, 1980-86.

Year	TC	Jan.	Feb.	Mar.	Apr.	May	June	July	Aug.	Sept.	Oct.	Nov.	Dec.	Total
1980	Ritto	29	36	15	13	11	16	49	24	44	10	17	19	283
	Miho	196	39	17	20	19	15	11	15	20	23	15	39	429
1981	Ritto	27	23	14	4	54	48	15	22	46	33	62	55	443
	Miho	100	59	27	26	74	38	15	14	19	66	66	43	547
1982	Ritto	60	75	29	43	42	27	38	40	46	25	39	36	500
	Miho	20	19	20	25	10	24	24	22	56	37	24	37	318
1983	Ritto	55	49	33	25	29	40	66	24	28	23	10	6	388
	Miho	80	44	26	14	6	10	21	33	27	27	17	14	319
1984	Ritto	34	15	11	16	17	31	11	1	13	16	17	5	187
	Miho	17	17	12	10	11	18	7	0	7	3	6	2	110
1985	Ritto	10	4	21	15	16	23	57	18	13	19	12	5	213
	Miho	5	4	4	11	14	5	16	11	18	7	10	7	112
1986	Ritto	50	15	15	13	21	22	7	7	10	8	8	4	180
	Miho	22	17	9	7	8	6	8	2	6	3	14	11	113
Total	Ritto	265	217	138	169	190	207	243	136	200	134	165	130	2,194
Total	Miho	440	199	115	113	142	116	102	97	153	166	152	153	1,948
Combined	Total	705	416	253	282	332	323	345	233	353	300	317	283	4,142

Table 2. Monthly distribution of seroconversions to equid herpesvirus-1, equine rhinovirus type 1, rotavirus, and equine adenovirus at Ritto and Miho Training Centers

	Total no. of horses showing seroconversion, 1980-86												
Virus	Jan.	Feb.	Mar.	Apr.	May	June	July	Aug.	Sept.	Oct.	Nov.	Dec.	Total
EHV-1	305	142	30	22	9	0	0	0	0	0	0	35	543
ERhV-1	18	15	7	10	11	4	2	0	9	10	6	7	99
Rota	16	11	1	4	9	3	4	0	1	2	6	12	69
EAdV	3	1	0	1	3	3	3	1	2	1	3	3	24

Note: A total number of 4,142 racehorses showed pyrexia, of which 3,102 were tested serologically.

Kentucky) was detected by the VN test. The microtiter assay, essentially as described by Bibrack and Hartl (1971), contained 0.05 ml of virus (100 $TCID_{50}$) mixed with an equal amount of twofold serum dilution in flat-bottomed microplates (Nunc, Roskilde, Denmark). Vero cells (1×10^6 of cells in 0.075 ml) were added to the resulting mixture after incubation at 37°C for 1 hr. The antibody titer was expressed as the reciprocal of the highest serum dilution that had neutralized the virus completely.

Hemagglutination inhibition (HI). Antibody against PI-3 was detected by the HI test, using commercial antigen (Denka Sieken Co., Ltd., Tokyo). Serum was treated with recaptor destroying enzyme and absorbed by guinea pig red blood cells. It was then inactivated by heat to eliminate the inhibitor to hemagglutination. A mixture of 0.025 ml each of antigen (4 units) and treated serum (eightfold dilution) was incubated at room temperature for 60 min and then allowed to stand.

Status of infection. When a convalescent horse showed a serum antibody titer at least eight times as high as in the acute stage, the horse was regarded as being infected with the virus tested for.

RESULTS

Pyrexia. The maximum number of horses with pyrexia per year occurred in 1981 at the Miho TC and in 1982 at the Ritto TC (Table 1). It declined year by year thereafter.

EHV-1 infection. Outbreaks of EHV-1 infection occurred at both TCs during the winter and spring of each year (Table 2). The mean age of horses showing seroconversion was 2.96 years; 68.9% were three years old (Fig. 1).

ERhV-1 infection. The mean age of horses showing seroconversion to ERhV-1 infection was 2.44; 69.2% were two years old (Table 2).

Rotavirus infection. Epizootics of rotavirus infection occurred at the Miho TC during 1981 and 1983, and at the Ritto TC during 1982 and 1983 (Table 2). The number of horses infected with rotavirus was smaller than those with EHV-1 or ERhV-1. Of the seroconversions, 55.0% occurred in winter, December through February. The mean age of horses showing seroconversion was 2.73.

Table 3. Number of seroconversions to *Chlamydia psittaci*, equid herpesvirus-2, reovirus, and parainfluenza virus, 1980-86

Virus	No. of horses showing seroconversion	No. of sero-positive horses at acute stage	No. of horses tested
C. psi.	8	45	800
EHV-2	0	105	105
Reovirus	1	145	800
PI-3	0	0	800

Note: The horses were selected for testing because they had shown no seroconversion to equid herpesvirus-1, equine rhinovirus type 1, equine adenovirus, or rotavirus.

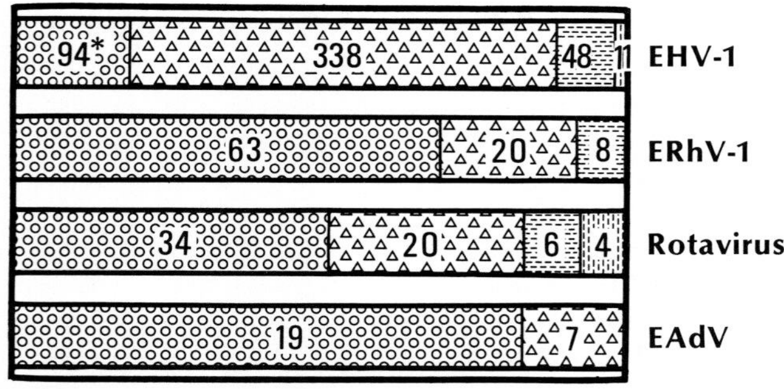

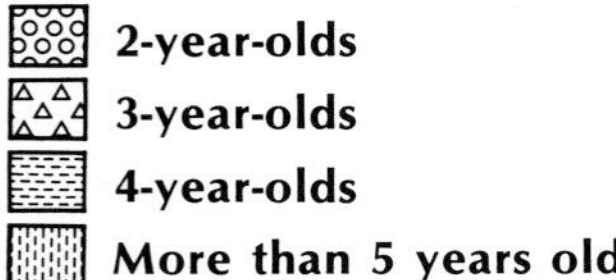

Fig. 1. Age distribution of horses showing seroconversion to viruses.

EAdV infection. A total of 24 horses seroconverted to EAdV (Table 2). The maximum number of seroconversions in any single month was three at the Ritto TC during December 1982.

Serological tests. Eight samples obtained from two- and three-year-old horses showed seroconversion to *C. psi* (Table 3). Forty-five horses were already positive in the acute-phase sample, with a titer of 1:8 or higher. Of the 105 horses tested for EHV-2 infection, all had antibody in the acute-phase sera, with no subsequent evidence of seroconversion.

Of 800 horses tested, 145 were positive to reovirus but only one three-year-old showed evidence of seroconversion. None of the horses tested had antibody to PI-3.

DISCUSSION

Seroconversion to a variety of infectious agents was observed in almost a quarter of the horses with pyrexia. Although the spread of viral infection did not threaten racing, it did influence training and the participation in races of individual horses. Since pyrexia is a symptom of respiratory or systemic infectious disease, determining the cause can help in preventing large-scale epizootics.

Of the horses showing seroconversion, 74.9% developed pyrexia attributable to EHV-1, which might have been prevented by vaccination. In Japan the authorized EHV-1 vaccine is intended to prevent abortion, not respiratory disease. EHV-1 subtype 1 was introduced into Japan after broodmares were imported from the United States in 1967 (Kawakami et al. 1970). Before that, only subtype 2 had been found in Japan (Shimizu et al., 1963). In the present survey, EHV-1 showed a seasonal occurrence from December to March, with a peak incidence in January, although EHV-1 was found during all seasons of the year on rearing or breeding farms (Matsumura et al. 1986; Sugiura et al. 1983a). Since EHV-1 infection occurs among young horses, most racehorses have antibodies to EHV-1. Clinical signs are rarely observed on the rearing farms even when antibody titers increase (Matsumura et al. 1986; Sugiura et al. 1983a). The virulence of the virus may be low but if a horse is exposed to stress from a change in the weather, clinical signs may develop.

Serological reactors against the Lincoln strain of bovine rotavirus have been found in 65.7% of foals and 27.0% of racehorses in Japan (Imagawa, Ando & Akiyama 1979), and rotavirus has been isolated from foals with diarrhea (Imagawa et al. 1979). Before the present survey, no epizootic had in fact been recorded among racehorses. In humans there is a tendency for repeated rotavirus infections (Mata et al. 1983), so reinfections may have been included among the horses showing seroconversion. A serological study of EAdV undertaken by Kamada (1978) at the Tokyo Racecourse showed that 44.3% of racehorses possessed CF antibody. The number of seropositive horses was very small in the present survey, suggesting that this virus has diminished in the past 13 years.

Serological reactors to *C. psi.* [Ogawa et al., oral presentation, 97th meeting, Japanese Society of Veterinary Science (JSVS), Tokyo]; EHV-2 (Kono & Kobayashi 1964; Sugiura et al. 1983b); and reovirus types 1 to 3 (Imagawa et al., oral presentation, 100th meeting, JSVS, Tokyo) have been detected in the Japanese horse population. No relationship has been reported between these agents and clinical disease in Japan. The present survey made it apparent that *C. psi* was not widely distributed among racehorses in Japan. On the other hand, 36.8% of the racehorses studied had antibody to reovirus and 100% had antibody to EHV-2, but only one animal showed seroconversion to reovirus. It is likely that the racehorses had been exposed to these viruses before entering the TCs.

The presence of serological reactors to PI-3 has been reported in Europe (Hofer et al. 1972; Zmudzinski et al. 1980), but no evidence of antibody to PI-3 was found among racehorses in this survey.

REFERENCES

Bibrack, B., and Hartl, G. (1971) Mikrotest zum Nachweiss neutralizierender Antikorpers gegen das Rhinopneumonititis-Virus der Pferde. *Zbl. Vet. Med. B.* **18,** 517-26.

Burrows, R., Goodridge, D.; Denyer, M.; Hutchings, G.; and Frank, C.J. (1982) Equine influenza infections in Great Britain, 1979. *Vet. Rec.* **110,** 492-97.

Conner, M.; Kalica, A.; Kita, J.; Quick, S.; Schiff, E.; Joubert, J.; and Gillespie, J. (1984) Isolation and characteristics of an equine reovirus type 3 and antibody prevalence survey to reoviruses in horses located in New York State. *Vet. Microbiol.* **9,** 15-25.

Fontaine, M.; Labe, J.; Legeay, Y.; and Durand, M. (1978) Outbreak of a cardiopulmonary disorder in horses. *Rev. Med. Vet.* **129,** 271-79.

Fretz, P.B.; Babiuk, L.A.; and McLaughlin, B. (1979) Equine respiratory disease on the Western Canadian racetracks. *Can. Vet. J.* **20,** 58-61.

Fukunaga, Y.; Ando, Y.; Kamada, M.; Imagawa, H.; Wada, R.; Kumanomido, T.; Akiyama, Y.; Watanabe, O.; Niwa, K.; Takenaga, S.; Shibata, M.; and Yamamoto, T. (1981) An outbreak of Getah virus infection in horses. Clinical and epizootiological aspects at the Miho Training Center in 1978. *Bull. Equine Res. Inst.* **18,** 94-102.

Hofer, B.; Stech, F.; Gerber, H.; Lohrer, J.; Nickolet, J.; and Paccaud, M.F. (1972) An investigation of the etiology of viral respiratory disease in a remount depot. *Proc. 3rd Int. Conf. Equine Infect. Dis.,* pp. 527-45.

Imagawa, H.; Ando, Y.; and Akiyama, Y. (1979) A survey on complement fixation antibody against bovine rotavirus in light horses in Japan. *Exp. Rep. Equine Hlth Lab.* **16,** 23-29.

Imagawa, H.; Ando Y.; Sugiura, T.; Wada, R.; Hirasawa, K.; and Akiyama, Y. (1981) Isolation of foal rotavirus in MA-104 cells. *Bull. Equine Res. Inst.* **18,** 119-28.

Inoue, S. (1978) Complement fixation test. In *Examination of Virus and Rickettsia,* 2d ed., pp. 73-83. Ed. K. Yanagisawa. Society for Japanese Public Health, Tokyo.

Kamada, M. (1978) Comparison of the four serological tests for detecting antibodies against equine adenovirus. *Exp. Rep. Equine Hlth Lab.* **15,** 91-96.

Kamada, M.; Ando, Y.; Fukunaga, Y.; Kumanomido, T.; Imagawa, H.; Wada, R.; and Akiyama, Y. (1980) Equine Getah virus infection: Isolation of the virus from racehorses during an enzootic in Japan. *Am. J. Trop. Med. Hyg.* **29,** 984-88.

Kawakami, Y.; Nakano, K.; Kume, T.; Hiramune, T.; and Murase, N. (1970) Abortion by equine rhinopneumonitis virus in Hidaka, Hokkaido, district in Japan. *Bull. Natl. Inst. Anim. Hlth* **61,** 9-16.

Kemen, M.J.; Frank, R.A.; and Babish, J.B. (1985) An outbreak of equine influenza at a harness horse racetrack. *Cornell Vet.* **75,** 277-88.

Kono, Y.; Ishikawa, K.; Fukunaga, Y.; and Fujino, M. (1972) The first outbreak of equine influenze in Japan. *Nat. Inst. Anim. Hlth Q. (Jpn)* **12,** 183-87.

Kono, Y., and Kobayashi, K. (1964) Cytopathogenic equine orphan (CEO) virus in horse kidney cell culture. II. Immunological studies of CEO virus. *Nat. Inst. Anim. Hlth Q.* (Jpn) **4,** 21-27.

Mata, L.; Simhon, A.; Urrutia, J.J.; Kronmal, R.A.; Fernandez, R.; and Garcia, B. (1983) Epidemiology of rotaviruses in a cohort of 45 Guatamalan Mayan Indian children observed from birth to the age of three years. *J. Infect. Dis.* **148,** 452-61.

Matsumura, T.; Komano, M.; Sugiura, T.; and Fukunaga, Y. (1986) Sero-epizootiological studies on viral diseases in horses on a breeding farm of Japan during a period from 1981 to 1985. *Bull. Equine Res. Inst.* **23,** 28-34.

Powell, D.G.; Burrows, R.; Spooner, P.R.; Goodridge, D.; Thomson, C.R.; and Mumford, J. (1978) A study of infectious respiratory disease among horses in Great Britain, 1971-1976. *Proc. 4th Int. Conf. Equine Infect. Dis.* pp. 451-59.

Sentsui, H., and Kono, Y. (1980) An epidemic of Getah virus infection among racehorses: Isolation of the virus. *Res. Vet. Sci.* **29,** 157-61.

Sherman, J.; Mitchell, W.R.; Martin, S.W.; Thorsen, J.; and Ingram, D.G. (1979) Epidemiology of equine upper respiratory tract disease on Standardbred racetracks. *Can. J. Comp. Med.* **43,** 1-9.

Shimizu, T.; Ishizaki, R.; and Matumoto, M. (1963) Survey of antibody to equine rhinopneumonitis virus in horse population in Japan. *Bull. Nat. Inst. Anim. Hlth* **44,** 11-17.

Sugiura, T.; Ando, Y.; Masuzawa, H.; Kuriyama, H.; Ogawa, A.; and Hirasawa, K. (1983a) Sero-epizootiological studies on rearing horses on the Hidaka Rearing Farm from 1980 to 1983. *Bull. Equine Res. Inst.* **20,** 48-54.

Sugiura, T.; Fukuzawa, Y.; Kamada, M.; Ando, Y.; and Hirasawa, K. (1983b) Isolation of equine herpesvirus type 2 from foals with pneumonitis. *Bull. Equine Res. Inst.* **20,** 148-153.

Sturm, R.T.; Lang, G.H.; and Mitchell, W.R. (1980) Prevalence of reovirus 1, 2 and 3 antibodies among Ontario racehorses. *Can. Vet. J.* **21,** 206-9.

Zmudzinski, J.; Baczynski, Z.; and Skukmowska-Kryazkowska, D. (1980) Serological examinations of horses for the presence of antibodies against pneumotropic viruses. *Bull. Vet. Inst. Pulawy* **24,** 49-51.

Monoclonal Antibodies to Equine Arteritis Virus

Ewan D. Chirnside, R. Frank Cook, M.W. Lock, and Jennifer A. Mumford

SUMMARY

Monoclonal antibodies (MAbs) raised to equine arteritis virus (EAV) were prepared to characterize and purify specific viral proteins, and to aid in rapid identification of EAV-infected cells and serological diagnosis of EAV by enzyme-linked immunoassays (ELISA). Specific antibody-producing hybridomas, derived from experiments in which mice were immunized with partially purified EAV, were screened in three ELISA systems, using purified virus, host cell proteins, and medium constituents as antigens. In Western blot analysis, selected MAbs showed exquisite activity to EAV proteins, confirming the existence of a 30-kilodalton (kdal) and a 14-kdal structural protein (p30 and p14, respectively). EAV infected RK13 cells were detectable 12 hr postinfection with a MAb directed at the virus nucleocapsid protein. A second MAb was used for chromatography on Sepharose 4B-MAb (D6) affinity columns to further purify sucrose gradient-prepared EAV. Enhanced purification of major viral proteins of the molecular weights 14, 16, 30, 42, and 59 kdal was achieved. Such preparations stimulate specific antibody to EAV in rabbits with no cross-reactivity to cell or medium contaminants.

INTRODUCTION

The outbreak of viral arteritis among Thoroughbreds in Kentucky (Timoney 1985) and the demonstration of an EAV carrier state in stallions (Timoney et al. 1986) have emphasized the need for rapid, more sensitive diagnostic techniques. The current method of detecting antibody is a complement-dependent virus neutralization test in microtiter plates, which requires at least 48 hr (Senne et al. 1985) and in some cases as long as five days (Moraillon & Moraillon 1978). The drawbacks are obvious when mares must be screened before covering, or when antibody levals must be established before horses are exported to EAV-free countries. Nor can the current test differentiate between antibody produced in response to a live vaccine and antibody generated by virus infection.

This study was undertaken to prepare reagents that would improve diagnostic techniques and could eventually differentiate between responses to vaccine and to infection. A panel of specific MAbs to EAV was raised to aid in identifying and purifying viral proteins; to serve as diagnostic tools in detecting antigen and antibody by fluorescence and ELISA; and in the future to to determine the extent of strain variation between EAV isolates.

MATERIALS AND METHODS

Virus and cells. The Bucyrus strain of EAV (Doll et al. 1957) was used throughout. Virus of passage level 12 (in rabbit kidney, RK13) was propagated in RK13 cells grown in Eagle's minimal essential medium (MEM), supplemented with 10% fetal calf serum and containing penicillin (100 i.u./ml), streptomycin (100 i.u./ml), and fungizone (2.5μg/ml) (all from Flow Laboratories, Rickmansworth, England).

Virus growth and purification. After washing for 2 hr in serum-free MEM (SF-MEM), RK13 cells growing in roller bottles were infected at a multiplicity of infection (m.o.i.) of 0.01 in 10 ml SF-MEM for 1 hr. After the addition of 40 ml of SF-MEM, rollers were incubated at 37°C until 80% of the RK13 cells showed cytopathic effect (40-45 hr postinfection). Each bottle was shaken vigorously and the tissue culture supernatant was pooled and centrifuged to pellet out cell debris (3,000 rpm, 10 min, 4°C). The virus pellet was harvested by centrifuging the supernatant at 21,000 rpm for 3 hr at 4°C. The pellet was then resuspended in STE buffer (10 mM Tris-HC1, 1 mM EDTA, 100 mM NaC1, pH 7.5) and centrifuged overnight through a 25-50% sucrose gradient (21,000 rpm, 10°C). The virus band was then recovered and washed in 1 mM phosphate buffer, pH 7.0, pelleted by centrifugation (24,000 rpm, 2 hr, 4°C), resuspended in TE buffer (10 mM Tris-HC1, 1 mM EDTA, pH 7.5), and aliquoted into stock vials for storage at −70°C.

Radiolabeled ^{35}S L-methionine virus was prepared as described, with the exception that methionine-free SF-MEM contained 2 μg/ml actinomycin D and 500 μCi^{35}S L-methionine (Amersham International, Amersham, England) was added to each roller bottle 6 hr postinoculation (p.i.).

MAb production. Female Balb/c mice were immunized with sucrose gradient-purified EAV to produce a virus neutralizing antibody titer greater than 1:32 prior to fusion. MAbs were produced by polyethylene glycol fusion of spleen lymphocytes with mouse myeloma cell line NSO and maintained as described by Campbell (1984). Hybridoma screening was by indirect ELISA using purified EAV as antigen, and secreted antibody was detected by a rabbit antimouse

Equine Virology Unit, Animal Health Trust, Lanwades Park, Kennett, Newmarket, Suffolk CB8 7PN, England.

Table 1. Properties of monoclonal antibodies to EAV

Monoclonal antibody	ELISA[a]	Titer[b]	Virus neutralizing activity	Fluorescence	Target Western blot (kdal)	Antigen immuno-precipitation (kdal)	Murine isotype
D6	0.7	1:2560	—	—	30.2	30	IgG1
D2	0.5	1:1280	—	—	13.2	ND[c]	IgG2A
F5	0.4	1:20	—	—	ND	ND	ND
B7	0.4	1:640	—	+ 12h	14	14	IgG2A

[a] Maximum O.D. 492 nm in indirect ELISA using sucrose gradient–purified EAV as antigen.
[b] Ascites dilution of maximum reactivity by endpoint titration.
[c] ND = not determined.

horseradish peroxidase conjugate (Dakopatts, Glostrup, Denmark). False positives to tissue culture contaminants were identified by parallel ELISA against an RK13 cell extract and fetal calf serum, both at 20µg/well. EAV-positive hybridomas were cloned twice by limiting dilution, screened for antibody production after each cloning by ELISA, and grown in pristane-primed mice as ascites tumors. Ascites fluid was purified by ammonium sulphate fractionation and desalting on PD10 columns (Pharmacia Ltd., Milton Keynes, England), then stored at −20°C. MAb isotyping was determined by indirect ELISA with peroxidase-conjugated antimouse subclass antisera (Miles-Yeda, Liverpool, England).

Virus neutralization (VN) test. Serial twofold dilutions of inactivated serum samples (56°C, 30 min) were carried out in a 96-well plate (25 µl/well) from an initial 1:4 dilution. To each well was added MEM (25 µl), supplemented with 5% foetal calf serum and 200 mM HEPES, followed by 25 µl of virus challenge dose containing $10^{2.0}$ $TCID_{50}$. After the plates were incubated for 60 min (37°C, 5% CO_2), 25 µl of a 1:2 dilution of guinea-pig complement was added, followed by incubation for 45 min. RK13 cells (150 µl, 1.2×10^5 cells/ml) were added, the plates were sealed, and the results were read after four days' incubation. Each test was standardized using known EAV-neutralizing rabbit and horse sera as controls, and virus was titrated to ensure a challenge dose of $10^{2.0 \pm 0.4}$ $TCID_{50}$ per well.

Immunofluorescence. Infected cultures of RK13 cells grown on coverslips were washed four times in phosphate-buffered saline (PBS), dried, and fixed for 10 min with ice-cold methanol at 4°C. After incubation for 3 hr with a 1:25 dilution of MAb, the coverslips were washed five times with PBS (5 min/wash). The procedure was repeated with 1:200 rabbit antimouse IgG serum, followed by FITC-labeled anti-rabbit IgG serum (Dakopatts). Counterstained with 0.005% Evans blue, the coverslips were mounted on PBS glycerol (1:9) and viewed under an epifluorescent microscope.

Immunoprecipitation. Ascites fluid (20 µl was incubated with unlabeled or ^{35}S-labeled cell lysate at 4°C overnight, and then mixed with 0.20g protein A-Sepharose 4B (Pharmacia) which had previously been swollen, washed, and incubated in SaC buffer (PBS, 0.5% NP40, 0.02% NaN_3) containing ovalbumin (1 mg/ml) (Jones 1980). After washing four times with SaC buffer, absorbed proteins were recovered by boiling for 5 min in SDS sample buffer and centrifuging at low speed for 10 min; the supernatant was then run through a 10-30% gradient polyacrylamide gel.

Electrophoresis and blotting. Polyacrylamide gel electrophoresis, Western blotting, and autoradiography were carried out following the methodology of Burnett (1981). The detection of ^{35}S-labeled viral proteins was enhanced by fluorography using diphenyloxazole in DMSO (Bonner & Laskey 1974). Immunoblots were performed after blocking non-specific binding sites with 4% bovine serum albumin in PBS with MAb or test antisera at 1:50 dilution. Nitrocellulose sheets were washed between steps with 0.1% NP40 in PBS. The detection of bound MAb was amplified with 1:200 rabbit antimouse IgG serum (Dakopatts) prior to addition of ^{125}I-protein A (2×10^6 cpm radiolabel per blot).

Purification of viral proteins by MAb affinity chromatography. MAb D6 was adjusted to a final protein concentration of 2mg/ml and coupled to CNBr-activated Sepharose 4B as described by the manufacturer. Prior to affinity chromatography, the column was prewashed with two column volumes each of PBS, 3 M NaSCN, 0.1 M acetate buffer pH4.0, and PBS again, to remove unbound material. Sucrose gradient-purified EAV was run into the affinity column in PBS followed by half a column volume of PBS, and allowed to bind overnight at 4°C. PBS was then run through the column to elute unbound material until a steady base line (O.D. 280 nm) was established, followed by specific elution of MAb-bound material by 3 M NaSCN and any other column contaminants by 0.1 M acetate buffer, pH 4.

RESULTS

In a total of 14 fusion experiments using sucrose gradient-purified virus for mouse immunization, four MAbs specific for EAV were produced and characterized (Table 1).

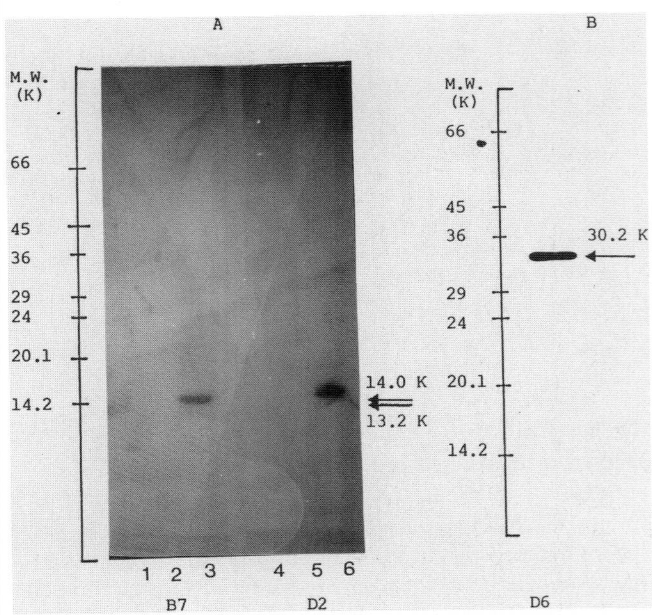

Fig. 1. A, Western blots of MAbs B7 and D2 against fetal calf serum (*Wells 1 and 4*); RK13 mock-infected cell preparation (*Wells 2 and 5*); and sucrose gradient-purified EAV (*Wells 3 and 6*). B, Western blot of MAb D6 against sucrose gradient-purified EAV. K = kilodalton.

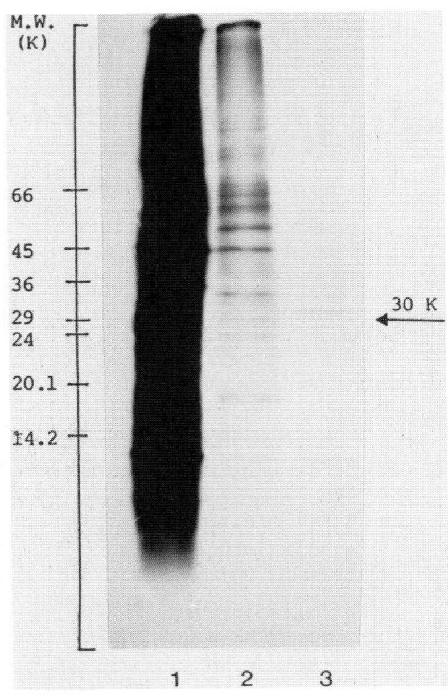

Fig. 2. Radioimmune precipitation of ^{35}S-methionine-labeled, sucrose gradient-purified EAV: *1*. ^{35}S-labeled virus; *2*. nonprecipitated proteins; *3*. D6 immunoprecipitate. K = kilodalton.

Properties of MAb to EAV. The ELISA titers of the four MAbs producing maximal O.D. 492nm on indirect ELISA ranged from 1:20 to 1:2560 in purified ascites (mean titers of at least two different ascites preparations). None of the MAbs neutralized EAV in VN tests.

In Western blotting experiments, two viral polypeptides were recognized, having molecular weights of 13.2-14 kdal (D2, B7) and 30.2 kdal (D6) (Fig. 1). MAb F5 was not further investigated because of its very poor ELISA titer. In the case of MAbs B7 and D6, the same protein was recognized in immunoprecipitation experiments as in Western blots (Fig. 2).

MAb B7 fluoresced on EAV-infected RK13 cell sheets 12 hr postinoculation (Fig. 3). No fluorescence was detected on mock-infected cell sheets used as controls or with MAbs D6, D2, or F5. Fluorescence with B7 was detectable in infected cells 12-36 hr postinoculation, after which the cytopathic effect completely destroyed the cell sheet.

Affinity purification of EAV. Highly purified EAV antigen is a requirement for diagnostic techniques based on antigen/antibody binding assays, such as ELISA or radioimmunoassay.

In affinity chromatography of whole sucrose gradient-purified ^{35}S-methionine-labeled virus on Sepharose 4B-linked MAb D6, a peak of radiolabeled protein was eluted from the column with 3 M NaSCN (Fig. 4). Indirect ELISA of collected fractions with D6 showed a coincident peak of viral protein eluted. Fluorographs of these fractions separated on a 10-30% gradient polyacrylamide gel resulted in enhanced recovery of labeled polypeptides with molecular weights of 59, 42, 30, 16, and 14 kdal in fractions corresponding to the D6 ELISA peak (Fig. 5).

When a 2-ml D6 Sepharose 4B column was scaled up to 20 ml, a peak of viral protein was eluted by 3M NaSCN and detected by ELISA with MAbs D6, B7, and a polyclonal rabbit antiserum raised to EAV.

Immune response to affinity-purified viral proteins. Affinity-purified fractions from the ELISA peak were pooled and a rabbit given a course of two weekly subcutaneous injections of 1 ml distributed over five separate sites. The rabbit's immune response to injection was monitored by a virus neutralization test and by indirect ELISA to EAV (Fig. 6). Throughout the course of immunization, an EAV-specific response was indicated, with little cross-reaction in ELISA to tissue culture contaminants presented as a mock-infected cell extract. In Western blots to sucrose gradient-purified virus (Fig. 7), the rabbit serum (R21) specifically recognized polypeptides of the molecular weights 14, 16, 21, 30, 39, and 73 kdal in sucrose gradient-purified virus. However, this antiserum failed to neutralize EAV in microtiter VN tests.

DISCUSSION

This report describes the production of four MAbs specifically targeted to EAV. The MAbs recognized two distinct viral proteins, one of 13.2-14 kdal, corresponding to the EAV nucleocapsid protein C (Van Berlo et al. 1986; Hyllseth 1973) and another of 30 kdal, possibly the p30 polypeptide

Fig. 3. Immunofluorescence of MAb B7: EAV-infected RK13 cells (*left*); noninfected control (*right*).

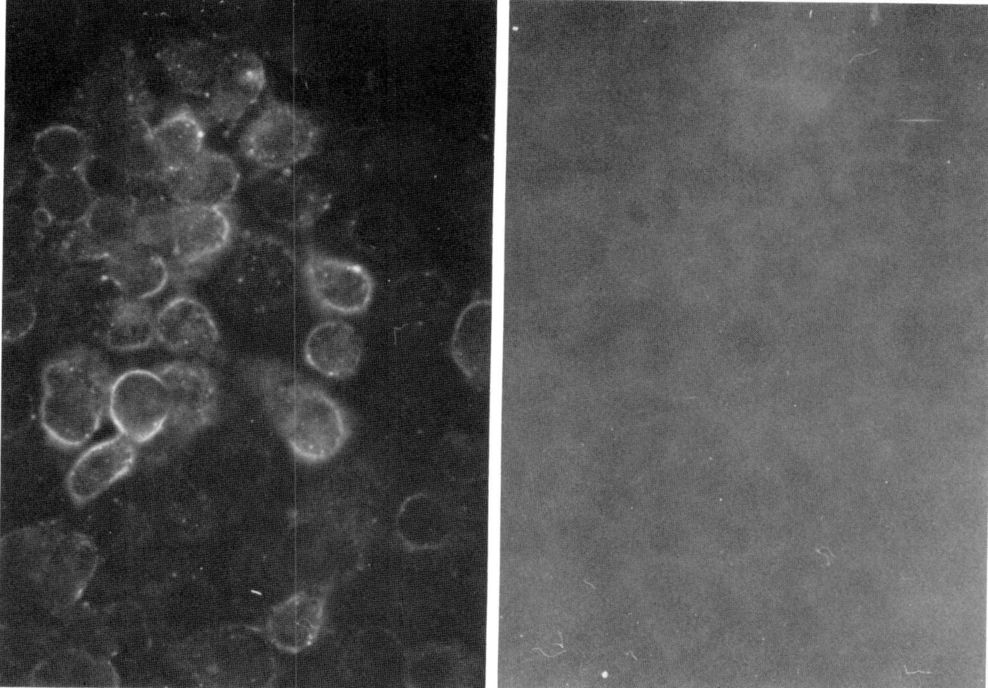

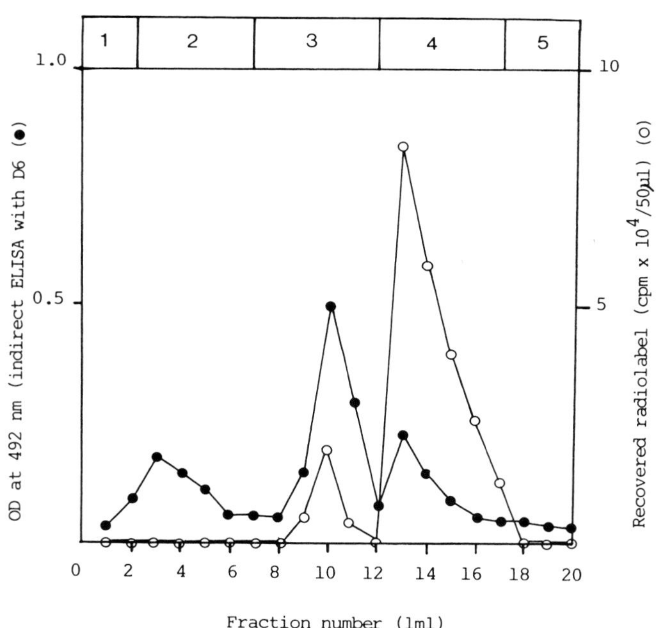

Fig. 4. Elution of ^{35}S-methionine-labeled EAV from D6-sepharose 4B. Labeled sucrose gradient-purified EAV (20 µl) was loaded onto a 2–ml column (*1*), left overnight at 4°C and eluted with PBS (*2*), followed by 3 M NaSCN (*3*), 0.1M acetate buffer pH 4 (*4*), and PBS (*5*). Eluate was collected in l-ml fractions and subjected to indirect ELISA with MAb D6 (*solid circles*) and counted for ^{35}S label (*open circles*).

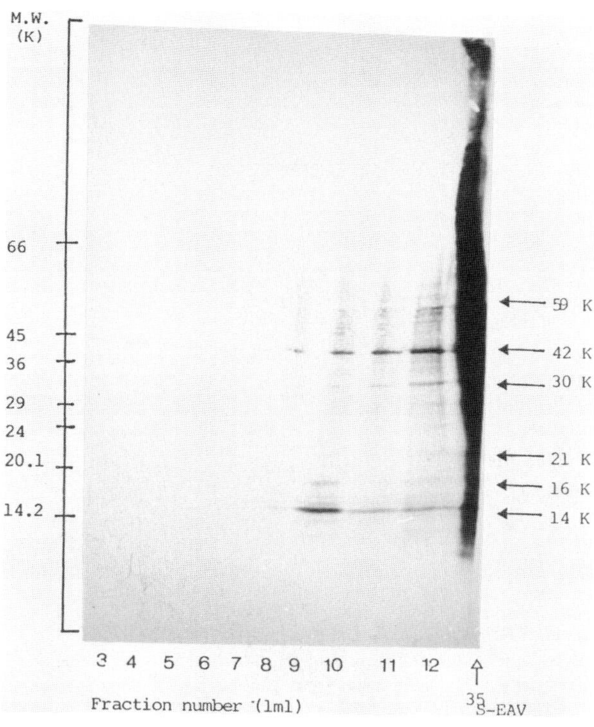

Fig. 5. Fluorograph of collected fractions from a D6 sepharose 4B affinity column; *Nos. 8-12* corresponding to D6 ELISA peak. (fraction numbers correspond to those in *Fig. 4*). K = kilodalton.

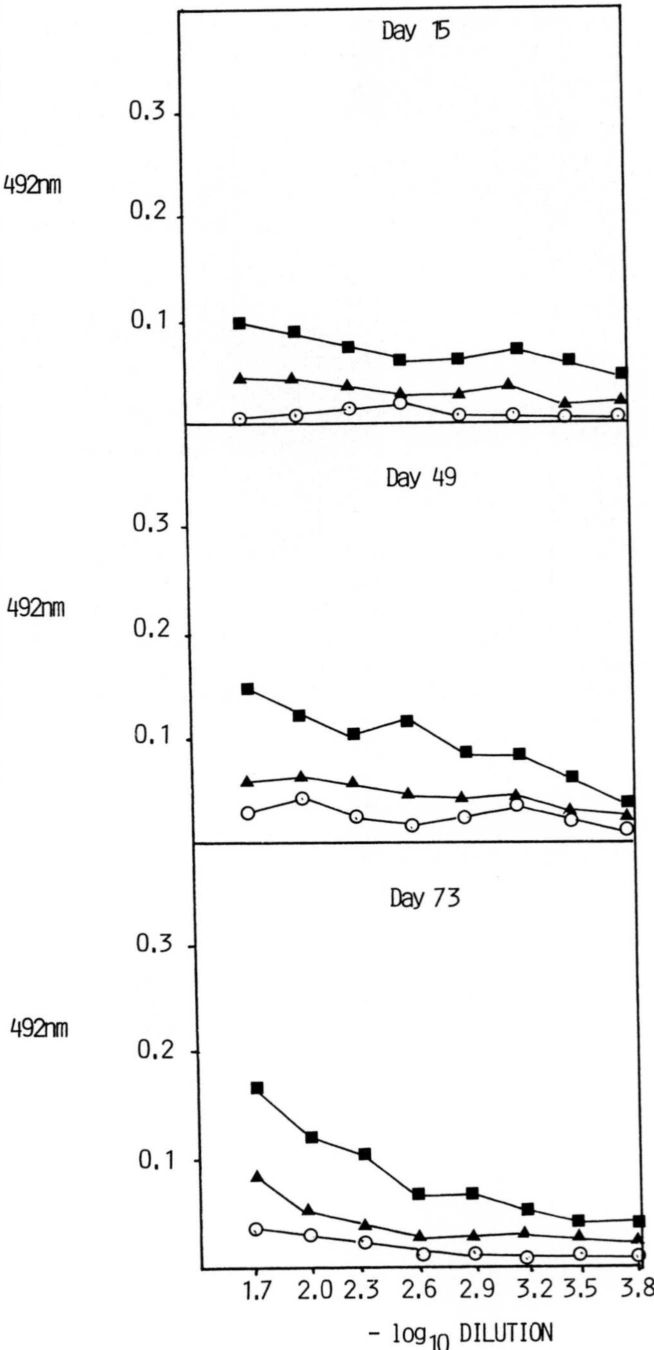

Fig. 6. Effect of sequential immunizations with affinity-purified EAV: *squares*, test bleed sera in indirect ELISA to sucrose gradient-purified EAV (1:400); *triangles*, EAV-infected RK13 supernatant (1:10); *circles*, mock-infected RK13 cell prep (1:10). Rabbit antiserum was amplified with a goat antirabbit horseradish peroxidase conjugate (Dakopatts).

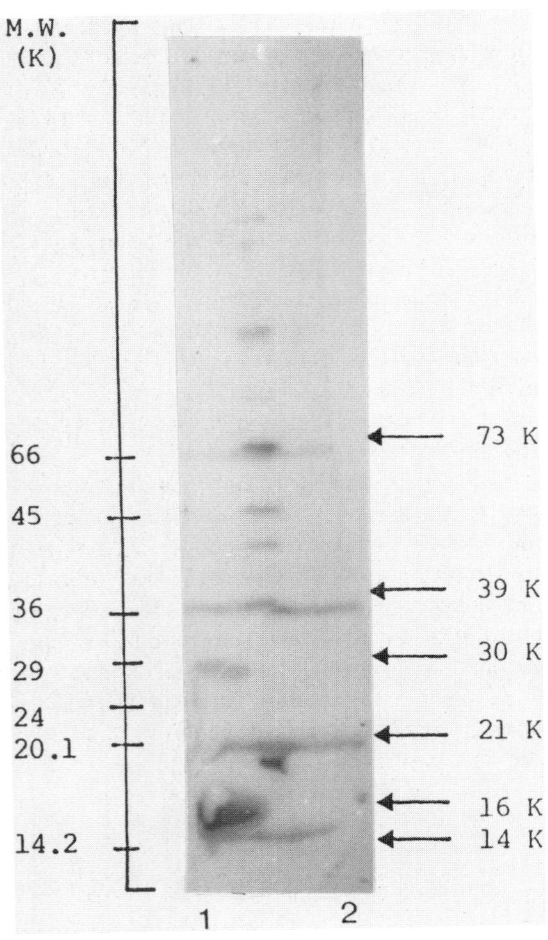

Fig. 7. Western blot of rabbit 21 serum against: *1*. sucrose gradient-purified EAV; *2*. EAV-infected RK13 supernatant. K = kilodalton.

previously reported in in vitro RNA translation studies of genomic RNA (Van Berlo et al. 1986).

MAb D6 is specific in both Western blotting and immunoprecipitation for a 30-kdal viral protein. When bound to Sepharose 4B as affinity ligand, D6 provided a receptor that enhanced the purification from sucrose gradient preparations of proteins of 59, 42, 30, 16, and 14 kdal, all which have previously been reported as virus-specific (Van Berlo et al. 1986; Zeegers, Van der Zeijst & Horzinek 1976; Hyllseth 1973). These properties suggest that the 30-kdal protein is an integral viral component. A 30-kdal protein has been reported as required in Togavirus replication in complex with other viral proteins (Westway 1980) and was found in both membrane and nuclear fractions of virus preparations. The recovery of a range of virus polypeptides in fractions produced by affinity chromatography showed that D6 binds whole virus, indicating the availability of the p30 protein at the virion surface. Virus polypeptide fractions produced by affinity chromatography induced a specific immune response to EAV in rabbits, providing antisera that recognized purified virus in indirect ELISA, and virus-specific polypeptides in immunoblotting experiments. The proteins recognized by this antiserum have molecular weights of 73, 39, 30, 21, 16, and 14 kdal, correlating with those reported during in vitro translation of genomic RNA (Van Berlo et al. 1986). The antiserum prepared against affinity-purified viral proteins did not neutralize EAV in VN tests, possibly due to the destruction of a neutralization epitope on a major protein during column elution with 3M NaSCN.

MAb B7 fluorescense on infected cells by its recognition of the 14-kdal viral nucleocapsid protein provides a rapid and efficient means of detecting virus in infected tissue samples. B7 may also serve as a ligand for affinity chromatography in purifying the nucleocapsid protein for use as an antigen in an EAV ELISA.

An EAV-specific ELISA would serve as a more rapid diagnostic tool than the EAV VN test, which although specific for infected and vaccinated horses can take as long as five days to complete. An ELISA using MAbs raised to EAV could be designed to detect antibody titer accurately and possibly to discriminate between seropositives resulting from infection and those resulting from a live attenuated vaccine, based on differential recognition of the altered epitope. With a large enough panel of MAbs, detection of strain variation could be built into such a test system.

ACKNOWLEDGMENTS

The authors would like to thank the European Breeders Fund and the New York Jockey Club for their support of this work.

REFERENCES

Bonner, W.M., and Laskey, R.A. (1974) A film detection method for tritium-labelled proteins and nucleic acids in polyacrylamide gels. *Eur. J. Biochem.* **46,** 83-88.

Burnett, W.M. (1981) "Western blotting": electrophoretic transfer of proteins from sodium dodecyl sulphate-polyacrylamide gels to unmodified nitrocellulose and radiographic detection with antibody and radioiodinated protein A. *Analyt. Biochem.* **112,** 195-203.

Campbell, A.M. (1984) Monoclonal Antibody Technology. *Laboratory Techniques in Biochemistry and Molecular Biology,* Vol. 13. Eds. R.H. Burdon and P.H. Knippenberg. Elsevier, Amsterdam.

Doll, E.R.; Bryans, J.T.; McCollum, W.H.; Crowe, M.E.W. (1957). Isolation of a filterable agent causing arteritis of horses and abortion by mares. Its differentiation from the equine abortion (influenza) virus. *Cornell Vet.* **47,** 3-41.

Hyllseth, B. (1973) Structural proteins of equine arteritis virus. *Arch. Ges. Virusforsch.* **40,** 177-88.

Jones, P.P. (1980) Analysis of radiolabelled lymphocyte proteins by one- and two-dimensional polyacrylamide gel electrophoresis. In *Selected Methods in Immunology,* pp. 398-440. Eds. B.B. Mishell and S.M. Shiigi. W.H. Freeman, New York.

Moraillon, A., and Moraillon, R. (1978) Results of an epidemiological investigation on (equine) viral arteritis in France and some other European and African countries. *Ann. Rech. Vet.* **9,** 43-54.

Senne, D.A.; Pearson, J.E.; and Carbrey, E.A. (1985) Equine viral arteritis: a standard procedure for the virus neutralisation test and comparison of results of a proficiency test performed at five laboratories. *Proc. U.S. Anim. Hlth Assoc.,* pp. 29-34.

Timoney, P.J. (1985) Epidemiological features of the 1984 outbreak of equine viral arteritis in the thoroughbred population in Kentucky, USA. *Proc. Soc. Vet. Epidemiol. Prev. Med.,* pp. 84-89.

Timoney, P.J.; McCollum, W.H.; Roberts, A.W.; and Murphy, T.W. (1986) Demonstration of the carrier state in naturally acquired equine arteritis virus infection in the stallion. *Res. Vet. Sci.* **41,** 279-80.

Van Berlo, M.F.; Rottier, P.J.M.; Spaan, W.J.M.; and Horzinek, M.C. (1986) Equine arteritis virus-induced polypeptide synthesis. *J. Gen. Virol.* **67,** 1543-49.

Westaway, E.G. (1980) Replication of flaviviruses. In *The Togaviruses,* pp. 531-81. Ed. R.W. Schlesinger. Academic Press, London.

Zeegers, J.J.W.; Van der Zeijst, B.A.M.; and Horzinek, M.C. (1976) The structural proteins of equine arteritis virus. *Virology* **73,** 200-5.

The Relationship of Air Hygiene in Stables to Lower Airway Disease during an Outbreak of Equid Herpesvirus-1 Infection

A.F. Clarke, T.M. Madelin, and R.G. Allpress

SUMMARY

This study assessed the relationship between air hygiene and the incidence of lower airway disease in two types of identically managed stabling for horses. The construction of the first type ensured good ventilation, while the other type was heavily insulated, with inadequate ventilation. The wood shavings in the poorly ventilated boxes were heavily contaminated with fungus, and there were greater amounts of mucopus in the tracheas of the horses stabled there than in the well-ventilated boxes. The amounts of tracheal mocupus rose in both yards during an outbreak of equid herpesvirus-1 (EHV-1) infection, but the increase was less in the "clean" environment.

The study highlights the importance of air hygiene for the respiratory well-being of horses, and the potential role of environmental factors in infectious respiratory disease.

INTRODUCTION

Lower respiratory tract disease has been identified as a cause of poor performance in Thoroughbred horses (Burrell 1985; Burrell et al. 1985). Some episodes of the disease in horses have been associated with seroconversion to known viruses, including EHV-1, and environmental factors have also been implicated in the etiology (Clarke 1987a; Clarke, Madelin & Allpress 1987). Interactions between the host's environment and the outcome of episodes of herpesviruses have been reported in farm animals (Wiseman et al. 1978), but no such reports regarding horses are known to us.

Lower respiratory tract disease, frequently covert, can be diagnosed using a fiber-optic endoscope to grade the mucopus present in the horse's trachea. In this study, clinical endoscopic examinations of Thoroughbred horses housed in two different types of structures were compared over a two-year period, 1985-86. In the first year there was an outbreak of EHV-1 respiratory disease. The results of the endoscopic examinations were compared statistically to detect possible associations between lower airway disease, EHV-1 infection, and the difference in environment.

Clarke, Madelin: Department of Animal Husbandry, University of Bristol, Langford House, Langford, Bristol BS18 7DU, England. Allpress: Tortington Centre, Arundel, West Sussex BN18 OBG, England.

MATERIALS AND METHODS

This study was carried out in two yards under the management of the same trainer, with accomodation for 140 horses at Yard A and 65 at Yard B. Horses were housed mainly in individual boxes at both yards. However, one barn at Yard B could house 16 horses as a group. The boxes in Yard A were designed for efficient ventilation in all weather conditions, whereas those in Yard B were poorly ventilated and heavily insulated. All horses were bedded on wood shavings and vaccinated at three-month intervals with Pneumobort K (Fort Dodge Labs, Fort Dodge, Iowa). Boxes were mucked out daily, with deep litter being avoided.

Airborne particle counts were monitored using a Rion KC01A particle counter (Hawksley, Lancing, Sussex). Readings were taken before mucking out the boxes and immediately after, when particle release from beddings into stable air was at a maximum (Clarke 1987a).

The ventilation of buildings was assessed by releasing smoke pellets (Smoke Products Ltd., Eldwick, England) into a building and measuring the clearance of the smoke from the building using the Rion particle counter. Ventilation rates (in air changes per hour) were calculated from first order kinetic theory, which assumes log linear decline of the tracer with time.

An Andersen sampler (Andersen 1958; Gelman Sciences Ltd., Northampton, England) was used to deposit airborne particles onto petri dishes containing media selective for fungi and actinomycetes (Table 1). Samples were collected immediately after mucking out. The sampling time was 10 seconds, and plates were incubated for up to 10 days prior to examination.

A Burkard single-stage impactor air sampler (Equigiene; Wrington, Avon, England) was used to collect dust samples on microscope slides, which were examined and graded using light microscopy, according to the method described by Clarke and Madelin (1987):

Grade I. Negligible quantities of mold spores present, the principal dust constituents being plant hairs, pollen grains, and other vegetable and miscellaneous fragments.

Grade II. Mold spores present, primarily of large-spored, "fair weather air" types, such as Alternaria and Cladosporium; small numbers of the respirable species may be present; much plant material.

Table 1. Media for sampling mycoflora

Fungal medium	Actinomycete medium
Malt extract, 20.0 g	Oxoid nutrient agar, 14.0 g
Agar, 20.0 g	Casein hydrolysate, 2.0 g
Distilled H_2O, 1 liter	Agar, 10.0 g
[a]Penicillin, 20 units ml^{-1}	Distilled H_2O, 1 liter
[a]Streptomycin, 40 units ml^{-1}	[c]Actidione, 50 μg ml^{-1}
[b]Triton N101, 0.05%	

Note: Incubation temperatures = 25°C, 38°C, and 55°C. (After Madelin 1987.)

[a] Suppress bacteria.

[b] Alkylphenolpolyetheleneglycol prevents overgrowth of plate by rapidly spreading species of fungi (Fleuka Ag; Fluorochem Ltd., Glossop, England).

[c] Actidione (cyclohexinide) 50 μg ml^{-1} inhibits fungi.

Table 2. Airborne particle counts (per ml air) and ventilation rates

	Yard A		Yard B	
	Box 1	Box 2	Box	Barn
Quiet	5.4	9	7.3	13.6
Busy	11.8	16.2	104	610
Mixed activity	2.2	1.8	14.3	45
Ventilation rates[a]	19	17	5	7
Outside weather conditions	Windy	Windy	Windy	Windy

[a] Air changes per hour.

Table 3. Species of actinomycetes and fungi cultured

	Yard A	Yard B[a]
Actinomycetes, 38°C	Streptomyces[b]	*Saccharomonspora viridis* Streptomyces
Actinomycetes, 55°C	—	*Micropolyspora faeni* *S. viridis* *Thermoactinomyces vulgaris*
Fungi, 25°C	*Alternaria alternata* *Aspergillus candidus* *Botrytis cinera* *Cladosporium herbarum* *Mucor racemosus* *Penicillium chrysogenum* *P. citrinum*	*Paecilomyces variotti* *Rhizomucor pusillus* *Mucor racemosus*
Fungi, 38°C	*Paecilomyces variotti*[c]	*Paecilomyces variotti* *Rhizomucor pusillus*

[a] Heavily overloaded with >400 colonies on each plate.

[b] 15 colonies.

[c] 7 colonies.

Grade III. Dust consists primarily of large numbers of respirable spores (2-5 μm fungal spores and 1 μm actinomycete spores); may include evidence of heavy dust mite infestation.

Air hygiene analyses using the particle counter, the Andersen sampler, and the impactor sampler were carried out in two boxes at each yard. The particle counter and the Andersen sampler were positioned on a 76-cm-high table in the center of each box during testing. The single-stage impactor was used to collect samples from six other boxes at each yard and from fresh wood shavings.

A 1,330-mm-long 11.3-mm-wide Olympus PCF pediatric colonscope was used for the endoscopic examinations. The presence and the amount of mucoid exudate on the floor of the trachea was graded from 0 to 3 as described by Burrell (1985): 0 = minimal exudate, 1 = isolated globules, 2 = a thin continuous stream less than 15 mm wide, and 3 = a thick continuous stream more than 15 mm wide. Horses were regularly examined by the same veterinarian as part of a clinical monitoring program. During 1985, 693 examinations were performed on 179 horses at Yard A and 110 on 47 horses at Yard B. Between January and June 1986, 279 examinations were performed on 163 horses at Yard A and 48 on 38 horses at Yard B.

Contingency tables were established to compare tracheal mucopus gradings of the horses in both environments for the two years. Chi-squared tests of independence were used for the analysis of data. Significant levels were set at 0.05.

RESULTS

From the beginning of the 1985 racing season, horses at Yards A and B "failed to thrive" and some performed below expectations. The problems culminated in May, when several horses were "disappointing" on the racecourse. Regular monitoring of temperatures revealed increasing numbers of horses to be suffering from pyrexia. There was little external evidence of respiratory disease, as few horses coughed, although some had clear serous nasal discharges and enlarged submandibular lymph nodes. During June the cantering and fast work of all horses was canceled for two weeks.

Three or more serum samples were collected from 38 horses during 1985. Thirteen of the 38 demonstrated a fourfold or greater change in serum neutralizing antibody to EHV-1 subtype 2. There was no such outbreak during the 1986 season. Between January and September 1986, only two of 39 horses from which three or more serum samples were collected revealed changes as high as fourfold in serum neutralizing antibody titer levels to EHV-1 subtype 2.

Mucking out of boxes in Yard A was associated with a doubling of airborne particles 0.5 to 5.0 μm in size (Table 2). In sharp contrast there was a 14-fold increase in the box examined at Yard B and a 45-fold increase in the 16-horse barn.

Mesophilic fungal species were the primary constituents of the airborne spores at Yard A (Table 3). Several species of

Table 4. Comparison of tracheal mucopus gradings during 1985 racing season

Mucopus grading[a]	Yard A	Yard B
0	266	33
1	282	40
2	126	32
3	19	5

[a] Grade 0 = minimal exudate; 1 = isolated globules; 2 = thin continuous stream <15 mm wide; 3 = thick continuous stream >15 mm wide.

Table 5. Comparison of tracheal mucopus gradings between January 1 and June 30, 1986

Mucopus grading[a]	Yard A	Yard B
0	153	15
1	92	13
2	28	13
3	6	7

[a] Grade 0 = minimal exudate; 1 = isolated globules; 2 = thin continuous stream <15 mm wide; 3 = thick continuous stream >15 mm wide.

thermotolerant and thermophilic fungi and actinomycetes were cultured from air samples at Yard B.

Microscopic examination of dust samples collected at Yard A revealed small numbers of respirable spores, and all samples were categorized as Grade II. All dust samples collected from boxes at Yard B were Grade III, with large numbers of respirable fungal and actinomycete spores being present. The samples collected from fresh wood shavings stored at both yards were categorized as Grade I.

In comparing the mucopus gradings of horses in both yards during 1985 and 1986 (Tables 4 and 5), significantly more ($P < 0.05$) tracheal mucopus was found at Yard B than at Yard A. At Yard A, more high gradings ($P < 0.001$) were recorded in the 1985 season than the 1986 season. A similar comparison for Yard B showed no statistically significant difference between the two years.

DISCUSSION

Respiratory disease associated with EHV-1 infection is a well-recognized problem for Thoroughbred horses in training (Allen & Bryans 1986). Since episodes of the disease are often clinically silent, they may go unnoticed while horses are at rest. However, in the galloping horse, which has a respiratory rate in excess of 150 breaths per minute and tidal volume of approximately 12 liters (Hornicke, Meixner & Pollman 1983), even small changes in the potency of the airways can have a marked effect on the mechanics of respiration. The relatively minor forms of disease in early life may be precursors of chronic respiratory disease later (Viel 1985; Clarke 1987a).

In the present study, both EHV-1 infection and environmental factors were identified as having etiological roles in lower respiratory tract disease. A synergistic relationship between EHV-1, the environmental factors described, and lower respiratory disease can be inferred from the results of this study. However, the design of the study precludes the establishment of absolute causal relationships.

Horses housed in the insulated, poorly ventilated housing at Yard B were exposed to greater challenges of respirable dust than those at Yard A. The increased numbers of airborne particles at Yard B were associated with the proliferation of mold species that produce large numbers of respirable spores. The species of molds cultured from Yard A are typical of those found in fresh wood chips, while the airborne spores of Yard B are consistent with the degradation of wood chips (Hoover-Litty & Hanlin 1985; Thornqvist & Lundstrom 1982; Jorgensen & Fjellheim 1982; Pellikka & Kotimaa 1983). Well-managed wood shavings appear to be relatively resistant to fungal contamination (Clarke 1987b). However, contamination similar to that in Yard B has been observed where deep litter management is practiced (Clarke 1987a). A number of factors, including humidity, temperature, and the length of time between changes of bedding, are likely to affect the molding of plant-based bedding materials. After improvements in the ventilation of the boxes at Yard B, the air hygiene improved.

Of the species cultured only *Micropolyspora faeni* has been definitely implicated in small airway disease of horses, although other fungi and actinomycetes are also suspected. Horses with chronic obstructive pulmonary disease failed to develop symptoms on exposure to *M. faeni* or *Aspergillus fumigatus* but did develop signs of the disease when exposed to the dust from moldy hay and straw (McPherson et al. 1979). All of the mold species isolated have been implicated as causative agents of allergic respiratory disease in man, and may be a pathogen in other diseases of both horses and humans.

The difference in tracheal mucopus measured in the two environments concurs with the results of a three-day examination of 78 two-year-old Thoroughbreds at the same two yards (Clarke et al. 1987). Lower respiratory tract disease has been reported to be significantly longer in duration among horses bedded on straw than those bedded on shredded newspaper (Burrell 1986). The threshold limiting value of respirable dust to which a horse may be safely exposed is likely to vary from horse to horse and within a single animal, depending on individual susceptibilities and extenuating factors, including infectious disease. Because the exposure to even minor levels of respirable dust may cause some degree of irritation, the horse's exposure to dust should be minimized.

Gerber (1973) reported an increased risk of chronic obstructive pulmonary disease among horses following respiratory infections. Burrell (1985) observed seroconversions to respiratory viruses in episodes of lower respiratory tract inflammation. The present study implicates EHV-1 in the etiology of lower respiratory tract disease, with the amount of tracheal mucopus rising during an episode of EHV-1 infection. Environmental factors also played a role, since horses housed in the contaminated environment had more mucopus in their tracheas than occurred in the clean environment.

There are several means by which an infectious disease may initiate lower airway disease and decrease the horse's tolerance for respirable dust. For example, EHV-1 respiratory infections adversely affect the mucociliary escalator, damage epithelial surfaces, and alter the immune responses to antigenic challenges (Bryans 1981a; Allen & Bryans 1986).

The immune competence of the horse is the primary limiting factor for the development of respiratory disease following exposure to highly infectious agents such as EHV-1. Unfortunately, the immunity to respiratory tract infection with EHV-1 conferred by currently available vaccines is not particularly long-lasting or effective (Allen & Bryans 1986). Until a more effective vaccine is developed, attention to the horse's environment can minimize the duration and severity of episodes of respiratory disease that can cause the equine athlete to lose training days. A clean environment can also reduce the incidence of more debilitating conditions such as chronic obstructive pulmonary disease.

There has been a tendency to consider infectious disease as a two-way interaction limited to the parasite and the immune status of the host. The results of the present field study indicate the role of environmental factors should be considered in future studies of the pathogenesis, treatment, and prevention of infectious respiratory disease. In some instances, environmental factors may be responsible for episodes of the virus.

ACKNOWLEDGMENTS

The generosity of the Home of Rest for Horses in providing a research grant is gratefully acknowledged. Serological examinations were carried out at the Animal Health Trust, Newmarket. This study would not have been possible without the cooperation and assistance of Mr. John Dunlop and his staff.

REFERENCES

Allen, G.P., and Bryans, J.T. (1986) Molecular epizootiology, pathogenesis and prophylaxis of Equine Herpes Virus-1 infection. *Prog. Vet. Microbiol. Immunol.* **2,** 78-144.

Andersen, A.A. (1958) New sampler for the collection, sizing and enumeration of viable airborne particles. *J. Bacteriol.* **76,** 471.

Bryans, J.T. (1981a) Application of management procedures and prophylactic immunisation to control of equine rhinopneumonitis. *Proc. 26th Am. Assoc. Equine Practnr.*, pp. 259-72.

———. (1981b) Control of equine influenza. *Proc. 26th Am. Assoc. Equine Practnr.*, pp. 279-87.

Burrell, M.H. (1985) Endoscopic and virological observations on respiratory disease in a group of young thoroughbred horses in training. *Equine Vet. J.* **17,** 99-103.

———. (1986) Aetiological aspects of respiratory disease. *Annual Report of Animal Health Trust,* pp. 54-57.

Burrell, M.H.; Mackintosh, M.E.; Mumford, J.A.; and Rossdale, P.D. (1985) A two-year study of respiratory disease in a Newmarket stable: Some preliminary observations. *Proc. Soc. for Vet. Epidemiol. and Prev. Med.*, pp. 74-83.

Clarke, A.F. (1987a) Chronic pulmonary disease—a multifaceted disease complex in the horse. *Irish Vet. J.* **41,** 258-64.

———. (1987b) Stable environment in relation to the control of respiratory disease. In *Horse Management,* 2d ed., pp. 125-74, Ed. J. Hickman. Academic Press, London.

Clarke, A.F., and Madelin, T.M. (1987) Technique for assessing respiratory health hazards from hay and other source materials. *Equine Vet. J.* **19,** 442-47.

Clarke, A.F.; Madelin, T.M.; and Allpress, R.G. (1987) The relationship of air hygiene in stables to lower airway disease and pharyngeal lymphoid hyperplasia in two groups of Thoroughbred horses. *Equine Vet. J.* **19,** 524-30.

Gerber, H. (1973) Chronic pulmonary disease in the horse. *Equine Vet. J.* **5,** 26-33.

Hoover-Litty, H., and Hanlin, R.T. (1985) The mycoflora of wood chips to be used as mulch. *Mycologia* **77,** 721-31.

Hornicke, H.; Meixner, R. and Pollmann, U. (1983) Respiration in exercising horses. *Proc. 1st Int. Conf. Equine Exercise Physiol.*, pp. 7-16.

Jorgensen, H. and Fjellheim, B. (1982) Allergic alveolitis due to exposure to fungal spores from fuel chips. A variant of "Farmer's Lung." *Tidsskrift for den Norske Laeget orening* **102,** 737-39.

Madelin, T.M. (1987) The effect of a surfactant in media for the enumeration, growth and identification of airborne fungi. *J. Appl. Bact.* **63,** 47-52.

McPherson, E.A.; Lawson, G.H.K.; Murphy, J.R.; Nicholson, J.M.; Breeze, R.G.; and Pirie, H.M. (1979) Chronic obstructive pulmonary disease (COPD) in horses: Aetiological studies: Responses to intradermal and inhalation antigenic challenge. *Equine Vet. J.* **11,** 159-66.

Pellikka, M., and Kotimaa, M. (1983) The mould dust concentration caused by the handling of fuel chips and its modifying factor. *Folia Forestalia* No. **563.**

Thornqvist, T., and Lundstrom, H. (1982) Health hazards caused by fungi in stored wood chips. *Forest Products J.* **32,** 29-32.

Viel, L. (1985) Diagnostic procedures, prognosis and therapeutic approaches of chronic respiratory diseases in horses. *Can. Vet. J.* **26,** 33-35.

Wiseman, A.; Msolla, P.M.; Selman, I.E.; Allan, E.M.; Cornwell, H.J.C.; Pirie, H.M.; and Imray, W.S. (1978) An acute severe outbreak of infectious bovine rhinotracheitis: Clinical, epidemiological, microbiological and pathological aspects. *Vet. Rec.* **103,** 391-97.

Association between Predisposition to Equine Sarcoid and MHC in Multiple-Case Families

Heinz Gerber, Marie-Louise Dubath, and Sandor Lazary

SUMMARY

The distribution of equine leucocyte antigens (ELAs) in sarcoid-affected Swiss warmblood horses ($N = 102$) was determined and compared with that in unaffected controls ($N = 361$). The ELA first-locus alleles A5 and W20 were represented at higher frequencies in the affected group ($P < 0.005$ and < 0.05, respectively). Of the second-locus ELAs, W13 showed a strong association with susceptibility to sarcoid disease ($P < 0.0005$).

Further studies on multiple sarcoid cases in equine families showed that predisposition is associated with certain haplotypes within families. However, the disease–associated ELA haplotype can contain various equine leucocyte antigens (A3, A5, and W20, with or without W13), varying from family to family.

This study provides further evidence that the equine major histocompatibility complex (MHC) plays a role in the pathogenesis of sarcoid in horses.

INTRODUCTION

Associations between the MHC and diseases have been clearly demonstrated in mice (Lilly 1967), chickens (Briles, Stone & Cole 1977), and humans (Tiwari & Terasaki 1985).

In recent years, two series of allelic, serologically detectable ELAs have been recognized as gene products of the equine MHC (Lazary et al. 1986; Bernoco et al. 1987). The study by Lazary and colleagues (1985) of the ELA distribution in sarcoid-affected unrelated animals demonstrated that in Swiss-, French-, and Irish-bred warmblooded horses, susceptibility to sarcoid is associated with certain ELAs. The study by Meredith and colleagues (1986) of the ELA system and predisposition to sarcoid in Thoroughbreds resulted in a similar finding: a strong relationship between equine MHC and susceptibility to sarcoid. We report here the frequency distributions of the allelic ELA markers in healthy and sarcoid-diseased Swiss warmblood horses. The first part of the experiment compared healthy and diseased animals, while the second part analyzed the typing results in multiple-sarcoid-case families.

Klinik für Nutztiere und Pferde (Gerber, Dubath) and Division of Immunogenetics (Lazary), Institute for Animal Husbandry, University of Berne, Switzerland.

MATERIALS AND METHODS

Horses. The multiple-sarcoid-case families studied were all Swiss-bred horses, of three breeds: Swiss Warmbloods ($N = 102$), Thoroughbreds ($N = 5$), and Shagya Arabs ($N = 3$), including the 55 Swiss Warmbloods from our previous report (Lazary et al. 1985). The Swiss warmblood is a hunter-type light horse close to the French *Selle français*, but some families also carry Swedish and German blood. English Thoroughbred is used to some extent to improve the breed.

The affected group included approximately equal numbers of females and males, ranging in age from two to 18 years. The samples from the affected horses and the controls were collected at our clinic and private equine practices. The horses were selected on the basis of the clinical appearance of tumors and the biopsy findings.

Clinically diagnosed sarcoids were confirmed histologically only when the tumors were operated upon conventionally. Later on, the animals in the diseased populations were examined for family relationships. When such relationships were found, the horses were selectively included in the investigation of family groups. Samples of venous blood were drawn into heparinized tubes at the authors' clinic and in private practices.

Serology. ELA typing was performed using the two-stage complement-dependent microlymphocytotoxicity test (Terasaki & McClelland 1964). Before isolation of cells, a pinch of iron powder was added to the 10-ml heparinized blood samples, and the tubes were incubated at 37°C for 30 min to remove phagocytic cells. The mononuclear cells were then isolated by the Ficoll/Ronpacon technique (sp.g 1.077; Böyum 1968) from anticoagulated (50 i.u. heparin/ml) blood, taken one or two days before testing. Pooled serum from young rabbits, frozen in small portions at −70°C, was the source of complement.

The antisera for the detection of ELAs were prepared locally (Lazary et al. 1980) and tested in four international comparison workshops (Bernoco et al. 1987). The serum clusters recognize the following internationally accepted ELA specificities: A1-A10 and W14-W20 class I antigens, belonging to the first locus, and W12 and W13 (earlier B2 and B1). The W12 and W13 antigens belong to the second locus of the equine MHC and probably represent class II antigens (Lazary et al. 1986).

Table 1. Distribution of equine leucocyte antigens in Swiss warmblood horses, with and without sarcoids

ELA	Gene frequencies Sarcoid (N = 102)	Controls (N = 361)	Relative risk (RR)	Etiological fraction	X^2 test	Significance (P)
Locus 1						
A1	0.01	0.04				
A2	0.07	0.14	0.4	−0.18	7.54	0.006
A3	0.20	0.16				
A4	0.00	0.01				
A5	0.21	0.12	2.1	0.19	9.54	0.002
A6	0.01	0.03				
A7	0.00	0.00				
A8	0.01	0.01				
A9	0.02	0.01				
A10	0.05	0.05				
W14	0.00	0.00				
W15	0.09	0.11				
W16	0.03	0.03				
W18	0.05	0.06				
W19	0.03	0.04				
W20	0.09	0.05	1.9	0.08	4.26	0.04
Be22	0.00	0.01				
Be25	0.00	0.00				
Be26	0.02	0.01				
"Blanks"	0.11	0.12				
Locus 2						
W12	0.01	0.03				
W13	0.25	0.13	2.3	0.24	12.82	0.0003

Typing criteria. In the population study, the typing results on all Swiss warmbloods were computed according to Svejgaard, Platz, and Ryder (1983) for each ELA specificity. The frequencies of the representatives of the two allelic ELA series were calculated separately. The following formulas were used:

$$\text{Phenotype frequency for antigen (P)} = \frac{na}{N}$$

$$\text{Gene frequency for antigen} = 1 - \sqrt{1 - P}$$

$$\text{Relative risk } (RR) = \frac{a \times d}{b \times c}$$

$$\text{Etiological fraction } (EF) = \frac{RR - 1}{RR} \cdot \frac{a}{a + b}$$

$$X^2 \text{ test} = \frac{N(ad - bc)^2}{(a+b)\,(c+d)\,(a+c)\,(b+d)}$$

where a = antigen carrier, affected; b = antigen absent, affected; c = antigen carrier, unaffected; d = antigen absent, unaffected; na = number of antigen carriers; N = total number of population examined; RR = risk of developing the disease in an antigen carrier, expressed in multiples of the risk in horses lacking the antigens; EF = the degree of a disease that is due to the disease-associated factor. Significance *(P)* is reported without correction for the number of comparisons.

In multiple-case families, at least three members (parent(s), full- and/or half-siblings) were affected by sarcoid. In most cases the "families" consisted of half-siblings. In these cases, only the two ELA alleles (or haplotypes) of the common parent were analyzed for an association with disease susceptibility. Since the antigens A5, W20, and W13 occurred with increased frequencies in affected animals, suggesting contribution to the pathogenesis of the disease, offspring that inherited any one of these antigens (haplotypes) from a nonshared parent were excluded from the statistical analysis as noninformative. Apparent homozygotes—those horses for which the nonshared parent could not be typed—were included in our calculations.

The X^2 test was carried out separately on affected and healthy informative offspring on the basis of the number of observed/expected haplotypes transmitted. Offspring from families with common ELAs were combined for calculation. In the chi-square analysis performed for the control population, the distribution of ELA phenotypes demonstrated a good fit to Hardy-Weinberg expectation: $P>0.4$.

RESULTS

In the Swiss warmblood horse population, sarcoid-affected animals ($N = 102$) displayed statistically significant differences in the distribution of the first-locus ELA antigens A2 ($P>0.01$), A5 ($P>0.01$), and W20 ($P>0.05$), as well as in the second-locus gene product ELA W13 ($P>0.001$),

Table 2. Distribution of transmitted ELA haplotypes in informative offspring, tested for distortion of haplotype segregation

Parents	Parental haplotypes No. 1	Parental haplotypes No. 2	Ratio, sarcoid: healthy offspring	No. of sarcoid offspring with parental haplotype: No. 1	No. 2		No. of healthy offspring with parental haplotype: No. 1	No. 2	
Stallion 1	A3+W13	A2	3:6	3	0		4	2	
Stallion 2	A3+W13	A3+W12	2:16	2	0		8	8	
Stallion 3	A5+W13	W15	4:3	4	0		1	2	
Stallion 6	A5+W13	W15	4:16	3	1		4	12	
Total (Group 1)			13:41	12	1	$P<0.02$	17	24	n.s.
Stallion 4	A5	W19	11:14	9	2		8	6	
Mare 1	A5	A6	2:3	2	0		1	2	
Stallion 7 (Thoroughbred family)	A5	A2	4:4	3	1		2	2	
Stallion 8	A5	A2	3:4	3	0		2	2	
Total (Group 2)			20:25	17	3	$P<0.02$	13	12	n.s.
Stallion 5	W20	W16	5:8	4	1		5	3	
Mare 2 (Shagya Arab)	W20	A1	2:2	2	0		0	2	
Total (Group 3)			7:10	6	1	$P<0.2$	5	5	n.s.

Note: n.s. = not significant.

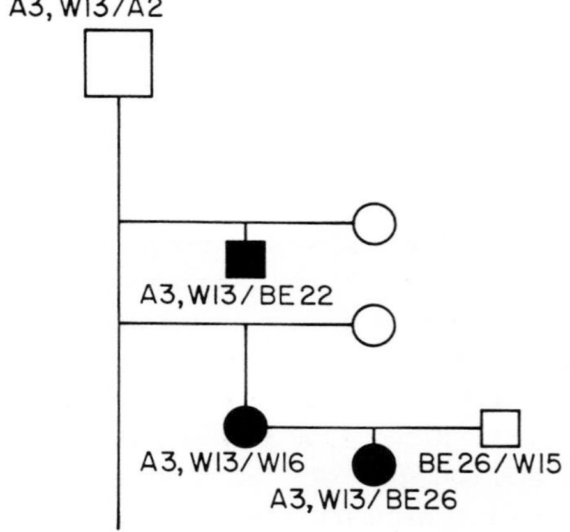

Fig. 1. Typing results of affected offspring of stallion No. 1: *circle*, female; *square*, male; *black symbol*, sarcoid-diseased.

compared with the distribution in the controls ($N=361$) (Table 1). While A5, W20, and W13 antigens showed association with susceptibility to sarcoid, the A2 antigen occurred with lesser frequency in this group. The W13 gene product occurred frequently in combination with A3, A5, or W15 first-locus antigens as a haplotype in both groups of animals. On the other hand, in no case did the W20 antigen form a haplotype with W13. In the following families, the segregtion of the associated antigens (haplotypes) was demonstrated.

Offspring of Stallion No. 1. This stallion transmitted the ELA-haplotypes A3 + W13 or A2 to his offspring. Three sarcoid-affected offspring were found, two of them being half-siblings that shared the informative paternal haplotype A3 + W13 (Fig. 1). One of them transmitted this haplotype to a daughter, together with the susceptibility to sarcoid disease.

Six other offspring of stallion No. 1, which were unaffected by sarcoid disease, inherited in four cases the haplotype A3 + W13 and in two cases the haplotype A2 (Table 2).

Offspring of stallion No. 2. Sire No. 2 was homozygous for the ELA first-locus antigen A3, but heterozygous for the second-locus antigens W13 and W12. His sarcoid-affected offspring, two half-siblings and two full siblings, shared the paternal haplotype A3 + W13 (Fig. 2). However, the inheritance of A3 + W13 haplotype can be accepted as informative only in the half-siblings. The inheritance of the maternal haplotype with W20 antigen in the full siblings prevents them from being informative.

Stallion 2 transmitted the A3 + W13 and the A2 + W12 haplotypes to non-sarcoid affected offspring in eight out of eight cases (Table 2).

Offspring of stallion No. 3. Sire No. 3 possessed the A5 + W13 and W15 haplotypes, and his sarcoid-affected offspring shared the paternal haplotype A5 + W13 (Fig. 3). The inheritance of the haplotype was informative in all four cases.

Non-sarcoid affected offspring of this stallion inherited W15 in one case and the A5 + W13 haplotype in two cases (Table 2).

Offspring of stallion No. 4. Stallion No. 4 transmitted either the haplotype A5 or W19 to his offspring. Of the 16 descen-

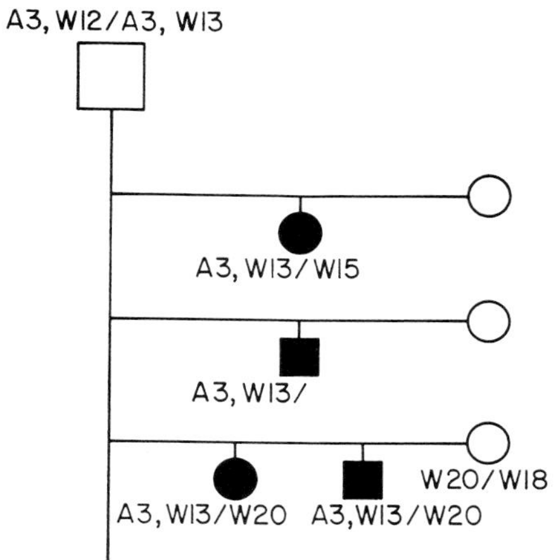

Fig. 2. Typing results of affected offspring of stallion No. 2: *circle*, female; *square*, male; *black symbol*, sarcoid-diseased.

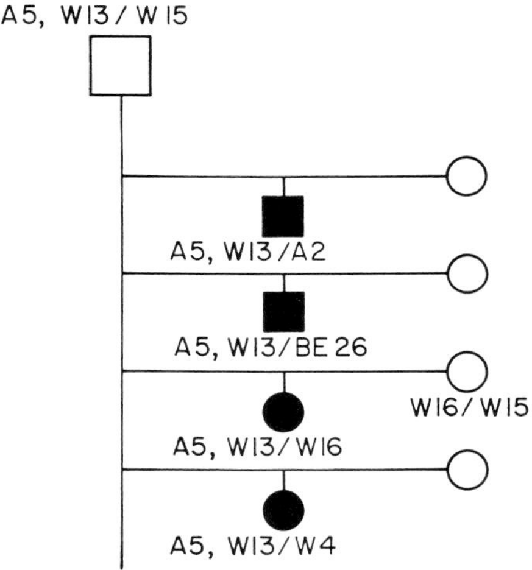

Fig. 3. Typing results of affected offspring of stallion No. 3: *circle*, female; *square*, male; *black symbol*, sarcoid-diseased.

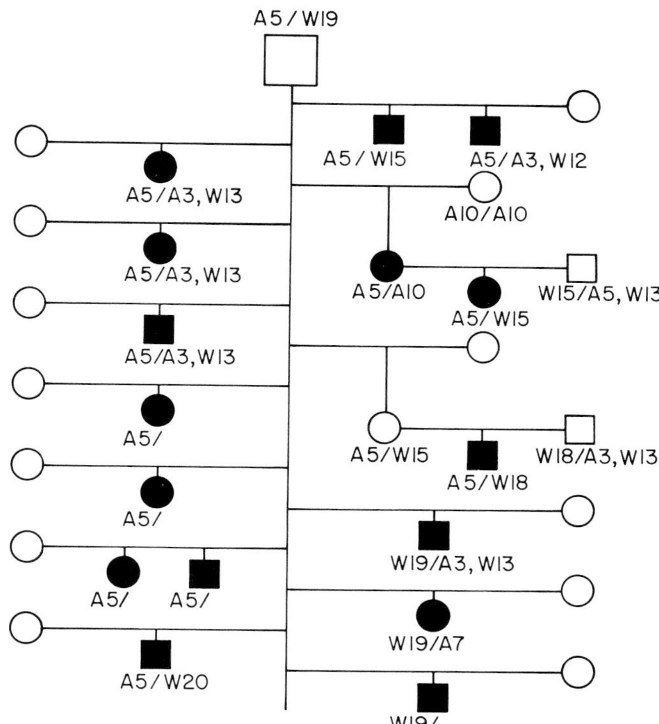

Fig. 4. Typing results of affected offspring of stallion No. 4: *circle*, female; *square*, male; *black symbol*, sarcoid-diseased.

dants affected by sarcoid that we tested, 13 inherited the paternal haplotype A5, and the other three W19 (Fig. 4). The transmission of the A5 haplotype to the grandchildren was also followed.

One of the daughters of sire No. 4 was not affected by sarcoid but nevertheless transmitted haplotype A5 to a son, together with the disposition to sarcoid disease. Informative inheritance of the paternal haplotype A5 together with the susceptibility trait was shown in nine cases. The disposition to disease in the two offspring displaying haplotypes W19/A7 and W19, respectively, cannot be explained by the inherited haplotypes.

The distribution of the two paternal haplotypes A5 and W19 in healthy offspring was 8 to 6 (Table 2).

Offspring of mare No. 1. Dam No. 1 was carrier of the haplotypes A5 and A6. All three of her sarcoid-affected progeny inherited the maternal haplotype A5. In one of her affected sons, the paternal haplotype showed a recombination within the MHC; the stallion with the Be26/A3, W13 haplotypes in all cases ($N = 12$) transmitted the haplotype B26 without the second-locus antigen W13 to his offspring. On the other hand, the stallion transmitted A3 together with W13 to his offspring in nine cases. The sarcoid-free son with the maternal haplotype A5 is three years old. The other two healthy half-siblings carrying the A6 maternal haplotype are the oldest descendants of mare No. 1.

Offspring of stallion No. 5. Stallion No. 5 was heterozygous for the ELA haplotypes W20 and W16. We typed six sarcoid-affected offspring, of which four inherited, informatively, the W20 haplotype. In one case (W16/A9), susceptibility to sarcoid could not be explained by the inherited ELA haplotypes. In nondiseased offspring ($N = 8$), inheritance of haplotypes W20 and W16 was in the ratio of 5:3.

Other animals. Besides the animals cited in Figures 1-6, three other stallions (Nos. 6, 7, and 8), one mare (No. 2), and their affected offspring met the criteria for statistical analysis. The ELA typing results of these ancestors and the distribution of their haplotypes in the informative affected offspring are summarized in Table 2. In the first group were offspring from ancestors carrying the second-locus ELA W13 in different

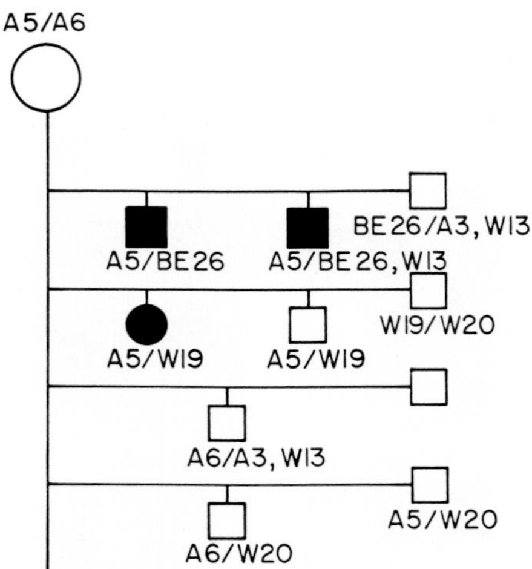

Fig. 5. Typing results of affected offspring of mare No. 1: *circle,* female; *square,* male; *black symbol,* sarcoid-diseased.

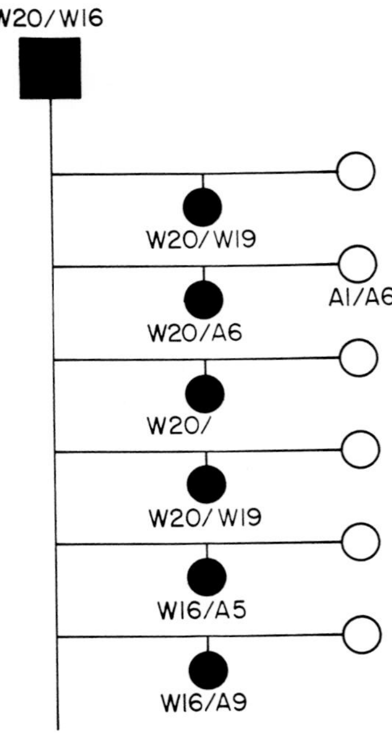

Fig. 6: Typing results of affected offspring of stallion No. 5: *circle,* female; *square,* male; *black symbol,* sarcoid-diseased.

combinations with first-locus ELA antigens (A3 or A5). The informative sarcoid-affected offspring showed a distorted inheritance in favor of the W13-containing haplotypes in the ratio of 12:1. This was significantly different (P>0.02) from the expected distribution (6.5:6.5).

In the second group, the affected informative offspring of horses carrying ELA A5 antigen without W13 in one haplotype inherited this haplotype in a distorted ratio of 17:3, compared with the expected 10:10. This distortion was also statistically significant (P>0.02).

In the third group, the sarcoid-affected offspring of W20-carrying ancestors, a distorted inheritance was observed in favor of the W20 (ratio 6:1). The results in this group were not significant, due to the small number of animals.

In none of the groups did the sarcoid-free offspring of the same ancestors show any significant differences from expected frequencies in haplotype distribution.

DISCUSSION

The association of certain ELAs with susceptibility to sarcoid in Swiss warmblood horses has been confirmed, as shown in Table 1. The first published report (Lazary et al. 1985), as well as the paper presented here, shows a positive association with more than one antigen. Of primary importance is the finding that the increased frequency of ELA W13 antigen in different combinations with first-locus alleles in the affected group is highly significant. Meredith and colleagues (1986) reported the same findings when studying the distribution of ELA antigens in sarcoid-affected Thoroughbreds. As many Swiss warmblood pedigrees show Thoroughbred crosses in earlier generations, W13 may have been introduced and maintained in the Swiss population by the Thoroughbreds. W13 is rarely seen in Arabs, nor is it frequent in the Swiss draft horse (Freiberger). Sarcoids, however, occur in association with other antigens.

The role of ELA W13 in the affected population is expressed by the high etiological fraction (0.24). On the other hand, a high proportion of affected animals carried the first-locus antigens A5 or W20 combined with unknown second-locus gene product(s) in the haplotype (in cases where W13 was absent). This finding suggests that the ELA W13 is not the exclusive determinant in the pathogenesis of sarcoid. The main question raised by the data from the population study is, how do the ELA antigens segregate in diseased family members?

The segregation data from the single families strongly suggest that a certain parental ELA as a haplotype, in combination with known or unknown genes, is associated with the disease. This observation may mean that the detected ELA has only a marker function for the haplotype and that the disease is due to a susceptibility gene(s) in linkage disequilibrium with the particular ELA alleles. The other possibility is that the ELA in question is itself involved in the pathogenesis of sarcoid.

It remains to be seen whether a specific, as yet unrecognized, MHC gene or separate susceptibility gene(s) are involved in the pathogenesis of equine sarcoid.

ACKNOWLEDGMENTS

This work was supported by the Swiss National Fund for Scientific Research, grant No. 3.982-1.84.

REFERENCES

Bernoco, D.; Antczak, D.F.; Bailey, E.; Bell, K.; Bull, R.W.; Byrns, G.; Guerin, G.; Lazary, S.; McClure, J.; Templeton, F.; and Varewyck, H. (1987) Joint report of the Fourth International Workshop on lymphocyte alloantigens of the horse. *Anim. Genet.* **18,** 81-94.

Böyum, A. (1968) Isolation of leukocytes from human blood. Further observations. Methylcellulose, dextran and ficoll as erythrocyte-aggregating agents. *Scand. J. Clin. Lab. Invest.* **21** (Suppl. 97), 77-85.

Briles, W.E.; Stone, H.A.; and Cole, R.K. (1977) Marek's disease effects of B histocompatibility of alloalleles in resistant and susceptible chicken lines. *Science* **195,** 193-95.

Lazary, S.; De Weck, A.L.; Bullen, S.; Straub, R.; and Gerber, H. (1980) Equine leucocyte antigen system I. Serological studies. *Transplantation* **30,** 203-9.

Lazary, S.; Gerber, H.; Glatt, P.A.; and Straub, R. (1985) Equine Leucocyte Antigens (ELA) in Sarcoid-Affected Horses. *Equine Vet. J.* **17,** 283-86.

Lazary, S.; Dubath, M.-L.; Luder, C.; and Gerber, H. (1986) Equine leucocyte antigen system IV. Recombination within the major histocompatibility complex (MHC). *J. Immunogenet.* **13,** 315-25.

Lilly, F. (1967) Susceptibility to two strains of friend leukemia virus in mice. *Science* **155,** 461-62.

Meredith, D.; Elser, A.H.; Wolf, B.; Soma, L.R.; Donawick, W.J.; and Lazary, S. (1986) Equine leucocyte antigens: relationships with sarcoid tumors and laminitis in two pure breeds. *Immunogenet.* **23,** 221-25.

Svejgaard, A.; Platz, P.; and Ryder, L.P. (1983) HLA and disease 1982. A Survey. *Immunol. Rev.* **70,** 193-218.

Terasaki, P.I., and McClelland, J.D. (1964) Microdroplet assay of human serum cytotoxins. *Nature* **204,** 998-1000.

Tiwari, J.L., and Terasaki, P.I. (1985) *HLA and Disease Associations.* Springer-Verlag, New York.

Participants

Conference Chairman

David G. Powell
Department of Veterinary Science
College of Agriculture
University of Kentucky

Scientific Review Committee

John T. Bryans
George P. Allen
William H. McCollum
David G. Powell
Peter J. Timoney

AUSTRALIA

Graham D. Bailey
Dept. of Veterinary Pathology
University of Sydney
New South Wales 2006

Peter John Huntington
Dept. of Agriculture & Rural Affairs
Attwood Veterinary Research Lab
Michleham Road, Westmeadows
Victoria 3047

Paul B. Kavenagh
29 Scott Street
Camperdown
Victoria 3260

Jean Margaret Sabine
Dept. of Veterinary Pathology
University of Sydney
New South Wales 2006

Michael J. Studdert
Dept. of Veterinary Paraclinical Sciences
University of Melbourne
Parkville, Victoria 3052

James Millar Whalley
School of Biological Sciences
Macquarie University
Sydney, New South Wales 2109

BRAZIL

Orencio Maximo de Carvalho, Jr.
Instituto Biologico
Av. Conselheiro Rodrigues Alves
#1252, Vila Mariana
P.O. Box 7119
Sao Paulo 01051

CANADA

Victor Bermudez
Ontario Veterinary College
University of Guelph
Department of Pathology
Guelph, Ontario N1G 2W1

Laurent Viel
University of Guelph
Clinical Studies
Guelph, Ontario N1G 2W1

Russ Willoughby
Equine Research Center
University of Guelph
Guelph, Ontario NIG 2W1

ENGLAND

Ewan D. Chirnside
Equine Virology Unit
Animal Health Trust
Lanwades Park
Newmarket, Suffolk CB8 7PN

Yen-Chung Chong
University of Cambridge
School of Clinical Veterinary Medicine
Madingley Road
Cambridge, CB3 OES

Andrew Clarke
Dept. of Animal Husbandry
Langford House
Langford, Bristol BS18 7DU

R. Frank Cook
Equine Virology Unit
Animal Health Trust
Lanwades Park
Newmarket, Suffolk CB8 7PN

Rodney Stuart Daniels
National Institute for
Biological Standards & Control
Virology Division
Blanche Lane, South Mimms
Potters Bar, Hertfordshire EN6 3QG

Neil Edington
Dept. of Microbiology & Parasitology
Royal Veterinary College
University of London
Royal College Street
London NW1 0TU

Ian William Halliburton
University of Leeds
Department of Microbiology
Leeds LS2
West Yorkshire, LS2 95T

Duncan Hannant
Equine Virology Unit
Animal Health Trust
Lanwades Park
Newmarket, Suffolk CB8 7PN

Andrew James Higgins
Animal Health Trust
P.O. Box 5
Newmarket, Suffolk CB8 7DW

R. A. Killington
Dept. of Microbiology (Virology)
The University of Leeds
Leeds
West Yorkshire LS2 9JT

Margaret H. Lucas
Central Veterinary Laboratory
New Haw
Weybridge
Surrey KT15 3NB

Mary E. Mackintosh
Bacteriology Unit
Animal Health Trust
Lanwades Park, Kennett
Newmarket, Suffolk CB8 7PN

Timothy Stephen Mair
University of Bristol
Langford House
Department of Veterinary Medicine
Langford, Nr. Bristol BS18 7DU

Claire Myfanwy Morris
University of Cambridge
Dept. of Clinical Veterinary Medicine
Madingley Road
Cambridge CB3 OES

J. A. Mumford
Equine Virology Unit
Animal Health Trust
Lanwades Park
Newmarket, Suffolk CB8 7PN

Walter Plowright
Equine Virology Research Foundation
Whitehill Lodge, Reading Road
Goring-on-Thames
Reading RG8 OLL

E. J. Lawson Soulsby
University of Cambridge
Dept. of Clinical Veterinary Medicine
Madingley Road
Cambridge CB3 OES

Katherine E. Whitwell
Animal Health Trust
P.O. Box 5
Snailwell Road, Balaton Lodge
Newmarket, Suffolk CB8 7DW

John M. Wood
National Institute for
Biological Standards & Control
Virology Division
Blanche Lane, South Mimms
Potters Bar, Hertfordshire EN6 3QG

FRANCE

Andre Brun
Rhone Merieux Laboratoire Iffa
254 rue Marcel Merieux, B.P. 7009
Lyon Cedex 07
Lyon 69342

Claire Collobert
Institut de Pathologie due Cheval
Goustranville Dozule F-14430

Aime Jacquet
Federation Nationale Des
Societes de Courses de France
11 Rue du Cirque
Paris 75008

Eric Plateau
Lab Cent Recherches Veterinaire
Ministere de l'Agriculture
22 rue Pierre Curie
Maisons-Alfort
Cedex Paris B. P. 67 94703

Edouard Pouret
Aunou-le-Faucon
Argentan 61200

HOLLAND

G. A. Berghuis
Gist-Brocades Animal Health
Wateringseweg 1, P.O. Box 1
2600 Ma Delft

K. J. Breukink
Gist-Brocades Animal Health
Wateringseweg 1, P.O. Box 1
2600 Ma Delft

J. W. Greve
Gist-Brocades Animal Health
Wateringseweg 1, P.O. Box 1
2600 Ma Delft

M. E. Keij
Gist-Brocades Animal Health
Wateringseweg 1, P.O. Box 1
2600 Ma Delft

G. Meursing
Gist-Brocades Animal Health
Wateringseweg 1, P.O. Box 1
2600 Ma Delft

B. Prinsen
Gist-Brocades Animal Health
Wateringseweg 1, P.O. Box 1
2600 Ma Delft

H.M.B.J. Schiffeles
Gist-Brocades Animal Health
Wateringseweg 1, P.O. Box 1
2600 Ma Delft

J.G.W. Schror
Gist-Brocades Animal Health
Wateringseweg 1, P.O. Box 1
2600 Ma Delft

W. Vaal
Gist-Brocades Animal Health
Wateringseweg 1, P.O. Box 1
2600 Ma Delft

Jan Vaarten
Duphar B. V.
C. J. Van Houtenlaan 36
Weesp 1380 AA

G. Van Bokhorst
Gist-Brocades Animal Health
Wateringseweg 1, P.O. Box 1
2600 Ma Delft

J. Th. M. Van Schie
Gist-Brocades Animal Health
Wateringseweg 1, P.O. Box 1
2600 Ma Delft

A. A. Van Unen
Gist-Brocades Animal Health
Wateringseweg 1, P.O. Box 1
2600 Ma Delft

J.H.J. Vestjens
Gist-Brocades Animal Health
Wateringseweg 1, P.O. Box 1
2600 Ma Delft

R.J. Vink
Gist-Brocades Animal Health
Wateringseweg 1, P.O. Box 1
2600 Ma Delft

IRELAND

Ann Cullinane
Irish Equine Centre
Johnstown
Naas Co. Kildare

Ursula Fogarty
Irish Equine Centre
Johnstown
Naas Co. Kildare

Frank J. Hughes
Gist-Brocades (Ireland) Ltd.
Ballyboggan Road
Finglas
Dublin 11

James Charles Kelly
Sallins Road
Naas Co. Kildare

J. J. O'Brien
Veterinary Research Laboratories
Stoney Road
Stormont, Belfast BT4 3SD

Patrick Joseph O'Connor
Dept. of Agriculture and Food
Agriculture House
Kildare Street
Dublin 2

Kenneth L. Strickland
Veterinary Research Laboratory
Abbotstown
Castleknock
Dublin 15

ITALY

Mauro Quercioli
c/o Allevamento di Besnate.
C. Na Risaia-Besnate-Varese

Associazione Nazionale Allevatori
Cavalli Purosangue
20144 Milano-Via del Caravaggio 3

JAPAN

Masanobu Kamada
Epizootic Research Station
Japan Racing Association
Shiba 1400-4, Kokubunji-Machi
Shimotsuga-Gun Tochigi 329-04

Takumi Kanemaru
Epizootic Research Station
Japan Racing Association
Shiba 1400-4, Kokubunji-Machi
Shimotsuga-Gun Tochigi 329-04

Gihei Sato
Dept. of Veterinary Public Health
Obihoro University of Agriculture
& Veterinary Medicine
Obihiro Hokkaido 080

Hiroshi Sentsui
National Institute of Animal Health
Kannondai 3-1-1
Yatabe-Machi
Tsukuba-Gun Ibaraki 305

Chihiro Sugimoto
National Institute of Animal Health
Kannondai 3-1-1
Yatabe-Machi
Tsukuba-Gun Ibaraki 305

Takeo Sugiura
Epizootic Research Station
Japan Racing Association
Shiba 1400-4, Kokubunji-Machi
Shimotsuga-Gun Tochigi 329-04

NORWAY

Olav Gladhaug
Norwegian College of Veterinary
Medicine
Dept. of Microbiology & Immunology
P.O. Box 8146, Dep 0033
Oslo 1

Bjorn Hyllseth
Norwegian College of Veterinary
Medicine
Dept. of Microbiology & Immunology
P.O. Box 8146, DEP 0033
Oslo 1

REPUBLIC OF SOUTH AFRICA

Baltus J. Erasmus
Veterinary Res. Inst.
P. O. Box 12610
Onderstepoort 0110

SCOTLAND

Lesley Nicolson
Dept. of Veterinary Pathology
University of Glasgow
Bearsden Road
Glasgow G61 1QH

Marcello P. Riggio
Dept. of Veterinary Pathology
University of Glasgow Veterinary School
Garscube Estate, Bearsden Road
Bearsden, Glasgow G61 1QH

SWEDEN

Peter Forssberg
Oesta
S-755 90
Uppsala

Berndt W. Klingeborn
Department of Virology
The National Veterinary Institute
Biomedicum, Box 585
S-751 23
Uppsala

Clars Rulcher
Kistav 14
Sollentuna S-191 70

SWITZERLAND

Heinz Gerber
Klinik fur Nutztiere und Pferde
Universitat Bern
Bremgartenstrasse 109A
Bern

Marianne Weiss
Institute of Veterinary Bacteriology
Veterinary Faculty
University of Berne
Langgass-Str. 122, P.O.B. 2735
Berne CH-3001

UNITED STATES OF AMERICA

William M. Acree
Fort Dodge Laboratories
800 5th St., N.W.
Fort Dodge, IA 50501

Karen Affleck
Department of Veterinary Science
108 Gluck Equine Research Center
University of Kentucky
Lexington, KY 40546-0099

George P. Allen
Department of Veterinary Science
108 Gluck Equine Research Center
University of Kentucky
Lexington, KY 40546-0099

Ernest Bailey
Department of Veterinary Science
108 Gluck Equine Research Center
University of Kentucky
Lexington, KY 40546-0099

Henrique Balboza
c/o BET Farms
Jacks Creek Pike
Lexington, KY 40515

LaVerne Ballard
Special Programs
204 Frazee Hall
University of Kentucky
Lexington, KY 40506-0031

David R. Barnes
9175 Station Road
Erie, PA 16510

Jill Beech
University of Pennsylvania
School of Veterinary Medicine
382 W. Street Rd., New Bolton Ctr.
Kennett Square, PA 19348

William Bernard
Veterinary Medicine
University of Pennsylvania
382 West Street Road, New Bolton Ctr.
Kennett Square, PA 19348-1692

Harlan G. Bigbee
Scherine Corporation
1011 Morris Avenue
Union, NJ 07083

Tex Boggs
University Extension
114 Frazee Hall
University of Kentucky
Lexington, KY 40506-0031

Christopher M. Brown
Michigan State University
Dept. of Large Animal Clinical Science
Veterinary Clinical Center
East Lansing, MI 48824-1314

Karen K. Brown
Mobay Corporation
Animal Health Division
9009 West 67th Street
Merriam, KS 66202

J. T. Bryans
Department of Veterinary Science
108 Gluck Equine Research Center
University of Kentucky
Lexington, KY 40546-0099

Elizabeth C. Burgess
School of Veterinary Medicine
University of Wisconsin
2015 Linden Drive West
Madison, WI 53706

Nicolas Carrillo
Nicolas Carrillo Correa, Inc.
Box 836
Hato Rey, PR 00919

Leroy Coggins
Pathology & Parasitology
School of Veterinary Medicine
North Carolina State University
4799 Hillsborough Street
Raleigh, NC 27606

Linda Coogle
Department of Veterinary Science
108 Gluck Equine Research Center
University of Kentucky
Lexington, KY 40546-0099

Gillian Ann Comyu
Equine Veterinary Services
Justin Morrill Highway
South Stratford, VT 05070

H. Steve Conboy
P.O. Box 11889
Castleton Farm
Lexington, KY 40578

Margaret E. Conner
Dept. of Virology & Epidemiology
Baylor College of Medicine
1 Baylor Plaza
Houston, TX 77030

Bill Cooney
Rhone Merieux Inc.
117 Rowe Road
Athens, GA 30601

Barbara Cordell
California Biotechnology, Inc.
2450 Bayshore Parkway
Mountain View, CA 94043

Carol M. Cottrill
Pediatrics
University of Kentucky Medical Center
Room MN 472
Lexington, KY 40536-0091

Judy H. Cox
Dept. of Surgery & Medicine
College of Veterinary Medicine
Kansas State University
Manhattan, KS 66506

Susan Ann Crane
University of Pennsylvania
Veterinary School
382 West Street Road, New Bolton Ctr.
Kennett Square, PA 19348

M. Ward Crowe
Department of Veterinary Science
108 Gluck Equine Research Center
University of Kentucky
Lexington, KY 40546-0099

Timothy A. Cudd
Rood & Riddle Equine Hospital
P.O. Box 12070
Lexington, KY 40580

Beverly Dale
California BioTechnology, Inc.
2450 Bayshore Parkway
Mountain View, CA 94043

Benjamin J. Darien
Dept. of Large Animal Clinical Services
Michigan State University
East Lansing, MI 48824-1314

Jane Davis
261 Large Animal Clinic
College of Veterinary Medicine
University of Illinois
1102 West Hazelwood Drive
Urbana, IL 61801

Ronald L. Dawe
Apex Veterinary Hospital, P.A.
Route 4, Box 342-D
Apex, NC 27502

Jacqueline E. Dawson
2803 VMBSB, Veterinary Medicine
University of Illinois
2001 S. Lincoln Avenue
Urbana, IL 61801

R. H. Douglas
BET Farms
Jacks Creek Pike
Lexington, KY 40515

James E. Dowd
5833 Bullard Road
Fenton, MI 48430

Bernard Drissen
Equine Services
P.O. Box 464
Simpsonville, KY 40067

Edward J. Dubovi
Cornell University
New York State College of Veterinary Medicine
Diagnostic Laboratory
Ithaca, NY 14850

Wendy M. Duckett
North Carolina State Veterinary School
4700 Hillsborough Street
Raleigh, NC 27606

Douglas Durham
Centaur, Inc.
108A South Columbus Street
Alexandria, VA 22314

Roberta Dwyer
Department of Veterinary Science
108 Gluck Equine Research Center
University of Kentucky
Lexington, KY 40546-0099

Kenneth Jack Easley
Equine Services
P.O. Box 464
Simpsonville, KY 40067

Barry Fitzgerald
Department of Veterinary Science
108 Gluck Equine Research Center
University of Kentucky
Lexington, KY 40546-0099

Lane D. Foil
Dept. of Entomology
Louisiana State University
402 Life Sciences Building
Baton Rouge, LA 70803

Barbara D. Forney
Broodmare Association
Box 195A, Rd. 2
Cochranville, PA 19330

Jorge Enrique Galan
Department of Biology
Campus Box 1137
Washington University
St. Louis, MO 63130

E. Paul J. Gibbs
College of Veterinary Medicine
Box J-137, JHMHC
University of Florida
Gainesville, FL 32610

Ralph C. Giles
Livestock Disease Diagnostic Center
University of Kentucky
1429 Newtown Pike
Lexington, KY 40511

Michael A. Gill
Norden Laboratories
Box 80809
Lincoln, NB 68501

James H. Gillespie
Dept. of Microbiology,
Immunology & Parasitology
Schurman Hall
Cornell University
Ithaca, NY 14853

Chester Gipson
U.S. Department of Agriculture
6505 Bellecrest Road, Room 845
Hyattsville, MD 20782

John C. Gordon
Dept. of Veterinary Preventative Medicine
1900 Coffey Road
Ohio State University
Columbus, OH 43210-1092

Nina Hahn
College of Veterinary Medicine
Virginia Tech
Blacksburg, VA 24061

Donna A. Hall
204 Frazee Hall
University of Kentucky
Lexington, KY 40546

Elaine P. Hammel
University of Pennsylvania
382 West Street Rd., New Bolton Center
Kennett Square, PA 19348

Kim Herbert
The Blood Horse
1736 Alexandria Drive
Lexington, KY 40504

William P. Higgins
P.O. Box 351
Culpeper, VA 22701

Donald G. Hildebrand
Rhone Merieux Inc.
117 Rowe Road
Athens, GA 30601

Cynthia J. Holland
Dept. of Veterinary Pathobiology
University of Illinois
2001 S. Lincoln Avenue
Urbana, IL 61801

Dorothy F. Holmes
Dept. of Microbiology, Immunology
& Parasitology
Cornell University
Schurman Hall
Ithaca, NY 14853

Chuen B. Hong
Livestock Disease Diagnostic Center
University of Kentucky
1429 Newton Pike
Lexington, KY 40511

John P. Hughes
Dept. of Reproduction
School of Veterinary Medicine
University of California
Davis, CA 95616

Charles J. Issel
Dept. of Veterinary Science
Louisiana State University
Dalrymple Building
Baton Rouge, LA 70803

R. J. Jacob
Dept. of Microbiology & Immunology
University of Kentucky Medical Center
Lexington, KY 40536-0091

Donald C. Johnson
3537 Forest Avenue
Brookfield, IL 60513

Robert L. Jones
Colorado State University
Diagnostic Laboratory
Fort Collins, CO 80523

Yoshihiro Kawaoka
St. Jude Children's Hospital
P.O. Box 318
332 North Lauderdale
Memphis, TN 38101-0318

Charles H. Keiser
Animal Hospital of Danville
Route 4, Lebanon Road
Danville, KY 40422

Cathryn Kohn
Veterinary Clinical Sciences
Ohio State University
1935 Coffey Road
Columbus, OH 43210-1089

Lucinda M. Lamb
New York State College of Veterinary
Medicine
Schurman Hall
Cornell University
Ithaca, NY 14853

Donald H. Lein
Diagnostic Laboratory
NYSCVM
Cornell University
P.O. Box 786
Ithaca, NY 14851

Pierre Lessard
College of Veterinary Medicine
Virginia Tech
Blacksburg, VA 24061

Michel Levy
Dept. of Large Animal Clinics
Lynn Hall
Purdue University
West Lafayette, IN 47907

Irwin K. M. Liu
Dept. of Reproduction
School of Veterinary Medicine
University of California
Davis, CA 95616

Ted F. Lock
1102 W. Hazelwood Drive
261 Large Animal Clinic
Urbana, IL 61801

Richard A. Lyons, Jr.
Bratt Animal Hospital
2401 Crawford Street
Terre Haute, IN 47803

Brad MacKinnon
Agritech Systems, Inc.
100 Fore Street
Portland, ME 04101

Lawrence T. Maddren
12 North Pennington Road
New Brunswick, NJ 08901

John Madigan
School of Veterinary Medicine
University of California
Davis, CA 95616

Michael Joseph Mallay
Muhlenberg County Animal Clinic
815 North Second Street
Central City, KY 42330

W. H. McCollum
Department of Veterinary Science
108 Gluck Equine Research Center
University of Kentucky
Lexington, KY 40546-0099

Michael J. McDonald
2001 Old St. Augustine, E102
Tallahassee, FL 32304

Anne Micka
Department of Veterinary Science
108 Gluck Equine Research Center
University of Kentucky
Lexington, KY 40546-0099

Bobby O. Moore
Fort Dodge Laboratories
Fort Dodge, IA 50501

Jim P. Morehead
Rood & Riddle Equine Hospital
P.O. Box 12070
Lexington, KY 40580

Carl D. Morrison III
Stone Farm, Inc.
1873 Winchester Road
Paris, KY 40361

Todd W. Murphy
Department of Veterinary Science
108 Gluck Equine Research Center
University of Kentucky
Lexington, KY 40546-0099

Beth Myhre
Route 1, Box 92
Ronan, MT 59864

Suzanne Neu
Department of Veterinary Science
108 Gluck Equine Research Center
University of Kentucky
Lexington, KY 40546-0099

Louis E. Newman
Livestock Disease Diagnostic Center
University of Kentucky
1429 Newton Pike
Lexington, KY 40511

Sidney R. Nusbaum
Department of Agriculture
Division of Animal Health
201 Health & Agriculture Bldg.
Trenton, NJ 08625

Dennis J. O'Callaghan
Dept. of Microbiology & Immunology
Louisiana State University Medical Center
P.O. Box 33932
1501 Kings Highway
Shreveport, LA 71130-3932

Thomas P. S. Oliver
P.O. Box 454
Lahaska, PA 18931

Eileen Ostlund
Department of Veterinary Science
108 Gluck Equine Research Center
University of Kentucky
Lexington, KY 40546-0099

Elizabeth E. Pantzer
P.O. Box 13545
Lexington, KY 40583

David Parrish
Hagyard-Davidson-McGee Associates
848V Nandino Blvd.
Lexington, KY 40511

J. E. Pearson
P.O. Box 844
USDA, APHIS
National Veterinary Services Laboratories
Ames, IA 50010

Rachel A. Pemstein
Hagyard-Davidson-McGee Associates
848V Nandino Blvd.
Lexington, KY 40511

Arnold Guy Pessin
P.O. Box 23860
Lexington, KY 40523

K. B. Poonacha
Livestock Disease Diagnostic Center
University of Kentucky
1429 Newtown Pike
Lexington, KY 40511

David G. Powell
Department of Veterinary Science
108 Gluck Equine Research Center
University of Kentucky
Lexington, KY 40546-0099

Jeff L. Pumphrey
Hagyard-Davidson-McGee Associates
848V Nandino Blvd.
Lexington, KY 40511

Beverly J. Purswell
Virginia-Maryland Regional College
of Veterinary Medicine
Virginia Tech, Phase 11
Blacksburg, VA 24061

Charles Chandler Randall
Dept. of Microbiology
Univ. of Mississippi Medical Center
2500 North State Street
Jackson, MS 39216-4505

Yasuko Rikihisa
Dept. of Veterinary Pathobiology
Ohio State University
1925 Coffey Road
Columbus, OH 43210-1092

Miodrag Ristic
Dept. of Veterinary Pathobiology
University of Illinois
2001 S. Lincoln Avenue
Urbana, IL 61801

Alice T. Robertson
Louisiana State University Medical Center
Dept. of Microbiology & Immunology
1501 Kings Highway
Shreveport, LA 71130-3932

James R. Rooney
Department of Veterinary Science
108 Gluck Equine Research Center
University of Kentucky
Lexington, KY 40546-0099

Jon B. Rosenberg
Elon Animal Hospital
P.O. Box 155
Elon College, NC 27244

Linda Kelley Schlater
National Veterinary Services Laboratories
P.O. Box 844
Ames, IA 50010

Kathleen Ann Schmit
College of Veterinary Medicine
University of Minnesota
216 Veterinary Science Bldg.
1971 Commonwealth Ave.
St. Paul, MN 55108

John A. Schnackel
Fort Dodge Laboratories
Fort Dodge, IA 50501-0518

Jean E. Sessions
Glenvilah Veterinary Clinic
12948-E Travilah Road
Potomac, MD 20854

Pam Silvia
Department of Veterinary Science
108 Gluck Equine Research Center
University of Kentucky
Lexington, KY 40546-0099

James D. Smith
Hagyard-Davidson-McGee Associates
848V Nandino Blvd.
Lexington, KY 40511

Tony C. Smith
P.O. Box 400
Naches, WA 98937

Janice E. Sojka
Large Animal Clinic
Purdue University
Lynn Hall
West Lafayette, IN 47907

Michael S. Spensley
Department of Medicine
School of Veterinary Medicine
University of California
Davis, CA 95616

Sharon J. Spier
School of Veterinary Medicine
University of California
Davis, CA 95616

Phillip J. Sprino
Salsbury Laboratories, Inc.
2000 Rockford Road
Charles City, IA 50616

Paul J. Strzemienski
Section of Reproduction
School of Veterinary Medicine
University of Pennsylvania
New Bolton Center
Kennett Square, PA 19348

T. W. Swerczek
Livestock Disease Diagnostic Center
University of Kentucky
1429 Newtown Pike
Lexington, KY 40511

Robert J. Tashjian
American Quarterhorse Association
29 Prospect Street
West Boylston, MA 01583

Deborah W. Taylor
Kentucky Equine Research Foundation
University of Kentucky
Lexington, KY 40546

Robert Eugene Taylor
1305 Owen Street
Saginaw, MI 48601

Kent Thompson
Department of Veterinary Science
108 Gluck Equine Research Center
University of Kentucky
Lexington, KY 40546-0099

Susannah Thompson
Ranch Jonata
P.O. Box 5
Buellton, CA 93427

John F. Timoney
Dept. of Veterinary Microbiology,
Immunology & Parasitology
C 324 Schurman Hall
Cornell University
Ithaca, NY 14853

Peter J. Timoney
Department of Veterinary Science
108 Gluck Equine Research Center
University of Kentucky
Lexington, KY 40546-0099

Thomas Tobin
Department of Veterinary Science
108 Gluck Equine Research Center
University of Kentucky
Lexington, KY 40546-0099

Robert Tramontin
Livestock Disease Diagnostic Center
University of Kentucky
1429 Newtown Pike
Lexington, KY 40511

Patricia A. Tuttle
Livestock Disease Diagnostic Center
University of Kentucky
1429 Newtown Pike
Lexington, KY 40511

Elaine D. Watson
University of Pennsylvania
Section of Reproductive Studies
382 West Street Road, New Bolton Ctr.
Kennett Square, PA 19348

Julia Hall Wilson
Box J-126
Health Sciences Center
University of Florida
Gainesville, FL 32610

W. David Wilson
Department of Medicine
School of Veterinary Medicine
University of California
Davis, CA 95616

Michelle Yeargan
Department of Veterinary Science
108 Gluck Equine Research Center
University of Kentucky
Lexington, KY 40546-0099

Walter W. Zent
Hagyard-Davidson-McGee Associates
848V Nandino Blvd.
Lexington, KY 40511

WEST GERMANY

Klaus Petzoldt
Institut fur Mikrobiologie und
Tierseuchen der Tierarztlichen
Hochschule Hannover
Bischofshofar
Damm 15 Hannover 1, D-3000

Peter Michael Steinle
Loewensteiner Str. 6
Ludwigsburg 7140

Peter Thein
Bayer AG, GB VT-FE Biologie
Postfach Lo 17 09
5600 Wuppertal 1

Geert Vanden Bossche
Institute of Virology, Fu Berlin
Diagnostik, Domane Dahlem
Konigin-Luise-Strasse 49,
1000 Berlin 33

WEST INDIES

Ernest Radcliffe Ceasar
c/o Ministry of Agriculture
Animal Division
Trinidad & Tobago Port of Spain
Trinidad

Index